P9-DIF-369

Handbook of Pediatric Nutrition

Third Edition

Patricia Queen Samour, MMSc, RD
Clinical Nutrition Director
Nutrition Services
Beth Israel Deaconess Medical Center
Boston, Massachusetts

Kathy King, RD, LD
Private Practitioner
Publisher
Helm Publishing
Lake Dallas, Texas

JONES AND BARTLETT PUBLISHERS
Sudbury, Massachusetts
BOSTON TORONTO LONDON SINGAPORE

World Headquarters
Jones and Bartlett Publishers
40 Tall Pine Drive
Sudbury, MA 01776
978-443-5000
info@jbpub.com
www.jbpub.com

Jones and Bartlett Publishers Canada
2406 Nikanna Road
Mississauga, ON L5C 2W6
CANADA

Jones and Bartlett Publishers
International
Barb House, Barb Mews
London W6 7PA
UK

Jones and Bartlett's books and products are available through most bookstores and online booksellers. To contact Jones and Bartlett Publishers directly, call 800-832-0034, fax 978-443-8000, or visit our website www.jbpub.com.

Substantial discounts on bulk quantities of Jones and Bartlett's publications are available to corporations, professional associations, and other qualified organizations. For details and specific discount information, contact the special sales department at Jones and Bartlett via the above contact information or send an email to specialsales@jbpub.com.

Production Credits
Chief Executive Officer: Clayton Jones
Chief Operating Officer: Don W. Jones, Jr.
President, Higher Education and Professional Publishing: Robert W. Holland, Jr.
V.P., Sales and Marketing: William J. Kane
V.P., Design and Production: Anne Spencer
V.P., Manufacturing and Inventory Control: Therese Bräuer
Publisher: Michael Brown
Production Director: Amy Rose
Associate Production Editor: Renée Sekerak
Editorial Assistant: Kylah McNeill
Composition: Auburn Associates, Inc.
Cover Design: Kristin Ohlin
Cover Image: © Photos.com
Printing and Binding: Malloy, Inc.
Cover Printing: Malloy, Inc.

Library of Congress Cataloging-in-Publication Data

Handbook of pediatric nutrition / [edited by] Patricia Queen Samour, Kathy King
— 3rd ed.
p. ; cm.
Includes bibliographical references and index.
ISBN 0-7637-8356-0 (casebound)
1. Children—Nutrition—Handbooks, manuals, etc.
[DNLM: 1. Child Nutrition. 2. Child Nutrition Disorders. 3. Diet Therapy—Child. 4. Diet Therapy—Infant. 5. Infant Nutrition Disorders. 6. Infant Nutrition. WS 115 H2363 2005] I. Samour, Patricia Queen. II. Kathy King.
RJ206.H23 2005
618.92—dc22

2004029265

Printed in the United States of America
08 07 06 05 04 10 9 8 7 6 5 4 3 2 1

Dedication

This book is dedicated to children, their caretakers, and to the healthcare professionals who care for them.

Acknowledgments

I'd like to thank my husband Charlie for all his love, support, and patience while I worked on this book. *Patt Samour*

I'd like to thank my sweet daughters, Savannah and Cherokee, for being the flowers in my garden. *Kathy King*

We would like to thank our Jones & Bartlett editors and all of our contributing authors to this exciting third edition, especially the twelve who have shared their expertise on all three editions. You are truly our foundation. What a great wealth of knowledge and expertise!

Table of Contents

Contributors

Phyllis B. Acosta, PhD, RD
Nutrition Consultant
Grayson, Georgia

Susan Akers, RD, LD
Pediatric Nutrition Specialist
MetroHealth Medical Center
Cleveland, Ohio

Diane M. Anderson, PhD, RD, CSP
Baylor College of Medicine
Section of Neonatology
Department of Pediatrics
Houston, Texas

Karen V. Barale, MS, RD, CD, FADA
Washington State University
Extension Educator, Pierce County
Tacoma, Washington

Susan Bessler, MS, RD, CSP
Clinical Dietitian
Department of Clinical Nutrition
Children's Hospital and Research Center at Oakland
Oakland, California

Vanessa Cavallaro, MS, RD
Cambridge, Massachusetts

Karen Hanson Chalmers, MS, RD, CDE
Director
Nutrition Services
Joslin Diabetes Center
Boston, Massachusetts

Paula M. Charuhas, MS, RD, FADA, CD, CNSD
Nutrition Education Coordinator
Pediatric Nutrition Specialist
Seattle Cancer Care Alliance
Seattle, Washington

Lynn Christie, MS, RD
Pediatric Allergy and Immunology
Arkansas Children's Hospital
Little Rock, Arkansas

Wm. Cameron Chumlea, PhD
Fels Professor
Departments of Community Health and Pediatrics
Lifespan Health Research Center
Wright State University School of Medicine
Dayton, Ohio

Harriet H. Cloud, MS, RD
Owner, Nutrition Matters
Pediatric Nutrition Consultant
Professor Emeritus
University of Alabama at Birmingham
Birmingham, Alabama

Kattia M. Corrales, MS, RD, LDN
Nutrition and Diabetes Educator
Pediatric and Adolescent Unit
Joslin Diabetes Center
Boston, Massachusetts

Janice Hovasi Cox, MS, RD
Neonatal/Pediatric Dietitian
The Children's Hospital at Bronson
Kalamazoo, Michigan

Lauren R. Furuta, RD, MOE
Clinical Dietitian Specialist
Clinical Nutrition Service
Children's Hospital
Boston, Massachusetts

Michele Morath Gottschlich, PhD, RD, LD, CNSD
Director
Nutrition Services
Shriners Hospitals for Children
Associate Professor
University of Cincinnati
Cincinnati, Ohio

Sharon Groh-Wargo, PhD, RD
Assistant Professor
Nutrition and Pediatrics
Case Western Reserve University School of Medicine
MetroHealth Medical Center
Cleveland, Ohio

Mary L. Hediger, PhD
Division of Epidemiology, Statistics and Prevention Research
National Institute of Child Health and Human Development
National Institutes of Health
Bethesda, Maryland

Laurie Anne Higgins, MS, RD, LDN, CDE
Nutrition and Diabetes Educator
Pediatric and Adolescent Unit
Joslin Diabetes Center
Boston, Massachusetts

Bridget Klawitter, PhD, RD, CD, FADA
Director
Clinical Nutrition and Diabetes Services
All Saints Healthcare Systems, Inc.
Racine, Wisconsin
Nutrition Consultant
Nutrition Management & Consultations
Salem, Wisconsin

Lynne Lewis, RN, MS, CPNP
Children's Hospital
Boston, Massachusetts

Betty Lucas, MPH, RD, CD
Nutritionist
Center on Human Development and Disability
University of Washington
Seattle, Washington

Barbara Luke, ScD, MPH, RD
Professor
School of Nursing and Health Studies
University of Miami
Coral Gables, Florida

Theresa Mayes, RD
Shriners Hospitals for Children
Cincinnati, Ohio

Ingrida Mara Melbardis, RD
Pediatric Dietitian
The Children's Hospital at Bronson
Kalamazoo, Michigan

Virginia Messina
Port Townsend, Washington

Myrna Miller, RN, BSN
Nurse Clinician
Gastroenterology
The Children's Medical Center
Dayton, Ohio

Nancy Nevin-Folino, MEd, RD, CSP, LD, FADA
Clinical Nutrition Specialist
The Children's Medical Center
Dayton, Ohio

Beth Ogata, MS, RD, CD
Nutritionist
Center on Human Development and Disability
University of Washington
Seattle, Washington

Bonnie Spear, PhD, RD
Associate Professor Pediatrics
Co-Director, Leadership in Adolescent Health Training Project
University of Alabama at Birmingham
Birmingham, Alabama

Nancy S. Spinozzi, RD, LDN
Pediatric Dietitian Specialist
Clinical Nutrition Service
Children's Hospital
Boston, Massachusetts

Sherri L. Utter, MS, RD, LDN
Clinical Nutrition Specialist
Children's Hospital Boston
Boston, Massachusetts

Janet Washington, MPH, RD, LDN
Instructor, Nutrition Department
Coordinator, Sports Nutrition Certificate
Simmons College
Boston, Massachusetts

Jacqueline Jones Wessel, MEd, RD, CNSD, CSP, CLE
Nutrition Support Consultant
Pediatric Gastroenterology and Nutrition
Children's Hospital and Medical Center
Cincinnati, Ohio

John Westerdahl, MPH, RD, CNS
Director
Health Promotion Department
Nutritional Services Department
Castle Medical Center
Kailua, Hawaii

Nancy H. Wooldridge, MS, RD, LD
Co-Director and Nutrition Faculty Member
Pediatric Pulmonary Center
Department of Pediatrics
University of Alabama at Birmingham
Birmingham, Alabama

Preface

Commonly used by dietetic practitioners studying for their Pediatric Specialty certification, the *Handbook of Pediatric Nutrition* is considered the last word in pediatric nutrition. This third edition is written by registered dietitians, a nurse, and researchers who are experts in their respective areas of clinical pediatric practice. It covers the latest clinical research, accepted practice protocols, and study of the normal child from preconception through adolescence. It addresses the needs of infants and children with various diseases or conditions affecting their growth and nutritional status. There is a strong focus on practice with numerous references cited throughout each chapter and the appendices. This resource can be used in many practice settings such as acute/chronic care, ambulatory clinics, rehabilitation, community, private practice, and research.

What's New

This third edition is a first in many ways. It has a new publisher, new chapters, new appendix materials, and many new authors, as well as returning contributing experts from the previous editions. All chapters and appendices have been reviewed, revised, and updated. Not only is more evidence based-outcome data available in the literature, but also other areas affecting practice have changed, such as enteral formulas, pharmaceuticals, and newer treatment modalities. This edition contains numerous tables, exhibits, charts, and forms for practitioners to use in their everyday practice.

This edition offers revised vegetarian diets (birth through adolescence), the newest diabetes guidelines, transplant nutrition concerns, and botanicals. Due to the increased prevalence of overweight children in the United States, a new expanded chapter on weight management was added that covers a range of issues, from obesity to eating disorders, including polycystic ovary and metabolic syndromes. A new chapter on prenatal nutrition discusses preconceptual nutrition, weight goals for women from different ethnic populations, pregnancy concerns, and pregnant teens.

Appendices

The appendices have been totally revised with new growth charts, the 2005 dietary guidelines, new data on the "Tanner" sexual stages of development, and new arm measurement data from the World Health Organization (WHO) Bulletin. The new growth chart by Babson and Benda assesses the growth of premature infants based on more recent data.

The NCHS growth charts are the gold standard for measuring the height/length, weight, and head circumference of infants and children in the United States. These charts have many practical uses for assessing normal growth, failure to grow, obesity, and diseases or conditions which may affect growth (such as patients with renal disease, cystic fibrosis, diabetes, or on enteral/parenteral nutrition). The BMI charts are now available for the first time for children and young adults up to 20 years of age. These charts are being used in public health, schools (as part of a "health card"), and other settings in an effort to alert parents and children of being overweight (or underweight with anorexia/bulemia).

The new 2005 USDA dietary guidelines are included with a clear message—that Americans need to eat more fruits, vegetables, whole grain high fiber foods, and exercise more. By adhering to these guidelines we have a chance of reducing the incidence of overweight children, and reducing the complications associated with excess weight and its impact on quality of life and health care costs.

The mid upper arm circumference (MUAC) data for boys and girls from ages 6 to 59 months was published in the WHO Bulletin in 1997. These tables are another tool to use in assessing the MUAC in relation to other infants and young children.

The "Tanner" stages of sexual development has been updated with new tables on sexual development. One of our book authors, Dr. William Chumlea, was one of the authors on this new publication. These tables and figures include data on the timing of sexual maturation and racial differences among United States children including non-Hispanic white, non-Hispanic black, and Mexican American. Much of this data have statistically significant differences from earlier versions.

In 2002, the Institute of Medicine's Food and Nutrition Board released the Daily Reference Intakes (DRIs) for energy, carbohydrates including sugars, proteins, amino acids, fiber, fat, fatty acids, and cholesterol. The DRIs updated the Recommended Daily Allowances (RDA). The DRIs represent a new conceptual approach to nutrient-based reference standards, necessitating new approaches by practitioners and researchers.

We Hope You Enjoy this New Edition

The *Handbook of Pediatric Nutrition, 3rd edition*, is practical and detailed, while providing cutting edge research and resources on the most important pediatric practice issues and therapies. From counseling strategies for children to burn therapies, and from the newest diabetes medications to the newest parenteral feedings, you will be able to find guidelines and answers to your pediatric nutrition questions.

Patt Queen Samour and Kathy King

Chapter 1

Physical Growth and Maturation

Wm. Cameron Chumlea

WHAT IS GROWTH?

Physical growth is the increase in the mass of body tissues that occurs in set patterns, but at different rates and ages as an infant becomes an adult. Good nutrition and exercise are necessary for growth and maturation. Normal, healthy children grow and mature with few problems; however, society is presently faced with an epidemic of obesity that affects the growth and the current and future health of children.[1,2] This chapter provides an overview of child growth and maturation and their assessment and a brief discussion of children with abnormal growth.

How Is Growth Measured?

Accurate and reliable measurements of body size describe a child's growth status. The most useful are recumbent length from birth to 3 years of age, stature after age 3 years, head circumference from birth to age 3 years (see Figures 1–1 to 1–3) and weight at every age.[3] Recumbent length and stature describe linear growth, and weight measures the mass of all body tissues. Descriptions of these measurements are available on videotapes from the National Center for Health Statistics[4,5] and the World Health Organization.[6] These media demonstrate standardized measurement techniques similar to those in the *Anthropometric Standardization Reference Manual.*[3]

Weight and stature are important measures, but weight indexed for stature is descriptive of the level of overweight or obesity. The body mass index or BMI is an indicator of the degree of overweight or obesity in children.[7] BMI is weight divided by stature squared, with all measures in the metric system ($kg/m^2 \times 10{,}000$). Additional measures related to body fatness are limb and trunk circumferences and skinfold thickness. Mid-arm circumference is an index of the underlying fat and muscle tissue; abdominal circumference is an indicator of abdominal obesity;[8] and skinfold measures subcutaneous adipose tissue thickness. Two common skinfold sites are on the back of the arm over the triceps muscle and just below the scapula. Large values for midarm and abdominal circumferences, and triceps and subscapular skinfolds are positively correlated with total and percent body fat in children.[9]

It is important to measure a child's level of fatness because obesity is the most prevalent disease of childhood. Today, a big child is potentially overweight or obese rather than healthy. Childhood obesity is frequently linked with Type II diabetes among children and subsequent overweight, obesity, and cardiovascular disease in adulthood.[2,7] It is also important to measure bone mineral content and bone mineral density in children in order to identify those with low levels (due to low calcium and protein intakes) who are at risk for osteoporosis in old age.[10] Measuring a child's body composition can identify risk factors for some chronic adult diseases early when treatment will be most effective.

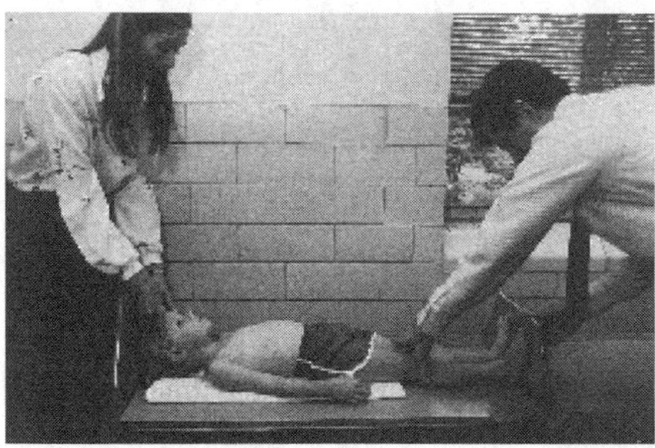

Figure 1–1 Measurement of Recumbent Length

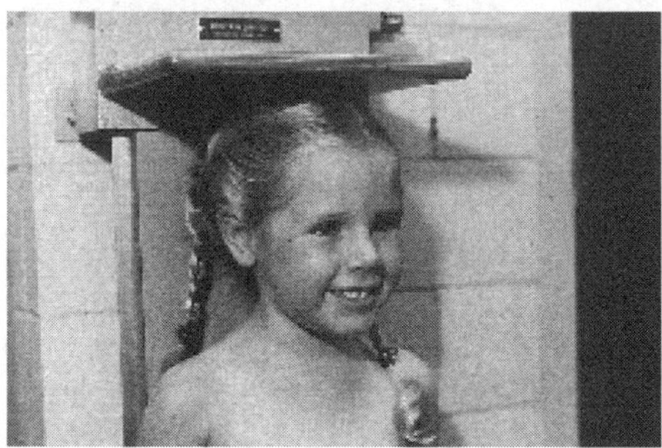

Figure 1–2 Measurement of Stature

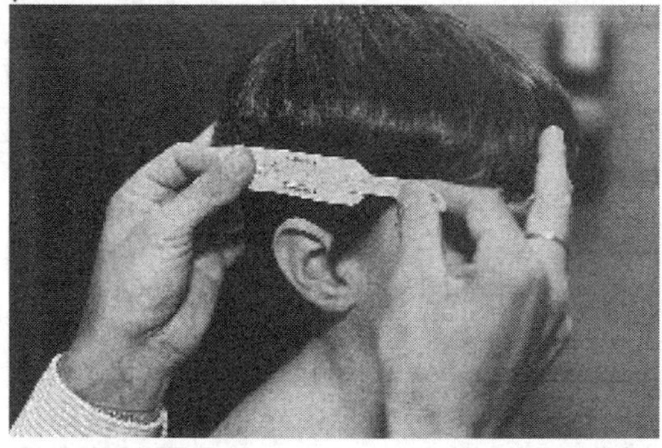

Figure 1–3 Measurement of Head Circumference

PERIODS AND PATTERNS OF GROWTH

A child's growth can be divided into four periods: infancy from birth to 2 years of age, the preschool years from about 3 to 6 years of age, the middle childhood years from about 7 to 10 years of age, and adolescence from about 11 to 18 years of age. Growth patterns and levels of maturation differ during these periods, but can overlap because of variation among children in the timing of their growth and maturation. A child's size and growth are related to his or her level of maturity and also reflect his or her genetic potential. At the same age, early-maturing children are taller and heavier than late-maturing children, while tall parents tend to have tall children and short parents tend to have short children. Weight has a genetic component that can explain familial aspects of obesity, but environmental factors affect the development of obesity also.

Infancy: Birth to 2 Years of Age

Infancy is distinguished by rapid growth as body dimensions increase faster than at any other time in postnatal life. Many infants lose weight shortly after birth, but regain their birth weight after about a week.[11] Most normal infants double their birth weight by 5 months and triple it by the age of 1 year. During the first year of life, weight increases 200%, body length 55%, and head circumference 40%. Similar changes occur in the trunk, arms, and legs. Between 1 and 2 years of age, the average infant grows about 12 cm in length and gains about 2.5 kg in weight.

An infant's head is disproportionately large. At birth, its diameter exceeds that of the chest, and its length is about a quarter of the body's total length. Head circumference increases from an average of about 35–36 cm at birth to an average of about 45–46 cm at 1 year of age. Head circumference measurements reflect brain growth, and the brain doubles its birth weight by 1 year of age.

Preschool Years: 3 to 6 Years of Age

During the preschool years, the rate of growth slows and stabilizes somewhat by about 4 to 5 years of age. By the age of 4 years, the average increase in stature is about 6 to 8 cm per year and about 2 to 4 kg per year in weight. Head circumference remains an important measure during the preschool years because the brain more than triples its birth weight by 6 years of age. Sex differences in size and weight during the preschool years are slight, but the pattern of more adipose tissue in girls than boys appears by 6 years of age. This is also a critical period for the development of overweight and an increased risk for subsequent obesity later in childhood and adulthood. Based upon their BMI percentiles, overweight children during this period should be monitored closely.[7,12]

Middle Childhood: 7 to 10 Years of Age

Middle childhood growth is at a steady rate. The average child at age 7 years grows about 5 to 6 cm per year in stature and about 2 kg per year in weight, but the increase in weight is about 4 kg per year by 10 years of age. The legs grow at a greater rate during middle childhood than the trunk, so that while the trunk accounts for about 55% of total stature at age 7 years, it accounts for only about 45% by 10 years of age. During this period, the average girl, as a function of her increasing maturity, grows slightly more per year in stature and weight than the average boy, which contributes, in part, to the larger size of girls at the start of adolescence. At 7 years of age, boys are, on average, only about 2 cm taller than girls, but there is little difference in weight. By 10 years of age, the average girl is 1 cm taller, 1 kg heavier, and the thickness of subcutaneous adipose tissue is about 25% greater than that of the average boy. Middle childhood is again a critical period for increased risk for the development of subsequent obesity. Based on their BMI percentiles, overweight and obese children during this period are at an ever-increasing risk for being obese as adults.[7]

Adolescence: 11 to 18 Years of Age

Adolescence starts before puberty and spans the years until growth and maturation are mostly completed, which is around 16 to 18 years of age in girls and 18 to 20 years of age in boys. A final increase in body size, shape, and weight transform a child into an adult. Between 11 and 14 years of age, most girls have their pubescent growth spurts and are taller than boys the same age. Boys, on average, enter their pubescent growth spurts about 2 years after girls, so that they have an additional 2 years of prepubertal growth. In addition, the pubescent growth spurt lasts for a longer time in boys than girls, and the amount of growth is larger. In boys, the average peak height velocity, the maximum rate of growth in stature during the growth spurt, ranges from about 9.5 to 10.5 cm per year, while in girls the maximum velocity is about 8.5 to 9.0 cm per year. These sex differences produce the larger average body size in men than in women. During adolescence, girls add more total body fat than boys, but boys develop more muscle tissue than girls, which results in the increased physical ability and performance of the average boy.[13]

HOW TO ASSESS GROWTH STATUS

Recumbent length, stature, and weight along with head circumference and BMI describe a child's growth status. These measures should be collected at regular intervals and plotted on the Centers for Disease Control, National Center for Health Statistics (CDC/NCHS) growth charts (see Appendix B).[14] These charts provide an assessment or comparison of the stature or length, weight, head circumference, and BMI of an infant, child, or adolescent with the percentile distribution of other children at the same ages. In the future, growth charts by the World Health Organization will be available from exclusively breast-fed infants.[15] There are also growth reference data for triceps and subscapular skinfold thicknesses and midarm circumference (see Appendix E).[11,16,17,18] The reference data from the Third National Health and Nutrition Examination Survey (NHANES III) for children is not recommended for general use because of the increased prevalence of obesity.[1]

A child's percentile position on the growth charts is a function of the difference in his or her genetic background compared to that of the children used to construct the charts. There are growth differences among black, white, and Mexican-American children, but these differences tend to be small.[14] There are also differences in the growth of Chinese- or Japanese-American children or American children of other racial or ethnic groups compared with that of white, black, and Mexican-American children represented on the CDC/NCHS growth charts. In the United States, the secular trend in stature (where each generation of children is taller as adults than the previous generation) has stopped for the majority of the population, but weight continues to increase. The trend in stature may still appear for children of some ethnic groups whose parents are recent immigrants.

Most healthy children maintain their growth percentile on the charts as they grow from one year to the next. For example, a child whose stature is at the 75th percentile at age of 4 years will have a stature at approximately the same percentile at age 10 years and again at age 16 years. However, some healthy children grow irregularly, reflecting the variation in growth and sexual maturation that occur among children at the same chronologic age. Significant deviations in a child's plotted position on the growth charts can be due to a recent illness or over- or under-nutrition.

It is important to account for the gestational age of premature infants or those small at birth when plotting their growth on the CDC/NCHS growth charts.[11] The amount of prematurity is subtracted from an infant's chronological age; for example, for an infant with a gestational age of 28 weeks, this is a correction of 12 weeks or 3 months of chronological age. After about 2.5 years of age, it is no longer necessary to make the adjustment for most healthy children who were premature. Growth charts for preterm low-birth-weight infants include weight, recumbent length, and head circumference (see Appendix A1–A4).[19]

GROWTH VELOCITY

When growth is measured at repeated visits, the amount of change or the rate of growth per unit of time in a measurement can be quantified. This provides additional information; for example, growth velocity can describe a child's response to nutritional intervention. Increment growth reference data (see Appendix C1–C8)[20,21] supplement the status growth charts by determining if a child's rate of growth is normal or unusual. Both assess the growth of children and monitor the results of nutritional therapy.

Maturation

The central nervous system integrates the activities of the endocrine system coordinating growth and sexual maturation. Before puberty, the central nervous system inhibits hormone production, but this inhibition decreases near puberty when the sex hormones reach adult concentrations. Endocrine and adrenal androgens influence growth, sexual maturation, and the development of secondary sex characteristics. Puberty is the age at which the reproductive system matures, and sexual reproduction is possible. Puberty is identified in girls by the onset of menstruation or menarche, but there is no similar marker in boys. The ages of individual children at the onset and completion of growth and sexual maturation are highly variable.

The progression of sexual maturation is assessed using Tanner stages as indicators of the development of breasts in girls, genitals in boys, and pubic hair in each sex (see Appendix F1–F4). Breast buds in girls (Tanner stage B-2) and genital enlargement in boys (Tanner stage G-2) indicate the onset of sexual maturation, which is followed by the appearance of pubic hair (Tanner stage PH-2) in both sexes. For girls, the 25th to the 75th percentiles for the age at onset of sexual maturation, Tanner stage B-2, range from 8.5 to 10.5 years in non-Hispanic blacks, 8.6 to 11.2 years in Mexican-Americans, and 9.5 to 11 years for non-Hispanic whites. The 25th to the 75th percentiles for the age at onset of sexual maturation, Tanner stage G-2 for boys, range from 7.5 to 10.9 years in non-Hispanic blacks, 8.9 to 11.7 years in Mexican-Americans, and 8.6 to 11.4 years for non-Hispanic whites. The onset of sexual maturation is significantly earlier in non-Hispanic black girls and boys than in non-Hispanic white and Mexican-American girls and boys.[22]

A girl attains menarche or starts to menstruate about 2 years after her breasts start to grow and about 12 to 18 months after her peak height velocity. Approximately 80% of non-Hispanic white girls start to menstruate between about 11.3 and 13.8 years of age with a median age of 12.55 years, while 80% of non-Hispanic black girls start to menstruate between about 10.5 and 13.6 years of age with a median age of 12.06 years, and 80% of Mexican-American girls start to menstruate between about 10.8 and 13.7 years of age with a median age of 12.25 years.[23] The ages at menarche for 50% of non-Hispanic black girls and 25% of the Mexican-American girls are significantly earlier than those of white girls, but there are no significant differences between the black and Mexican-American girls in their ages at menarche. Girls who attain menarche before 10.5 to 11.0 years are relatively "early" and those who attain menarche after 13.75 years are relatively "late." Peak height velocity (the age at the most rapid growth in stature) occurs in girls about a year or two before it does in boys, but the sex difference in age between sexual maturity stages can be less than half a year.

Recently, it has been reported that the onset of puberty is possibly occurring earlier among U.S. children than in the past several decades[24] based on the prevalence of Tanner stage 2 breast and/or pubic hair development. Despite slight declines in age, there is no conclusive evidence of an earlier age at menarche among non-Hispanic white girls and black girls.[23,24] Analysis of U.S. national health survey data indicates that sexual maturation among U.S. children has not become earlier, but more recent national survey data are needed to answer this health concern.

The sequence of Tanner stages between paired indicators is concordant for about 60% of healthy children. However about 30% of healthy children are discordant, i.e., they enter or are in a stage for one indicator and at the same time enter or are in earlier or later stages for the other indicator, and this discordance affects their growth. Boys whose pubic hair stages are more advanced than their genital stages and girls whose breast development stages are more advanced than their pubic hair stages are heavier and have higher BMI percentiles than concordant children. Children with the opposite discordance have lesser weights and BMI percentiles than concordant children. This variation in weight and BMI among healthy concordant and discordant children is greater than that among early and late maturing children.

BODY COMPOSITION

Muscle, adipose tissue, and bone are the primary body tissues that change during growth. These tissues are frequently quantified using a model that divides the body into fat and fat-free components based upon assumptions that the densities of fat and lean tissues are constant.[25] The density of fat varies little at any age, but the density of lean tissue varies depending upon its hydration, and the relative proportions of muscle and bone, which change among children with age, gender, race, and level of maturation.[26] Accurate body composition estimates are calculated from measures of body density, bone density, and the volume of total body water in a model that accounts for differences among growing children in their levels of fatness, muscle mass, age, ethnicity, and sex.[27] There are numerous methods for estimating body composition, but dual energy X-ray absorptiometry or DXA is the easiest for most children and even infants. There is a growing reference literature on the body composition of children and adolescents including fat-free mass (FFM), total body fat (TBF), and percent body fat (%BF),[28] but body composition references for infants and very young children remain limited. Reference averages for FFM and %BF estimates available from teenagers in the NHANES III are presented in Figures 1–4 and 1–5 respectively. There are differences in average values between non-Hispanic white and non-Hispanic black and Mexican-American children for FFM and %BF. It is not possible to determine if these differences are significant at this time because of the limitations of the method used to produce these estimates. In the next 5 years, NHANES national reference data for body composition from DXA will become available for U.S. children.

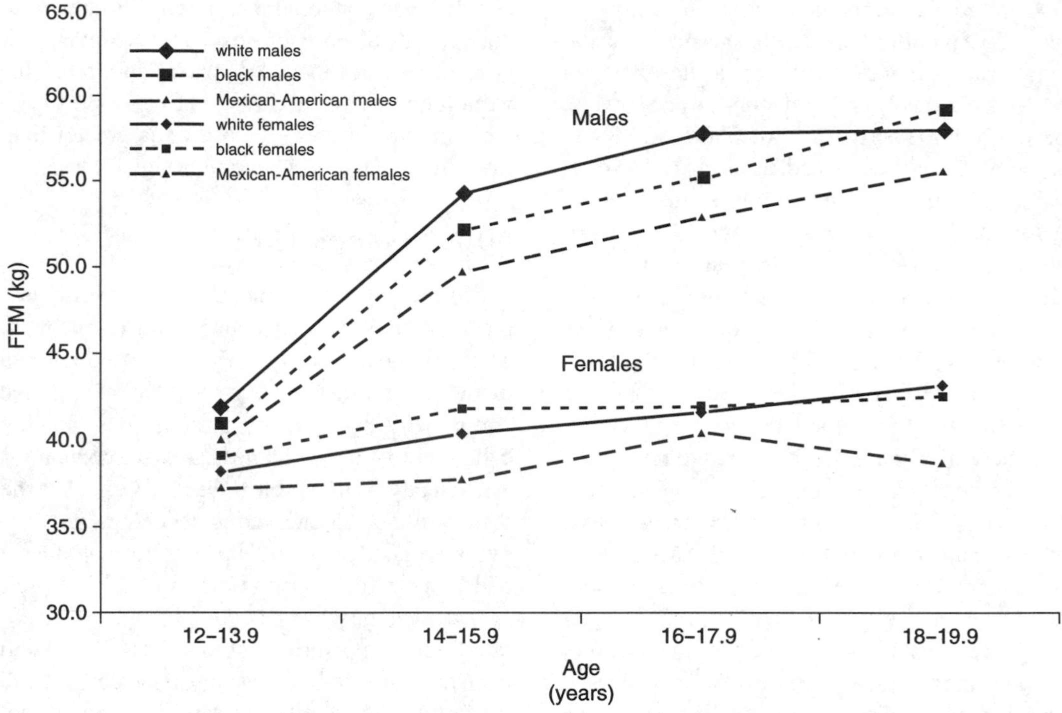

Figure 1–4 NHANES III FFM Estimates in Children. *Source:* Data from Chumlea Wm C, Guo SS, Kuczmarski R, Flegal KM, Johnson CL, Heymsfield SB, Lukaski HC, Schoeller D, Friedl K, Hubbard VS. Body composition estimates from NHANES III bioelectrical impedance data. *Int J Obes.* 2002;16:1596–1609.

GROWTH OF MUSCLE

Lean body mass (LBM) is metabolically active and is composed of muscle tissue, the internal organs, and the skeleton. Lean body mass contains a small amount of fat while FFM is LBM without any fat. Growth in FFM and LBM is primarily due to an increase in muscle mass, which is the largest single tissue component of the body, the major constituent of which is body water. At birth, 25% of body weight is muscle, and this increases to about 50% of body weight at adulthood. FFM, LBM, and muscle mass are positively associated with stature; for instance, a tall child has a greater amount of these than a shorter child at the same level of maturity. Muscle mass increases in boys and girls during childhood, and is roughly equal between them until about 13 to 14 years of age (Figure 1–6). In girls, muscle continues to grow into adolescence, but stop around 16 years of age. In boys, muscle grows rapidly after 13 years of age and well into late adolescence. This growth period in boys is about twice as long as in girls, and as a result, boys have several times as much muscle as girls, which is located primarily in the shoulders and arms. Men have greater absolute amounts of FFM and LBM than women, irrespective of stature.

GROWTH OF BODY FAT

Body fat stores energy, and in children, the majority of the body's fat is subcutaneous, but adipose tissue is also deposited in the visceral parts of the body. Internal adipose tissue deposition occurs in middle-aged adults, but now also appears in obese children. However, the majority of total body fat among obese children remains subcuta-

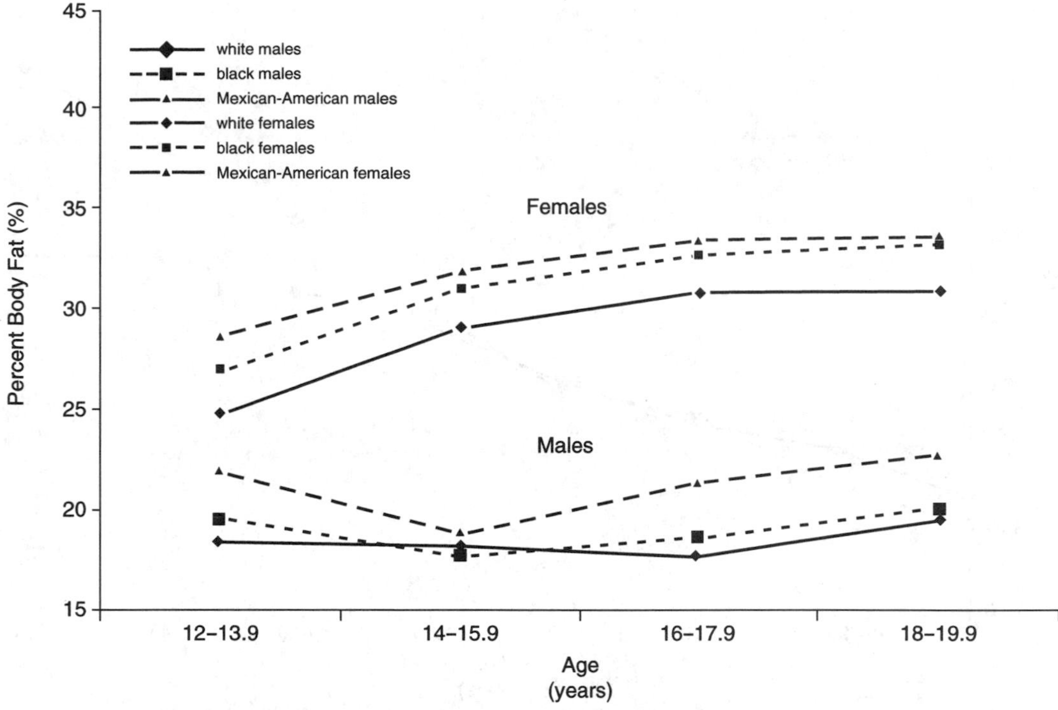

Figure 1–5 NHANES III %BF Estimates in Children. *Source:* Data from Chumlea Wm C, Guo SS, Kuczmarski R, Flegal KM, Johnson CL, Heymsfield SB, Lukaski HC, Schoeller D, Friedl K, Hubbard VS. Body composition estimates from NHANES III bioelectrical impedance data. *Int J Obes.* 2002;16:1596–1609.

---

neous. Over the past several decades, the increased prevalence of obesity in the U.S. population has included children. More children are obese today than in the past, and they are at greater levels of obesity than children were 10 to 20 years ago.

Girls have significantly more subcutaneous adipose tissue than boys, and this is not an artifact of their earlier maturation during adolescence. Boys and girls also differ in the deposition and patterning of adipose tissue. Both sexes deposit adipose tissue on the torso during childhood and adolescence, but adolescent girls add adipose tissue to breasts, buttocks, thighs, and across the back of the arms which accentuates the adult sex differences in body shape. Adipose tissue thickness on the arms and legs of boys increases during childhood but decreases after about 13 years of age because the underlying muscle grows at a greater rate at this time. Similar measures in girls show a continuous increase in adipose tissue thickness.

SKELETAL GROWTH

Skeletal growth is a continuous process, and the bones of the legs and the vertebrae are the major locations of growth in stature. Bone growth is rather steady until the adolescent growth spurt, but slows afterward. By about 18 years of age for girls and around 20 to 22 years of age for boys, the epiphyses or growth plates at the ends of long bones have fused to the shaft or diaphysis and the skeleton is mature. Assessment of skeletal maturation from radiographs of the hand-wrist or knee provides an index of a child's biological age known as *skeletal age.* Two chil-

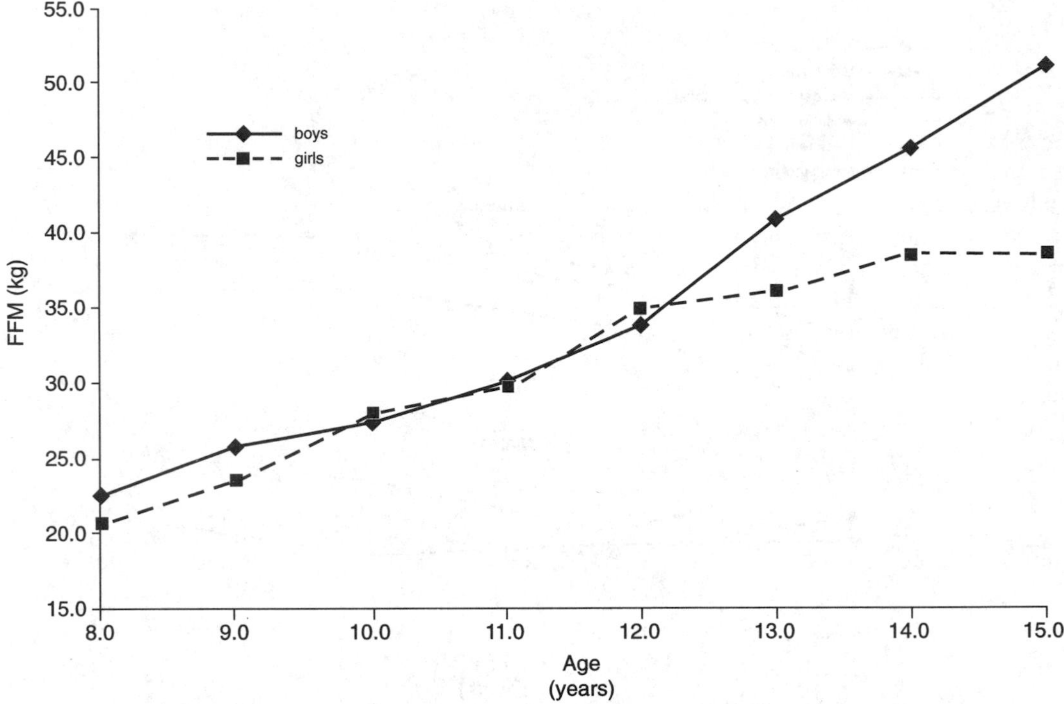

Figure 1–6 FFM in Fels Children. *Source:* Data from Guo S, Chumlea WC, Roche AF, Siervogel RM. Age- and maturity-related changes in body composition during adolescence into adulthood: The Fels Longitudinal Study. *Int J Obes*. 1997;21:1167–1175.

dren of the same chronological age may have different levels of skeletal maturation or skeletal ages, as they may also have different levels of sexual maturation.

The skeleton is the body's reserve of calcium, and an important aspect of skeletal growth is the building of this calcium reserve. The importance of this reserve for children is that those who end growth with a low bone mass (a low calcium reserve), are at an increased risk for developing osteoporosis. Peak bone mass is the maximum mineral mass attained by the skeleton. This peak occurs sometime in the third decade of life, but by maturity, the majority of peak bone mass has been reached. With DXA, it is possible to measure the amount of calcium or bone mineral content and bone mineral density of the skeleton of children. Limited reference data for bone mineral content and density are now available for children at many ages,[29] and will also be available from the National Health and Nutrition Survey in the future. These data and the use of DXA along with calcium supplementation provide mechanisms for monitoring the growth of the skeleton and its calcium content. This information can help children with low bone mass and density and low calcium intakes to attain their peak bone mass and reduce the prevalence of osteoporosis in the future.

SPECIAL CHILDREN

Assessing the growth status of children with Down's syndrome, cerebral palsy, contractures, braces, mental retardation, and so forth is difficult. The heterogeneity of these conditions limits recommended standard methodology, and there is limited or no specific reference data.[30] If the child can stand, standard methods can be used. If the child is nonambulatory, then recumbent methods are recommended. Reference data from the NCHS needs to be interpolated depending upon the condition of the child in question.

In a growth assessment of a handicapped child, one measurement is probably not sufficient. It may be necessary to take several measurements, especially the more difficult the measurement or the more uncooperative the child. Several Web sites provide useful information about measuring handicapped children, see Appendix B. Accurate records are important, and the CDC/NCHS growth charts can be used. A child may be at the 3rd percentile or less, but these growth charts can still provide information about a child's status, especially over time. For children with some specific conditions such as Trisomy 21, there are available growth charts.[31] For other groups of children, such as those with cerebral palsy, specific growth charts are being developed.

ACKNOWLEDGMENTS

I sincerely appreciate the input, assistance, and support of Michele Cannon in completing this work. This work was also supported by grants HL-72838 and HD-12252 from the National Institute of Health, Bethesda, Maryland.

REFERENCES

1. Troiano RP, Flegal KM, Kuczmarski RJ, Campbell SM, Johnson CL. Overweight prevalence and trends for children and adolescents. *Arch Pediatr Adolesc Med.* 1995; 149:1085–1091.
2. Dietz WH, Franks AL, Marks JS. The obesity problem. *N Engl J Med.* 1998;338:1157–1158.
3. Lohman TG, Roche AF, Martorell R, eds. *Anthropometric Standardization Reference Manual.* Champaign, IL: Human Kinetics Publishers; 1988.
4. USDHHS. NHANNES III *Anthropometric procedures* [videotape]. US Dept of Health and Human Services–Public Health Services. Washington DC; 1996.
5. NHANES III. *Analytic and reporting guidelines: The third health and nutrition examination survey (1988–94).* [CD-ROM]. National Centers for Health Statistics Centers for Disease Control and Prevention; 1997.
6. de Onis M, Onyangoa AW, Van den Broeck J, Chumlea WC, Martorell R, for the WHO Multicentre Growth Reference Study Group. Measurement and standardization protocols for anthropometry used in the construction of a new international growth reference. *Food Nutr Bull.* 2004;25:S27–S36.
7. Guo SS, Wu W, Chumlea Wm C, Roche AF. Predicting overweight and obesity in adulthood from body mass index values in childhood and adolescence. *Am J Clin Nutr.* 2002;76:653–658.
8. Goran MI, Gower BA. Relation between visceral fat and disease risk in children and adolescents. *Am J Clin Nutr.* 1999;70:149S–156S.
9. Roche A, Siervogel R, Chumlea W, Webb P. Grading body fatness from limited anthropometric data. *Am J Clin Nutr.* 1981;34:2831–2838.
10. Matkovic V, Jelic T, Wardlaw G. Timing of peak bone mass in Caucasian females and its implication for the prevention of osteoporosis- inference from a cross-sectional model. *J Clin Invest.* 1994;93:799–808.
11. Moore WM, Roche AF. *Pediatric Anthropometry,* 3rd ed. Columbus, OH: Ross Laboratories; 1987.
12. Whitaker RC, Wright JA, Pepe MS, Seidel KD, Dietz WH. Predicting obesity in young adulthood from childhood and parental obesity. *N Eng J Med.* 1997;337: 869–873.
13. Beunen G. Muscular strength development in children and adolescents. In: Froberg K, Lammert O, Hansen H, Blimkie CJR, eds. *Exercise and Fitness-Benefits and Risks.* Denmark: Odense University Press; 1997: 192–207.
14. Kuczmarski RJ, Ogden CL, Grummer-Strawn LM, et al. CDC Growth Charts: United States. *Advance Data.* 2000;314:1–28.
15. Garza C., de Onis M. A new international growth reference for young children. *Am J Clin Nutr.* 1999;70: 169S–172S.
16. Cronk CE, Roche AF. Race- and sex-specific reference data for triceps and subscapular skinfold and weight/ sataure 2. *Am J Clin Nutr.* 1982;35:347–354.
17. Ryan AS, Martinez GA, Baumgartner RN, Roche AF, Guo SS, Chumlea WC, Kuczmarski RJ. Median skinfold thickness distributions and fat-wave patterns in Mexican-American children from the Hispanic health and nutrition survey (HHANES 1982–1984). *Am J Clin Nutr.* 1990;51:925S–935S.
18. Frisancho AR. New norms of upper arm limb and fat and muscle areas for assessment of nutritional status. *Am J Clin Nutr.* 1981;34:2540–2545.
19. Guo SS, Roche AF, Chumlea WC, Casey PH, Moore WM. Growth in weight, recumbent length, and head circumference for preterm low-birthweight infants during

the first three years of life using gestation-adjusted ages. *Early Hum Dev.* 1997;47:305–325.

20. Roche AF, Himes JH. Incremental growth charts. *Am J Clin Nutr.* 1980;33:2041–2052.
21. Baumgartner RN, Roche AF, Himes JH. Incremental growth tables: Supplementary to previously published charts. *Am J Clin Nutr.* 1986;43:711–722.
22. Sun SS, Schubert CM, Chumlea WC, Roche AF, Kulin HE, Lee PA, Himes JH, Ryan AS. National estimates of the timing of sexual maturation and racial differences among U.S. children. *Pediatrics.* 2002;110:911–919.
23. Chumlea WC, Schubert CM, Roche AF, Kulin H, Lee PA, Himes JH, et al. Age at menarche and racial comparisons in U.S. girls. *Pediatrics.* 2003;111:110–113.
24. Herman-Giddens ME, J. SE, Wasserman RC, Bourdony CJ, Bhapkar MV, Koch GG, et al. Secondary sexual characteristics and menses in young girls seen in office practice: A study from the Pediatric Research in Office Settings Network. *Pediatrics.* 1997;99:505–512.
25. Siri W. Body composition from fluid spaces and density analysis of methods. In: Brozek J, Henshcel A, eds. *Techniques for Measuring Body Composition.* Washington, DC: National Academy Press; 1961:223–244.
26. Lohman TG. Applicability of body composition techniques and constants for children and youths. *Exer Sports Sci Rev.* 1986;14:325–357.
27. Guo S, Chumlea WC, Roche AF, Siervogel RM. Age- and maturity-related changes in body composition during adolescence into adulthood: The Fels Longitudinal Study. *Int J Obes.* 1997;21:1167–1175.
28. Chumlea Wm C, Guo SS, Kuczmarski R, Flegal KM, Johnson CL, Heymsfield SB, Lukaski HC, Schoeller D, Friedl K, Hubbard VS. Body composition estimates from NHANES III Bioelectrical impedance data. In: *Int J Obes.* 2002;16:1596–1609.
29. Maynard LM, Guo SS, Chumlea WC, et al. Total body and regional bone mineral content and area bone mineral density in children aged 8 to 18 years: From the Fels Longitudinal Study. *Am J Clin Nutr.* 1998;68:1111–1117.
30. Stevenson RD, Hayes RP, Cater LV, A. Blackman JA. Clinical correlates of linear growth in children with cerebral palsy. *Dev Med Child Neurol.* 1994;36:135–142.
31. Cronk C, Crocker AC, Pueschel SM, Shea AM, Zackai E, Pickens G, et al. Growth charts for children with Down Syndrome: 1 month to 18 years of age. *Pediatrics.* 1988;81:102–110.

SUGGESTED READINGS

Malina RM, Bouchard C, Bar-Or O. *Growth, Maturation, and Physical Activity*, 2nd ed. Champaign, IL: Human Kinetics; 2004.

Roche AF, Sun SS. *Human Growth Assessment and Interpretation.* Cambridge, UK: Cambridge University Press; 2003.

Roche AF, Chumlea WC, Thissen D. *Assessing Skeletal Maturity of the Hand-Wrist: Fels Method.* Springfield, IL: Charles C Thomas; 1988.

CHAPTER 2

Nutritional Assessment

Susan Bessler

The assessment of nutritional status is an integral component of pediatric health care. It identifies nutritionally depleted or at-risk infants and children, provides essential information for developing achievable nutritional care plans, and serves as a mechanism for evaluating the effectiveness of nutritional care.

SCREENING

The completion of in-depth nutritional assessments on all children served by a health care system is neither practical nor essential for providing quality nutrition care. Well-designed nutritional screening performed by trained personnel is effective in identifying children who are at an elevated nutritional risk and therefore may require a more comprehensive nutritional assessment.[1–5] Nutritional screenings can also function to predict outcome in specific diagnoses.[6] The information gathered for screening includes indices of nutritional status routinely collected during scheduled health care appointments or upon admission to a health care facility.[7,8]

Nutritional screening protocols must be adapted to the needs of the specific population served, staff and facility resources, and accrediting standards.[9] The participation of administrative, medical staff, nursing staff, and often family members is essential in developing a nutritional screening program because the measurement and documentation of many of the parameters involve nonnutrition personnel and equipment. The success of the program depends upon the coordinated efforts of the multidisciplinary team in completing assigned responsibilities.[1,10]

Key issues to be resolved when planning a nutritional screening program include designation of team member responsibilities, selection of nutritional parameters to be screened, timing of the screening, determining how the data will be analyzed, and the intended action once the data has been evaluated. In the hospital setting, a dietetic technician may collect the selected data by interview and from the patient's medical record whereas a clinic or extended care facility may have nursing complete nutritional screening. Family-administered screening instruments that have the child's primary caretaker report data have been developed for use in the community setting.[11] Most pediatric nutrition screening tools routinely include age, weight, length or height, and head circumference. Information about the child's medical history as well as diet and feeding ability is also routinely queried. The routine collection of lab values depends on the needs of the population and the laboratory support available. Once the nutritional data has been obtained, the child is assessed for nutrition risk and the appropriate referral or action plan is made. Exhibit 2–1 is an example of a hospital screening form that weighs the criteria and dictates the next appropriate step in the care plan. Nutrition screening process generally takes place at or soon after a clinic visit or hospital admission. Additionally, extended care facilities and hospitals with long-term patients may perform periodic re-screening to monitor changes in nutritional risk status.[12]

NUTRITIONAL ASSESSMENT

The assessment of a child's nutritional status is based on pertinent information collected from the medical history, anthropometric data, laboratory data, physical findings, and dietary interview. The forthcoming indices vary in time, invasiveness, and expense. Based on the patient and clinical setting, the practitioner needs to weigh the cost of the assessment tool with its potential benefit.

Medical History

Approximately 10–15% of children in the United States have special health care needs as defined as "having, or being at risk for congenital or acquired conditions that affect physical and/or cognitive growth and development."[13] These children may be at risk for associated nutrition sequelae as summarized in Table 2–1. A child's medical history should include a review of social history, growth, acute or chronic illnesses, history of pre-existing nutrient deficiencies, history of surgical or diagnostic procedures, and history of relevant therapies such as chemotherapy or radiation.[14] Medications should be reviewed for possible drug-nutrient interactions.

GROWTH DATA

Weight, Height and Head Circumference

Age appropriate growth is the hallmark of adequate nutrition. Monitoring growth through measurement of weight, length or height, and head circumference (in children 3 years of age or less) is a routine practice in most pediatric health care systems. These measurements are plotted on growth charts according to age for comparison with growth of a reference population of healthy normal infants and children. The most common charts used are those developed by the National Center for Health Statistics (NCHS)[15] based mostly on data from the National Health and Nutrition Examination Survey (NHANES)[16] (see Chapter 1 and Appendix B).

Upper Arm and Skinfold Measurements

Upper arm measurements and skinfold measurements (that include those on the triceps, biceps, subscapular, and abdomen) are used to predict and monitor body fat and muscle stores, clarify other anthropometric findings, and in some settings, predict morbidity and mortality.[17] The upper arm measurements most commonly evaluated include triceps skinfold (TSF, in millimeters), midarm circumference (MAC, in centimeters), and midarm muscle circumference (MAMC, in centimeters). MAMC is calculated using the following equation.

$$\text{MAMC (cm)} = \text{MAC (cm)} - (.314 \times \text{TSF (mm)})$$

MAMC can be determined using the nomogram in Appendix G.

The standards most commonly used for ages 1 to 75 are those revised by Frisancho[18] based on data from the HANES survey.[16] Standards for children under 1 year of age have been published based on data from children in the United States[19] and England.[20,21] Oakly and associates' standards for children 37 to 42 weeks gestation are based on both age and weight.[22] Mid-upper-arm-circumference standards (MUAC) have been developed by a World Health Organization (WHO) expert committee based on data from the NHANES I and II data (see Appendix E). The committee also developed MUAC standards for height when age is unknown.[23] Along with comparison to reference standards, skinfold measurements can be monitored using a child as his or her own control.

Although useful, these measurements have limitations. Caution must be used in comparing a child to the reference data. The data published by Frisancho[18] includes measurements for a solely Caucasian population and therefore use with other ethnic populations that may have different body compositions[24–27] may be erroneous. Even within the same reference population (i.e., ethnicity) mean body composition measurements can change over time.[20] Accurate skinfold measurements require both precise instruments that need to be checked

Exhibit 2–1 Nutrition Screening Profile

Children's Hospital Oakland

NUTRITION SCREENING PROFILE

CATEGORY		POINTS
ADMITTING DIAGNOSIS		______
Group 1 (8 points)	Group 2 (4 points)	
Burns ≥ 20%, Eating disorders DM(new), FTT, Immunodeficiency, Inborn Errors of Metabolism Inflammatory Bowel Disease, CF Short Bowel Syndrome, Malnutrition, Nutritional Rickets	Anemia, BPD, Burns < 20% CP, Cranial-Facial Surgery, CHD, DM(f/u), GE Reflux, Malabsorption, Liver Disease Pregnancy, Renal Disease Oncologic Disease	
DIET ORDER		______
TPN, Tube Feeding or *NPO/CL >3 Days	(8 points)	
Modified/ Special Diet	(3 points)	
Food Allergies	(1 point)	
Mechanical Feeding Problems	(1 point)	
ANTHROPOMETRICS wt: kg %, ht:	cm %	______
wt/ht: %, HC:	cm %	
wt, ht, wt : ht ≤ 5% (NCHS Percentiles)	(5 points)	
wt : ht ≥ 95% (NCHS Percentiles)	(0 points)**	
Recent wt loss / gain ≥ 10% BW	(5 points)	
Recent wt loss / gain ≥ 5 % BW	(2 points)	
wt% & ht% disparity > 2 percentile bands	(2 points)	
HC < 5%	(1 point)	
LABORATORY STUDIES Hgb: g/dl (nl=	)	______
Hgb 3 g/dl less than normal	(1 point)	
Albumin ≤ 3 g/dl	(3 points)	
ADDITIONAL INFORMATION		______
Age < 2 years old	(1 point)	
Diarrhea or Emesis > 5 days	(3 points)	
	TOTAL POINTS	______

CONCLUSION

______ PRIORITY #1 (8 or more points) Patient at high nutritional risk.
NUTRITION INTERVENTION RECOMMENDED

______ PRIORITY #2 (5 to 7 points) Patient at some nutritional risk.
Registered Dietitian to monitor nutritional status.

______ PRIORITY #3 (0 to 4 points) Patient at low nutritional risk.
Dietetic Technician to monitor nutritional status.

* ______ Recheck in 2 days.
** ______ Consider outpatient nutrition clinic for weight counselling

______________________, DT; Date: ______

______________________, RD: Date: ______

8345-019 (10/94)

White: Patient's Medical Record Pink: Nutrition Care Record

Source: Courtesy of the Clinical Nutrition Service, Children's Hospital Oakland, Oakland, California.

Table 2–1 Examples of Nutritional Risk Factors Associated with Selected Disorders

	Growth			*Diet*			*Medical*	
	Under-weight	*Over-weight*	*Short Stature*	*Low Energy Needs*	*High Energy Needs*	*Feeding Problems*	*Constipation*	*Chronic Medications*
Autism	✓[a]					✓		✓
Bronchopulmonary dysplasia	✓				✓			✓
Cerebral palsy	✓	✓	✓	✓	✓	✓	✓	✓
Cystic fibrosis	✓		✓		✓			
Down syndrome		✓		✓		✓		
Fetal alcohol syndrome	✓		✓					
Heart disease (congenital)	✓				✓			
HIV/AIDS[b]	✓				✓			✓
Prader-Willi syndrome		✓	✓	✓				
Premature birth	✓		✓		✓	✓		
Seizure disorder								✓
Spina bifida	✓	✓	✓	✓			✓	

[a]May be present
[b]HIV = human immunodeficiency virus; AIDS = acquired immunodeficiency syndrome

Source: Baer MT and Harris AB. Pediatric nutrition assessment: Identifying children at risk. Copyright The American Dietetic Association. Reprinted by permission from *Journal of the American Dietetic Association,* Vol. 97 (suppl 2): S107–S115, 1997.

and calibrated frequently and trained anthropometrists. Therefore, even under favorable conditions, varying compressibility of fat may make these measurements challenging to obtain and reproduce[28] especially in an obese or active child.

Body Mass Index

The most widely used standard to evaluate adiposity and proportionality in children greater than 2 years of age is the body-mass-index (BMI). The BMI, also known as the Quetelet Index,[9] is derived from dividing weight in kilograms by height in meters squared (wt/ht^2). For example, the BMI of a 14-year-old female who is 5'1" and 110 lb. is $50/(1.54)^2$ or 21. Standardized BMI curves are included on the most recent NCHS growth charts[15,30,31] (see Appendix B) and have been developed in other countries.[32–37] Based on the NHANES data,[16] mean BMI decreases from age 1 year to age 4 to 6 years at which point it increases. There is some evidence that children who rebound from this trough at earlier ages are at a higher risk for obesity later in life.[38] The American Academy of Pediatrics (AAP) considers a child greater than the 85th percentile at risk for overweight and greater than the 95th percentile at risk for obesity.[39] A child crossing BMI percentile boundaries should be further evaluated. BMI doesn't consistently quantitate adiposity in an individual. Two children with similar BMIs may have different proportions of fat and muscle mass.[40] Also, BMI may under predict adiposity in some children with disease states.[41]

Other Considerations

Obtaining and interpreting anthropometric indices of premature infants and children with developmental disorders may require specialized equipment and standards. This is detailed further in Chapter 14.

The developmental maturity of the child needs to be considered when interpreting anthropometric data. Correction for gestational age at birth is essential in the assessment of infants born prematurely (refer to Chapter 3). Children evaluated for delayed or precocious growth often have bone age assessments based on radiographic studies, which should be considered. For the older child, data relating to the stage of sexual maturity can alter assessment findings.[42,43] See Chapters 1 and 6 for more detail and Appendices F1–F4 for tables on sexual development.

Laboratory Measurements

Some laboratory measurements of nutritional status are routinely collected as part of a normal health care evaluation. Others are performed when the diagnosis, medical history, or nutritional history indicates nutritional risk. Appendix H lists laboratory norms based on age categories for selected tests of nutritional status.[44] The interpretation of laboratory findings must take into consideration the present and past medical status of the child. Many biochemical indices of nutritional status for normal individuals are altered by acute or chronic disease.

Serum Proteins

Albumin is the serum protein most commonly measured for assessment of nutritional status because it is inexpensive and readily available. However, due to a relatively long half-life of approximately 2 weeks and reduced degradation during periods of low protein intake, diagnosis of nutritional depletion can be missed or delayed if based solely on serum albumin levels. Likewise, serum albumin level serves as a relatively late indicator of nutritional repletion. Serum albumin may be decreased during malnutrition due to inadequate availability of precursors.[45] However, independent of nutritional status albumin can be depressed during infection, trauma, enteropathy, liver disease, or renal disease and elevated in dehydration, third spacing, and after administration of exogenous albumin.[45,46] Serum proteins with shorter half-lives including transferrin, retinal-binding protein, and thyroxin-binding pre-albumin more rapidly assess response to nutritional therapy though like serum albumin, may also be low during stress, sepsis and acute illnesses secondary to fluid shifts and preferential synthesis of acute phase proteins.[45,47,48] Measurement of the acute phase protein C-reactive protein (CRP) may help determine whether a low serum protein level is caused by stress or nutritional deficiency.[49,50] Fibronectin and somatomedin have half-lives less than 1 day but may not be ideal indicators of nutritional repletion once adequate protein and caloric intake is attained. They are more useful in the research rather than the clinical setting.[50,51] Table 2–2 lists half-life and normal reference values for serum proteins commonly used for nutritional assessment.

Iron Status

Iron deficiency anemia is a common pediatric nutritional problem in the United States[52–54] and is routinely assessed in the inpatient and community setting. Hemoglobin and/or hematocrit measurements are commonly used to assess iron nutrition. These are easily and relatively inexpensive to monitor. However, they are decreased only during later stages of iron deficiency and may be decreased for reasons other than iron deficiency. Other reasons for low hemoglobin and hematocrit include acute blood loss, acute or chronic infections, chronic inflammation, other micronutrient deficiencies such as B12 or Folate, or hereditary defects in red blood cell production; for example, thalasemia major or sickle cell disease.[55–56] Serum ferritin level is highly correlated with total body stores of iron and is the most sensitive index of iron status among healthy individuals. An elevated free erythrocyte protoporophyrin level and a decreased serum iron/total iron-binding capacity ratio and transferin saturation occur when iron stores are depleted. These biochemical findings are present before changes in hemoglobin and red blood cell morphology. With the exception of serum ferritin level, which rises, laboratory indicators for iron deficiency decrease during infection and chronic inflammation.[57–59] Table 2–3 summarizes iron status and hematologic abnormalities in states of negative iron balance.

Table 2–2 Serum Proteins Used in Assessing Nutritional Status

Protein	*Half-Life*	*Normal Value*	*Factors Known to Alter Concentration**
Albumin	18–20 days	Preterm: 2.5–4.5 g/dL Term: 2.5–5.0 g/dL 1–3 mo.: 3.0–4.2 g/dL 3–12 mo.: 2.7–5.0 g/dL > 1 year: 3.2–5.0 g/dL	↓inflammation, infection, trauma, liver disease, renal disease, protein-losing enteropathy; altered by fluid status
Transferrin†	8–9 days	180–260 mg/dL	↓inflammation, liver disease; ↑iron deficiency; altered by fluid status
Prealbumin	2–3 days	20–50 mg/dL	↓liver disease, cystic fibrosis, hyperthy roidism, infection, trauma
Retinol binding protein	12 hours	30–40 μg/mL	↓liver disease, zinc or vitamin A deficiency, infection; ↑renal disease

*Any condition that can alter a protein's rate of synthesis, degradation, or excretion has potential to alter the serum concentration.
†Transferrin may be calculated from total iron binding capacity (TIBC): (0.8 × TIBC) − 43.

Sources: Data from endnote references 33, 47, and 101.

Immunologic Function

Protein-energy malnutrition as well as subclinical deficiencies of one or more nutrients can impair immune response and increase risk for infection. The measurement of functional parameters of the immune system can therefore be useful to assess nutritional status. Among the immunologic indexes that are associated with nutritional status are levels of T-lymphocytes and leukocyte terminal deoxynucleotidyl transferase, appearance of delayed cutaneous hypersensitivity, opsonic function, salivary IgA, and total lymphocyte count. These tests vary in sensitivity for detecting nutritional depletion.[60] The total lymphocyte count (TLC) is the index of immune function most readily available for hospitalized patients. This value can be calculated from white blood cell (WBC) counts as follows:

$$\text{WBC/mm}^3 \times \%\ \text{lymphocytes} = \text{TLC/mm}^3$$

Values less than 1500 are associated with nutritional depletion. In infants less than 3 months of age, values of less than 2500 may be abnormal.[61] Independent of nutritional status, values of immunologic function may be altered during trauma, chemotherapy, immunosuppressant drug therapy, and lack of previous exposure to antigen (in the case of delayed cutaneous hypersensitivity).[60]

Clinical Evaluation

Examination and evaluation of general appearance and specific systems is an essential part of the nutritional assessment. In most cases, severe nutritional deprivation is easily detectable. Milder, nonspecific signs of malnutrition are more commonly observed but may be harder to detect. The presence of a suspected clinical deficiency is often reflected in the diet history and should be further supported by biochemical evaluation.[60,62] Table 2–4 lists clinical signs associated with nutrient deficiencies and specifies laboratory findings recommended to substantiate the diagnosis.

DIETARY EVALUATION

Components of a Pediatric Diet Evaluation

The thorough collection of dietary data should include the quantity and quality of

Table 2–3 Iron Status and Hematologic Abnormalities in States of Negative Iron Balance*

				Iron Deficiency Anemia	
	Normal	*Iron Depletion*	*Iron Deficiency*	*Early*	*Advanced*
Storage iron	NL	DECR	DECR	DECR	DECR
Erythron iron	NL	NL	DECR	DECR	DECR
Hemoglobin, Hematocrit, RBC count	NL	NL	NL	DECR	DECR
RBC indices	NL	NL	NL	NL	DECR

*NL, normal; DECR, decrease; RBC, red blood cell

Source: Adapted with permission from Cecalupo AJ and Cohen HJ, Nutritional anemias, in *Pediatric Nutrition Theory and Practice,* R.J. Grand, J.L. Sutphen and W.H. Dietz, eds, p. 491, © 1987, Newton, MA: Butterworth Heinemann.

Table 2–4 Clinical Signs and Laboratory Findings in the Malnourished Child and Adult*

Clinical Sign	*Suspect Nutrient*	*Supportive Objective Findings*
Epithelial		
Skin		
Xerosis, dry scaling	Essential fatty acids	Triene/tetraene ratio >0.4
Hyperkeratosis, plaques around hair follicles	Vitamin A	↓Plasma retinol
Ecchymoses, petechiae	Vitamin K	Prolonged prothrombin time
	Vitamin C	↓Serum ascorbic acid
Hair		
Easily plucked, dyspigmented, lackluster	Protein-calorie	↓Total protein ↓Albumin ↓Transferrin
Nails		
Thin, spoon-shaped	Iron	↓Serum Fe ↑TIBC
Mucosal		
Mouth, lips, and tongue	B vitamins	
Angular stomatitis (inflammation at corners of mouth)	B2 (riboflavin)	↓RBC glutathione reductase
Cheilosis (reddened lips with fissures at angles)	B2	See above
	B6 (pyridoxine)	↓Plasma pyridoxal phosphate†
Glossitis (inflammation of tongue)	B6	See above
	B2	See above
	B3 (niacin)	↓Plasma tryptophan ↓Urinary N-methyl nicotinamide†
Magenta tongue	B2	See above
Edema of tongue, tongue fissures	B3	See above
Gums		
Spongy, bleeding	Vitamin C	↓Plasma ascorbic acid
Ocular		
Pale conjunctivae secondary to anemia	Iron	↓Serum Fe, ↑TIBC, ↓serum folic acid, or ↓RBC folic acid
	Folic acid	
	Vitamin B12	↓Serum B12
	Copper	↓Serum copper
Bitot's spots (grayish, yellow, or white foamy spots on the whites of the eye)	Vitamin A	↓Plasma retinol
Conjunctival or corneal xerosis, keratomalacia (softening of part or all of cornea)	Vitamin A	↓Plasma retinol

continues

Table 2–4 continued

Clinical Sign	*Suspect Nutrient*	*Supportive Objective Findings*
Musculoskeletal		
Craniotabes (thinning of the inner table of the skull); palpable enlargement of costochondral junctions ("rachitic rosary"); thickening of wrists and ankles	Vitamin D	↓25-OH-vit D ↑Alkaline phosphatase ± ↓Ca, ↓PO_4 Long bone films
Scurvy (tenderness of extremities, hemorrhages under periosteum of long bones; enlargement of costochondral junction; cessation of osteogenesis of long bones)	Vitamin C	↓Serum ascorbic acid Long bone films
Skeletal lesions	Copper	↓Serum copper X-ray film changes similar to scurvy because copper is also essential for normal collagen formation
Muscle wasting, prominence of body skeleton, poor muscle tone	Protein-calorie	↓Serum proteins ↓Arm muscle circumference
General		
Edema	Protein	↓Serum proteins
Pallor 2° to anemia	Vitamin E (in premature infants)	↓Serum vitamin E ↑Peroxide hemolysis Evidence of hemolysis on blood smear
	Iron	↓Serum Fe, ↑TIBC
	Folic acid	↓Serum folic acid
	Vitamin B12	Macrocytosis on RBC smear ↓Serum B12
	Copper	Macrocytosis on RBC smear ↓Serum copper
Internal systems		
Nervous		
Mental confusion	Protein	↓Total protein, ↓albumin, ↓transferrin
	Vitamin B1 (thiamine)	↓RBC transketolase
Cardiovascular	Vitamin B1	Same as above
Beriberi (enlarged heart, congestive heart failure, tachycardia)		

continues

Table 2–4 continued

Clinical Sign	*Suspect Nutrient*	*Supportive Objective Findings*
Tachycardia 2° to anemia	Iron Folic acid B12 Copper Vitamin E (in premature infants)	See above
Gastrointestinal		
Hepatomegaly	Protein-calorie	↓Total protein, ↓albumin, ↓transferrin
Glandular		
Thyroid enlargement	Iodine	↓Total serum iodine: inorganic, PBI†

*Fe, iron; PBI, protein-bound iodine; RBC, red blood cells; TIBC, total iron-binding capacity
†Bio Science Laboratories, 7600 Tyrone Avenue, Van Nuys, CA 91405

Source: Reprinted with permission from Kerner A, *Manual of Pediatric Parenteral Nutrition,* pp. 22–23, © 1983, W.B. Saunders Company.

foods, psychosocial factors impacting food selection and intake, and clinical/physical factors related to nutritional status. Specific factors include:[61–63]

Food-related factors

- Chronological feeding history from birth or onset of nutritional problem
- Current nutrient intake
- Feeding skills
- History of prescribed or self-imposed diets or outcome
- Food allergies or intolerances

Psychosocial factors

- Family history and dynamics
- Socioeconomic status including use of supplemental food programs
- Patient's self-perception of nutritional status and/or caretaker's perception of child's nutritional status
- Religious or cultural beliefs impacting food intake

Clinical/physical factors

- Vitamin supplements and medication
- Stooling habits and characteristics
- Activity
- Sleep patterns

See Exhibit 2–2 for a sample dietary interview worksheet.

Complementary and Alternative Medicine

During the last one-and-a-half decades, the interest in and practice of complementary and alternative medicine (CAM) has increased.[64] CAMs may include, but are not limited to, homeopathic medicine, natural products, macrobiotics, megavitamins, and herbal medicine.[65] Families whose children have an acute or chronic condition may especially be seeking CAMs to augment routine medical treatment. Information on a family's past or present use of a CAM is important, however, may not be readily volunteered by the family. Specific ques-

Exhibit 2–2 Dietary Interview Summary Portion of a Nutrition Clinic Evaluation

NUTRITION CLINIC EVALUATION

Date of Visit: ______ Age: ______
Diagnosis: ______ Onset: ______
Concomitant Conditions: ______
______ Ref. Phys. ______
Problem: ______

Concerns of Parents or Patient: ______

Nutrition History: ______

Recent Nutrition History: ______

Formula: Kind ______ Amount ______ Cal. Density ______
Food Intake: ______

Food Summary (no. of servings/day):
Meat ______ Milk ______ Fr/Veg ______ Grains ______

Fever/Vomiting: ______ Elimination: ______
Appetite: ______
Feeding Ability/Concerns: ______

Vitamin Mineral Supp: ______
Activity level 1–8, 8 high ______

Social Setting in Regard to Meal Prep: ______

Social History: ______

Pertinent Family Medical/Weight History: ______

Source: Courtesy of the Clinical Nutrition Services, Children's Hospital Medical Center, Cincinnati, OH.

tions as are outlined in Exhibit 2–3 may be useful to elicit this information. Any appearance of being judgmental may inhibit disclosure and discussion (see also Chapter 26).[66]

Collection of Current Intake Data

The diet history can be comprehensive, encompassing most of the aforementioned factors, or specific to support a suspected diagnosis. Several approaches to quantitate nutrient intake data. A diet history is designed to determine pattern of usual food intake. This type of history requires a detailed interview by a trained nutritionist.[67,68] From the collected data, an estimate of nutrient intake is calculated. Studies indicate this method yields higher estimated values than the 24-hour recall and diet record.

A 24-hour recall provides an estimate of nutrient intake based on the individual's recollection of food consumed over the previous day. This method has been used successfully for groups or individuals. However, it is less valid in evaluating diet adequacy for an individual because the 24-hour period assessed may not be representative of the usual diet. Nutrient intakes calculated from 24-hour recalls are lower than those based on dietary histories or food records.[69–73]

Three-day to 7-day food records provide prospective food intake data. These are recorded by the parent, child, or other caregiver (and therefore require literacy) and are returned to the nutritionist for analysis. Food records encompassing 7-days may provide more accurate information than one of shorter duration due to the inclusion of both weekend and weekday meal patterns; however, accuracy of diet record keeping often deteriorates over time. When a 7-day food record is not possible, use of shorter time periods including selected days of the week is an adequate alternative.[74]

In inpatient facilities, nutrient intake analyses (calorie counts) are frequently ordered to assess a child's food intake. These are used to determine the ability of a child to consume a sufficient amount of food for growth or to verify the achievement and adequacy of a prescribed feeding regimen. These records, however, do not provide data representative of intake within the home environment.

Food frequencies estimate the frequency and amount of specific foods eaten. These often consist of questionnaires that can be self-administered and therefore reduce professional interview time. However, the questionnaire generally cannot retrieve unique details of an individual's diet unless designed to do so.[75] Overreporting of food intake is common with this method.[69,70,76,77] New methods of capturing dietary intake are being explored using such technology as portable computers, videotapes, and tape recorders.[77–80]

Exhibit 2–3 Sample Questions to Elicit Information on Use of Complementary Medicine

1. Is your child receiving any herbal preparations? If yes:
   - What is the name (if known)?
   - For what purpose is it given?
   - How is it administered (tea, tincture, fluid extract, tablet, or capsule)?
     - How much? How often?
     - Is it prescribed/recommended? Where is it purchased?
     - How is it tolerated? Any side effects noted?
2. Is your child receiving any additional vitamins or minerals? (if yes, the bulleted questions apply)
3. Are there any foods or vitamins you specifically avoid for your child?
4. Who are the people involved in your child's health care (caretakers and health providers)?
5. Do you have any questions regarding complementary or alternative health care?

Dietary Intake Evaluation

Estimated intakes of specific nutrients are calculated using values derived from food composition tables or computerized nutrient analysis programs. The calculated intake is evaluated for adequacy by comparing it with a reference intake. The recently revised *Dietary Reference Intakes* (DRIs) (see Appendix I) are the most commonly used reference allowances in the United States (replacing the 1989 Recommended Daily Allowances [RDAs]).[81–86] DRIs are based on contemporary studies that address not only preventing classical nutritional deficiencies but reducing the risk of chronic diseases, promoting optimal health, and preventing nutrient toxicities.[87]

The DRIs actually refer to at least six types of reference values: RDAs, Adequate Intake (AIs), Estimated Average Requirement (EARs), Estimate Energy Requirement (EER), Acceptable Macronutrient Distribution Range (AMDR), and Tolerable Upper Intake Level (TUL). The RDA is the dietary intake level that is sufficient to meet the nutrient requirements of nearly all healthy persons and is designed to include a wide margin of safety above amounts required to prevent deficiency.[88] Therefore, a healthy child whose estimated intake for a nutrient falls below the RDA may not have a nutritional deficiency or even a nutritional risk unless this intake is substantially below the RDA for a sufficient length of time. When assessing the adequacy of diets for infants and children with acute or chronic disease, potential alterations in nutrient requirements should be considered. In cases where sufficient scientific evidence is not available to estimate an average requirement, AIs have been set and should be used as a goal for intake where no RDAs exist. The EAR is the intake value that is estimated to meet the requirement defined by a specified indicator of adequacy in 50% of an age- and gender-specified group. The EER is the dietary energy intake predicted to allow for a level of physical activity consistent with normal health and development. The AMDR is the range of macronutrient intakes for a particular energy source that are associated with reduced risk of chronic disease while providing adequate intakes of essential nutrients. The TUL is the maximum level of daily nutrient intake that is unlikely to pose risks of adverse health effects to almost all of the individuals in a life stage and/or gender group.

CALCULATION OF ENERGY REQUIREMENTS

Overview

Accurate prediction of energy requirements is important for the healthy child and magnified in such clinical situations as treating the obese or failure-to-thrive child, and implementing enteral or parenteral nutrition support in the acute or chronically ill child.[89] Energy needs can be estimated by using the DRIs,[81–86] however they are based on populations of normal healthy subjects and may not be applicable to the child with altered activity or with potential alterations in needs related to clinical status.

Many equations have been generated to predict basal or resting energy needs and to which the clinician can add factors accounting for activity and stress. In a subgroup of children with illnesses and concomitant malnutrition, energy expenditure may be most accurately predicted by the use of indirect calorimetry.[90]

Definition of Terms

Total energy expenditure (TEE) consists of the energy required to meet the basal metabolic rate (BMR), diet-induced thermogenesis, activity, and growth.[91] BMR assumes the following basal conditions:[92]

1. fasting (at least 10–12 hours after the last meal)
2. awake and resting in a lying position (measurements are taken shortly after awakening)
3. normal body and ambient temperature
4. absence of psychological or physical stress

Diet-induced thermogenesis, also referred to as the specific dynamic action of food, is the energy necessary for digestion, transport, and storage of nutrients. It accounts for 5–10% of daily energy expenditure.[93]

Resting-energy expenditure (REE) is the energy expenditure of an individual at rest and in conditions of thermal neutrality. REE may include the thermal effect of a previous meal. BMR and REE usually differ by less than 10%.[92]

Standardized Equations

Equations have been developed to predict the BMR and REE of infants and children. A sampling of these equations are summarized in Table 2–5. BMR and REE estimates using standard calculations are based on the assumption that the individual is free of pathology and fever that affect energy expenditure and therefore, applying these equations to the ill pediatric patient requires an additional stress factor. Table 2–6 highlights a sampling of current findings in potential alterations in energy expenditure with different disease states. Regular reevaluation of energy needs should be completed as clinical status changes. Caution must be taken not to overfeed a critically ill child because excess nutritional delivery can potentially increase pulmonary and hepatic pathophysiology.[114]

The final factor in determining energy needs is activity. This can be accomplished by determining the amounts of time spent performing various types of activities and calculating an activity factor based on a 24-hour time period. Activity factors of 1.3 are associated with sedentary lifestyles, whereas activity factors equal to or greater than 2.0 represent lifestyles high in physical activity. Children under normal unconstrained conditions are considered to be active with activity factors ranging from 1.7 to 2.0 X REE. Table 2–7 lists the approximate energy expenditure for various activities in relation to REE. Table 2–8 demonstrates the method of calculating an activity factor and the TEE.

Individual variation in true energy expenditure may exist largely due to differences in lean body

Table 2–5 Equations for Predicting Energy Requirements of Children

Origin	*Energy Determination*	*Gender*	*Age*	*Equation*
Harris-Benedict[94]	BMR	Male	unspecified	66.47 + 13.75 W + 5.0 H − 6.76 A
		Female		655.1 + 9.56 W + 1.85 H − 4.68 A
World Health Organization (WHO)[95]	REE	Male	0–3 y	60.9 W − 54
			3–10 y	22.7 W + 495
		Female	0–3 y	61 W − 51
			3–10 y	22.5 W + 499
Schofield[96]	REE	Male	<3 y	0.17 W + 1.517 H − 617.6
			3–10 y	19.6 W + .1303 H + 414.9
			10–18 y	16.3 W + .1372 H + 515.5
		Female	<3 y	16.25 W + 1.0232 H − 413.5
			3–10 y	16.97 W + 161.8 H + 371.2
			10–18 y	8.365 W + 4.65 H + 200.0
Altman and Dittmer[97]	REE	Male	3–16 y	19.56 W + 506.16
		Female		18.67 W + 578.64
Maffeis et al.[98]	REE	Male	6–10 y	1287 + 28.6 W + 23.6 H − 69.1 A
		Female		1552 + 35.8 W + 15.6 H − 36.3 A
Piero et al. (for surgical infants)[99]	REE	unspecified	Infants	Cal/min = −74.436 + 34.661 W + 4.96 × HR + (0.78 × age in days)

W = weight in kilograms; A = age in years; H = height in centimeters; HR = heart rate in beats per minute

Source: See data from individual endnote references.

Table 2–6 Potential Changes in Energy Expenditure Associated with Different Diagnoses

Diagnosis	*Research*	*Population*	*Potential Stress Factor*
Closed Head Injury Postinjury day 1–14	Phillips et al. (1987)[100]	2–17 Years	Measured energy expenditure averaged 1.3 times Harris and Benedicts predicted value.
Sickle Cell Anemia	Williams et al. (2002)[101]	5–11 Years	Measured REE was 15% greater than predicted REE.
Inflammatory Bowel Disease	Kushner et al. (1991)[102]	19–40 Years	No significant increase in energy needs.
Cancer	Barale and Charuhas (1999)[103]	Unspecified	Supports adding 60–80% BEE to calculated BEE.
Allogeneric Stem Cell Transplantation Week 3 post transplant	Duggan et al. (2003)[104]	3–15 Years	Measured REE was .90–.95 predicted REE.
Extrahepatic Biliary Atresia	Pierro et al. (1989)[105]	2–73 Months	Energy expenditure was 29% higher than normal.
Spastic Quadriplegic Cerebral Palsy	Stallings et al. (1996)[106]	2–18 Years	Nonbasal energy expenditure was minimal.
Burns	Mayes et al. (1996)[107]	0.5–10 Years mean 30% BSA burns	Supports application of a factor 30% REE.
Post Surgery	Powis et al. (1998)[108]	0–3 Years major abdominal surgery	No increase in metabolic rate after major abdominal operations.
	Jones et al. (1993)[109]	0–4 Months various surgeries	Mean increase of 15 % REE following surgery.
Congenital Heart Defects	Barton et al. (1994)[110]	Less than 6 months severe congenital heart disease	Needs 40% greater than RDA for age.
HIV	Various	Mostly adult	Results of adult literature inconclusive with some studies showing increased REE[111] and others decreased.[112] No evidence that pediatric HIV disease in and of itself increases REE. See Chapter 21.
Fevers	Dubois EF (1954)[113]		REE increases 13% for each degree Centigrade of fever (7.2% for each degree Fahrenheit).

Source: See data from individual footnote references.

mass. The person with the higher lean body mass will have the higher energy expenditure.[115] In numerous studies, researchers have concluded that these standardized formulas may not be accurate in predicting individual energy needs for children with FTT, obesity, and some acute or chronic illnesses.[90,93,116,117]

Indirect Calorimetry

Indirect calorimetry is used to predict the energy needs for the subset of patients whose energy needs are elusive. This subset includes, but is not limited to, patients who are failing to thrive despite meeting predicted needs, obese patients, critically ill patients on nutrition support, and patients unable to be weaned from the ventilator. Indirect calorimetry measures oxygen consumption (VO_2) and carbon dioxide production (VCO_2). Most indirect calorimeters are open-circuit systems in which the patient breathes room air or air supplied from a mechanical ventilator and expires into a gas sampling system that eventually vents the expired air back into the room.[118] Indirect calorimetry provides two pieces of information: REE and a measure of substrate utilization as reflected in the respiratory quotient (RQ).

The following abbreviated Weir Equation calculates REE:[119]

$$\text{REE (kcal/min)} = 3.94 \times VO_2 + 1.11 \times VCO_2$$

Measured REE may need additional activity; stress added to accurately predict total energy needs. Also, measured REE does not account for anabolism or growth. In the adult or older child,

Table 2–7 Approximate Energy Expenditure for Various Activities in Relation to Resting Needs for Males and Females of Average Size*

Activity Category†	*Representative Value for Activity Factor per Unit Time of Activity*
Resting	REE × 1.0
Sleeping, reclining	
Very light	REE × 1.5
Seated and standing activities, painting trades, driving, laboratory work, typing, sewing, ironing, cooking, playing cards, playing a musical instrument	
Light	REE × 2.5
Walking on a level surface at 2.5 to 3 mph, garage work, electrical trades, carpentry, restaurant trades, house-cleaning, child care, golf, sailing, table tennis	
Moderate	REE × 5.0
Walking 3.5–4 mph, weeding and hoeing, carrying a load, cycling, skiing, tennis, dancing	
Heavy	REE × 7.0
Walking with load uphill, tree felling, heavy manual digging, basketball, climbing, football, soccer	

*Data from references 26 and 34.

†When reported as multiples of basal needs, the expenditures of males and females are similar.

Source: Reprinted with permission from *Recommended Dietary Allowances,* 10th ed., © 1989 by the National Academy of Sciences. Published by National Academy Press.

Table 2–8 Example of Calculation for Total Energy Expenditure in an 11-Year-Old Boy*

Activity Type	*REE Multiple*	*Duration (h)*	*Weighted REE Factor*
Resting	1.0	9	9
Very light	1.5	8	12
Light	2.5	4	10
Moderate	5.0	2	10
Heavy	7.0	1	7
TOTALS		24	48

Activity factor = weighted REE ÷ hours
= 48 ÷ 24
= 2.0

Total energy expenditure:

Gender	*Age (yr)*	*Wt (kg)*	*REE*† *(kcal/d)*	×	*Activity Factor*	=	*TEE (kcal/d)*
Male	11	35	1263.5	×	2.0	=	2527

*Hypothetical activity pattern
†Calculated from equations in Table 2–5

Source: Reprinted from Krug-Wispé S, Nutritional Assessment, in *Handbook of Pediatric Nutrition,* P. Queen and C.E. Lang, eds., p. 45, © 1993, Aspen Publishers, Inc., Gaithersburg, MD.

this represents a fraction of total energy needs. In the very young infant, this potential energy has been measured to be 2.73kcal/g tissue synthesized[115] though in the very sick or traumatized child, growth may be inhibited and applying growth factors may result in overfeeding.

Indirect calorimetry can also evaluate how the body is using fuel as reflected by the RQ. RQ is the ratio of carbon dioxide produced to oxygen consumed;

$$VCO_2/VO_2$$

Glucose oxidation is associated with an RQ of 1.0, fat oxidation with an RQ of 0.7, and protein metabolism with an RQ of 0.8. Alcohol or ketone metabolism may reduce the RQ to 0.67 while overfeeding with lipogenesis may increase the RQ to 1.3. Knowledge of inefficient substrate utilization and subsequent reduction of RQ through alteration of energy substrates can be medically advantageous.[120–122]

DATA EVALUATION AND PLAN

The assessment of nutritional status is based on the careful evaluation of all gathered information. Interrelationships between the health status of the child, feeding abilities, eating habits, anthropometric data, and laboratory findings need to be considered.[123–125]

Protein–Energy Malnutrition

The identification of the presence and severity of protein-energy malnutrition (PEM) among children in hospitals and clinics is a valuable function of nutritional assessment. An estimated 20–40% of hospitalized pediatric patients may have PEM.[126] Table 2–9 outlines anthropometric indices that have been developed to quantitate the severity of chronic and acute PEM. Children may present with one or both forms of PEM. Acute, but not chronic, PEM may increase morbidity and increase length of hospital stay.[126] For more information on "standard" reference values, refer to Chapter 18, Growth Failure.

Marasmus and Kwashiorkor

Marasmus and kwashiorkor are two classifications of severe, acute PEM. Marasmus develops over a period of weeks or months and is characterized by a wasted appearance due to diminished subcutaneous fat. Infants and children with marasmus have normal or low levels of serum albumin and other transport proteins and no evidence of edema. Liver size is normal.[123–126]

Conversely, kwashiorkor develops acutely, often in conjunction with an infection. Levels of serum albumin, other transport proteins, and lymphocytes are reduced. Edema is present over the trunk, extremities, and face. These infants and children often have subcutaneous fat stores that mask muscle wasting. Dermatitis and hair changes (flag sign) are usually present. In severe cases, fatty infiltration of the liver occurs.[123–126]

Marasmic kwashiorkor is the classification used to describe the presence of symptoms of kwashiorkor in a child with a weight for height less than 70% of standard or weight for age less then 60% of standard. This condition often develops following acute stress and is associated with high mortality.[126]

Other Nutritional Diagnoses

Other nutritional diagnoses such as obesity and growth failure as well as other diagnoses requiring therapeutic diet intervention will be further discussed in the forthcoming chapters.

Table 2–9 Anthropometric Indexes Associated with Protein-Energy Malnutrition

		Degree of PEM			
Type PEM	*Anthropometric Index*	*Normal*	*Mild*	*Moderate*	*Severe*
Chronic (stunting)					
	Height for age as % standard*	95	90–94	85–89	<85
Acute (wasting)					
	Weight for age as % standard*	90	75–89	60–74	<60
	Weight for height as % standard*	90	80–89	70–79	<70
	Arm circumference/ head circumference ratio†	>0.31	0.28–0.31	0.25–0.28	<.25

*Original data for determining degree of PEM used the 50th percentile of Boston growth data as standard. The 50th percentile on NCHS growth charts is now commonly used as the standard with these assessments.

†Ratio has been found to correlate with weight for age in children 3 months to 4 years of age.

Sources: Adapted with permission from Gomez F, Galvan R, Frenks, Munoz JC, Chavez R, Vasquez J. Mortality in second and third degree malnutrition. *J Trop Pediatr.* 1956;2:77 and Waterlow J. Classification and definition of protein calorie malnutrition. In Beaton G, Bengoa X, eds. *Nutrition in Preventive Medicine.* WHO monograph series No. 62. Geneva: WHO; 1976.

Care Plan

The nutritional care plan is developed to correct nutritional problems or reduce nutritional risks identified through the assessment. Basic information included in the medical and dietary histories provides a foundation for designing a plan that is reasonable and achievable within a given setting. The effectiveness of the nutritional intervention is determined through periodic nutritional reassessment. The care plan is modified as needed for changes in nutritional status/risk.

CONCLUSION

The provision of quality nutritional services to children is dependent on identifying those who are nutritionally depleted or at nutritional risk. In-depth nutritional assessments include a medical history and clinical evaluation, evaluation of anthropometric indices, and dietary evaluation. Biochemical indices may be evaluated as part of a routine nutritional screen or to confirm a suspected nutritional aberration. Assessment data are used to identify specific nutritional problems and to develop workable care plans targeted to improve nutritional status.

REFERENCES

1. Shapiro LR. Streamlining and implementing nutritional assessment. The dietary approach. *J Am Diet Assoc.* 1979;75:230–237.
2. Hunt DR, Maslovitz A, Rowlands BJ, Brooks B. A simple nutrition screening procedure for hospital patients. *J Am Diet Assoc.* 1985;85:332–335.
3. Christensen KS, Gstundtner KM. Hospital-wide screening improves basis for nutrition intervention. *J Am Diet Assoc.* 1985;85:332–335.
4. DeHoog S. Identifying patients at nutritional risk and determining clinical productivity: Essentials for an effective nutrition care program. *J Am Diet Assoc.* 1985;85:1620–1622.
5. Hedberg AM, Garcia N, Trejus IJ, Weinmann-Winkler S, Gabriel ML, Lutz AL. Nutrition risk screening: Development of a standardized protocol using dietetic technicians. *J Am Diet Assoc.* 1988;88:1553–1556.
6. Mezoff A, Gamm L, Konek S, Beal KG, Hitch D. Validation of a nutritional screen in children with respiratory syncytial virus admitted to an intensive care complex. *Pediatrics.* 1996;97:543–546.
7. Fomon SJ. *Nutritional Disorders of Children.* Rockville, MD: US Department of Health and Human Services, Education and Welfare; 1976:1–610, PHS publication no. (HAS) 75-5612.
8. Christakis G. Nutritional assessment in health programs. *Am J Public Health.* 1973;63(suppl):1–56.
9. *Comprehensive Accreditation Manuel for Hospitals 2004* CAMH. Oakbrook Terrace, IL: Joint Commission of Accreditation of Healthcare Organizations, 2004.
10. Kamath SK, Lawler M, Smith AE, Kalat T, Olson R. Hospital malnutrition: A 33 hospital screening study. *J Am Diet Assoc.* 1986;86:203–206.
11. Campbell MC, Kelsey KS. The PEACH Survey: A nutrition screening tool for use in early intervention programs. *J Am Diet Assoc.* 1994;99:1156–1158.
12. Noel MB, Wojnarosk SM. Nutrition screening for long-term care patients. *J Am Diet Assoc.* 1987;87: 1557–1558.
13. Baer MT, Farnan S, Mauer AM. Children with special health care needs. In: Shorbaugh CO, ed. *Call to Action: Better Nutrition for Mothers, Children, and Families.* Washington DC: National Center for Education in Maternal and Child Health; 1991:191–208.
14. Klawittler BM. Nutrition assesment of infants and children. In: Williams CD, ed. *Pediatric Manual of Clinical Dietetics.* Library of Congress, 1998:19–34.
15. *2000 CDC Growth Charts: United States.* Available at www.CDC.gov/growthcharts/.
16. National Center for Health Statistics. *Plan and operation of the Health and Nutrition Examination Survey,* United States, 1971–73, Vital Health Stat. 1973; No. 10a and 10b.
17. Alam N, Wojtyniak B, Rahaman MM. Anthropometric indicators and risk of death. *Am J Clin Nutr.* 1989;49: 884–888.
18. Frisancho AR. New norms of upper limb fat and muscle areas for assessment of nutritional status. *Am J Clin Nutr.* 1981;34:2540–2545.
19. Ryan AS, Martinez GA. Physical growth of infants 7–12 mos of age: Results from a national survey. *Am J Phys Anthropol.* 1987;73:449–457.
20. Paul AA, Cole TJ, Ahmed EA, Whithead RG. The need for revised standards for skinfold thickness in infancy. *Arch Dis Child.* 1998;78:354–358.
21. Tanner JM, Whitehouse RH. Revised standards for triceps and subscapular skinfolds in British children. *Arch Dis Child.* 1975;50:142–145.
22. Oakley RR, Parsons RJ, Whitelaw AOC. Standards for skinfold thickness in British newborn infants. *Arch Dis Child.* 1977;52:287–290.

23. The development of MUAC-for-age reference data recommended by a WHO expert committee. *WHO Bull.* 1997;75:11–18
24. Cronk CE, Roche AF. Race-and sex-specific reference data for triceps and subscapular skinfolds and weight/ stature. *Am J Clin Nutr.* 1982;35:347–354.
25. Owen GM, Lubin AH. Anthropometric differences between black and white preschool children. *Am J Dis Child.* 1973;168–169.
26. Ryan AS, Martinez GA, Baumgartner RN, Roche AF, Guo S, Chumlea WC, Kuczumarski RJ. Median skinfold thickness distributions and fat-wave patterns in Mexican-American children from the Hispanic Health and Nutrition Examination Survey (HHANES 1982–1984). *Am J Clin Nutr.* 1990;51:925S–935S.
27. Ryan AS, Martinez GA, Roche AF. An evaluation of the associations between socioeconomic status and the growth of Mexican-American children data from the Hispanic Health and Nutrition Examination Survey (HHANES 1982–1984). *Am J Clin Nutr.* 1990;51: 944S–952S.
28. Bray GA, Greenway FL, Molitech ME. Use of anthropometric measures to assess weight loss. *Am J Clin Nutr.* 1978;31:769–773.
29. Quatelet LAJ. *Physique Sociale,* vol 2. Brussels: C Muquardt; 1869.
30. Hammer LD, Kraemer HC, Wilson DM, Ritter PL, Dornbusch SM. Standardized percentile curves of body-mass index for children and adolescents. *AJDC.* 1997;145: 259–263.
31. Rosner B, Prineas R, Loggie J, Daniels SR. Percentiles for body mass index in US children 5 to 17 years of age. *J Pediatr.* 1998;132:211–222.
32. Leung SS, Cole TJ, Tse LY, Lou JT. Body mass index reference curves for Chinese children. *Ann Hum Bio.* 1998;25:169–174.
33. Cole TJ, Freeman JV, Preece MA. Body mass index reference curves for the UK 1990. *Arch Dis Child.* 1995;73:25–29.
34. Luciano A, Bressan F, Zoppi G. Body mass index reference curves for children ages 3–19 years from Verona, Italy. *Euro Clin Nutr.* 1997;51:6–10.
35. Bhalla AK, Walia BN. Percentile curves for body-mass index of Punjabi infants. *Indian Pediatr.* 1996;33: 471–476.
36. Aurelius G, Khan NC, True DB, Ha TT, Lindren G. Height weight and body mass index (BMI) of Vietnamese (Hanoi) schoolchildren aged 7–11 years related to parents' occupation and education. *Trop Pediatr.* 1996;42:21–26.
37. Lindgren G, Strandell A, Cole T, Healy M, Tanner J. Swedish population reference standards for height, weight, and body mass index attained at 6–16 years (girls) or 19 years (boys). *Acta Paediatrica.* 1995; 84:1019–1028.
38. Rolland-Cachera MF, Deheeger M, Bellisle F, Semp M, Guilloud-Bataillem M, Patois E. Obesity rebound in children: A simple indicator for predicting obesity. *Am J Clin Nutr.* 1984;39:129–135.
39. Kleinman RE, ed. *Pediatric Nutrition Handbook,* 5th ed. American Academy of Pediatrics; 2004.
40. Pietrobelii A, Faith MS, Allison DB, Gallagher D, Chiumello G, Heymsfield SB. Body mass index as a measure of adiposity among children and adolescents: A validation study. *J Pediatr.* 1998;132:204–210.
41. Warner JT, Cowan FJ, Dunstan FDJ, Gregory JW. The validity of body mass index for the assesment of adiposity in children with disease states. *Ann Human Bio.* 1997;24:209–215.
42. Hannan WJ, Wrate RM, Cowen SJ, Freman CPL. Body mass index as an estimate of body fat. *Inter J Eating Disorders.* 1995;18:91–97.
43. Tanner JM. Issues and advances in adolescent growth and development. *J Adolesc Health Care.* 1987;8: 470–478.
44. Behrman RE, Vaughan, VC, eds. *Nelsons Textbook of Medicine,* 13th ed. Philadelphia: WB Saunders Company; 1987.
45. Russell MS. Serum proteins and nitrogen balance: Evaluating response to nutrition support. In: *Dietetics in Nutrition Support Newsletter* (practice group for the American Dietetic Association). 1995;17:3–7.
46. Dowliko J, Nomplegsi DJ. The role of albumin in human physiology and pathophysiology. III. Albumin and disease states. *J Parenter Enter Nutr.* 1991; 15:477–487.
47. Golden MHN. Transport proteins as indices of protein status. *Am J Clin Nutr.* 1982;35:1159–1165.
48. Yoder MC, Anderson DC, Gopalakrishna GS, Douglas SD, Polin RA. Comparison of serum fibronectin, prealbumin and albumin concentrations during nutritional repletion in protein-calorie malnourished infants. *J Pediatr Gastroenterol Nutr.* 1987;6:84–88.
49. Joyce DL, Waites KB. Clinical applications of c-reactive protein in pediatrics. *Pediatr Infect Dis J.* 1997; 16:735–747.
50. Collier SB, Hendricks KM. Nutrition assessment. In: Baker RD, Baker SS, Daris AY, eds. *Pediatric Parenteral Nutrition.* New York:1997:42–63.
51. Buopane EA, Brown RO, Boucher BA, Fabian TC, Luther RW. Use of fibronectin and somatomedin C as nutritional markers in the enteral support of traumatized patients. *Crit Care Med.* 1989;17:126–132.
52. Merritt RJ, Blackburn GL. Nutritional assessment and metabolic response to illness of the hospitalized child.

In: Suskind R, ed. *Textbook of Pediatric Nutrition.* New York: Raven Press; 1981:296.

53. Cecalupo AJ, Cohen HJ. Nutritional anemias. In: Grand RJ, Sutphen JL, Dietz WH. *Pediatric Nutrition.* Stoneham, MA: Butterworth Publishers; 1987:489–499.
54. Expert Scientific Working Group. Summary of a report on assessment of the iron nutritional status of the United States population. *Am J Clin Nutr.* 1985; 42:1318–1330.
55. CDC. *Recommendations to Prevent and Control Iron Deficiency in the United States.* CDC MMWR. 1983;47 (RR-3):1–25.
56. Dallman RR, Yip R, Johnson C. Prevalence and causes of anemia in the United States, 1976–1980. *Am J Clin Nutr.* 1984;39:437–445.
57. Yip R, Johnson C, Dallman PR. Age-related changes in laboratory values used in the diagnosis of anemia and iron deficiency. *Am J Clin Nutr.* 1984;39:427–436.
58. Yip R, Dallman PR. The roles of inflammation and iron deficiency as causes of anemia. *Am J Clin Nutr.* 1988;48:1295–1300.
59. Cecalupo AJ, Cohen HJ. Nutritional anemias. In: Grand RJ, Sutphen JL, Dietz WH Jr, eds. *Pediatric Nutrition: Theory and Practice.* Boston, MA: Butterworth Publishing; 1987:489–491.
60. Puri S, Chandra RK. Nutritional regulation of host resistance and predictive value of immunologic tests in assessment of outcome. *Pediatr Clin North Am.* 1985;32:499–515.
61. Hattner JT, Kerner JA Jr. Nutritional assessment of the pediatric patient. In: Kerner JA Jr., ed. *Manual of Pediatric Parenteral Nutrition.* New York: John Wiley & Sons; 1983:19–60.
62. Christakis G. Nutritional assessment in health programs. *Am J Public Health.* 1973;63(suppl):1–56.
63. Pipes PL, Bumbalo J, Glass RP. Collecting and assessing food intake information. In: Pipes P, ed. *Nutrition in Infancy and Childhood.* St. Louis, MO: Times Mirror Mosby; 1989:58–85.
64. Barrocas A. Complementary and alternative medicine: Friend, foe or OWA. *J Am Diet Assoc.* 1997:1373–1376.
65. Workshop on Alternative Medicine. *Alternative Medicine: Expanding Medical Horizons.* Pittsburgh, PA: Government Printing Office; 1994; GPO No. 017-040-00537–7.
66. Eisenberg DM. Advising patients who seek alternative medical therapies. *Ann Intern Med.* 1997;127:61–67.
67. Burke BS. The dietary history as a tool in research. *J Am Diet Assoc.* 1947;23:1041.
68. Frank GC, Hollatz AT, Webber LS, Berenson GSS. Effect of interviewer recording practices on nutrient intake—Bogalusa Heart Study. *J Am Diet Assoc.* 1984; 84:1432–1439.
69. Medlin C, Skinner JD. Individual dietary intake methodology: A 50-year review of progress. *J Am Diet Assoc.* 1988;88:1250–1257.
70. Block G. A review of validations of dietary assessment methods. *Am J Epidemiol.* 1982;114:492–504.
71. Persson LA, Carlgren G. Measuring children's diets: Evaluation of dietary assessment techniques in infancy and childhood. *Internation J Epidemiol.* 1984;113: 506–517.
72. Carter RL, Sharbaugh CO, Stapell CA. Reliability and validity of the 24 hour recall. *J Am Diet Assoc.* 1981;79:542–547.
73. Emmons L, Hayes M. Accuracy of 24-hr recalls of young children. *J Am Diet Assoc.* 1973;62:409–415.
74. St Jeor SR, Guthrie HA, Jones MB. Variability in nutrient intake in a 28-day period. *J Am Diet Assoc.* 1983:155–162.
75. Rockett HRH, Colditz GA. Assessing diets of children and adolescents. *Am J Clin Nutr.* 1997;65:1116–1122.
76. Willett WC, Sampson L, Stampfer MJ, et al. Reproducibility and validity of a semiquantitative food frequency questionnaire. *Am J Epidemiol.* 1985;122: 51–65.
77. Larkin FA, Metzner HL, Thompson FE, Flegal KM, Guire KE. Comparison of estimated nutrient intakes by food frequency and dietary records in adults. *J Am Diet Assoc.* 1989;89:215–223.
78. Fong AK, Kretsch MJ. Nutrition evaluation scale system reduces time and labor in recording quantitative dietary intake. *J Am Diet Assoc.* 1990;90:664–670.
79. Brown JE, Tharp TM, Dahlber-Luby EM, et al. Videotape dietary assessment: Validity, reliability and comparison of results with 24-hour dietary recalls from elderly women in a retirement home. *J Am Diet Assoc.* 1990;90:1675–1679.
80. Ammerman AS, Kirkley BG, Dennis B, et al. A dietary assessment for individuals with low literacy skills using interactive touch-scan computer technology. *Am J Clin Nutr* 1994;59:289S.
81. Institute of Medicine, Food and Nutrition Board. *Dietary Reference Intakes: Energy, Carbohydrate, Fiber, Fat, Fatty Acids, Cholesterol, Protein and Amino Acids.* Washington, DC: National Academy Press; 2002.
82. Institute of Medicine, Food and Nutrition Board. *Dietary Reference Intakes: Dietary Reference Intakes for Vitamin A, Vitamin K, Arsenic, Boron, Chromium, Copper, Iodine, Iron, Magnanese, Molybedenum, Nickel, Silicon, Vanadium, and Zinc.* Washington, DC: National Academy Press; 2002.
83. Institute of Medicine, Food and Nutrition Board. *Dietary Reference Intakes for Vitamin C, Vitamin E, Selenium, and Carotenoids.* Washington, DC: National Academy Press; 2000.

84. Institute of Medicine, Food and Nutrition Board. *Dietary Reference Intakes for Calcium, Phosphorus, Magnesium, Vitamin D, and Fluoride.* Washington, DC: National Academy Press; 1997.

85. Institute of Medicine, Food and Nutrition Board. *Dietary Reference Intakes for Thiamin, Riboflavin, Niacin, Vitamin B6, Folate, Vitamin B12, Pantothenic Acid, Biotin, and Choline.* Washington, DC: National Academy Press; 2000.

86. Institute of Medicine, Food and Nutrition Board. *Dietary Reference Intakes for Sodium, Potassium, and Water.* Washington, DC: National Academy Press; 2004.

87. Yates AA, Schlicker SA, Suitor CW. Dietary reference intakes: The new basis for recommendations for calcium and related nutrients, B vitamins, and choline. *J Am Diet Assoc.* 1998:98:699–706.

88. Guthrie HA. The 1985 Dietary Allowance Committee: An overview. *J Am Diet Assoc.* 1985;85:1646–1648.

89. Garrel DR, Jobin N, De Jorge LHM. Should we still use the Harris and Benedict equations? *Nutr Clin Prac.* 1996;11:99–103.

90. Kaplan AS, Zemal BS, Neiswender KM, Stallings VA. Resting energy expenditure in clinical pediatrics: Measured versus prediction equations. *J Pediatr.* 1995;127;200–205.

91. World Health Organization. *Energy and protein requirements.* Report of a joint FAO/WHO/ UNU Expert Consultation. WHO Technical Report Series No. 724. Geneva: World Health Organization; 1985.

92. Bursztein S, Elwyn DH, Askanazi J, Kinney JM. The theoretical framework of indirect calorimetry and energy balance. In: *Energy Metabolism, Indirect Calorimetry and Nutrition.* Baltimore, MD: William & Wilkins; 1989;27–83.

93. Pencharz PB, Azcue MP. Measuring resting energy expenditure in clinical practice. *J Pediatr.* 1995;127: 269–271.

94. Harris JA, Benedict FG. *A Biometric Study of Basal Metabolism in Men.* Publication no. 279. Washington, DC: Carnagie Institute of Washington; 1919.

95. WHO. *Energy and Protein Requirements.* WHO Tech Rep Ser No. 724. Geneva; 1985.

96. Schofield WN. Predicting basal metabolic rate, new standards and review of previous work. *Hum Nutr Clin Nutr.* 1985;39c(1s):5–42.

97. Altman P, Dittmer D, eds. *Metabolism.* Bethesda, MD: Federation of American Societies for Experimental Biology; 1968.

98. Maffeis C, Schutz Y, Micciolo R, Zoccante L, Pinelli L. Resting metabolic rate in six-to ten-year-old obese and nonobese children. *J Pediatr.* 1993;122:556–562.

99. Pierro MO, Hammond JP, Donnell SC, Lloyd DA. A new equation to predict the resting energy expenditure of surgical infants. *J Ped Surg.* 1994;29:1103–1105.

100. Phillips R, Ott K, Young B. Nutritional support and measured energy expenditure of the child and adolescent with head injury. *J Neuro Surg.* 1987;67:846–851.

101. Williams R, Olivi, S, Mackert P, Fletcher L, Tian, G, Wang W. Comparison of energy prediction equations with measured resting energy expenditure in children with sickle cell anemia. *J Am Diet Assoc.* 2002; 102:956–961.

102. Kushner RF, Schoeller DA. Resting and total energy expenditure in patients with inflammatory bowel disease. *Am J Clin Nutr.* 1991;53:161–165.

103. Barale K, Charuhas P. Oncology and marrow transplantation. In: *Handbook of Pediatric Nutrition.* Gaithersburg, MD: Aspen Publishing; 1999:480.

104. Duggan C, Bechard L, Donovan K, Vangel M, O'Leary A, Holmes C, Le L, Guinan E. Changes in resting energy expenditure among children undergoing allogeneic stem cell transplantation. *Am J Clin Nutr.* 2003; 78(1):104–109.

105. Pierro A, Koletzko B, Carnielli V, Superine RA, Roberts EA, Filler RM, Smith J, Heim T. Resting energy expenditure is increased in infants and children with extrahepatic biliary atresia. *J Ped Surg.* 1989;24:534–538.

106. Stallings VA, Zemol BS, Davies JC, Cronk CE, Charney EB. Energy expenditure of children and adolescents with severe disabilities; a cerebral palsy model. *Am J Clin Nutr.* 1996;64:627–634.

107. Mayes, TM, Gottschlich MM, Khoury J, Warren GD. Evaluation of predicted and measured energy requirements in burned children. *J Amer Diet Assoc.* 1996;96: 24–29.

108. Powis MR, Smith K, Renii M, Halliday D, Pierro A. Effect of major abdominal operatons on energy and protein metabolism in infants and children. *J Ped Surg.* 1998;33:49–53.

109. Jones MO, Pierro P, Hammond P, Lloyd DA. The metabolic response to operative stress in infants. *J Ped Surg.* 1993;28:1258–1262.

110. Barton JS, Hindmarsh PC, Scrimseour CM, Rennie MJ, Preece MH. Energy expenditure in congenital heart disease. *Arch Dis Child.* 1994;70:5–9.

111. Grunfeld C, Feingold RR. Metabolic disturbances and wasting in the acquired immunodeficiency syndrome. *N Eng J Med.* 1992;327:329–337.

112. Kotler DP, Tierney AR, Brenner SK, Couture S, Wang J, Pierson RM. Of short-term energy balance in clinically stable patients with AIDS. *Am J Clin Nutr.* 1990;51:7–13.

113. Dubois EF. Energy metabolism. *Ann Rev Physiol.* 1954;16:125–134.

114. Chwals WJ. Overfeeding the critically ill child: fact or fantasy? *New Horizons.* 1994;2:147–155.

115. Subcommittee on the tenth edition of the RDAs, Food and Nutrition Board, National Research Council. *Recom-*

mended Dietary Allowances, 10th ed. Washington, DC: National Academy Press; 1989.

116. Coss-Bu JA, Jefferson LS, Walding D, Yadin D, Smith EO, Klish W. Resting energy expenditure in children in a pediatric intensive care unit: Comparison of Harris-Benedict and Talbot predictions with indirect calorimetry values. *Am J Clin Nutr.* 1998;67:74–80.

117. Bandini LG, Morelli JA, Must A, Dietz WH. Accuracy of standardized equations for predicting metabolic rate in premenarchal girls. *Am J Clin Nutr.* 1995;62: 711–714.

118. Matarese LE. Indirect calorimetry: technical aspects. *J Am Diet Assoc.* 1997;97:s154–s160.

119. Porter C, Cohen NH. Indirect calorimetry in critically ill patients. Role of the clinical dietitian in interpreting results. *Am J Diet Assoc.* 1996;96:49–57.

120. Weir JB. New methods for calculating metabolic rate with special reference to protein metabolism. *J Physiol.* 1949;109:1–9.

121. Bursztein S, Elwyn DH, Askanazi J, Kinney JM. The theoretical framework of indirect calorimetry and energy balance. In: *Energy Metabolism, Indirect Calorimetry and Nutrition.* Baltimore, MD: William and Wilkins; 1989:27–83.

122. Ireton-Jones CS, Turner WW Jr. The use of respiratory quotient to determine the efficacy of nutrition support systems. *J Am Diet Assoc.* 1987;87:180–183.

123. Waterlow JC. Classification and definition of protein-calorie malnutrition. *Br Med J.* 1972;3:566–569.

124. McLaren DS, Read WWC. Classification of nutritional status in early childhood. *Lancet.* 1972;2:146–148.

125. Waterlow JC. Note on the assessment and classification of protein-energy malnutrition in children. *Lancet.* 1973;2:87–89.

126. Pollack MM, Ruttimann UE, Wiley JS. Nutritional depletions in critically ill children: Associations with physiologic instability and increased quantity of care. *J Parenter Enter Nutr.* 1985;9:309–313.

CHAPTER 3

Prenatal Nutrition

Barbara Luke, Mary L. Hediger, and Janet Washington

INTRODUCTION

Nutrition in maternity is an area of research and clinical practice that has received renewed interest, as prevention becomes the universal standard of care. As part of the health care reform in the United States, medical nutrition therapy has gained acceptance, particularly during pregnancy.[1–4] The benefits of nutrition therapy during pregnancy are both immediate and far-reaching, from reducing maternal susceptibility to infections and nutrient deficiencies, minimizing the iron and calcium drain on the mother's reserves, and improving intrauterine growth and ultimate birthweight to preventing preterm birth and its adverse health consequences into childhood and beyond. In addition to translating research into clinical practice, an important component of medical nutrition therapy during pregnancy is consumer education and improving consumer dietary behavior.[5–7] The most recent *Guidelines for Perinatal Care* (5th edition, 2002), issued jointly by the American Academy of Pediatrics and the American College of Obstetricians and Gynecologists, places a strong emphasis on the importance of maternal and newborn nutrition.[8]

PRECONCEPTIONAL NUTRITION

Preconceptional nutritional status and the mother's dietary intake during the early weeks of pregnancy can critically influence the course and outcome of pregnancy. Although it would be beneficial for all women to receive preconceptional nutrition counseling to improve their health before beginning a pregnancy, it is of even greater importance for women who are underweight, have recently recovered from major illnesses or surgery, have diabetes or metabolic disorders such as phenylketonuria (PKU), or those who smoke or have had a previous infant with a neural tube defect. The goals of preconceptional nutrition counseling are to improve body weight to be within a normal range for the woman's height and body build and to correct any nutritional imbalances such as iron-deficiency and to help establish healthy eating patterns.

Each year in the United States, there are about 4,000 pregnancies affected by neural tube defects, including spina bifida or anencephaly. The scientific evidence from randomized trials around the world indicates that folic acid can reduce the occurrence of these congenital anomalies by at least 50% when taken daily before conception and during early pregnancy.[9,10] As the result of this strong evidence, in 1992 the U.S. Public Health Service issued the recommendation that all women of childbearing age who are capable of becoming pregnant consume 400 mcg of folic acid daily, in addition to intake of folate from a varied diet.[11] The recommended daily requirement for folate during pregnancy and lactation is 600 mcg and 500 mcg, respectively. Less than 10% of U.S. women have diets that meet this level of folate.[12] Good dietary sources of folic acid include oranges, asparagus, beans, beets, broccoli, spinach, romaine lettuce, fortified breakfast cereals, and beef liver.

As part of preconception counseling, as well as good health practice during pregnancy and lactation, women should avoid alcohol, smoking, recreational or illegal drug use, and take only those medications approved by her physician. Alcohol use during pregnancy is associated with Fetal Alcohol Syndrome (FAS), a syndrome of mental retardation and a specific array of facial malformations, which was first identified by French scientists in 1968. In the United States, FAS affects approximately 5,000 babies every year, making it the leading cause of mental retardation and learning and behavioral problems.[13] In addition, even moderate drinking—as little as three drinks per week during pregnancy—more than doubles the risk of low birth weight (less than 5.5 pounds).[14] Smoking during pregnancy is associated with increased risks for miscarriages, birth defects, and placental complications.[15,16] Expectant mothers who smoke are far more likely to deliver prematurely, 3 or more weeks before their due date. An estimated 27% of all premature births in the United States are due to smoking.[17,18] Environmental toxins should also be avoided during the preconception period, as well as during pregnancy and lactation. This includes exposure to pesticides, paints, and solvents, as well as household chemicals, lead in the water supply, cat feces (which can carry a parasite that causes toxoplasmosis), and saunas and hot tubs (because the high temperatures can be harmful to the unborn baby).

DIET DURING PREGNANCY

Both the quality and quantity of the diet during pregnancy critically influence the health of the mother and her unborn child. Energy and nutrient requirements increase during pregnancy to assure appropriate maternal adaptation to pregnancy and optimal fetal growth. In singleton pregnancies, the daily caloric requirement is approximately 27–30 kcal per kg maternal prepregnancy weight during the first trimester, and 30 kcal per kg maternal prepregnancy weight plus 200–300 kcal during the second and third trimesters. In underweight women, these caloric prescriptions would need to be adjusted upwards. The recommended caloric distribution of macronutrients during pregnancy is the same as for all healthy adults, 20% of kcal from protein, 30–35% of kcal from fat, and the remainder (45–50% of kcal) from carbohydrates. A summary of recommended dietary allowances (RDAs) and dietary reference intakes from the Food and Nutrition Board, the Institute of Medicine (IOM), is given in Table 3–1.

Use of Vitamin-Mineral Supplements

Ideally, pregnant women should get the level and range of required nutrients through a balanced diet. Recent national dietary surveys indicate, though, that adult women fail to meet the RDAs for five nutrients: calcium, magnesium, zinc, and vitamins E and B6.[19] In addition, prenatal use of vitamin-mineral supplements among low-income women has been shown to reduce the risks of preterm delivery and low birthweight, particularly, if initiated during the first trimester.[20] Data from national surveys indicates that the majority of Americans, including one-half to two-thirds of women of childbearing age, takes some form of vitamin-mineral supplements.[21–23] Vitamin-mineral supplement use is more common among women than men, among individuals with one or more health problems, and among older individuals.[21]

Supplementation in excess of twice the RDA (see Table 3–1) should be avoided, due to the potential for birth defects. The fat-soluble vitamins, particularly vitamins A and D, are the most potentially toxic during pregnancy. The pediatric and obstetric literature includes case reports of kidney malformations in children whose mothers took between 40,000 and 50,000 IU of vitamin A during pregnancy. Even at lower doses, excessive amounts of vitamin A may cause subtle damage to the developing nervous system, resulting in serious behavioral and learning disabilities in later life. The margin of safety for vitamin D is smaller for this vitamin than for any other. Birth defects of the heart, particularly aortic stenosis, have been

Table 3–1 Summary of Recommended Dietary Allowances and Adequate Intakes for Females by Age and Pregnancy and Lactation Status

Nutrient	*Nonpregnant*			*Pregnancy*			*Lactation*		
	14–18 yrs.	*19–30 yrs.*	*31–50 yrs.*	*18 yrs.*	*19–30 yrs.*	*31–50 yrs.*	*18 yrs.*	*19–30 yrs.*	*31–50 yrs.*
Macronutrients									
Carbohydrate (g)	130	130	130	175	175	175	210	210	210
Total fiber (g)	26	25	25	28	28	28	29	29	29
Total fat (g)	25–35	20–35	20–35	20–35	20–35	20–35	20–35	20–35	20–35
Protein (g)	46	46	46	71	71	71	71	71	71
Vitamins									
Biotin (μg)	25	30	30	30	30	30	35	35	35
Choline (mg)	400	425	425	450	450	450	550	550	550
Folate (μg)	400	400	400	600	600	600	500	500	500
Niacin (mg)	14	14	14	18	18	18	17	17	17
Pantothenic acid (mg)	5	5	5	6	6	6	7	7	7
Riboflavin (mg)	1.1	1.1	1.1	1.4	1.4	1.4	1.6	1.6	1.6
Thiamin (mg)	1.1	1.1	1.1	1.4	1.4	1.4	1.4	1.4	1.4
Vitamin A (μg)	700	700	700	750	770	770	1,200	1,300	1,300
Vitamin B6 (mg)	1.2	1.3	1.3	1.9	1.9	1.9	2.0	2.0	2.0
Vitamin B12 (μg)	2.4	2.4	2.4	2.6	2.6	2.6	2.8	2.8	2.8
Vitamin C (mg)	65	75	75	80	85	85	115	120	120
Vitamin D (μg)	5	5	5	5	5	5	5	5	5
Vitamin E (mg)	15	15	15	15	15	15	19	19	19
Vitamin K (μg)	75	90	90	75	90	90	75	90	90
Minerals									
Calcium (mg)	1,300	1,000	1,000	1,300	1,000	1,000	1,300	1,000	1,000
Chromium (μg)	24	25	25	29	30	30	44	45	45
Copper (μg)	890	900	900	1,000	1,000	1,000	1,300	1,300	1,300
Fluoride (mg)	3	3	3	3	3	3	3	3	3
Iodine (μg)	150	150	150	220	220	220	290	290	290
Iron (mg)	15	18	18	27	27	27	10	9	9
Magnesium (mg)	360	310	320	400	350	360	360	310	320
Manganese (mg)	1.6	1.8	1.8	2.0	2.0	2.0	2.6	2.6	2.6
Molybdenum (μg)	43	45	45	50	50	50	50	50	50
Phosphorus (mg)	1,250	700	700	1,250	700	700	1,250	700	700
Selenium (μg)	55	55	55	60	60	60	70	70	70
Zinc (mg)	9	8	8	12	11	11	13	12	12

Source: Dietary Reference Intakes, Institute of Medicine, National Academy of Sciences, www.nap.edu, 2004.

reported in both humans and experimental animals with doses as low as 4,000 IU, which is 10 times the RDA during pregnancy.

There are no requirements for routine supplementation with the possible exception of iron. In instances in which inadequacies cannot be remedied through diet or if a woman has unique nutritional requirements, such as multiple gestation, diagnoses of hemoglobinopathies or seizure disorders, or other circumstances, daily supplementation may be the most reasonable alternative. The IOM 1990 report[24] recommends daily iron supplementation with 30 mg per day during the second and third trimesters, as prophylaxis for iron deficiency. The treatment of iron-deficiency anemia requires daily doses of 60–120 mg of elemental iron to be taken between meals or at bedtime to facilitate absorption. Iron should not be taken as part of a vitamin-mineral supplement, due to the inhibition by other minerals, as well as poor iron release.[25] To minimize their side effects, iron supplements should be taken with a nondairy snack.

MATERNAL-INFANT WEIGHT RELATIONSHIPS

Infant birthweight and length of gestation are important indicators of health status at birth, with the proportions of low birth weight (LBW, <2500 g), very low birth weight (VLBW, <1500 g), and preterm births (<37 completed weeks' gestation) being primary measures of the nation's reproductive health. Compared to infants with birth weights under 2500 g, the risk of dying during the first year of life is six-fold greater for LBW infants and ninety-fold greater for VLBW infants.[26] Based on all live births in the United States in 2002,[27] 7.8% of infants are LBW, up 16% from 1980 (6.7%); 1.46% of infants are VLBW, up 8% since 1980 (1.35%). In absolute terms, 314,077 infants were born LBW, including 58,544 infants who were born VLBW. Twelve percent of all live births in 2002 were preterm, totaling 480,812 infants. This percent has risen by 14% since 1990. The two strongest predictors of infant birth weight, after length of gestation, are maternal prepregnancy weight and gestational weight gain. The landmark studies in this area are from the National Collaborative Perinatal Project, which was conducted between 1959–64.[28–31] Based on term, singleton pregnancies, these studies demonstrated that,

1. A progressive increase in weight gain paralleled an increase in mean birth weight and a decline in the incidence of low birth weight.
2. Increasing prepregnancy weight diminishes the effect of weight gain on birth weight.
3. There is an inverse relationship between weight gain and perinatal mortality, with gains up to 30 pounds.
4. Higher gestational weight gains are related to higher birth weights and better growth and development during the first postnatal year.

The following section puts the results of this pivotal study into historical context, and reviews the subsequent clinical nutrition literature and recommendations to date.

Historical Issues

One of the earliest large studies linking maternal weight gain to fetal growth and size, the National Collaborative Perinatal Project (NCPP), was conducted between 1959 and 1964, when tight restriction on weight gain was in force.[32,33] However, based on the information collected by the NCPP, the National Academy of Sciences concluded in their 1970 study that perinatal mortality rates were actually lowest at weight gains of 24 to 27 lbs., thereby beginning to refocus weight gain concerns away from the mother and onto the fetus.[34]

In the 1980s, the focus shifted almost completely to the well-being of the fetus and infant. New emphasis was placed on low or inadequate weight gains, dietary deficiencies, and their consequences for fetal growth and pregnancy outcome. It was in this context that the Committee on Nutritional Status During Pregnancy and Lactation of the Institute of Medicine revised the recommendations for weight gain during pregnancy. Their report, *Nutrition During Pregnancy*,[24] released in 1990, has proven to be the benchmark for current recommendations and research. Studies evaluating the IOM recommendations have been fairly uniform in agreeing that the weight gain target ranges (Table 3–2) are reasonable. Gains within the ranges are likely to be associated with a reduced risk of LBW, but gains above that range may increase the risk of an LGA or high birth weight (> 4,500 g) delivery. The recommendation that black women gain at the upper end of the range is questionable, and there are lingering questions about the ranges for overweight and particularly an upper limit for obese women.

The IOM Findings and Recommendations

The central recommendation of the IOM with regard to weight gain is that appropriate weight gain during pregnancy (Table 3–2) should be encouraged (by dietary intervention and counseling)—especially among high-risk groups, such as young adolescents (within 2 years of menarche), black women, women with low prepregnancy weight, and mothers of twins and higher order multiples (triplets, quadruplets, or quintuplets)—to enhance fetal growth and to diminish the risk of LBW and perinatal morbidity.[24] A unique feature of the IOM recommendations was that the suggested target weight gain ranges were specific to maternal prepregnancy weight status, using the body mass index (BMI, kg/m^2) as the preferred index of maternal prepregnancy status. BMI is a better indicator of nutritional status than weight alone. At a prepregnancy BMI of less than 19.8, a woman was considered to be underweight, at 19.8 to 26.0 normal weight, over 26.0 to 29.0 overweight, and over 29.0 obese.

The IOM established that:

1. In both developed and developing countries and for all racial and ethnic groups, there is a positive relationship between weight gain and birth weight.
2. Maternal prepregnancy weight or BMI (kg/m^2) and weight gain have independent and additive effects on birth weight outcome.
3. The average magnitude of the effect on birth weight (in women with a normal BMI) is, assuming a base birth weight of about 3,000 g, approximately 20 g of birth weight for every 1 kg of total gain.[35]
4. Prepregnancy BMI is a strong effect modifier; that is, the effect of gestational

Table 3–2 Institute of Medicine Categories of Pregravid Body Mass Index (BMI) and Suggested Weight Gain Ranges for Singleton Pregnancies

Weight status	*BMI range (kg/m^2)*	*Total gain at 40 weeks*	*Weight gain trimester 1*	*Rate of gain trimesters 2 & 3*
Underweight	<19.8 kg/m^2	12.5–18.0 kg (28–40 lb)	2.3 kg (5.1 lb)	0.49 kg/wk (1 lb/wk)
Normal weight	19.8–26.0 kg/m^2	11.5–16.0 kg (25–35 lb)	1.6 kg (3.5 lb)	0.44 kg/wk (1 lb/wk)
Overweight	26.1–29.0 kg/m^2	7.0–11.5 kg (15–25 lb)	0.9 kg (2.0 lb)	0.30 kg/wk (1/2 – 3/4 lb/wk)
Obese	>29.0 kg/m^2	≥6.8 kg (≥15 lb)	no recommendation	

The suggested range for twin pregnancies was 16.0–20.0 kg (35–45 lb). It was suggested that pregnant adolescents who were within 2 years of menarche and black women should strive for gains at the upper end and shorter women (< 157 cm or 62 in) at the lower end of the ranges.

Source: Adapted from Subcommittee on Nutritional Status and Weight Gain During Pregnancy, Committee on Nutritional Status During Pregnancy and Lactation, Institute of Medicine. ***Nutrition During Pregnancy.*** Washington, DC: National Academy Press, 1990.

weight gain is modified by maternal prepregnancy BMI. The effect of a given weight gain is greatest in thin women and least in the overweight and obese.

The IOM also concluded that low gestational weight gain is strongly associated with increased risk for LBW and fetal growth restriction (FGR). In so concluding, the IOM relied heavily on its deliberations on original analyses of data from the 1980 National Natality Survey.[36] Adjusting for maternal age, parity, height, cigarette smoking, and education, there was a greater than twofold risk of term LBW with a low total weight gain of 10 kg (22 lb) or less for both underweight women and normal weight women. For overweight women (BMI > 26.0 kg/m^2), the relationship was less.[36]

Although the IOM recommended target ranges of weight gain and did not develop growth curves based on empirical data, the shape of the gestational weight gain curves in adults was described. Weight gain is least in the first trimester (about 1 kg/mo),[36] and then accrues at around 0.45 kg/wk (1 lb/wk) for the duration of pregnancy.[24] The weight that is gained early in pregnancy appears to represent primarily maternal body fat. In a study of 20 middle-class white women from Burlington, Vermont, it was estimated that 75% of the nearly 3.3 kg gained in the first 15 weeks of pregnancy was attributable to increases in fat tissue, particularly that localized in the abdominal and suprailiac regions.[37]

Longitudinal studies through pregnancy done subsequent to the IOM study have confirmed this pattern. In a racially mixed sample (38% white, 39% black, 23% Puerto Rican) of 1,419 adolescents aged 18 years or less with uncomplicated term pregnancies from Camden County, New Jersey, the adolescents were found to exhibit a weight gain curve similar to that of adults. However, the median gains and rates of gain were higher throughout gestation, but especially from mid-pregnancy on (0.51 kg/wk).[38] Further, the average weight gain at term of 14–15 kg (31–33 lb) was at the high end of the range (11.5–16 kg) currently recommended for women with normal BMI (19.8–26.0). In a racially mixed sample (45% white, 17% black, 15% Hispanic, 13% Asian, 9% other) of 10,418 women, including both preterm and term deliveries, from San Francisco, Abrams and associates[39] found that the average rate of weight gain was lowest in the first trimester (0.17 ± 0.27 kg/wk), highest in the second trimester (0.56 ± 0.24 kg/wk), and just slightly slower in the third (0.52 ± 0.23 kg/wk).

Weight Gain and Preterm Delivery

Studies conducted since the release of the IOM report have shown that although total weight gain is an important predictor of birth weight, the pattern of weight gain and rates appear significant in predicting preterm delivery.[40] One of the first studies relating weight gain late in pregnancy to preterm delivery was a study of 1,790 adolescent pregnancies from Camden County, New Jersey.[41] Although a low early weight gain (<4.3 kg by 24 weeks' gestation) was associated with an increased risk of having an SGA infant (<10th birth weight for gestational age), preterm delivery at less than 37 completed weeks' gestation was associated instead with low weight gain rates (<400 g/wk) after 24 weeks. There was an increased risk of preterm delivery both when weight gain was less than 400 g/wk after 24 weeks and when weight gain was low both before and after 24 weeks. Further, the low rates after 24 weeks was associated with preterm delivery even when the total pregnancy weight gain was within targets set in clinical standards. Other subsequent studies of adults have confirmed that low rates of weight gain, either in the latter half of pregnancy or the second and third trimesters, are associated with preterm delivery.[42–47]

A case-control study in Italy has also confirmed for a European sample that gestational weight gain late in pregnancy is associated with preterm delivery. Spinillo and associates[46] studied the joint effects of both low prepregnancy BMI (≤19.5 kg/m^2) and a low rate of weight gain (≤0.37 kg/wk) in the second and third trimesters among 230 women who delivered preterm compared with 460 controls. Both low prepregnancy

BMI and a low rate of weight gain in the second and third trimesters were associated with an increased risk of preterm delivery, and the effects were mostly additive. The risk of preterm delivery associated with a low rate of gestational weight gain was greater among those with low prepregnancy BMI than those with a prepregnancy BMI above 19.5 kg/m^2.

That low rates of weight gain late in pregnancy appear now firmly associated with preterm delivery does not imply causation. Low rates of maternal weight gain late in pregnancy may be an indirect reflection of maternal nutritional status.[40] Poor nutrition in the first and early second trimester may affect placental development and vascularization, leading to fetal growth restriction. Early poor nutrition, whether characterized or not by low weight gain, might also affect the integrity of the chorioamniotic membranes, leading to preterm premature rupture of membranes (PPROM)[48] or increased susceptibility to vaginal or urinary tract infection. For example, studies of zinc nutriture have found that low intakes of zinc are related to an increased risk of preterm delivery,[49] and the risk of preterm delivery with low dietary zinc intake was nearly tripled for those with PPROM. Zinc has well-known antiseptic effects, so that low levels of intake might indicate an increased susceptibility to infection. On the other hand, the low rates of gestational gain may also reflect a slowed fetal growth associated with preterm delivery and be a marker for impending preterm birth. Several studies have demonstrated that birth weights of preterm infants were significantly smaller than the estimated fetal weight of same-aged fetuses that later delivered at term.[50–53] Infants delivered preterm after PPROM or with spontaneous preterm labor were smaller in all dimensions, implying an overall slowing of growth originating early in pregnancy and demonstrating more chronic stress.

Patterns of Maternal Weight Gain and Their Implications

The changes in body composition are reflected in patterns of weight gain and how the patterns are related to birth weight. The studies that have looked at patterns of weight gain by trimester have found that weight gain rates are highest in the second trimester (14–26 weeks) and most predictive of birth weight.[39,43,54,55] In a study of 2,994 nonobese white women with singleton pregnancies from San Francisco, Abrams and associates[39] found that first trimester gain averaged 2.1 ± 3.3 kg, second trimester gain 7.7 ± 2.9 kg, and third trimester gain 6.6 ± 2.7 kg. Further, in models including gestational age, weight gain by trimester, maternal height, infant sex, parity, smoking, prepregnancy BMI, and maternal age, second trimester weight gain was the strongest predictor of infant birth weight next to gestational age. In a study of 1,015 nonobese black and white women from Alabama, Hickey and associates[43] found that first trimester weight gain averaged 2.48 ± 3.36 kg, second trimester rates of gain averaged 0.49 ± 0.21 kg/wk, and third trimester 0.45 ± 0.28 kg/wk, and again low second trimester gains were most closely associated with decreased birth weight.

Weight Gain in Groups with Special Recommendations

Young Adolescents

The IOM recommended in its report that young adolescents (within 2 years of menarche) be targeted at the upper end of the weight gain ranges for their prepregnancy BMI.[24] At the time, given the lack of information on adolescent pregnancy outcomes and their relationship to weight gain, this was seen as merely a prudent recommendation based on the fact that young adolescents within 2 years of menarche are likely to still be biologically immature and may possibly compete with their fetus for nutrients. However, the weight gain recommendations for adolescent pregnancy have been one of the most debated points arising out of the IOM report.[56–60]

Complicating the development of weight gain recommendations for adolescents is the fact that there are no reliable markers for maternal growth during adolescent pregnancy that do not involve specialized techniques of assessment.[56,57] In addition, pregnant teenagers are at high risk for low weight gain and poor pregnancy outcomes by virtue of their demographic and social circumstances.[61] It is well-known that adolescent pregnancy is more common among minorities (blacks, Puerto Ricans, Mexican-Americans) and in low-income communities. It has been shown that the risk of low weight gain (<20 lb) and subsequently lower birth weight was also significantly increased when the adolescent had a sexually transmitted disease, was battered during the pregnancy, or if the pregnancy was unplanned.[61]

Nevertheless, it may be necessary for all adolescents to gain at the upper end of the IOM ranges. In a study of 459 teenagers, Rees and colleagues[62] found that for adolescents, the rates of weight gain in the second and third trimesters averaged 0.50 kg/week when birth weight was <3,000 g, but averaged 0.57 kg/week when birth weight was between 3,000–4,000 g. In producing infants of optimal size (3,000–4,000 g), then, the adolescents may need to have higher rates of weight gain than adults. This is undoubtedly because a substantial proportion of adolescents are biologically immature and still growing.

Black Women

The recommendation that black women gain at the upper end of the IOM ranges, however, does not seem to be supported by the most recent studies that have evaluated the recommendations. In particular, the studies of Caulfield and colleagues[63,64] have shown that although black women were at increased risk overall for SGA (<10th percentile) and at decreased risk for an LGA birth (>90th percentile) compared with white women, there were no significant differences in the effect of weight gain by ethnic group. Having black women gain more weight may not appreciably affect rates of SGA and LGA. Given that black women, at comparable weight gains, tend to retain more weight in the postpartum,[65–67] high weight gain for black women may only increase the risks for obesity while not significantly improving outcome.

Women with Low Prepregnancy Weight

Maternal size (weight, height, and BMI) is often taken to reflect prepregnancy nutritional status, although these indicators are not very specific. Women who are underweight (BMI <19.8) are thought to have low nutritional reserves and, even at comparable weight gains, give birth to infants who are smaller.[24] The IOM recommendation for underweight women is that they be targeted at a slightly higher total gain. Particularly these gains should be early in pregnancy to compensate for their low nutritional reserves.

The most direct evidence for the importance of weight gain to underweight women is from a study by Rosso and associates,[68] where placental weight and plasma volume were compared between 12 normal weight and 12 underweight women in Santiago, Chile. The underweight women gained less weight during pregnancy (10.8 ± 1.1 kg) compared with the normal weight women (12.0 ± 1.3 kg), and had both placental weights (473 ± 29 versus 646 ± 30 g, $p<.001$) and plasma volumes (2,731 ± 84 versus 3,227 ± 103 mL, $p<.002$) that were significantly smaller. At similar gestations, the infants of underweight women were also smaller (2,837 ± 125 versus 3,362 ± 106, $p<.005$). Thus, given what is known about weight gain and the timing of expansion of maternal compartments, better early weight gain in underweight women may be related to improved placental growth and a greater expansion of plasma volume, thereby improving fetal growth.

Establishing an Upper Limit for Obese Women

Obese women are known to be at increased risk for a number of pregnancy complications, including infection, gestational diabetes, pregnancy-induced hypertension, cesarean delivery, and postpartum morbidity.[69] Obese women have infants with larger birth weights and are at risk for large-for-gestational age infants. Such overly large infants are, in turn, also at risk for delivery complications (such as shoulder dystocia) and postpartum morbidity. Whether these complications and outcomes are also related to or exacerbated by weight gain is still unclear. The IOM has recommended that overweight women (26.1–29.0 kg/m^2) gain in the range of 7.0–11.5 kg, while obese women (BMI >29.0) gain at least 6.8 kg (15 lb), which is equivalent to the amount accounted for by the products of conception. No upper limit of weight gain was identified for obese women by the IOM.

Three studies have examined weight gain among obese women with the intent of establishing an upper limit for the range.[70–72] In a study of 53,541 singleton pregnancies from the Pregnancy Nutrition Surveillance System, Cogswell and associates[71] evaluated the risk of LBW and high birth weight (HBW >4,500 g) by weight gain for normal weight, overweight, and obese women defined using IOM criteria. For normal weight women, the risk of LBW was increased with a weight gain less than 15 lb and the risk of HBW was increased at gains of 40 lb or more. At gains greater than 30 lb the risk of LBW was decreased. However, among obese women, gains less than 15 lb were not associated with an increased risk of LBW, and gains greater than 20 lb were not associated with a decreased risk of LBW. At gains greater than 25 lb, the risk of HBW was significantly increased. Cogswell and colleagues[71] concluded that gestational weight gains of more than 25 lb may carry a significantly increased risk of HBW for obese women.

Two other studies have similarly concluded that an upper limit of 25 lb (11.5 kg) is probably a prudent upper limit for weight gain among obese women.[70,72] Edwards and associates[72] studied the outcomes of 660 normal weight women and 683 obese women from St. Paul, Minnesota. They found that compared with obese women who gained from 7–11.5 kg, obese women who lost or gained no weight were at increased risk for delivery of an infant of less than 3,000 g or SGA. Obese women that gained more than 16 kg (35 lb) were twice as likely to deliver infants who weighed 4,000 g or less. In their study of 613 morbidly obese women (BMI >35.0 kg/m^2), compared with 11,313 nonobese women, Bianco and colleagues[70] confirmed that an upper limit of 25 lb for obese women is associated with a reduction in risk for LGA and supported the suggestion that the upper limit be set at 25 lb.

Multiple Gestations

Multiple births have risen dramatically over the past 20 years in the United States, primarily due to the increasing use of assisted reproductive technologies. Women pregnant with multiples are more likely to be hospitalized for antenatal complications, contributing substantially to the overall costs of these high-risk pregnancies.[73] The most common antenatal complications include:

preterm premature rupture of membranes (PPROM, 12–25%)
preterm labor (60–86%)
anemia (19–58%)
preeclampsia (8–33%)

Mothers of multiples are also at increased risk for postpartum hemorrhage (12–35%).[74–79] In the March of Dimes Prematurity and Prevention Study of 33,873 twin births between 1982 and 1986, causes of iatrogenically (medically) induced preterm delivery included maternal hypertension (44%), fetal distress or growth retardation (33%), placental complications (9%), or fetal death (7%).[76]

Although infants of multiple births account for only 2.5% of all births, they are disproportionately represented among the low birth weight (<2,500 g) and very low birth weight (<1,500 g) infant populations. Seventy percent of triplet and higher order multiples and 50% of twins are LBW, compared with 6% of singletons; 12% of triplets and higher order multiples and 10% of twins are VLBW, compared with less than 1% of singletons.[27] Preterm birth (<37 weeks' gestation) occurs in 92% of triplet and higher order births and 53% of twin births, compared with less than 10% of singleton births. Early preterm births (<32 weeks' gestation) occurs in 35% of triplet and higher order births and 11% of twin births, compared with less than 2% of singleton births.[21,80] Of the VLBW infants born between 1989 and

1994 at the 12 centers of the National Institute of Child Health and Human Development Neonatal Research Network, twins comprised 19–20%.[81–83] However, when matched for gestational age, appropriately grown twins and singletons do not differ in their morbidity or mortality.[84–86]

The IOM report suggested a range of maternal weight gain of 35–45 lbs for term (38–41 week) twin pregnancies or a rate of weight gain of 1.5 pounds per week during the second and third trimesters (13–41 weeks).[24] Several studies have evaluated weight gain in twin and triplet pregnancies. Pederson and colleagues[87] reported total weight gains of 44 lbs (20 kg) at 37 or less weeks' gestation and both twin birth weights at 2,500 g or less. Based on birth certificate data, Brown and Schloesser[88] reported that for term gestations with both twin birth weights between 3,001–3,500 g, weight gains averaged 41 lbs (18.6 kg) for underweight women and 44 lbs (20 kg) for normal weight women. Lantz and associates[89] reported that among underweight women, a rate of gain of 1.0 lb or less per week before 20 weeks' gestation and less than 1.75 lb/wk after 20 weeks' gestation was associated with twin birth weights of 2,500 g or less. Comparable outcomes were observed among normal weight women with weight gains of at least 1.5 lb/wk after 20 weeks' gestation.

Several studies have been conducted by Luke and associates on the association between maternal weight gain and the intrauterine growth and birth weight of twins and triplets.[90–97] Average twin pair birth weights of 2,500 g or less were associated with maternal gains of 40–45 lbs (18.2–20.5 kg), as 24 lbs by 24 weeks.[96,97] A low rate of gain before 24 weeks (<0.85 lb/wk), regardless of the rate of gain after 24 weeks, was significantly associated with poor intrauterine growth and higher morbidity.[94] Luke and Leurgans[94] reported that physician-advised weight gain for twin gestations averaged 30 lbs, while actual gains averaged 40–45 lbs. This study also evaluated the IOM guidelines of 35–45 lb gain for twin gestations and concluded that weight gains above this range were associated with twin birth weights of 2,500 to 2,800 g at 35–38 weeks, the optimal birth weight for gestational age associated with the lowest morbidity and mortality for twins.[98]

Two studies confirmed the importance of maternal weight gain before 20 weeks' gestation on twin birth weights.[91,95] The first study, based on 646 twin pregnancies from three study sites, demonstrated that twin birth weight was significantly associated with weight gain before 20 weeks' gestation in underweight women, before 20 weeks and after 28 weeks in overweight women, and during all three gestational periods in normal weight women.[91] The second study, based on 1,564 twin pregnancies at four study sites, confirmed and expanded these findings and showed that both early maternal weight gain (before 20 weeks' gestation) and mid-maternal weight gain (between 20–28 weeks' gestation) significantly affect the rates of fetal growth between 20–28 weeks and 28 weeks to birth.[95] More recently, Luke and colleagues[99] published BMI-specific weight gain guidelines associated with optimal twin birth weights.

Summary of Maternal Weight Gain Recommendations

Studies of maternal weight gain, using the IOM recommendations as guidelines (Table 3–2), have confirmed their usefulness, particularly for underweight and normal weight women. Gains within the IOM range for underweight and normal weight women should reduce the risk of low birth weight or having a growth-restricted infant, while gaining below the upper limit should reduce the risk of high birth weight.

The patterns of changes in maternal body composition and pattern of weight gain that have been described also have implications for assessment and the interpretation of weight gain. The efficacy of nutritional interventions (when to encourage gains, when to be concerned about low or excessive gains) may be dependent upon consideration of the pattern. For example, it may be more effective for women who tend to have low prepregnancy weight (at whatever height) to encourage weight gain early in pregnancy and thereby enhance maternal nutritional stores. Low rates of gain in the third trimester, when the fetus should be growing most rapidly, may reflect suboptimal fetal growth even if earlier gains had been within acceptable ranges, and total weight gain was still essentially on target. At this point in the pregnancy (third trimester), an intervention to increase weight gain may not be particularly effective in increasing birth weight.

However, the initial IOM recommendations for young adolescents, black women, and obese women have elicited some suggested modifications:

1. All pregnant adolescents, not just those within 2 years of menarche, should be targeted toward the upper end of the ranges appropriate for their prepregnancy BMI. This is because menarche is an insensitive indicator of biological maturity. Adolescents up to 18 years of age and beyond may still be actively developing, particularly expanding their fat-free mass.
2. The IOM recommends that black women gain at the upper end of the ranges for their BMI. However, evaluations by race of the IOM recommendations have shown that additional weight gain among black women has little effect on reducing the risk of low birth weight and instead contributes to greater postpartum weight retention and may contribute to the development of obesity in parous black women.
3. Although a minimum weight gain of 6.8 kg (15 lb) is reasonable for obese women, the upper limit of the range should be set at 11.5 kg (25 lb). Weight gains over 11.5 kg for obese women are associated with a dramatically increased risk of having a high birth weight or LGA infant, without benefit in reducing LBW.
4. The IOM recommendations of 35–45 lbs for term twin pregnancies is probably conservative, since half of all twin births are preterm and research has demonstrated improved birth weights by patterns of gain rather than absolute amounts. Women with pregravid BMIs within the normal range (19.8–26.0) who are pregnant with twins should strive to gain at least 24 lb by 24 weeks' gestation and maintain a rate of gain of 1.0–1.5 lb/wk thereafter. Women with pregravid BMIs above the normal range (>26.0) can gain at slightly lower rates. Women with pregravid BMIs below the normal range (<19.8) should strive for a weight gain equal to their pregravid weight deficit plus 24 lb by 24 weeks and maintain a rate of gain in the upper range (1.5 lb/wk) thereafter. Women pregnant with triplet and higher-order gestations should probably strive for gains of closer to 40 lb by 24 weeks and rates of gain of 2.0–2.5 lb/wk thereafter.

SPECIAL PREGNANCY CIRCUMSTANCES

Nausea and Vomiting

Food intake can be affected in an adverse way during pregnancy by gastrointestinal motility disorders such as nausea, vomiting, heartburn, constipation, and diarrhea.[100] Nausea and vomiting are the most common of these disorders with nausea effecting 70% of pregnant women during the first trimester and vomiting effecting 30–50% of pregnant women.[101] Incorrectly labeled as "morning sickness," nausea and vomiting may occur at any time of day or night. Nausea, a frequent discomfort of early pregnancy, can last well into the second trimester and vary greatly in severity.

Management of nausea and vomiting depends on the severity of the symptoms. Dietary manipulation may resolve mild cases. First trimester nausea may improve with small meals, bland food, and the avoidance of fried, spicy, and fatty foods. Some women respond to avoiding the smells of the kitchen, getting out of bed slowly in the morning, and drinking small amounts of liquid between meals.[102]

Current dietary recommendations shown to have beneficial nausea-reducing effects and considered safe and effective include taking a multivitamin early in the pregnancy-planning process, supplementing the diet with Vitamin B6, and treating nausea with ginger as a nonpharmacologic option.[103]

For some, this discomfort may progress to more serious prolonged nausea and excessive vomiting defined as hyperemesis gravidarum. In order to prevent excessive pregnancy weight loss and infants born with low birth weight, specialized treatment is recommended. Such treatment may require hydration with hospitalization, antiemetic medications, correction of electrolyte or metabolic disturbances, and nutritional support.[102,103]

Gestational Diabetes

With diabetes on the rise in the general population, the incidence of diabetes occurring in pregnancy is expected to increase.[104] The current estimate is that 7% of pregnant women become diabetic; however, the percentage varies within given populations or ethnic groups.[105] Gestational diabetes (GDM) is defined as glucose intolerance occurring during pregnancy.[104] Women at risk for GDM typically have a personal history of GDM, may exhibit obesity, and have a strong family history of diabetes. To diagnose GDM, women are screened with an oral glucose challenge test between weeks 24 and 28 of gestation.[106]

A consequence of GDM includes fetal macrosomia, large fetal size for weeks of gestation.[105] The pregnant woman may experience an increased risk of a difficult labor and delivery.[107] Intensive treatment of hyperglycemia in women with GDM lessens the risk of adverse outcomes.[108] This intensive treatment can reduce the risk of fetal macrosomia and provides the best outcome for normal or large for gestational age infants with poorer outcomes observed for small-for-gestational-age infants.[109]

Intensive treatment consists of optimal nutrition management including nutrition counseling and individualization of medical nutrition therapy (MNT) by a registered dietitian. Carbohydrates are less tolerated at breakfast than at other meals so carbohydrate and calories are adjusted in meal plans based on monitoring weight, blood sugar, and ketones.[110] Diets that contain 40% carbohydrates reduce postprandial glucose levels.[111] In addition, moderate exercise is recommended. If MNT does not provide for the maintenance of blood sugar at the desirable levels, insulin may be needed.[105,112]

Women with GDM tend to return to normal glucose tolerance in the postpartum period. Postpartum counseling should highlight the importance of attaining normal weight for height and regular physical activity in an effort to reduce the lifetime risk of subsequent diabetes.

Preeclampsia

Preeclampsia is a pregnancy-specific syndrome observed after 20 weeks of pregnancy with systolic blood pressure greater than 140 or diastolic blood pressure greater than 90 accompanied by significant proteinuria and resolves with delivery.

Eclampsia is the occurrence of seizures with preeclampsia that does not have another cause. Gestational hypertension is defined as elevated blood pressure detected for the first time after 20 weeks of gestation without proteinuria.[113]

Risk factors include preeclampsia in a previous pregnancy, a maternal age that is younger (<20 years) or older (>40 years), obesity, insulin resistance, and diabetes and genetic factors.[104,114]

The incidence of preeclampsia is greater in twins than single births.[115] Preeclampsia is associated with preterm delivery, small infants, neonatal death, and maternal morbidity and mortality.[116,117]

Theories abound concerning prevention or therapy in preeclampsia. The role of diet and nutrient supplementation has not been adequately studied. Sodium restriction and calcium, zinc, and magnesium supplementation have not been proven effective.[118] More recently, vitamins C and E looked promising, but their effectiveness has not been proven.[113]

Pica

Many women crave certain food items or have aversions to food items during pregnancy.[119] Pica is defined as the craving for nonfood substances.[120] The most common nonfood cravings include starch (amylophagia), dirt or clay (geophagia), and ice or freezer frost (pagophagia). Other substances may include soap, ashes, chalk, and food items such as baking soda or cornstarch.[104]

The etiology is poorly understood. When women crave nonfood substances, there is always the concern that these nonfood substances will replace nutrients and calories for fetal growth. The nutrition assessment and screening for pregnant women should include questions about cravings for nonfood items or foods not usually consumed. Pica is associated with iron deficiency, therefore screening for nutrient deficiencies and assessing the possible exposure to toxic substances is recommended. Counsel women on the importance of consuming nutrient-dense foods during their pregnancy and suggest possible food substitutions for the nonfood items.

Mercury

Mercury, a metallic element, naturally occurs in the environment.[121] Typically, small amounts of mercury do not pose a problem, however, mercury and mercury-containing chemicals from pollutants can contaminate the waters supporting marine life. Microorganisms convert mercury to methylmercury. Fish accumulate and store this contaminant, which binds to fish protein and is not excreted. Larger fish consuming smaller fish may contain additional methylmercury.[122] The contamination from methylmercury varies with fish age, size, diet, species, and water location.[123] The mercury contained in seafood products readily crosses the placental barrier and has the potential to damage the developing fetal nervous system.[122,121]

To educate the public about the hazards of methylmercury, the FDA and the EPA issued a joint consumer advisory about mercury in fish and shellfish and recommends that pregnant women, women of childbearing age, and young children avoid eating shark, swordfish, mackerel, and tilefish.[123]

Key parts of the advisory are as follows:[124]

Fish and shellfish are an important part of a healthy diet. Fish and shellfish contain high-quality protein and other essential nutrients, are low in saturated fat, and contain omega-3 fatty acids. A well-balanced diet that includes a variety of fish and shellfish can contribute to heart health and children's proper growth and development. Thus, women and young children in particular should include fish or shellfish in their diets due to the many nutritional benefits.

By following these three recommendations for selecting and eating fish or shellfish, women and young children will receive the benefits of eating fish and shellfish and be confident that they have reduced their exposure to the harmful effects of mercury.

1. Do not eat shark, swordfish, king mackerel, or tilefish because they contain high levels of mercury.
2. Eat up to 12 ounces (2 average meals) a week of a variety of fish and shellfish that are lower in mercury.
   - Five of the most commonly eaten fish that are low in mercury are shrimp, canned light tuna, salmon, pollock, and catfish.
   - Another commonly eaten fish, albacore ("white") tuna has more mercury than canned light tuna. So, when choosing your two meals of fish and shellfish, you may eat up to 6 ounces (one average meal) of albacore tuna per week.
3. Check local advisories about the safety of fish caught by family and friends in your local lakes, rivers, and coastal areas. If no advice is available, eat up to 6 ounces (one average meal) per week of fish you catch from local waters, but don't consume any other fish during that week. Follow these same recommendations when feeding fish and shellfish to your young child, but serve smaller portions.

To keep abreast of current food-related information call the FDA toll-free food hotline: 1.800.SAFEFOOD or visit the following Web site: www.epa.gov/ost/fish.

REFERENCES

1. Brown JE. Improving pregnancy outcomes in the United States: The importance of preventive nutrition services. *J Am Dietet Assoc.* 1989:631–633.
2. Brown JE, Kahn ESB. Maternal nutrition and the outcome of pregnancy: A renaissance in research. *Clin Perinatology.* 1997;24:433–449.
3. Coulston AM, Rosen C. American health care reform: Implications for medical nutrition therapy. *Am J Clin Nutr.* 1994;59:1275–1276.
4. Jensen GL, Lee P, Bothe A, Blackburn G, Hambridge KM, Klein S. Clinical nutrition: Opportunity in a changing health care environment. *Am J Clin Nutr.* 1998;68:983–990.
5. Crawford P. The nutrition connection: Why doesn't the public know? *Am J Public Health.* 1988;78:1147–1148.
6. Angell M, Kassirer J. Clinical research—What should the public believe? *N Engl J Med.* 1994;331:189–190.
7. Heaney RP. Food: What a surprise! *Am J Clin Nutr.* 1996;64:791–792.
8. AAP/ACOG. *Guidelines for Perinatal Care*, 5th ed. Elk Grove Village: American Academy of Pediatrics, and Washington, DC: American College of Obstetricians and Gynecologists, 2002.
9. Czeizel AE. Prevention of congenital abnormalities by periconceptional multivitamin supplementation. *Brit Med J.* 1993;306:1645–1648.
10. MRC Vitamin Study Research Group. Prevention of neural tube defects: Results of the Medical Research Council Vitamin Study. Lancet. 1991;338:131–137.
11. USDHHS, Public Health Service. Recommendations for the use of folic acid to reduce the number of cases of spina bifida and other neural tube defects. *Morbidity and Mortality Weekly Report* 1992;41(RR-14);1–7.
12. Block G, Abrams B. Vitamin and mineral status of women of childbearing potential. *Ann NY Acad Sci.* 1993;678:244–254.
13. Jones KL, Smith AW. Recognition of the fetal alcohol syndrome in early infancy. *Lancet.* 1973;2:999–1001.
14. Windham GC, Fenster L, Hopkins B, Swan SH. The association of moderate maternal and paternal alcohol consumption with birthweight and gestational age. *Epidemiology.* 1995;6:591–597.
15. Armstrong BG, McDonald AD, Sloan M. Cigarette, alcohol, and coffee consumption and spontaneous abortion. *Am J Public Health.* 1992;82:85–87.
16. Kallen K. Multiple malformations and maternal smoking. *Paediatric and Perinatal Epidemiology.* 2000; 14:227–233.
17. Peacock JL, Bland JM, Anderson HR. Preterm delivery: Effects of socioeconomic factors, psychological stress, smoking, alcohol, and caffeine. *Britsh Med J.* 1995;311:531–535.
18. Shaw NR, Bracken MB. A systematic review and meta-analysis of prospective studies on the association between maternal cigarette smoking and preterm delivery. *Am J Obstet Gynecol.* 2000;182:465–472.
19. Enns CW, Goldman JD, Cook A. Trends in food and nutrient intakes by adults: NFCS 1977–78, CSFII 1989–91, and CSFII 1994–95. *Family Economics and Nutrition Review.* 1997;10:2–15.
20. Scholl TO, Hediger ML, Bendich A, Schall JI, Smith WK, Krueger PM. Use of multivitamin/mineral prenatal supplements: Influence on the outcome of pregnancy. *Am J Epidemiol.* 1997;146:134–141.
21. Bender MM, Levy AS, Schucker RE, Yetley EA. Trends in prevalence and magnitude of vitamin and mineral supplement usage and correlation with health status. *J Am Diet Assoc.* 1992;92:1096–1101.
22. Block G, Cox C, Madans J, et al.Vitamin supplement use by demographic characteristics. *Am J Epidemiol.* 1988;127:297–309.
23. Koplan JP, Annest JL, Layde PM, Rubin GL. Nutrient intake and supplementation in the United States (NHANES II). *Am J Public Health.* 1986;76:287–289.
24. Subcommittee on Nutritional Status and Weight Gain During Pregnancy, Committee on Nutritional Status During Pregnancy and Lactation, Institute of Medicine. *Nutrition During Pregnancy.* Washington, DC: National Academy Press, 1990.
25. Seligman PA, Caskey JH, Frazier JL, Zucker RM, Podell ER, Alen RH. Measurements of iron absorption from prenatal multivitamin-mineral supplements. *Obstet Gynecol.* 1983;61:356–362.
26. MacDorman MF, Atkinson JO. *Infant Mortality Statistics from the Linked Birth/Infant Death Data Set—1995 Period Data.* Monthly Vital Statistics Report; vol. 46, no. 6, suppl. 2. Hyattsville, MD: National Center for Health Statistics; 1998.
27. Martin JA, Hamilton BE, Sutton PD, Ventura SJ, Menacker F, Munson ML. *Births: Final Data for 2002.* National Vital Statistics Reports; vol. 52, no. 10. Hyatttsville, MD: National Center for Health Statistics, 2003.
28. Eastman NJ, Jackson E. Weight relationships in pregnancy: The bearing of maternal weight gain and pre-pregnancy weight on birthweight in full term pregnancies. *Obstet Gynecol Survey.* 1968;23:1003–1025.
29. Niswander KR, Singer J, Westphal M, Weiss W. Weight gain during pregnancy and prepregnancy weight: Association with birth weight of term gestations. *Obstet Gynecol.* 1969;33:482–491.
30. Niswander K, Jackson E. Physical characteristics of the gravida and their association with birth weight and perinatal death. *Am J Obstet Gynecol.* 1974;119:306–313.

31. Singer JE, Westphal M, Niswander K. Relationship of weight gain during pregnancy to birth weight and infant growth and development in the first year of life. *Obstet Gynecol.* 1968;31:417–423.
32. Niswander RK, Gordon M. *The Women and Their Pregnancies.* Philadelphia, PA: WB Saunders Co., 1972.
33. Naeye RL. Weight gain and the outcome of pregnancy. *Am J Obstet Gynecol.* 1979;135:3–9.
34. National Research Council, National Academy of Sciences. *Maternal Nutrition and the Course of Pregnancy.* Washington, DC: National Academy of Sciences, 1970.
35. Abrams BF, Laros RK. Prepregnancy weight, weight gain, and birth weight. *Am J Obstet Gynecol.* 1986; 154:503–509.
36. Kleinman JC. *Maternal Weight Gain During Pregnancy: Determinants and Consequences.* NCHS Working Paper Series No. 33. Hyattsville, MD: National Center for Health Statistics, Public Health Service, US Department of Health and Human Services, 1990.
37. Clapp JF, Seaward BL, Sleamaker RH, Hiser J. Maternal physiologic adaptations to early human pregnancy. *Am J Obstet Gynecol.* 1988;159:1456–1460.
38. Hediger ML, Scholl TO, Ances IG, Belsky DH, Salmon RW. Rate and amount of weight gain during adolescent pregnancy: Associations with maternal weight-for-height and birth weight. *Am J Clin Nutr.* 1990; 52:793–799.
39. Abrams B, Carmichael S, Selvin S. Factors associated with the pattern of maternal weight gain during pregnancy. *Obstet Gynecol.* 1995;86:170–176.
40. Carmichael SL, Abrams B. A critical review of the relationship between gestational weight gain and preterm delivery. *Obstet Gynecol.* 1997;89:865–873.
41. Hediger ML, Scholl TO, Belsky DH, Ances IG, Salmon RW. Patterns of weight gain in adolescent pregnancy: Effects on birth weight and preterm delivery. *Obstet Gynecol.* 1989;74:6–12.
42. Abrams B, Newman V, Key T, Parker J. Maternal weight gain and preterm delivery. *Obstet Gynecol.* 1989;74: 577–583.
43. Hickey CA, Cliver SP, McNeal SF, Hoffman HJ, Goldenberg RL. Prenatal weight gain patterns and spontaneous preterm birth among nonobese black and white women. *Obstet Gynecol.* 1995;85:909–914.
44. Hickey CA, McNeal SF, Menefee L, Ivey S. Prenatal weight gain within upper and lower recommended ranges: Effect on birth weight of black and white infants. *Obstet Gynecol.* 1997;90:489–494.
45. Siega-Riz AM, Adair LS, Hobel CJ. Maternal underweight status and inadequate rate of weight gain during the third trimester of pregnancy increase the risk of preterm delivery. *J Nutr.* 1996;126:146–153.
46. Spinillo A, Capuzzo E, Piazzi G, Ferrari A, Morales V, Di Mario M. Risk for spontaneous preterm delivery by combined body mass index and gestational weight gain patterns. *Acta Obstet Gynecol Scand.* 1998;77:32–36.
47. Wen SW, Goldenberg RL, Cutter GR, Hoffman HJ, Cliver SP. Intrauterine growth retardation and preterm delivery: Prenatal risk factors in an indigent population. *Am J Obstet Gynecol.* 1990;162:213–218.
48. Allen SR. Epidemiology of premature rupture of the fetal membranes. *Clin Obstet Gynecol.* 1991;34:685–693.
49. Scholl TO, Hediger ML, Schall JI, Fischer RL, Khoo CS. Low zinc intake during pregnancy: Its association with preterm and very preterm delivery. *Am J Epidemiol.* 1993;137:1115–1124.
50. Weiner CP, Sabbagha RE, Vaisrub N, Depp R. A hypothetical model suggesting suboptimal intrauterine growth in infants delivered preterm. *Obstet Gynecol.* 1985;65:323–326.
51. Ott WJ. Intrauterine growth retardation and preterm delivery. *Am J Obstet Gynecol.* 1993;168:1710–1717.
52. Secher NJ, Kern Hansen P, Thomsen BL, Keiding N. Growth retardation in preterm infants. *Br J Obstet Gynaecol.* 1987;94:115–120.
53. Hediger ML, Scholl TO, Schall JI, Miller LW, Fischer RL. Fetal growth and the etiology of preterm delivery. *Obstet Gynecol.* 1995;85:60–64.
54. Abrams B, Selvin S. Maternal weight gain pattern and birth weight. *Obstet Gynecol.* 1995;86:163–169.
55. Carmichael S, Abrams B, Selvin S. The pattern of maternal weight gain in women with good pregnancy outcomes. *Am J Public Health.* 1997;87:1984–1988.
56. Scholl TO, Hediger ML. A review of the epidemiology of nutrition and adolescent pregnancy: Maternal growth during pregnancy and its effect on the fetus. *J Am Coll Nutr.* 1993;12:101–107.
57. Scholl TO, Hediger ML, Schall JI, Khoo CS, Fischer RL. Maternal growth during pregnancy and the competition for nutrients. *Am J Clin Nutr.* 1994;60:183–188.
58. McAnarney ER, Stevens-Simon C. First, do no harm. Low birth weight and adolescent obesity. *Am J Dis Child.* 1993;147:983–985.
59. Stevens-Simon C, McAnarney ER. Adolescent pregnancy: Gestational weight gain and maternal and infant outcomes. *Am J Dis Child.* 1992;146:1459–1464.
60. Stevens-Simon C, McAnarney ER, Roghmann KJ. Adolescent gestational weight gain and birth weight. *Pediatrics.* 1993;92:805–809.
61. Berenson AB, Wiemann CM, Rowe TF, Rickert VI. Inadequate weight gain among pregnant adolescents: Risk factors and relationship to infant birth weight. *Am J Obstet Gynecol.* 1997;178:1220–1227.
62. Rees JM, Engelbert-Fenton KA, Gong EJ, Bach CM. Weight gain in adolescents during pregnancy: Rate

related to birth-weight outcome. *Am J Clin Nutr.* 1992; 56:868–873.

63. Caulfield LE, Witter FR, Stoltzfus RJ. Determinants of gestational weight gain outside the recommended ranges among black and white women. *Obstet Gynecol.* 1996;87:760–766.
64. Caulfield LE, Stoltzfus RJ, Witter FR. Implications of the Institute of Medicine weight gain recommendations for preventing adverse pregnancy outcomes in black and white women. *Am J Public Health.* 1998; 88:1168–1174.
65. Keppel KG, Taffel SM. Pregnancy-related weight gain and retention: Implications of the 1990 Institute of Medicine guideline. *Am J Public Health.* 1993; 83:1100–1103.
66. Lederman SA. The effect of pregnancy weight gain on later obesity. *Obstet Gynecol.* 1993;82:148–155.
67. Parker JD, Abrams B. Prenatal weight gain advice: An examination of the recent prenatal weight gain recommendations of the Institute of Medicine. *Obstet Gynecol.* 1992;79:664–669.
68. Rosso P, Donoso E, Braun S, Espinoza R, Salas SP. Hemodynamic changes in underweight pregnant women. *Obstet Gynecol.* 1992;79:908–912.
69. Abrams B, Parker J. Overweight and pregnancy complications. *Int J Obesity.* 1988;12:293–303.
70. Bianco AT, Smilen SW, Davis Y, Lopez S, Lapinski R, Lockwood CJ. Pregnancy outcome and weight gain recommendations for the morbidly obese woman. *Obstet Gynecol.* 1998;91:97–102.
71. Cogswell ME, Serdula MK, Hungerford DW, Yip R. Gestational weight gain among average-weight and overweight women—What is excessive? *Am J Obstet Gynecol.* 1995;172:705–712.
72. Edwards LE, Hellerstedt WL, Alton IR, Story M, Himes JH. Pregnancy complications and birth outcomes in obese and normal-weight women: Effects of gestational weight change. *Obstet Gynecol.* 1996;87:389–394.
73. Haas JS, Berman S, Goldberg AB, Lee LWK, Cook EF. Prenatal hospitalizations and compliance with guidelines for prenatal care. *Am J Public Health.* 1996; 86:815–819.
74. Albrecht JL, Tomich PG. The maternal and neonatal outcome of triplet gestations. *Am J Obstet Gynecol.* 1996;174:1551–1556.
75. Ellings JM, Newman RB, Hulsey TC, Bivins HA, Keenan A. Reduction in very low birth weight deliveries and perinatal mortality in a specialized, multidisciplinary twin clinic. *Obstet Gynecol.* 1993;81:387–391.
76. Gardner MO, Goldenberg RL, Cliver SP, et al. The origin and outcome of preterm twin pregnancies. *Obstet Gynecol.* 1995;85:553–557.
77. Newman RB, Jones JS, Miller MC. Influence of clinical variables on triplet birth weight. *Acta Genet Med Gemellol.* 1991;40:173–179.
78. Peaceman AM, Dooley SL, Tamura RK. Antepartum management of triplet gestations. *Am J Obstet Gynecol.* 1992;167:1117–1120.
79. Syrop CH, Varner MW. Triplet gestation: Maternal and neonatal implications. *Acta Genet Med Gemellol.* 1985; 34:81–88.
80. Martin JA, MacDorman MF, Mathews TJ. Triplet births: trends and outcomes, 1971–94. Vital Health Stat 21. 1997,Jan(55):1–20.
81. Donovan EF, Ehrenkranz RA, Shankaran C, et al. Outcomes of very low birth weight twins cared for in the National Institutes of Child Health and Human Development Neonatal Research Network's intensive care units. *Am J Obstet Gynecol.* 1998;179:742–749.
82. Faranoff AA, Wright LL, Stevenson DK, et al. Very-low-birth-weight outcomes of the National Institute of Child Health and Human Development Neonatal Network, May 1991 to December 1992. *Am J Obstet Gynecol.* 1995;173:1423–1431.
83. Hack M, Wright LL, Shankaran S, et al. Very-low-birth-weight outcomes of the National Institute of Child Health and Human Development Neonatal Network, November 1989 to October 1990. *Am J Obstet Gynecol.* 1995;172:457–464.
84. Kilpatrick SJ, Jackson R, Crough-Minihane MS. Perinatal mortality in twins and singletons matched for gestational age at delivery at ≥30 weeks. *Am J Obstet Gynecol.* 1996;174:66–71.
85. Luke B, Minogue J, Witter FR. The role of fetal growth restriction and gestational age on length of hospital stay in twin infants. *Obstet Gynecol.* 1993;81:949–953.
86. Wolf EJ, Vintzileos AM, Rosenkrantz TS, et al. A comparison of pre-discharge survival and morbidity in singleton and twin very low birth weight infants. *Obstet Gynecol.* 1992;80:436–469.
87. Pederson AL, Worthington-Roberts B, Hickok DE. Weight gain patterns during twin gestation. *J Am Dietet Assoc.* 1989;89:642–646.
88. Brown JE, Schloesser PT. Prepregnancy weight status, prenatal weight gain, and the outcome of term twin gestations. *Am J Obstet Gynecol.* 1990;162:182–186.
89. Lantz ME, Chez RA, Rodriguez A, Porter KB. Maternal weight gain patterns and birth weight outcome in twin gestation. *Obstet Gynecol.* 1996;87:551–556.
90. Luke B, Bryan E, Sweetland C, Leurgans S, Keith LG. Prenatal weight gain and the birth weight of triplets. *Acta Genet Med Gemellol.* 1995;44:93–101.
91. Luke B, Gillespie B, Min S-J, Avni M, Witter FR, O'Sullivan MJ. Critical periods of maternal weight gain: Effects on twin birthweight. *Am J Obstet Gynecol.* 1997;177:1055–1062.

92. Luke B, Keith LG, Johnson TRB, Keith D. Pregravid weight, gestational weight gain and current weight of women delivered of twins. *J Perinatal Med.* 1991; 19:333–340.
93. Luke B, Keith LG, Keith D. Maternal nutrition in twin gestations: Weight gain, cravings and aversions, and sources of nutrition advice. *Acta Genet Med Gemellol.* 1997;46:157–166.
94. Luke B, Leurgans S. Maternal weight gains in ideal twin outcomes. *J Am Dietet Assoc.* 1996;96:178–181.
95. Luke B, Min S-J, Gillespie B, Avni M, Witter FR, Newman RB, Mauldin JG, Salman AF, O'Sullivan MJ. The importance of early weight gain on the intrauterine growth and birthweight of twins. *Am J Obstet Gynecol.* 1998;179:1155–1161.
96. Luke B, Minogue J, Abbey H, Keith LG, Feng TI, Johnson TRB. The association between maternal weight gain and the birth weight of twins. *J Maternal-Fetal Med.* 1992;1:267–276.
97. Luke B, Minogue J, Witter FR, Keith LG, Johnson TRB. The ideal twin pregnancy: Patterns of weight gain, discordancy, and length of gestation. *Am J Obstet Gynecol.* 1993;169:588–597.
98. Luke B. Reducing fetal deaths in multiple births: Optimal birth weights and gestational ages for infants of twin and triplet births. *Acta Genet Med Gemellol.* 1996;45:333–348.
99. Luke B, Hediger ML, Nugent C, Newman RB, Mauldin JG, Witter FR, O'Sullivan MJ. Body mass index-specific weight gains associated with optimal birth weights in twin pregnancies. *J Reprod Med.* 2003; 48:217–224.
100. Dundas ML, Taylor ML. Perinatal factors, motivation and attitudes concerning pregnancy affect dietary intake. *Top Clin Nutr.* 2002;17:71–79.
101. Kolasa KM, Weismiller DG. Nutrition during pregnancy. *Am Fam Physician.* 1997;56:205–212.
102. Nelson-Piercy C. Treatment of nausea and vomiting in pregnancy: When should it be treated and what can be safely taken. *Drug Safety* 1998;19155–19164.
103. American College of Obstetrics and Gynecology Practice Bulletin. Nausea and vomiting of pregnancy. *Obstet Gynecol.* 2004;103:803–814.
104. Position of the American Dietetic Association: Nutrition and lifestyle for a healthy pregnancy outcome. *J Am Diet Assoc.* 2002;102:1479–1490.
105. Gestational diabetes. ACOG Practice Bulletin No. 30. American College of Obstetricians and Gynecologists. *Obstet Gynecol.* 2001;98:525–538.
106. American Diabetes Association: Gestational Diabetes Mellitus Position Statement. *Diabetes Care.* 2004; 27:S88–90.
107. Casey BM, Lucas MJ, Mcintire DD, Leveno KJ. Pregnancy outcomes in women with gestational diabetes compared with the general obstetric population. *Obstet Gynecol.* 1997;90:869–873.
108. Franz MJ, Bantle JP, Beebe CA, Brunzell JD, Chiasson J-L, Garg A, Holzmeister LA, Hoogwerf B, Mayer-Davis E, Moordian AD, Purmell JQ, Wheeler M. Evidence-based nutrition principles and recommendations for the treatment and prevention of diabetes and related complications (Technical Review) *Diabetes Care.* 2002; 25:148–198.
109. Garcia-Patterson A, Corcoy R, Balsells M, Altirriba O, Adelantado JM, Cabero L, De Leiva A. In pregnancies with gestational diabetes mellitus and intensive therapy, perinatal outcome is worse in small-for-gestational-age newborns. *Am J Obstet Gynecol.* 1998;179:481–485.
110. Peterson CH, Jovanovic-Peterson L. Percentage of carbohydrate and glycemic response to breakfast, lunch and dinner in women with gestational diabetes. *Diabetes.* 1991;40:S172–S174.
111. Major CA, Henry MJ, De Veciana M, Morgan MA. The effects of carbohydrate restriction in patients with diet-controlled gestational diabetes. *Obstet Gynecol.* 1998; 91:600–604.
112. American Diabetes Association: Proceedings of the fourth international workshop: Conference on gestational diabetes. *Diabetes Care.* 1998;S2:B1–B167.
113. Roberts JM, Balk JL, Bodnar LM, Belizan JM, Bergel E, Martinez A. Nutrient involvement in preeclampsia. *J Nutr.* 2003:1684S–1692S.
114. Cedergren MI. Maternal morbid obesity and the pregnancy outcome. *Obstet Gynecol.* 2004;103:219–224.
115. Kametras, NA, McAuliffe F, Krampl E, Chambers J, Nicolaides, KH. Maternal cardiac function in twin pregnancy. *Obstet Gynecol.* 2003;102:806–815.
116. Sibai BM, Lindheimer M, Hauth J. et al. Risk factors for preeclampsia, abruption placentae and adverse neonatal outcomes among women with chronic hypertension. *N Eng J Med.* 1998;339:667–671.
117. Churchill D, Perry IJ, Beevers DG. Ambulatory blood pressure in pregnancy and fetal growth. *Lancet.* 1997; 349:7–10.
118. Dekker G, Sibai B. Primary, secondary and tertiary prevention of pre-eclampsia. *Lancet.* 2001;357:209–215.
119. Pope JF, Skinner JD, Carruth BR. Cravings and aversions of pregnant adolescents. *J Am Diet Assoc.* 1992; 92:1479–1482.
120. Horner RD, Lackey CJ, Kolasas K, Warren K. Pica practices of pregnant women. *J Am Diet Assoc.* 1991; 91:34–38.
121. Chan HM, Egeland GM. Fish consumption, mercury exposure and heart disease. *Nutrition Reviews.* 2004;62: 68–72.
122. Dey PM, Gochfeld M, Reuhl KR. Developmental

methylmercury administration alters cerebellar PSA-NCAM expression and Golgi sialytransferease activity. *Brain Research.* 1999;845:139–151.

123. Evans E. The FDA recommendations on fish intake during pregnancy. *JOGNN.* 2002;31:541–546.

124. US Department of Health and Human Services and US Environmental Protection Agency. *What You Need to Know About Mercury in Fish and Shellfish.* 2004; Retrieved June 9, 2004, from www.cfsan.fda.gov/~dms/admehg3.html.

CHAPTER 4

Nutrition for Premature Infants

Diane M. Anderson

Premature infants are defined as infants born before 37 weeks gestation as compared to full-term infants born from 37 to 42 weeks.[1] The physiologic immaturity of premature infants renders them susceptible to a number of problems (see Table 4–1), many of which imperil their nutrition and growth (see Table 4–2). Low birth weight (LBW) refers to infants with a birth weight of less than 2500 g; very low birth weight (VLBW) infants weigh less than 1500 g, and extremely low birth weight (ELBW) infants weigh less than 1000 g.[1,2] Infants can be LBW but yet be full term due to poor intrauterine growth.

Assessment of intrauterine growth is determined by plotting the infant's birth weight by gestational age on various charts. On the Lubchenco chart, small-for-gestational-age (SGA) infants have a birth weight of less than the 10th percentile.[3] Large-for-gestational-age (LGA) infants have a birth weight greater than the 90th percentile.[3] Appropriate-for-gestational-age infants are between the 10th and 90th percentiles (see Appendix A-2). On the Babson and Benda Growth Chart, SGA and LGA can be defined as two standard deviations from the mean birth weight (approximately the 3rd and the 97th percentiles).[4] Recently, Fenton has updated the Babson and Benda Growth Chart, both sets of classification definitions are available on this chart (see Appendix A-3).[5] This chart also may be downloaded from http://members.shaw.ca/growthchart. Table 4–3 lists the etiologies for SGA and Table 4–4 lists the factors associated with LGA infants. These assessments are used to anticipate medical and nutritional problems and management needs of the infant (see Table 4–5). For example, consider an infant born at 34 weeks' gestation whose birth weight is 1200 g. This infant is premature because the gestational age is less than 37 weeks. On the Lubchenco, the Babson and Benda, and the Fenton growth grids, the infant is SGA because birth weight is less than the 10th percentile or less than two standard deviations from the mean birth weight.

SGA infants are further classified by their body length and head circumference as symmetrically or asymmetrically growth retarded.[2] The symmetrically SGA infant's birth weight, head circumference, and body length are all classified as small, whereas the asymmetrically SGA infant has a small body weight but an appropriate head circumference and body length. Previously, it was assumed that infants who experience asymmetrical growth retardation, stood a better chance for catch-up growth.[2] The potential for catch-up growth is determined by the etiology of the poor fetal growth.[2,6] Those infants who have the insult late in gestation due to placental insufficiency or uterine restrictions will grow when provided appropriate nutrition.[6] Those infants who had an early perinatal insult related to congenital infection or genetic disorders remain small in physical size.[2,6]

Early studies suggested that catch-up growth for premature infants was limited to the first few years of life, but one recent report demonstrated

Table 4–1 Potential Problems of the Premature Infant

Undernutrition	Apnea
Glucose instability	Infection
Hypocalcemia	Hyperbilirubinemia
Fat malabsorption	Limited renal function
Decreased gastric motility	Necrotizing enterocolitis
Uncoordinated suck and swallow	Osteopenia
Asphyxia	Intraventricular hemorrhage
Respiratory distress syndrome	Periventricular leukomalacia
Hypotension	Bronchopulmonary dysplasia
Poor temperature control	Retinopathy of prematurity
Patent ductus arteriosus	Anemia

Sources: Data from endnote references 10 and 58.

that weight and length growth can continue through adulthood.[7,8] By 20 years of age, females have caught up in weight, height, and body mass index (BMI).[8] In contrast, males remain smaller than men who were born at term.[8] A suboptimal head circumference measurement at 8 months of age has been independently associated with decreased intellectual quotients, cognitive functioning skills, and behavior problems at school age.[9] Additional factors associated with poor developmental outcome include lower socioeconomic status, lower maternal education, and neurological impairment of the infant.[9]

Premature infants represent a heterogeneous population for nutrition management. Intrauterine growth establishes nutritional status at birth, and gestational age determines nutrient need and feeding modality employed. As the infant matures, postnatal nutrient needs and feeding modality will vary. Finally, the infant's clinical condition can acutely change and alter nutrition care. Due to these factors, their nutrition management is a day-to-day decision-making process regarding what to feed, what volume and nutrient density to provide, and how to administer nourishment. The goal is to provide nutrition for optimal growth and development to take place. The intrauterine growth rate and weight gain composition without metabolic complications has been advocated as the goal for premature infant nutrition.[10]

PARENTERAL NUTRITION

Parenteral nutrition is often indicated and initiated in the first few days of life to allow the premature infant to adapt to the extrauterine environment before enteral feedings are begun. It is also used to supplement enteral feedings, because premature infants have decreased enteral feeding tolerance and small gastric capacities, which limit volume intakes and advancements. Premature infants are at risk for necrotizing enterocolitis (NEC), and enteral feedings will be cautiously advanced.[10] For the VLBW infant, parenteral nutrition should be initiated within the first 24 hours of life to promote energy intake and glucose homeostasis, to establish nitrogen balance, and to prevent essential fatty acid deficiency.[11,12] The provision of amino acids as part of parenteral nutrition within the first 24 hours of life has been associated with nitrogen balance; improved glucose tolerance, which facilitates greater glucose administration; increased protein synthesis; and normal plasma amino acid levels.[11,13] Tables 4–6 and 4–7 give suggested guidelines for parenteral administration of specific nutrients. Table 4–8 briefly describes a protocol for parenteral nutrition management.

For the premature infant who is not fluid restricted, adequate nutrition can be provided by a peripheral line.[14] A central venous catheter is re-

Table 4–2 Premature Infant's Risk Factors for Nutritional Deficiencies

1. Decreased nutrient stores
   - Premature infants are born before anticipated quantities of nutrients are deposited.
   - Low stores include glycogen, fat, protein, fat soluble vitamins, calcium, phosphorus, magnesium, and trace minerals.
2. Rapid growth
   - Full-term infants often triple their birthweight by 1 year of age; for the preterm infant, a 10-fold increase may be needed to achieve optimal catch-up growth.
   - With rapid growth, energy and nutrient needs will be increased.
3. Immature physiological systems
   - Digestion and absorption capabilities are decreased due to low concentrations of lactase, pancreatic lipase, and bile salts.
   - Gastrointestinal motility and stomach capacity are decreased, which limits gastric emptying and feeding volume.
   - A coordinated suck and swallow is not developed until 32 to 34 weeks' gestation.
   - Hepatic enzymes are deceased, which may make specific amino acids conditionally essential (cysteine) or toxic (phenylalanine), due to the inability to synthesize or degrade.
   - Renal concentrating ability is limited.
4. Illnesses
   - Respiratory distress syndrome delays the introduction of enteral feedings because of the increased risk of aspiration. Gastrointestinal motility will also be decreased, and feedings may not be tolerated.
   - Patent ductus arteriosus often required fluid restriction, which limits caloric intake. Infants are usually made NPO when a ductus is treated with indomethacin because the clinically significant ductus alters mesenteric blood flow. The infant is at risk for necrotizing enterocolitis.
   - Necrotizing enterocolitis forces nutrition management to parenteral nutrition for bowel rest. With refeeding, an elemental infant formula is often indicated. Some infants may develop short-gut syndrome as a complication and require extensive nutritional management for malabsorption.
   - Bronchopulmonary dysplasia leads to an increased energy demand with fluid restriction. Calorically dense formulas are often utilized. Chronic diuretic use will create electrolyte and calcium depletion.
   - Hyperbilirubinemia may be treated by phototherapy, which increases the infant's insensible water loss and fluid requirement. If exchange transfusion is needed, introduction of enteral feedings will be delayed. Necrotizing enterocolitis has been reported as a complication of exchange transfusion therapy.
   - Sepsis and suspected sepsis will result in withholding all enteral fluids until it is established that the infant is stable. The affected infant may have an altered mesenteric blood flow, which can result in necrotizing enterocolitis, or may have apnea, which may cause aspiration of feedings.

Source: Klaus MH and Fanaroff AA. *Care of the High-Risk Neonate*, 5th ed. Philadelphia: W.B. Saunders; 2001:44.

---

quired for the infant who requires prolonged parenteral nutrition, has limited venous access, is fluid restricted, or has an increased nutrient demand that cannot be met by peripheral nutrition. Peripheral inserted central catheters (PICC) are frequently used with premature infants because the PICC line can be placed at an infant's bedside. A PICC line can reduce the stress to the infant from repeated insertion of peripheral lines and facilitate the delivery of concentrated parenteral nutrients.[14] A tunneled, central venous catheter must be placed surgically under anesthesia and is used when a PICC line cannot be inserted.

Table 4–3 Etiologic Factors for SGA Births

Normal variation	High altitude
Pregnancy-induced hypertension	Elevated maternal hemoglobin
Chronic hypertension	Multiple gestation
Chronic renal disease	Congenital malformations
Diabetes with vascular complications	Chromosomal abnormalities
Intrauterine infection	Placental insufficiency
Maternal malnutrition	Twin-to-twin transfusion
Cigarette smoking	Placental and cord defects
Drug or alcohol abuse	Short interpregnancy interval

Sources: Data from endnote references 2 and 6.

Management Concerns and Medical Problems

Fluid management is very individualized for the preterm infant. Insensible water losses will be high, and the infant's renal function and neuroendocrine control will be immature.[15] Fluid overload should be avoided to prevent the development of necrotizing enterocolitis (NEC), bronchopulmonary dysplasia, and patent ductus arteriosus.[15,16] Table 4–9 gives laboratory parameters that should be observed in guiding parenteral nutrition therapy.

Insensible fluid losses are high for many reasons.[15] First, the premature infant has a large surface area related to his or her weight, which facilitates easy heat and water losses. Secondly, the premature infant's skin offers little protection from evaporative losses. It has a high water content, and the epidermis is thin and highly permeable. Finally, environmental factors in the newborn intensive care unit increase insensible fluid losses, for example, the use of radiant warmers, phototherapy, and high or low ambient temperature.[15] These losses can be decreased by the use of humidified incubators, plastic shields, and plastic wraps or clothing.

Preterm infants have a limited ability to hydrolyze triglycerides. Elevated serum triglyceride levels are more frequently found with decreasing gestational age, infection, surgical stress, malnutrition, and with the SGA infant.[10,17] The serum triglyceride levels should be kept under 150 mg/dl.[10] Although the free fatty acids from intralipid compete with indirect bilirubin for binding onto albumin, intralipid may be provided during hyperbilirubinemia at the present recommended intakes. Intralipid should be administered at a maximum of 3 g/kg over a 24-hour infusion.[10,18] The concern is that free bilirubin may cross the blood-brain barrier and cause kernicterus. At this level of intake and rate of infusion, it appears to be safe.[19]

Several amino acid solutions are formulated for the pediatric patient.[20] These solutions contain a larger percentage of total nitrogen as essential

Table 4–4 Factors Associated with LGA Births

Infant of diabetic mother	Genetic predisposition
Beckwith's syndrome	High prepregnancy with large pregnancy weight gain
Transposition of the great vessels	Multiparity
Miscalculation of expected date of confinement	

Source: Data from endnote reference 2.

Table 4–5 Anticipated Problems for SGA and LGA Infants

Problems	*Issues*
Small for gestational age	
Hypoglycemia	Caused by Low glycogen stores Decreased gluconeogenesis Increased metabolic rate Decreased glycogenolysis Decreased counterregulatory hormones Hyperinsulinemia
Increased energy demand	Caused by Increased metabolic rate Increased growth rate Increased energy cost of growth
Heat loss	Caused by Large surface area Decreased subcutaneous fat
Large for gestational age	
Birth trauma	Shoulder dystocia, fractured clavicle, depressed skull fracture, brachial plexus palsy, facial paralysis
Hypoglycemia	Caused by hyperinsulinism

Sources: Data from endnote references 2, 6, and 59.

amino acids and branch chain amino acids, and they have a balanced pattern of nonessential amino acids instead of a single amino acid concentration.[14] The use a pediatric solution, as compared to an adult product, results in plasma amino acid levels that are similar to the breast-fed infant and improve weight gain and nitrogen balance.[21] The addition of cystine to Trophamine (Kendall McGraw Laboratories), one of the pediatric amino acid solutions, has suggested improved nitrogen balance.[11] The addition of cysteine hydrochloride has not consistently improved nitrogen balance.[22]

Transition to Enteral Feedings

Weaning to enteral feedings is a slow process that is necessary to facilitate feeding tolerance and prevent the development of necrotizing enterocolitis.[18,23] Enteral feedings are gradually increased in volume and strength as parenteral fluids are decreased at a similar volume. The two fluid types are coordinated to keep stable the total fluids provided until enteral feedings provide adequate nutrition for growth. Parenteral fluids are discontinued at approximately 100 to 120 ml/kg/day of enteral feedings.

ENTERAL NUTRITION

Premature infants are at risk for aspiration, NEC, and feeding intolerance, so enteral feedings are slowly introduced and advanced.[23] Infants with cardiovascular instability, which can present as severe acidosis, hypotension, or hypoxemia,[24] may not be fed. Trophic feedings have been advocated

Table 4–6 Parenteral Nutrition Guidelines: Energy, Protein and Minerals per Day

Nutrient	*Unit/kg*
Energy (kcal)	80–100
Glucose (mg/kg/min)	6–12
Fat (g)	0.5–3.0
Protein (g)	2.7–3.8
Sodium (mEq)	2–4
Potassium (mEq)	1.5–3
Chloride (mEq)	2–4
Calcium (mg)	60–100
Phosphorus (mg)	43–70
Magnesium (mg)	4.3–10
Zinc (μg)	400
Copper (μg)	20
Chromium (μg)	0.05–0.2
Manganese (μg)	1
Selenium (μg)	1.5–2.0
Molybdenum (μg)	0.25
Iodide (μg)	1

Sources: Data from endnote references 10 and 60.

for the first week of life to facilitate gut development and have not been associated with increasing the incidence of NEC.[10,18,25,26] Trophic feedings are small volumes of feedings given to nourish the gut, but do not serve as a major source of nutrition. Benefits are listed in Table 4–10. These feedings can consist of human milk or premature infant formula provided at 10–20 ml/kg/day for 4 to 7 days.[24] The use of umbilical artery catheters should not be a contraindication for starting trophic feedings.[10,27] When the infant's condition stabilizes feedings are advanced.[24] For the healthy premature infant, feedings can be initiated and advanced during the first week of life. Feeding advancement for the VLBW infant is often limited to 20 ml/kg/d or less because rapid feeding advancement has been associated with NEC.[18,28] In one study, the feeds advancement of 35 versus 15 ml/kg/day were both tolerated.[29] The optimal volume of advancement needs to be further studied.[30] The use of standardized feeding schedule, which includes time to initiate feeds, feeds volume advancement, and milk strength, has been associated with a decreased incidence of NEC.[31]

The type of milk selected depends on individual factors and can sometimes involve complex decisions. Table 4–11 lists factors that must be considered. Whatever milk is chosen, it should provide appropriate amounts of energy, protein, minerals, and vitamins (see Table 4–12). The goal is to promote growth and to prepare the infant for discharge. In Table 4–13, selected nutrients are compared (at 150 ml of milk or formula). This value represents the average volume intake for a premature infant on full enteral feedings. Fortified human milk or premature infant formulas will meet the needs of most premature infants.

The premature infant's vitamin needs will be met by the use of fortified human milk or premature infant formula, and no additional supplementation is indicated.[10] Iron needs will be met by the consumption of 120 kcal/kg of an iron-fortified premature infant formula, because this will provide 2 mg/kg or iron, which is the goal.[10] For the infant receiving human milk, iron supplementation can be initiated at 2 mg/kg/d once full-volume feedings have been achieved or 1 month of age.[10] The fortifiers vary in their iron

Table 4–7 Parenteral Vitamin Guidelines per Day

Vitamin	*Dose/kg*	*Maximum Dose per Day**
Vitamin A (IU)	920	2300
Vitamin E (IU)	2.8	7
Vitamin K (μg)	80	200
Vitamin D (IU)	160	400
Vitamin C (mg)	32	80
Thiamin (mg)	0.48	1.2
Riboflavin (mg)	0.56	1.4
Niacin (mg)	6.8	17
Vitamin B6 (mg)	0.4	1
Folate (μg)	56	140
Vitamin B12 (μg)	0.4	1
Biotin (μg)	8	20
Pantothenic Acid (mg)	2	5

*Preterm infants receive 40% of the daily dose MVI Pediatric (Astra Pharmaceuticals) per kg until the maximum daily dose is achieved at 2.5 kg.

Sources: Data from endnote references 10 and 61.

content and extra iron supplements should be limited to those that have low iron content. When erythropoietin therapy is employed, iron supplementation at 6 mg/kg/d to facilitate red cell production is recommended.[10] Erythropoietin therapy is not indicated for most premature infants, nor has it been shown to be effective in preventing the need for blood transfusions.[32]

Pharmacological dosage of vitamin E (50 to 100 mg/kg/d) for premature infants to prevent retinopathy of prematurity, bronchopulmonary dysplasia (BPD), or intraventricular hemorrhage, is not recommended.[10] Although vitamin E is an antioxidant, it has not consistently prevented these illnesses and complications associated with its pharmacological dosing including NEC, sepsis, intraventricular hemorrhage, and death.[33]

To prevent BPD in the ELBW infant, vitamin A supplementation has been suggested due to its role in cell differentiation and tissue repair.[34] Providing 5000 IU of vitamin A intramuscularly (IM) three times per week for the first month of life will lower oxygen requirements at 36 weeks' gestation.[34] It is recommended that physicians must decide the use of vitamin A supplementation in their nurseries.[10] Considerations include the variation in the incidence of BPD among nurseries, the lack of additional benefits by vitamin A supplementation, and the acceptance of IM therapy.[10,35] Additional factors associated with the occurrence of BBP are antenatal steroids, exogenous surfactant, mode of ventilation, postnatal steroids, and criteria to prescribe oxygen.[35]

Osteopenia or poor bone mineralization is commonly reported for premature infants when the intake of calcium and phosphorus is inadequate, and this is superimposed on top of their poor nutrient stores at birth.[36] Risk factors include prolonged parenteral nutrition and/or diets of unfortified human milk. A diet of fortified human milk or premature infant formula will meet the infant's needs.[10] Vitamin D intake at 200 to 400 IU per day with the calcium- and phosphorus-enriched premature formula is adequate.[37] Perhaps prolonged immobility may contribute by increasing calcium losses and decreasing mineralization.[36] Chronic diuretic use can increase urinary calcium losses.[36]

Premature infants are at risk for trace mineral deficiency due to their poor nutrient stores at

Table 4–8 Parenteral Nutrition Progression

	DOL to Begin*	*Beginning Quantity*	*Increase*	*Maximum or Goal*	*Considerations*
Fluid (ml/kg/day)	1	80–100	10–20	140–160	• Fluid needs will vary by birth weight, gestational age, postnatal age, and environmental conditions. • The ELBW* neonate may require 200–300 ml/kg/day to maintain normal hydration the first week of life. • Fluids should be provided to keep the infant in normal hydration status. Refer to Table 4–9 for monitoring guidelines.
Glucose (mg/kg/min)	1	4.5–6	1–2	11–12	• Begin on DOL 1 to prevent hypoglycemia. • Decrease glucose load for hyperglycemia. Glucose homeostasis will usually improve in 1 to 2 days. • Insulin infusions should be used with caution. Insulin usage may result in unstable blood glucose levels, hypoglycemia, and acidosis. The dose is 0.001 to 0.01 U/kg/min.
Protein (g/kg/day)	1	1–3	–	3–3.8	• Advance protein to meet needs. There is no documentation that gradual protein advancement is needed.
Lipids (g/kg/day)	1	0.5–1	1	3	• Provide over an 18 to 24 hr period. • Twenty percent intralipid is preferred over the 10% emulsion. Serum levels of cholesterol, triglycerides, and phospholipids levels are lower with use of the 20% emulsion.
Sodium chloride (mEq/kg/day)	2–4	1–3	–	2–4	• Allow diuresis to occur the first few days of life to decrease extracellular blood volume. • Start sodium to prevent hyponatremia.
Potassium (mEq/kg/day)	2	1.5–3	–	2–3	• Add potassium after urine flow is established and serum potassium level is normal. • Check for hyperkalemia as the ELBW infant has a decreased glomerular filtration rate, acidosis, and the release of nitrogen and potassium secondary to negative balance.
Magnesium (mg/kg/day)	1	6–10	–	6–10	• Remove from parenteral nutrition when mother has received magnesium.
Vitamins and Minerals	1				

*DOL = day of life; ELBW = extremely low birth weight

Parenteral nutrition progression may be slowed with fluid and electrolyte imbalance, glucose imbalance, renal failure, the anticipation of enteral feedings, or the initiation and tolerance of enteral feedings.

Sources: Data from endnote references 10, 15, 18, 24, and 62.

Table 4–9 Fluid and Electrolyte Monitoring Parameters

Parameter	Value
Fluid intake	80–150 ml/kg†
Urine output	2–4 ml/kg/h
Daily body weights	Allow 1–3% daily weight loss or 10–20% maximum total weight loss
Serum sodium	134–146 mmol/L
Serum potassium	3–7 mmol/L
Serum chloride	97–110 mmol/L
Serum creatinine	0.3–1.0 mg/dl
Blood urea nitrogen	3–25 mg/dl
Urine specific gravity	1.008–1.012
Urine osmolality	300 mOsm

†The critically ill premature infant has highly variable fluid needs. This range represents the usual volume of fluid administered. To prevent over- or underhydration, fluids should be provided so as to keep the other monitoring parameters within normal levels.

Sources: Data from endnote references 15, 63, and 64.

birth, rapid growth, and the dependence on adequate intake. With use of today's parenteral guidelines, premature infant formula or fortified human milk, deficiencies should be uncommon. Infants who have excessive losses via an ileostomy drainage or high urine output related to renal failure, could need two to three times the recommended guidelines for zinc.[38] Additional case reports of zinc deficiency have been reported when the mother's milk had an extremely low zinc content or the infant had been provided with copper and/or iron supplements that will compete with zinc for absorption.[39]

The feeding method employed will depend on the infant's gestational age, clinical condition, and nursery staff experience.[10] Table 4–14 describes methods in use and Table 4–15 gives guidelines for amounts and rates of feedings. Due to the infant's constantly changing clinical condition and development, several methods will be used. Both continuous and bolus infusions are used with gavage feedings.[10] A recent study

Table 4–10 Benefits of Trophic Feedings

1. Feeding
   - Improved feeding tolerance
   - Achieve full feedings sooner
   - Achieve full PO sooner
2. Gastrointestinal
   - Increased plasma gastrin
   - Decreased intestinal transit time
   - More mature intestinal motor pattern
   - Increased calcium, copper, and phosphorus retention
3. Clinical
   - Decreased serum bilirubin and days of phototherapy
   - Decreased incidence of cholestasis
   - Lower serum alkaline phosphatase activity levels
4. Decreased length of stay

Sources: Data from endnote references 18, 23–26.

Table 4–11 Milk and Formula Selection Indications and Concerns

Milk	*Indications*	*Concerns*
Human Milk	• Nutrients are readily absorbed. • Anti-infective factors are present. • Decreased incidence in necrotizing and sepsis. • Nutrient composition is unique. • Maternal-infant attachment enhanced. • Maternal emotional support by family and health care team is indicated to facilitate lactation. • Quicker achievement of full enteral feedings versus premature infant formula. • Slower weight gain, but earlier discharge has been demonstrated on fortified human milk feedings versus premature infant formula.	• Milk from mothers who deliver prematurely will often contain a higher protein concentration than that found in the milk from mothers who deliver at term. This elevated protein concentration decreased by 28 days of lactation and may not meet the protein needs of the rapidly growing premature infant. • The concentration of protein, calcium, phosphorous, and sodium is too low to meet the needs of many premature infants. To increase nutrient density, human milk fortifiers should be added to the milk. • Iron supplementation at 2 mg/kg is needed for those infants receiving the low iron containing fortifier. For those who are provided the fortifier with iron, no iron supplementation is needed. • Milk volume production may be inadequate to nourish the infant.
Formulas for premature infants	• Glucose polymers comprise 50–60% of the carbohydrate calories, which decreases the lactose load presented to the premature infant for digestion. Glucose polymers also decrease the osmolality of the formula. • Lactose comprises 40–50% of the carbohydrate calories. • Medium chain triglycerides (MCTs) are 40–50% of the fat calories. MCTs do not require pancreatic lipase or bile salts for digestion and absorption. • Protein is at a higher concentration than that incorporated into standard infant formula to meet the increased protein needs of the preterm infant. • The protein is a 60/40 whey/casein ratio as compared with the 18/82 ratio found in bovine milk. This whey predominance prevents the elevation of plasma phenylalaine and tyrosine levels.	• Feeding volumes should be advanced slowly with the very low birthweight infant. • Vitamin and iron supplements are not indicated for the infant receiving iron-fortified premature infant formula.

	• Calcium and phosphorous are two to three times the concentration found in standard infant formulas. These levels will maintain normal serum calcium and phosphorous levels, prevent osteopenia, and promote calcium and phosphorous accretion at the fetal rate. • Sodium, potassium, and chloride concentrations are greater than in standard infant formulas to meet the increased electrolyte needs of the premature infant. • Vitamins, trace minerals, and additional minerals are incorporated into these formulas at high concentration to meet the infant's increased nutrient need while facilitating a limited volume intake. • Iron-fortified formulas are available, which eliminated the need for iron supplementation. • Formula osmolarity is within the physiologic range at 211–260 mOsm/L, which facilitates formula tolerances and decreases the risk of necrotizing enterocolotis. • Premature formulas can be used until the infant reaches 2.5–3.6 kg, depending on the formula vitamin concentration and volume intake.	
Transition Formulas (Premature Discharge Formulas)	• Designed for the premature infant at discharge. The infant should weigh at least 1.8 kg when this formula is provided. • Formula should be initiated at least 2 days prior to discharge to document formula tolerance and weight gain. • Formulas have the nutrient composition that is between the concentrated premature formulas and the standard infant formulas. • Glucose polymers comprise 50–60% of the carbohydrate calories, and lactose comprises 40–50%.	• Infants with a birth weight of less than 1250 grams and those premature infants unable to consume adequate volumes of standard formula to support growth should received the premature discharge formula. • Transitional formulas should be provided up to 6 to 9 months of corrected age. • Formulas are iron fortified and vitamin dense such that nutrient supplementation is not needed.

continues

Table 4–11 continued

Milk	*Indications*	*Concerns*
	• MCTs are 20–25% of the fat calories. • The protein is either a 60/40 or 50/50 whey/casein ratio. • Improved bone mineral concentration and greater weight and length gains were documented with premature infants fed a transition formula for the first 9 months of life.	• Formulas are available as a powder and can be concentrated to meet the needs of the infant with bronchopulmonary dyplasia. This formula can be provided in the nursery and in the home setting.
Standard infant formulas	• Can be used at discharged for larger premature infants who can gain 20–30 g/day while consuming at least 180 ml/kg/day of this formula.	• Nutrient content is inadequate for the premature infant during the neonatal period. • During the early neonatal period, these formulas may not be tolerated well. Lactose is the sole carbohydrate source, and only long chain fatty acids are incorporated into these formulas.
Elemental infant formula	• Infants who are recovering or suffering from gastrointestinal disorders can benefit from elemental infant formula.	• Nutrient content is inadequate for the premature infant, with special reference to calcium and phosphorous levels. • The time to switch to a premature formula must always be considered to improve nutrient intake. Depending on the infant's feeding history, the formulas can be switched or the premature infant formula can be provided as one feed per day and advanced by one additional feed per day as tolerated.
Soy formulas		• These formulas are not indicted for premature infants who weigh less than 1.8 kg. • The premature infant is at risk for osteopenia. The phytates in the formula bind phosphorous and make it unavailable for absorption. The aluminum content may also interfere with appropriate bone growth. • The amino acid profile may be inappropriate for the premature infant. • Decreased weight gain and length growth have been reported when soy formulas were fed to premature infants.

Sources: Data from endnote references 10, 24, and 65–72.

Table 4–12 Enteral Nutrient Guidelines per kg/day

Nutrient	*Amount*	*Nutrient*	*Amount*
Energy (kcal)	105–130	Molybdenum (μg)	0.3
Protein (g)	3–4	Iodine (μg)	30–60
Carbohydrate (g)	10–14	Vitamin A (IU)	700–1500
Fat (g)	5–7	Vitamin D (IU)	150–400*
Sodium (mEq)	2–3	Vitamin E (IU)	6–12
Potassium (mEq)	2–3	Vitamin K (μg)	7–10
Chloride (mEq)	2–3	Vitamin C (mg)	18–24
Calcium (mg)	120–230	Thiamin (μg)	180–240
Phosphorus (mg)	60–140	Riboflavin (μg)	250–360
Magnesium (mg)	7.9–15	Niacin (mg)	3.6–4.8
Iron (mg)	2	Vitamin B6 (μg)	150–210
Zinc (μg)	1000	Folate (μg)	25–50
Copper (μg)	120–150	Vitamin B12 (μg)	0.3
Chromium (μg)	0.1–0.5	Biotin (μg)	3.6–6
Manganese (μg)	7.5	Pantothenic Acid (mg)	1.2–1.7
Selenium (μg)	1.3–3.0		

*Maximum of 400 IU/day

Sources: Data from endnote references 10 and 60.

demonstrated improved weight gain and feeding tolerance with the use of bolus versus continuous infusion.[25] The use of transpyloric feedings dictates the use of continuous infusion to prevent an osmotic load presented to the intestine and dumping from occurring.[40] The delivery of nutrients to the infant is decreased with continuous infusions.[10] Specifically, human milk fat and fat additives and minerals in the human milk fortifier adhere to or precipitate in the delivery system.[10,24,41] The use of a syringe pump with the syringe in an upright position will increase fat delivery.[24]

Breastfeeding

Mothers who want to breastfeed their premature infant must usually express their milk. During the infant's prolonged hospitalization, it will be difficult for the mother to be available for 24-hour breastfeeding. Further, their infants are too little and/or sick to nurse. Family members,

Table 4–13 Selected Nutrient Comparison per 150 ml of Milk or Formula

Guidelines (per kg)	*Human*	*Standard*	*Transition*	*Premature*
120 kcal	101	101	110	120
3.5–4.0 g protein	1.4	2.1	3.2	3.6
2.5–3.5 mEq sodium	1.2	1.1–1.2	1.7	2.3–3
210 mg calcium	42	80	117–134	200–219
110 mg phosphorus	23	42–54	69–74	101–122
270 IU vitamin D	3	62	78–89	183–293

Sources: Data from endnote references 67 and 68.

Table 4–14 Methods of Feeding

Type	*Considerations*
Breast/bottle	Most physiological methods Infant at least 32 to 34 weeks' gestation Infant medically stable Infant's respiratory rate less than 60 breaths per minute
Gavage	Supplement to breast/bottle feedings Suggested for infants less than 32 weeks' gestation Use when respiratory rate less than 80 breaths per minute Use for intubated infant Use for neurologically impaired neonate
Transpyloric	Employ when gavage feedings not tolerated Use when the infant is at risk for milk aspiration Infant intubated Use for the infant with decreased gut motility Must wait for passage of tube to begin feedings Requires radiographic assessment to check placement Complications include dumping syndrome, altered intestinal micro flora, nutrient malabsorption, perforation of intestine
Gastrostomy	Gastrointestinal malformation Infant neurologically impaired

Sources: Data from endnote references 10, 24, 40, and 43.

friends, and nursery staff must provide support for these women to enable them to be successful in providing milk during this stressful period (see Table 4–16). Kangaroo care (skin-to-skin contact between the parent and the infant) will facilitate parent-infant bonding and has been linked to a longer period of lactation by the mother who delivers prematurely.[42]

NUTRITIONAL ASSESSMENT

Dietary Considerations

Daily assessment is necessary to determine the need for changing feeding volume, solution strength, or feeding method. Intake is evaluated against nutrient guidelines. Finally, feeding technique needs to be advanced to the most physiological method possible for the infant. Breast or bottle feedings are introduced as the infant's coordination of sucking, swallowing, and breathing is developed at 32 to 34 weeks gestation.[10] The number of oral feedings should be increased per day as the infant demonstrates the ability to effectively feed. Feedings are usually limited to 20 minutes per feeding period to prevent fatigue and excessive energy expenditure.[43] Feedings may be limited to once a day until the infant demonstrates successful feeding.

Anthropometric Measurements

Anthropometric measurements are difficult to perform on premature infants, principally due to an infant's small size and clinical condition. Medical equipment can interfere with the measurement or can add to the recorded weight. Also, the infant is at risk for cold stress during these procedures which diverts energy from growth to heat production.

Table 4–15 Feeding Guidelines

Trophic Feedings	Provide to infants < 1250 grams BW* Consider for infants 1250–1500 grams BW 10–20 ml/kg/day Human milk or premature infant formula Bolus feedings
Feeds Advancement	< 1500 g BW and < 32 wks GA 10–20 ml/kg/day ≥ 1500 g < 2000 g BW and 32–33 wks GA 20–35 ml/kg/day ≥ 2000 g BW and ≥ 34 wks GA Initiate and advance at 25–50 ml/kg/day to ab lib depending on clinical status of infant
Milk Selection	< 2000 g BW or < 34 wks GA • Human milk: Fortify with two packs human milk fortifier/100 ml milk when 100 ml/kg feeds achieved. Next day increase to four packs human milk fortifier/100 ml of milk. • Premature infant formula ≥ 2000 g BW and ≥ 34 weeks GA • Human milk • Standard infant formula

*BW = birthweight, GA = gestational age

Source: Data from endnote reference 73.

Daily weights should be recorded on a premature infant growth grid (see Appendix A-1).[44] Weights will be influenced by the medical equipment attached to the infant, the use of different scales, the infant's hydration status, and total nutrient intake. Weights taken at the same time each day will avoid recording diurnal variations. Initial weight loss that reflects the loss of extracellular fluid ranges from 10 to 20% of birth weight during the first week of life.[15] After regaining birth weight, the weight gain goal is 10–20 g/kg/day for infants who weigh over 2000 g.[24,45] When the infant weighs 2 kg, a weight gain of 20 to 30 g/day is appropriate.[24,45]

Head circumference should be measured weekly. Alterations in measurement will occur from birth to week 1 of life due to head molding or edema. Additional errors are introduced when scalp intravenous lines are employed or the head has been shaved. Record the measurement on a premature growth grid (see Appendix A).[4,5,44] The goal is 0.7–1.0 cm/wk.[24,44,45] Length measurements are difficult to obtain accurately. Length should increase by 0.7–1.0 cm/wk.[24,44,45]

Skinfolds and mid-arm circumference measurements do not change rapidly enough to be more helpful than weight measurements for diet changes. These measurements are generally not employed for routine clinical care but are indicated for growth studies. There are limited standards.[46,47]

Assessing Inadequate Weight Gain

When a series of daily measurements indicate inadequate weight gain, a search must be made for the cause. Table 4–17 outlines areas to check.

Table 4–16 Steps to Support Lactating Women

1. Instruction
   - Methods of milk expression
   - Sterilization of expression equipment
   - Storage and transport of milk
   - Diet for lactation
   - Tips for relaxation
2. Tips to help with let down prior to expression
   - Showering
   - Hand massaging of the breasts
   - Applying warm washcloths to the breasts
   - Consuming warm beverages
   - Visiting the infant
   - Talking to the infant's nurse by phone
   - Placing the infant's picture on the pump
3. Nursery staff and nursery support
   - Availability of lactation consultant for mothers and staff
   - Education of nursery staff on milk expression
   - Electric pump and pumping room conveniently available to the nursery
   - Electric pumps available for rental and hand pumps for purchase
   - Mother's milk used to feed the infant whenever available
   - Nonnutritive breastfeeding (Milk expression prior to placing the infant to a "empty" breast) which facilitates milk supply and positive oral experience for infant. Utilize before infant is ready to breastfeed.
   - Help mother with the initiation of nursing
   - Promote kangaroo care
4. Initiation of breastfeeding
   - Wake baby up
   - Express a little milk prior to nursing so nipple is easier to grasp by the small infant
   - Position infant so mother and infant are stomach to stomach
   - Allow mother to room in with baby prior to discharge to establish breastfeeding pattern

Sources: Data from endnote reference 42 and 73–76.

Assessment of Feeding Tolerance

Feeding intolerance and clinical compromise are common for the premature infant, so constant surveillance is required to detect early signs of feeding intolerance, sepsis, or NEC.[45] Depending on the findings, feedings may be held, decreased, diluted, discontinued, or their frequency may be changed. Feedings will often be held with signs of illness including persistent apnea and bradycardia, temperature instability or lethargy. Clinical parameters are discussed later.

Gastric residuals are often present but what exactly constitutes an unacceptable volume is difficult to define. Residuals may be due to immature intestinal motor activity, as residuals are seen prior to feeds initiation.[18] Some infants have small aspirates no matter what the feeding volume, and yet are tolerating feedings.[48] With bolus feedings a residual up to 50% of the feeding volume or 1.5 times the hourly rate for continuous feeding is often accepted.[24] A fixed volume of 2–3 ml/residual has also been used.[49] Mucus residuals are not a concern and are present in the infant recovering from lung disease. Undigested formula may dictate that the feeding volume is too large, that the infant does not tolerate this formula, that the infant has poor gastrointestinal

Table 4–17 Possible Etiologies for Inadequate Weight Gain

1. Nutrient calculations are incorrect.
2. Parenteral nutrition not optimized.
3. Infant is not receiving ordered diet.
   - Intravenous fluid administration has been interrupted to give blood or drugs or the intravenous line has become infiltrated.
   - Infant is unable to consume what is ordered by bottle, and no gavage supplements were provided.
   - Feedings were held because the infant's respiratory rate increased or body temperature instability developed.
4. Infant does not tolerate given formula.
5. Calculated nutrient guidelines are inadequate for the infant due to growth retardation or illness.
6. Infant is cold stressed.
7. Infant has outgrown previous diet order.
8. Nutrition solution not prepared correctly.
9. Incorrect formula provided to infant.
10. Human milk issues
    - Continuous infusion will lead to fat separation in feeding syringe. Switch to bolus feedings or ensure feeding syringe facing upward to facilitate milk fat delivery to infant.
    - Ensure correct number of fortifier packets added to milk.
    - Ensure infant not receiving only the fore milk which is low in fat.
11. Metabolic issues
    - Acidosis
    - Electrolyte abnormality
12. Low hemoglobin

Sources: Data from endnote references 45 and 77.

motility, or that the infant has NEC or intestinal obstruction. Residuals containing bile are not uncommon when the infant is fed transpylorically.[45] Residuals are not a consistent marker of feeding intolerance or NEC, but should be noted in relation to other clinical parameters.[49,50]

Abdominal girth circumference increases will occur with growth, air swallowing, feeding intolerance, infrequent stooling, or NEC. When the abdomen is distended, an evaluation to rule out bowel obstruction is done.[51] A workup for sepsis and NEC may be considered with other signs of feeding intolerance or increase in abdominal tone is noted. Visible loops of bowel may indicate illness.

Blood in the stool is a concern and should be evaluated. Blood may be a sign of illness, feeding-tube irritation of the intestine, anal fissure, or swallowed blood during delivery.

Assessment of Nutrient Adequacy and Tolerance

Both the specific clinical signs of nutrient deficiency/toxicity and the associated laboratory values should be regularly assessed. Vitamin assays should be performed when pharmacological dosing of vitamins are being given to permit detection of vitamin toxicity or when a deficiency is suspected. Serial plasma trace mineral levels may be more helpful than one plasma level when assessing a trace mineral deficiency.[24] There are several reviews on clinical signs.[24,52–54] Acceptable standards for laboratory values are difficult to establish because premature infants differ by their physical maturity, clinical condition, and nutrient stores. For example, serum proteins will vary by the infant's hepatic maturity, energy and protein intake, vitamin and mineral nutritional status, and clinical condition.

During the first week of life, serum electrolytes, glucose, creatinine, and urea nitrogen are monitored daily or more frequently when values are abnormal. As these blood parameters stabilize, they can be examined twice a week for those infants receiving parenteral nutrition and as needed for infants on enteral feedings.[24,44] Serum electrolytes are assessed for those infants receiving diuretics or those with a history of abnormal values until values are normal. Additional parameters monitored when parenteral nutrition is being administered include serum triglycerides to check lipid tolerance, direct bilirubin to detect cholestasis, and serum alanine aminotransferase (ALT, serum glutamic-pyruvic transaminase) to evaluate hepatic function.[24,44] Serum calcium, phosphorus, and alkaline phosphatase levels may be monitored to detect osteopenia in the premature infant. Hematocrit and hemoglobin levels are checked as needed.

DISCHARGE CONCERNS

The premature infant is ready for discharge from the hospital when body temperature can be maintained, breastfeeding or bottle feeding supports growth, and cardiorespiratory function is mature and stable.[55] Most important, the caretaker must be ready to care for this high-risk infant. Twenty-four hour visitation allows the parents to become active in caring for their infant. Rooming in with the infant will help to facilitate care and give confidence to the parent.[56]

The infant should be evaluated for participation in the Special Supplemental Nutrition Program for Women, Infants, and Children (WIC), and enrollment into a developmental follow-up program for premature infants. The follow-up program should monitor the infant's growth and development, offer aid with chronic illness management, provide early detection of problems, make referrals to specialized services as indicated, and give the parents support and guidance in caring for their prematurely born infant.[57] These clinics not only aid with early detection of problems, but also evaluate the care that newborn intensive care units provide. A primary care physician must be identified to provide well-baby and sick care, and an appointment should be established prior to discharge to home.[55] Most infants will be discharged home on human milk, standard infant formula, or transition formula. The breast-fed infant should receive a multiple vitamin with iron supplement; the infant-fed formula with iron will not require additional iron supplementation. Infants receiving the premature discharge formula do not require extra vitamins, but the premature infant receiving term formula should receive a multivitamin until 3 kg of body weight is achieved.[10] Infants suffering from bronchopulmonary dysplasia may need a nutrient dense formula. The premature discharge formulas can be easily concentrated to 24 or 27 kilocaloric per ounce.

CONCLUSION

Although premature infants begin life in a compromised nutritional state, nutrition and medical therapies continue to evolve, which enhance the infant's potential for optimal growth and development.[18] Daily nutrition evaluation of the premature infant is necessary to ensure that appropriate nutrition therapy can be provided.

REFERENCES

1. American Academy of Pediatrics and American College of Obstetricians and Gynecologists. *Guidelines for Perinatal Care*, 5th ed. Elk Grove, IL: American Academy of Pediatrics; 2002.
2. Southgate WM, Pittard WB. Classification and physical examination of the newborn infant. In: Klaus MH, Fanaroff AA. *Care of the High-Risk Neonate*, 5th ed. Philadelphia: W.B. Saunders Co.; 2001:100–129.
3. Battaglia FC, Lubchenco LO. A practical classification of newborn infants by weight and gestational age. *J Pediatr*. 1967;71:159–163.
4. Babson SG, Benda GI. Growth graphs for the clinical assessment of infants of varying gestational age. *J Pediatr*. 1976;89:814–820.
5. Fenton TR. A new growth chart for preterm babies: Babson and Benda's chart updated with recent data and a new format. *BMC Pediatrics*. 2003;3:13.

6. Kliegman RM, Das U (S) G. Intrauterine growth retardation. In: Fanaroff AA, Martin RJ, eds. *Neonatal-Perinatal Medicine Diseases of the Fetus and Infant*, 7th ed. St. Louis, MO: Mosby; 2002:228–262.
7. Hack M, Merkatz IR, McGrath SK, Jones PK, et al. Catch-up growth in very-low-birth-weight infants. *Am J Dis Child*. 1984;138:370–375.
8. Hack M, Schluchter M, Cartar L, et al. Growth of very low birth weight infants to age 20 years. Available at www.pediatrics.org/cgi/content/full/112/1/e30. *Pediatrics*. 2003;112:e30–e38.
9. Hack M, Breslau N, Weissman B, Aram D, et al. Effect of very low birth weight and subnormal head size on cognitive abilities at school age. *N Engl J Med*. 1991;325: 231–237.
10. American Academy of Pediatrics Committee on Nutrition. Nutritional needs of preterm infants. In: Kleinman RE, ed. *Pediatric Nutrition Handbook*, 5th ed. Elk Grove Village, IL: American Academy of Pediatrics; 2004:23–54.
11. Rivera A, Bell EF, Bier DM. Effect of intravenous amino acids on protein metabolism of preterm infants during the first three days of life. *Pediatr Res*. 1993;33:106–111.
12. Murdock N, Crighton A, Nelson LM, Forsyth JS. Low birthweight infants and total parenteral nutrition immediately after birth. II. Randomised study of biochemical tolerance of intravenous glucose, amino acids, and lipid. *Arch Dis Child*. 1995;73:F8–F12.
13. Rivera A, Bell EF, Stegink LD, Ziegler EE. Plasma amino acid profiles during the first three days of life in infants with respiratory distress syndrome: Effect of parenteral amino acid supplementation. *J Pediatr*. 1989;115: 464–468.
14. Heird WC, Gomez MR. Parenteral nutrition in low-birth-weight infants. *Annu Rev Nutr*. 1996;16:471–499.
15. Bell EF, Oh W. Fluid and electrolyte management. In: Avery GB, Fletcher MA, MacDonald MG, eds. *Neonatology Pathophysiology and Management of the Newborn*, 5th ed. Philadelphia: Lippincott Williams & Wilkins; 1999:345–361.
16. Bell EF, Acarregui MJ. Restricted versus liberal water intake for preventing morbidity and mortality in preterm infants. (Cochrane Review). In: *The Cochrane Library*, Issue 4, available at www.nichd.nih.gov/cochrane.htm. 1998.
17. Shulman RJ, Phillips S. Parenteral nutrition in infants and children. *J Pediatri Gastro Nutr*. 2003;36:587–607.
18. Ziegler EE, Thureen PJ, Carlson SJ. Aggressive nutrition of the very low birthweight infant. *Clin Peri*. 2002; 29:225–244.
19. Putet G. Lipid metabolism of the micropremie. *Clin Peri*. 2000;27:57–69.
20. Thureen PJ, Hay WW. Intravenous nutrition and postnatal growth of the micropremie. *Clin Peri*. 2000;27:197–219.
21. Helms RA, Christensen ML, Mauer EC, Storm MC. Comparison of a pediatric versus standard amino acid formulation in preterm neonates requiring parenteral nutrition. *J Pediatr*. 1987;110:466–472.
22. Zlotkin SH, Bryan MH, Anderson GH. Cysteine supplementation to cysteine-free intravenous feeding regimens in newborn infants. *Am J Clin Nutr*. 1981;34:914–923.
23. Anderson DM. Feeding the ill or preterm infant. *Neonatal Network*. 2002;21:7–14.
24. Schanler RJ. The low birth weight infant. In: Walker WA, Watkins JB, Duggan C, ed. *Nutrition in Pediatrics: Basic Science and Clinical Applications*, 3rd ed. Hamilton, Ontario, Canada: BC Decker, Inc.; 2003:491–514.
25. Schanler RJ, Shulman RJ, Lau C, O'Brian Smith E, et al. Feeding strategies for premature infants: Randomized trial of gastrointestinal priming and tube-feeding method. *Pediatrics*. 1999;103:434–439.
26. Dunn L, Hulman S, Weiner J, Kliegman R. Beneficial effects of early hypocaloric enteral feeding on neonatal gastrointestinal function: Preliminary report of a randomized trial. *J Pediatr*. 1988;112:622–629.
27. Davey AM, Wagner CL, Cox C, et al. Feeding premature infants while low umbilical artery catheters are in place: A prospective, randomized trial. *J Pediatr*. 1994;124: 795–799.
28. Anderson DM, Kliegman RM. The relationship of neonatal alimentation practices to the occurrence of endemic necrotizing enterocolitis. *Am J Peri*. 1991;8:62–67.
29. Rayyis SF, Ambalavanan N, Wright L, et al. Randomized trial of "slow" versus "fast" feed advancements on the incidence of necrotizing enterocolitis in very low birth weight infants. *J Pediatr*. 1999;134:293–297.
30. Kennedy KA, Tyson JE, Chamnanvanakij S. Rapid versus slow rate of advancement of feedings for promoting growth and preventing necrotizing enterocolitis in parenterally fed low-birth-weight infants (Cochrane Review). In: *The Cochrane Library*, Issue 3, available at www.nichd.nih.gov/cochraneneonatal.
31. Kamitsuka MD, Horton MK, Williams MA. The incidence of necrotizing enterocolitis after introducing standardized feeding schedules for infants between 1250 and 2500 grams and less than 35 weeks of gestation. *Pediatrics*. 2000;105:379–384.
32. Ohls RK, Ehrenkranz RA, Wright LL, Lemons JA, et al. Effects of early erythropoietin therapy on the transfusion requirements of preterm infants below 1250 grams birth weight: A multicenter, randomized, controlled trial. *Pediatrics*. 2001;108:934–942.
33. Greer FR. Special needs and dangers of fat soluble vitamins A, E and K. In: Tsang RC, Zlotkin SH, Nichols BL, Hansen JW, eds. *Nutrition During Infancy Principles and Practice*, 2nd ed. Cincinnati, OH: Digital Educational Publishing, Inc.; 1997:285–312.

34. Tyson JE, Wright LL, Oh W, Kennedy KA, et al. Vitamin A supplementation for extremely-low-birth-weight infants. *N Eng J Med.* 1999;340:1962–1968.

35. Darlow BA, Graham PJ. Vitamin A supplementation for preventing morbidity and mortality in very low birthweight infants. (Cochrane Review). In: *The Cochrane Library*. Available at www.nichd.nih.gov/cochrane, August 26, 2002.

36. DeMarini S, Tsang RC. Disorders of calcium, phosphorus, and magnesium metabolism. In: Fanaroff AA, Martin RJ, eds. *Neonatal-Perinatal Medicine Diseases of the Fetus and Infant*, 7th ed. St. Louis, MO: Mosby; 2002:1376–1392.

37. Koo WWK, Krug-Wispe S, Neylan M, Succop P, et al. Effect of three levels of vitamin D intake in preterm infants receiving high mineral-containing milk. *J Pediatr Gastroenterol Nutr*. 1995;21:182–189.

38. Zlotkin SH, Atkinson S, Lockitch G. Trace elements in nutrition for premature infants. *Clin Peri.* 1995;22:223–240.

39. Atkinson SA, Zlotkin S. Recognizing deficiencies and excesses of zinc, copper, and other trace elements. In.: Tsang RC, Zlotkin SH, Nichols BL, Hansen JW, eds. *Nutrition During Infancy Principles and Practice*, 2nd ed. Cincinnati, OH; Digital Educational Publishing, Inc.; 1997:209–232.

40. Wessel JJ. Feeding methodologies. In: Groh-Wargo S, Thompson M, Cox JH, eds. *Nutritional Care for High-Risk Newborns*, 3rd ed. Chicago: Precept Press; 2000: 321–339.

41. Greer FR, McCormick A, Loker J. Changes in fat concentration of human milk during delivery by intermittent bolus and continuous mechanical pump infusion. *J Pediatr*. 1984;105:745–749.

42. Hurst NM, Valentine CJ, Renfro L, Burns P, et al. Skin-to-skin holding in the neonatal intensive care unit influences maternal milk volume. *J Peri*. 1997;17:213–217.

43. Kalhan SC, Price PT. Nutrition and selected disorders of the gastrointestinal tract. In: Klaus MH, Fanaroff AA. *Care of the High-Risk Neonate*, 5th ed. Philadelphia: W.B. Saunders Co.; 2001:147–194.

44. Ehrenkranz RA, Younes N, Lemons JA, Fanaroff AA, et al. Longitudinal growth of hospitalized very low birth weight infants. *Pediatrics*. 1999;104:280–289.

45. Anderson DM. Nutritional assessment and therapeutic interventions for the preterm infant. *Clin Peri*. 2002;29: 313–326.

46. Vaucher YE, Harrison GG, Udall JN, Morrow G. Skinfold thickness in North American infants 24–41 weeks gestation. *Hum Biol*. 1984;56:713–731.

47. Sasanow SR, Georgieff MK, Pereira GR. Mid-arm circumference and midarm/head circumference ratios: Standard curves for anthropometric assessment of the neonatal nutritional status. *J Pediatr*. 1986;109:311–315.

48. Rickard K, Gresham E. Nutritional considerations for the newborn requiring intensive care. *J Am Diet Assoc*. 1975;66:592–600.

49. Mihatsch WA, von Schoenaich P, Fahnenstich H, et al. The significance of gastric residuals in the early enteral feeding advancement of extremely low birth weight infants. *Pediatrics*. 2002;109:457–459.

50. Cobb, BA, Carlo WA, Ambalavanan N. Gastric residuals and their relationship to necrotizing enterocolitis in very low birth weight infants. *Pediatrics*. 2004;113:50–53.

51. Premji SS, Paes B, Jacobson K, et al. Evidence-based feeding guidelines for very low-birth-weight infants. *Advances in Neonatal Care*. 2002;2:5–18.

52. Schanler RJ. Who needs water-soluble vitamins? In: Tsang RC, Zlotkin SH, Nichols BL, Hansen JW, eds. *Nutrition During Infancy Principles and Practice*, 2nd ed. Cincinnati, OH: Digital Educational Publishing, Inc.; 1997:255–284.

53. Koo WWK, Tsang RC. Building better bones: Calcium, magnesium, phosphorus, and vitamin D. In: Tsang RC, Zlotkin SH, Nichols BL, Hansen JW, eds. *Nutrition During Infancy Principles and Practice,* 2nd ed. Cincinnati, OH: Digital Educational Publishing, Inc.; 1997: 175–208.

54. Atkinson SA, Zlotkin S. Recognizing deficiencies and excesses or zinc, copper and other trace elements. In: Tsang RC, Zlotkin SH, Nichols BL, Hansen JW, eds. *Nutrition During Infancy Principles and Practice*, 2nd ed. Cincinnati, OH: Digital Educational Publishing, Inc.; 1997:209–232.

55. American Academy of Pediatrics Committee on Fetus and Newborn. Hospital discharge of the high-risk neonate-proposed guidelines. *Pediatrics*. 1998;102;411–417.

56. Klaus MH, Kennell JH. Care of the mother, father, and infant. In: Fanaroff AA, Martin RJ, eds. *Neonatal-Perinatal Medicine: Diseases of the Fetus and Infant*, 7th ed. St. Louis, MO: Mosby; 2002:563–577.

57. Hack M. The outcome of neonatal care. In: Klaus MH, Fanaroff AA, eds. *Care of the High-Risk Neonate*, 5th ed. Philadelphia: W.B. Saunders Co.; 2001:528–535.

58. Klaus MH, Fanaroff AA. *Care of the High-Risk Neonate*, 5th edition. Philadelphia: W.B. Saunders Co; 2001.

59. Kliegman RM. Problems in metabolic adaptation: Glucose, calcium, and magnesium. In: Klaus MH, Fanaroff AA. *Care of the High-Risk Neonate*, 5th edition. Philadelphia: W.B. Saunders Co.; 2001:301–323.

60. Hansen JW. Consensus recommendations. In: Tsang RC, Lucas A, Uauy R, Zlotkin S, eds. *Nutritional Needs of the Preterm Infant*. Baltimore, MD: Williams & Wilkins; 1993:288–289.

61. Greene HL, Hambidge KM, Schanler R, Tsang RC. Guidelines for the use of vitamins, trace elements, calcium, magnesium, and phosphorus in infants and children receiving total parenteral nutrition: Report of the

Subcommittee on Pediatric Parenteral Nutrient Requirements from the Committee on Clinical Practice Issues of The American Society for Clinical Nutrition. *Am J Clin Nutr*. 1988;48:1324–1342.

62. Thureen PJ, Melara D, Fennessey PV, et al. Effect of low versus high intravenous amino acid intake on very low birth weight infants in the early neonatal period. *Pediatr Res*. 2003;53:24–32.
63. Nicholson JF, Pesce MA. Reference ranges for laboratory tests and procedures. In: Behrman RE, Kliegman RM, Jenson HB, eds. *Nelson Textbook of Pediatrics*, 17th ed. Philadelphia: Saunders; 2004:2396–2427.
64. Davis ID, Stork JE, Avner ED. Fluid and electrolytes management. In: Fanaroff AA, Martin RJ, eds. *Neonatal-Perinatal Medicine Diseases of the Fetus and Infant*, 7th ed. St. Louis, MO: Mosby; 2002:619–627.
65. Schanler RJ, Shulman RJ, Lau C. Feeding strategies for premature infants: Beneficial outcomes of feeding fortified human milk versus preterm formula. *Pediatrics*. 1999;103:1150–1157.
66. American Academy of Pediatrics Committee on Nutrition. Soy protein-based formulas: Recommendations for use in infant feeding. *Pediatrics*. 1998;101:148–153.
67. *Nutrient Levels of Mead Johnson Formulas*. Evansville, IN: Mead Johnson Nutritionals; 2003.
68. Ross Pediatrics. Formula Compare. *NEONOVA® Nutrition Optimizer.* Version 4.57. Columbus, OH: Ross Laboratories; 2004.
69. Lucas A, Bishop NJ, King FJ, Cole TJ. Randomized trial of nutrition for preterm infants after discharge. *Arch Dis Child*. 1992;67:324–327.
70. Bishop NJ, King FJ, Lucas A. Increased bone mineral content of preterm infants fed with a nutrient enriched formula after discharge from hospital. *Arch Dis Child*. 1993;68:573–578.
71. Carver JD, Wu PYK, Hall RT, et al. Growth of preterm infants fed nutrient-enriched or term formula after hospital discharge. *Pediatrics*. 2001;107:683–689.
72. Lucas A, Cole TJ. Breast milk and neonatal necrotising enterocolitis. *Lancet*. 1990;336:1519–1523.
73. Nutrition, Metabolic Management, and Gastroenterology Committee. In: Adams JM, Adcock LM, Anderson DM, et al. *Guidelines for Acute Care of the Neonate*. Houston, TX: Newborn Section Department of Pediatrics, Baylor College of Medicine; 2004:89–97.
74. Hurst NM, Myatt A, Schanler RJ. Growth and development of a hospital-based lactation program and mother's own milk bank. *JOGNN*. 1998;27:503–510.
75. Lau C. Effect of stress on lactation. *Pediatr Clin No Am*. 2001;48:221–234.
76. Kubit JG. Lactation issues. In: Groh-Wargo S, Thompson M, Cox JH, eds. *Nutritional Care for High-Risk Newborns*, 3rd ed. Chicago: Precept Press; 2000:303–319.
77. Anderson DM. Nutrition for premature infants. In: Samour PQ, Helm KK, Lang CE, eds. *Handbook of Pediatric Nutrition*, 2nd ed. Gaithersburg, MD: Aspen Publishers; 1999:43–63.

Chapter 5

Normal Nutrition During Infancy

Susan Akers and Sharon Groh-Wargo

At no other time in the lifecycle is nutrition delivery more important for health, growth, and development than during infancy. Most issues revolving around nutrient needs and delivery are consistent for all healthy infants. However, not all infants will develop or adapt to change at the same rate. The most positive feeding experiences are those that meet the nutrient demands of the infant while focusing on the individual developmental readiness of the infant. The objectives of this chapter are to cover current recommended feeding practices for healthy, full-term infants and to discuss common feeding problems encountered during the first year.

BREASTFEEDING

Breastfeeding is the recommended method of feeding for virtually all infants.[1,2] Both the American Academy of Pediatrics (AAP)[3] and the American Dietetic Association (ADA)[4] continue to promote breastfeeding as the best source of infant nutrition. The Healthy People 2010 goal for initiating breastfeeding during the early postpartum period is 75% of all newborn infants.[5] Recent studies looking at breastfeeding trends in the United States have revealed very promising data. Not only are more mothers choosing to breastfeed their newborns, averaging 70% at time of discharge from hospital, Mountain and Pacific regions have also already exceeded the Healthy People 2010 goal.[4,6]

The distribution of women choosing to breastfeed continues to vary among different cultures, ethnic backgrounds, education levels, and ages. Statistically, African-Americans, the poor, the less educated, those younger than 20 years of age, and those women participating in Women, Infants, and Children (WIC) have the lowest initiation rates for breastfeeding.[5] However, the greatest increases in initiation rates since the 1990s were observed in African-American women and mothers younger than 20 years old.[7] As positive as these initiation rates appear, there is still a significant decrease in the number of women breastfeeding their young through 6 months of age. The average rate of infants being exclusively breastfed at 6 months is only 33%, considerably lower than the goal of 50% for Healthy People 2010. Women returning to work and those participating in WIC are the most likely to wean from the breast before this age.[6,7]

Education and support can help these groups make informed choices. Health professionals must often fill this role and, therefore, need to be knowledgeable about both the science and art of breastfeeding, as well as understand the general nutrition needs of their patients.[8]

Informed Choice

In order to make an informed decision, each mother, together with the baby's father or other significant family member, need to weigh the implications of feeding choices. This process is ideally completed early in the pregnancy. Studies have shown that women's attitudes regarding breastfeeding are influenced more by familial and social opinions than by sociodemographic factors.[9] Nutritional and health advantages commonly listed for human milk and breastfeeding include:

- superior nutritional composition[2–4,10]
- provision of immunologic and enzymatic components[2,3]
- health benefits for mothers[2,3]
- lower cost and increased convenience[3]
- enhanced maternal-infant bonding[2]
- decreased incidence of respiratory and gastrointestinal infections[3,11]
- leaner body composition for infants at 1 year of age[12]
- decreased incidence of atopic dermatitis[13]
- controversial benefits of decreased risk for obesity in adulthood and[14,15] improved cognitive development[10]

Human Milk Composition

Human milk is not a uniform body of fluids but a secretion of the mammary gland with changing composition.[2] The composition of human milk varies from individual to individual, and also with stage of lactation, time of day, time into feeding, and maternal diet.[16] Laboratory techniques continue to improve, allowing the over 200 constituents of maternal milk to be analyzed and identified[2] (see Table 5–1). The four stages of human milk expression include colostrum, transitional milk, mature milk, and extended lactation, each containing its own significant biochemical components and properties.

1. *Colostrum* is the milk produced during the first several days following delivery. It is lower in fat and energy than mature milk but higher in protein, fat-soluble vitamins, minerals, and electrolytes.[2] This early stage of lactation also provides a rich source of antibodies.[2] Human milk has a ratio of about 80:20 casein to whey ratio[2] in colostrum and decreases to about 55:45 in mature human milk.
2. *Transition milk* begins from approximately 7 to 14 days postpartum, when the composition of human milk decreases in the concentration of immunoglobins and total proteins and increases in the amount of lactose, fat, and total calories.[2]
3. The third phase, beginning at about 2 weeks postpartum, referred to as *mature milk*, continues throughout lactation until about 7 to 8 months.[2]
4. *Extended lactation* (7 months to 2 years) results in milk different from colostrum, transitional, and mature human milk. Its carbohydrate, protein, and fat content remains relatively stable, but concentrations of vitamins and minerals continue to decrease gradually over time until weaning off breast milk. Some of these declining nutrients include calcium, zinc, and lactose.[2,17]

Maternal Diet During Breastfeeding

Throughout pregnancy, the maternal body is preparing for lactation by increasing the development of the breast tissue and storing additional nutrients and energy.[2] The nutritional requirements during lactation are at one of the highest levels of all human development.[16] In 1997, the Standing Committee on the Scientific Evaluation of Dietary Reference Intakes (DRI Committee) of the Food and Nutrition Board (Institute of Medicine, National Academy of Sciences) began publishing revisions of nutrient requirements for North Americans and Canadians, including lactating women. Requirements were established to meet the additional demands of lactation without compromising the nutrient stores of the mother. A review of the new DRIs can be found at www.nap.edu and in Appendix I of this book.

In general, the recommendations for maternal diet during lactation include a well-balanced diet comparable to that of a nonlactating woman, with an additional caloric demand of 300–400 calories per day for milk production. For those mothers

Table 5–1 Composition of Mature Human Milk and Cow Milk

Nutrient	*Human Milk (100 mL)*	*Cow Milk (100 mL)*
Macronutrients		
Energy (kcal)	62–70	61
Protein (g)	0.9	3.3
Carbohydrate (g)	7.3	4.7
Fat (g)	3–5	3.3
Vitamins		
Vitamin A (IU)	133–177	126
β-Carotene (μg)	16–21	N/A
Vitamin D (IU)	2.5–5.0	41*
Vitamin E (IU)	0.48	0.06
Vitamin K (μg)	0.1–0.23	6.0
Vitamin C (mg)	5.0–6.0	0.94
Thiamine (μg)	18.3–20	38
Riboflavin (μg)	31.0–50	162
Vitamin B6 (μg)	10.7–20	42
Vitamin B12 (μg)	0.02–0.06	0.36
Nicotinic acid (μg)	0.18	0.08
Folic acid (μg)	4.2–5.0	5.0
Pantothenic acid (μg)	261	314
Biotin (μg)	0.53	N/A
Minerals		
Calcium (mg)	29.4	119
Phosphorus (mg)	13.9	93
Magnesium (mg)	3.0	13
Iron (mg)	0.02–0.04	0.05
Zinc (mg)	0.15–0.25	0.38
Manganese (μg)	0.41	2–4
Copper (μg)	31	30
Chromium (μg)	0.03	0.8–1.3
Selenium (μg)	1.6	0.5–5.0
Fluoride (μg)	0.5–1.0	N/A
Sodium (mg)	11.2–14	49
Potassium (mg)	44.3	152
Chloride (mg)	37.3	N/A
Other composition data		
Protein source	80% whey; 20% casein	18% whey; 82% casein
% Calories protein	6	21
Carbohydrate source	Lactose	Lactose
% Calories carbohydrate	39	31
Fat source	Human	Butterfat
% Calories fat	55	48
Osmolality (mOsm/kg H_2O)	300	288

*Vitamin D added.

NA, not available

Sources: Data from endnote references 51, 70, 93–107.

not motivated to eat a well-balanced diet or for those avoiding primary food groups, continuation of prenatal vitamin and/or possibly calcium supplementation, is recommended. Lactation will not produce a net drain on the mother if the amount of energy available and the requirements of any given nutrient are replaced in the diet.[2,16] Energy requirements are greater if weight gain during the pregnancy was low, weight during lactation falls below standards for height and age, and/or more than one infant is being nursed. There is some evidence that successful lactation can be maintained at energy intakes somewhat lower than the DRIs, without adversely affecting lactation performance or infant growth.[2,16,18] It is suggested that iron supplementation of the mother be continued postpartum whether breastfeeding or not, in order to replenish iron stores depleted by pregnancy.[19]

Most breastfeeding women experience increased thirst. This should naturally result in additional intake of fluids. There is no evidence that forcing fluids will increase, or restricting fluids will decrease, milk production.[2,20] Regular exercise and weight loss up to 2kg per month should not affect milk production,[20] but both should be kept within moderate levels to help conserve the mother's energy to care for the infant (see Table 5–2).

In summary, the composition of breast milk remains stable even with significant variability in women's diets. The quantity and quality of breast milk can support growth and promote the health of infants, even when mother's supply of nutrients is limited.[16] However, maternal diet can affect composition in the following ways:

- alter some vitamins and minerals such as vitamins A, E, B12, iodine, and selenium
- decreased milk volume from a diet low in energy, carbohydrate, and/or protein[18,21]
- altered fatty acid composition, which mirrors maternal intake[10,16]
- appearance of colic symptoms in babies whose mothers drink a lot of cow milk, due to transmission of allergens in the milk[22]
- passage of caffeine, nicotine, and alcohol into milk, possibly causing adverse affects in the baby when maternal consumption is high[23–25]
- passage of medications, drugs, and environmental contaminants[1,2]

Management

Successful lactation is greatly influenced by the motivation and confidence of the mother, and by support from those around her, including the father, other family members, and medical professionals. The ability to lactate is a natural characteristic of all mammals, and infants have the capability to suckle even in utero. Infant

Table 5–2 Effect of Changes in Maternal Diet on Vitamin and Mineral Composition of Human Milk

Yes *Maternal Diet Can Change Composition*	*No* *Maternal Diet Cannot Change Composition*
Vitamins	
Vitamin A	
Vitamin D	
Vitamin C	
Thiamine	
Vitamin K	
Folate	
Riboflavin	
Niacin	
Vitamin E	
Pyridoxine	
Biotin	
Pantothenic Acid	
Cyanocobalamin	
Minerals	
Manganese	Sodium
Iodine	Calcium
Fluoride	Phosphorus
Selenium	Magnesium
	Iron
	Zinc
	Copper

Sources: Data from endnote references 20, 21, 70, 108, and 109.

suckling stimulates release of the hormones prolactin, responsible for milk production, and oxytocin, responsible for milk release, from the pituitary. In order to establish and sustain lactation, therefore, it is necessary to allow the baby access to the breast on demand. The more a mother nurses, the more milk she will produce. The following list offers some tips for ensuring breastfeeding success:

1. Initial breastfeeding: This should take place as soon after delivery as possible, ideally within the first hour of life.
2. Positioning: Find a comfortable position either lying down or sitting up. Use pillows to support the baby's body and the mother's back and arms. Change the position of the baby with every feeding during the first few weeks so that pressure on the mother's nipple is rotated allowing complete emptying of all milk ducts. The mother should use one hand to support and guide her breast and the other hand around the baby's back, cupping the infants' bottom to support and move the baby.
3. Latching on: Stimulate the rooting reflex by touching the baby's closest cheek. When the mouth is open wide, pull the baby close. Be sure that most of the mother's areola is in the baby's mouth, the baby's lower lip is turned out, and the tongue is under the mother's nipple. Rapid sucking, followed by slower, rhythmic sucking and swallowing, will stimulate the milk ejection reflex (MER), or the actual release of milk. Signs that let-down has occurred include rapid swallowing of the infant, tingling in the breast, tightening in the uterus, milk around the baby's mouth, or milk dripping from the other breast. Use the little finger to break the suction before moving the baby.
4. Timing: During the first few weeks, nurse the baby 8 to 12 times a day or about every 2 to 3 hours. The feedings will become less frequent after breastfeeding is established. It is more important to completely empty the first breast and get adequate hind milk than it is to breastfeed from both sides. Alternating breasts from feeding to feeding establishes good milk supply on both sides. The baby should dictate duration of feeding.
5. Assessing adequacy (or "How do I know if my baby is getting enough?"): A newborn who is receiving adequate fluid and calories will (1) have at least six to eight thoroughly wet diapers a day, (maybe only four to five heavy wet diapers if they are disposable); (2) have a bowel movement with most feedings; (3) nurse 8 to 12 times a day; (4) seem satisfied after nursing; and (5) gain approximately 1 oz a day in first 3 months of life.[2,26]

A number of situations arise during the early weeks of breastfeeding that, if unanticipated and poorly managed, can jeopardize a successful nursing experience. Table 5–3 points out the most frequent complaints from breastfeeding mothers and possible treatments. Many new mothers return to work or school after their babies are born. They can continue to breastfeed by

1. arranging to go to the baby or having the baby brought to them
2. pumping and saving the milk in a refrigerator for use within 48 hours or a freezer for up to 3 months
3. discontinuing the feeding(s) when they are away but continuing to nurse at other times

There are several good sources that discuss these alternatives, as well as issues related to milk storage.[2,27]

BOTTLE-FEEDING

Breast milk composition continues to be the gold standard by which infant formulas are modeled. However, when breastfeeding is not chosen, is unsuccessful, or is stopped before 1 year of age, bottle-feeding with a commercially prepared iron-fortified infant formula is the recommended alternative.[1] The infant formula market continues to expand and offers a wide variety of products.

Infant Formula Composition

The American Academy of Pediatrics[4] and the Food and Drug Administration (FDA)[28] have identified the importance of regulating the composition and safety of infant formulas. The Infant Formula Act of 1980 was reviewed and updated by an expert panel within the Life Science Research Office (LSRO) and focused on the minimum and maximums of nutrients present in infant formulas.[1,28] These desirable ranges for each nutrient must remain at optimal bioavailable levels throughout the shelf life of each product and provide complete nutrition for the first 4 to 6 months of life.[1] Formulas are grouped by the following categories: standard, soy, protein hy-

Table 5–3 Most Frequent Complaints from Breastfeeding Mothers

Problem	*Description*	*Treatment*
Sore Nipples	These are most often the result of improper positioning.	Involves nursing on the least sore nipple first and changing the position of the baby's mouth on the mother's nipple.
Engorgement	This painful swelling of the breast can occur as mature milk production begins and is accompanied by an increase in blood flow and fluid accumulation.	Frequent nursing may help to minimize the discomfort until the breast adjusts. Expressing more milk than is necessary to relieve the pressure will only result in increased milk production and should be discouraged.
Jaundice	In the newborn, this is associated with an elevated bilirubin level and is often the result of inadequate feeding.[2]	Early and frequent feedings will facilitate a good milk supply and stimulate increased gut motility, thus decreasing the absorption of bilirubin. Supplemental water has not been shown to be an effective treatment and may interfere with establishing breast-feeding skills in the baby and, therefore, a good milk supply in mother.
Poor Milk Supply	This is probably more a theoretical concern than an actual problem because many mothers are insecure with their ability to successfully provide adequate nutrition without tangible evidence of consumption.	Information about assessing adequacy should be presented in a positive and supportive manner. Frequent feedings and adequate rest will do more to promote milk production than forcing fluids or increasing calories in the mother, unless the diet is severely restricted. Overuse of pacifiers, swings, and other calming devices may deter the mother from offering the breast as comfort. If there is still concern regarding actual milk consumption, the infant can be weighed before and after a feeding to determine intake.

Sources: Adapted from S.L. Groh and K. Antonelli, Normal Nutrition During Infancy, in *Handbook of Pediatric Nutrition,* P.M. Queen and C.E. Lang, eds., © 1993, Aspen Publishers, Inc.

drolysate, elemental or amino acid, and follow-up formulas. This chapter will concentrate on formulas indicated for term infants. For formulas indicated for premature infants or infants greater than 1 year old, refer to the corresponding chapters in this book (see Tables 5–4 through 5–8 for composition of selected formulas).

Standard Formulas

The most common human milk substitute is standard cow's milk formula. These formulas are made from cow milk that is altered by removing the butterfat, adding vegetable oils and carbohydrate, and decreasing the protein. Standard formulas vary in their ratio of caseine to whey; Carnation's Good Start contains all whey. Although the addition of the demineralized whey appears to more closely mimic human milk, there is a lack of scientific data to support superior performance over other standard formulas when fed to babies.[1,29] The current requirements for protein in infant formulas range from 1.7 to 3.4 g per 100 calories.[28] Taurine, a free amino acid present in human milk, is often added to standard formulas.

Approximately 40–50% of energy provided by standard infant formula comes from vegetable fat blends in a balance of saturated and polyunsaturated fatty acids.[1] The source and amount of fats may vary from product to product impacting intended benefits of these fats. The recent addition of arachidonic (AA) and docosahexaenoic acids (DHA) in infant formulas has been recognized by the FDA as "generally regarded as safe" (GRAS), however, significant benefits are still controversial.[30] The addition of palm olein oils to infant formulas, rather than palm oils, has been found to decrease the absorption of calcium, effecting bone mineralization[31] and should be considered.

Although the incidence of primary lactose intolerance remains rare in infancy, the infant formula market has expanded standard formulas to include lactose-free products. The only indication for using a lactose-free formula is relief of temporary or secondary lactose intolerance following gastroenteritis. These formulas are not appropriate for infants diagnosed with milk protein intolerance or galactosemia. In either situation, soy formulas can be used instead of changing to a lactose-free product.

Standard formulas are marketed as iron fortified (12 mg/quart) and low iron (1 mg/quart). Only the iron-fortified formulas meet the iron requirements of infancy and the AAP has discouraged the use of low-iron formulas.[32] Despite this recommendation, low-iron formulas continue to be used by about 9–30% of those participating in WIC.[32]

Soy Formulas

In the 1960s, soy formulas were developed for infants who could not tolerate cow's milk protein or lactose. Soy formulas can also be useful for infants with galactosemia or who are born to families practicing vegetarianism. Although these indications are limited, the number of infants being fed soy formulas in the United States has nearly doubled in the last decade. Soy formulas currently represent 25% of the infant formula market.[33] Recent studies have discouraged the use of soy formulas for non-IgE-associated cow's milk protein (CMP) allergy, suggesting that at least 50–60% of infants with CMP intolerance will also have a soy intolerance.[34,35] These infants should use protein hydrolysates or amino acid–based formulas.

Soy formulas contain methionine, carnitine, and taurine-fortified soy protein isolate (2.45 to 3.1 g/100 kcal). The protein content of soy formula is higher than standard formula because the biologic value of soy protein is lower than cow's milk protein. Soy formulas contain a blend of vegetable oils, and recently the addition of ARA and DHA in some products.

Though all soy formulas are lactose free, some are also sucrose free or corn free. Soy phytates and fiber oligosaccharides contained in soy formulas have been found to interfere with the absorption of calcium, phosphorous, zinc, and iron. For this reason, calcium and phosphorous levels in soy formulas have been increased by 20% over those of cow's milk-based formulas and are fortified with zinc and iron.[32,33] These formulas then

Table 5–4 Standard Infant Formulas

	Enfamil with Iron per 100 kcals; Mead Johnson	*Similac with Iron per 100 kcals; Ross*	*Carnation Good Start per 100 kcals; Nestle*	*Parents Choice with Iron per 100 kcals; Wyeth-Ayerst*
Macronutrients				
Energy (kcals)	100	100	100	100
Protein (g)	2.1	2.07	2.2	2.2
Carbohydrate (g)	10.9	10.8	11.2	10.6
Fat (g)	5.3	5.4	5.1	5.3
Linoleic acid (mg)	860	1000	900	500
Vitamins				
Vitamin A (IU)	300	300	300	300
Vitamin D (IU)	60	60	60	60
Vitamin E (IU)	2	1.5	2	1.4
Vitamin K (IU)	8	8	8	8
Vitamin C (mg)	12	9	9	8.5
Thiamine (μg)	80	100	60	100
Riboflavin (μg)	140	150	140	150
Vitamin B6 (μg)	60	60	65	62.5
Vitamin B12 (μg)	0.3	0.25	0.22	0.2
Niacin (μg)	1000	1050	750	750
Folic acid (μg)	16	15	15	7.5
Pantothenic acid (μg)	500	450	450	315
Biotin (μg)	3	4.4	2.2	2.2
Choline (mg)	12	16	12	15
Inositol (mg)	6	4.7	15	4.1
Minerals				
Calcium (mg)	78	78	75	63
Phosphorus (mg)	53	42	42	42
Magnesium (μg)	8	6	7	7
Iron (mg)	1.8	1.8	1.5	1.8
Zinc (mg)	1	0.75	0.8	0.8
Manganese (μg)	15	5	7	15
Copper (μg)	75	90	80	70
Iodine (μg)	10	6	10	9
Sodium (mg)	27	24	23	22
Potassium (mg)	108	105	98	83
Chloride (mg)	63	65	59	55.5
Other Data				
Protein source	nonfat milk, whey	nonfat milk, whey	cow's milk, whey	nonfat milk, whey
% Calories protein	8.5	8	8.8	8.8
Carbohydrate source	Lactose	Lactose	Lactose	Lactose
% Calories carbohydrate	43.5	43	44.8	42.4

Sources: Data collected from manufacturers of specified formulas.

Table 5–5 Soy Infant Formulas

	Isomil per 100 kcals; Ross	*Prosobee per 100 kcals; Mead Johnson*	*Good Start Essentials Soy per 100 kcals; Nestle*	*Parents Choice Soy per 100 kcals; Wyeth-Ayerst*
Macronutrients				
Energy (kcals)	100	100	100	100
Protein (g)	2.45	2.5	2.8	2.7
Carbohydrate (g)	10.3	10.6	11.1	10.2
Fat (g)	5.46	5.3	5.1	5.3
Linoleic Acid (mg)	1000	860	920	500
Vitamins				
Vitamin A (IU)	300	300	300	300
Vitamin D (IU)	60	60	60	60
Vitamin E (IU)	1.5	2	3	1.4
Vitamin K (IU)	11	8	8	8.3
Vitamin C (mg)	9	12	16	8.3
Thiamine (μg)	60	80	60	100
Riboflavin (μg)	90	90	94	150
Vitamin B6 (μg)	60	60	60	62.5
Vitamin B12 (μg)	0.45	0.3	0.31	0.3
Niacin (μg)	1350	1000	1300	750
Folic acid (μg)	15	16	16	7.5
Pantothenic acid (μg)	750	500	470	450
Biotin (μg)	4.5	3	7.8	5.5
Choline (mg)	12	12	12	13
Inositol (mg)	5	6	18	4.1
Minerals				
Calcium (mg)	105	105	105	90
Phosphorus (mg)	75	83	63	63
Magnesium (μg)	7.5	11	11	10
Iron (mg)	1.8	1.8	1.8	1.8
Zinc (mg)	0.75	1.2	0.9	0.8
Manganese (μg)	25	25	34	30
Copper (μg)	75	75	120	70
Iodine (μg)	15	15	15	9
Sodium (mg)	44	36	35	30
Potassium (mg)	108	120	116	105
Chloride (mg)	62	80	71	56
Other Data				
Protein source	Soy protein isolate; L-Methionine	Soy protein isolate; L-Methionine	Soy protein isolate	Soy protein isolate
% Calories protein	10	10	11.2	10.8
Carbohydrate source	Corn syrup; sucrose	Corn syrup solids	Corn maltodextrin, Sucrose	Corn syrup solids; Sucrose
% Calories carbohydrate	41	42	44.4	40.8

Sources: Data collected from manufacturers of specified formulas.

Table 5–6 Protein Hydrolysate Formulas

	Nutramigen Lipil per 100 kcals; Mead Johnson	*Pregestimil per 100 kcals; Mead Johnson*	*Alimentum Advance per 100 kcals; Ross*
Macronutrients			
Energy (kcals)	100	100	100
Protein (g)	2.8	2.8	2.75
Carbohydrate (g)	10.3	10.2	10.2
Fat (g)	5.3	5.6	5.54
Linoleic acid (mg)	860	1040	1900
Vitamins			
Vitamin A (IU)	300	380	300
Vitamin D (IU)	50	50	45
Vitamin E (IU)	2	4	3
Vitamin K (IU)	8	12	15
Vitamin C (mg)	12	12	9
Thiamine (μg)	80	80	60
Riboflavin (μg)	90	90	90
Vitamin B6 (μg)	60	60	60
Vitamin B12 (μg)	0.3	0.3	0.45
Niacin (μg)	1000	1000	1350
Folic acid (μg)	16	16	15
Pantothenic acid (μg)	500	500	750
Biotin (μg)	3	3	4.5
Choline (mg)	12	12	12
Inositol (mg)	17	17	5
Minerals			
Calcium (mg)	94	115	105
Phosphorus (mg)	63	75	75
Magnesium (μg)	11	11	7.5
Iron (mg)	1.8	1.8	1.8
Zinc (mg)	1	1	0.75
Manganese (μg)	25	25	8
Copper (μg)	75	75	75
Iodine (μg)	15	15	15
Sodium (mg)	47	47	44
Potassium (mg)	110	110	118
Chloride (mg)	86	86	80
Other Data			
Protein source	Casein hydrolysate; Amino acids	Casein hydrolysate; Amino acids	Casein hydrolysate; Amino acids
% Calories protein	11	11	11
Carbohydrate source	Corn syrup solids; Modified corn starch	Corn syrup solids; Modified corn starch; Dextrose	Sucrose; Modified Tapioca Starch (70:30)
% Calories carbohydrate	41	41	41

Sources: Data collected from manufacturers of specified formulas.

meet the requirements for vitamins and minerals established by the AAP and FDA.[33]

Overall, studies have confirmed that soy formulas are adequate for promoting normal growth and development when fed to full-term, healthy infants. Soy formulas are not recommended for premature infants (see Chapter 4 regarding this topic).[33]

Protein Hydrolysates

Indications for using hydrolyzed protein formulas include CMP allergy, soy allergy, or significant malabsorption related to a variety of gastrointestinal or liver diseases.[1] To be labeled hypoallergenic, these formulas must demonstrate tolerance in 90% of infants with confirmed cow's milk protein allergy.[34] The level of protein hydrolysis varies from product to product. Some casein hydrolysates, such as Alimentum and Nutramigen, contain nonantigenic peptides of more than 1500 molecular weight[34] and have been used successfully for over 50 years. Enzymatic hydrolysates of whey contain some peptides of less than 2000 molecular weight, such as Carnation Good Start, and are an acceptable alternative for those infants who are sensitive but not truly allergic to cow's milk or soy.

Sources of carbohydrate and fat vary among the protein hydrolysates and should be considered when they are fed for indications other than protein allergy or hypersensitivity. The AAP does not promote the use of hypoallergenic formulas for the treatment of colic, sleeplessness, or irritability because of insufficient data connecting these common symptoms; however, a limited trial with a hypoallergenic should be considered.[34] Data does support the use of hypoallergenic formulas if exclusive breastfeeding is not possible during the first year of life for infants who are at risk for atopic disease.[34] Professionals need to keep in mind the low incidence of cow's milk allergy, less than 4%,[34] and the significantly higher cost of these specialized formulas. Making the recommendation of hydrolyzed formulas should be considered carefully.

Amino Acid–Based Formulas

In the last 10 years, the FDA has approved only two amino acid–based infant formulas, Neocate and Elecare, for meeting all nutrient needs during the first year of life. These products are indicated for infants with severe protein hypersensitivity and persistence of symptoms on other formulas. Amino acid–based formulas are extremely expensive and difficult for families to obtain. WIC participants in some states can obtain these formulas, while other families must pay out of pocket or fight for insurance coverage with limited success.

Follow-Up Formulas

"Follow-up formulas" are designed for infants older than 4 to 6 months who are taking solid foods but not enough to meet all essential nutrients needed for optimal growth and development. Infants can remain on these products up to 18 months of age. In the last several years, nearly every infant formula company has expanded to include a follow-up product. The AAP has stated that although nutritionally adequate, these formulas offer no clearly established superiority over traditional formulas or breast milk for infants.[1,36] In general, these products are higher in iron, protein, and some minerals and cost less than products designed to meet all nutrient needs for infants throughout the entire first year.

Evaporated Milk Formulas

The AAP does not currently support the use of evaporated milk preparations for infants because of their inadequate nutrient composition.[1] While not recommended, a home-prepared formula from evaporated milk is probably preferable to using unmodified cow's milk when commercial formula or breast milk is temporarily unavailable. The usual recipe is one can of evaporated whole milk (13 oz), 19.5 oz of water, and 3 tablespoons of sugar or corn syrup.[37] The evaporation process denatures the protein, rendering it softer and more digestible, and adding the sugar or corn syrup improves the protein:fat:carbohydrate ratio. Evaporated milk formula has the same disadvantages as unmodified cow's or goat's milk: poorly digested fat, low concentration of iron and vitamin C, and excessive amounts of sodium, protein and

Table 5–7 Amino Acid–Based Formulas

	Elecare per 100 kcals; Ross	*Neocate per 100 kcals; Scientific Hosp. Supplies*
Macronutrients		
Energy (kcals)	100	100
Protein (g)	4.76	3.7
Carbohydrate (g)	10.7	11.7
Fat (g)	3.01	4.5
Linoleic acid (mg)	800	677
Vitamins		
Vitamin A (IU)	273	409
Vitamin D (IU)	42	87
Vitamin E (IU)	2.1	1.14
Vitamin K (IU)	6	9
Vitamin C (mg)	9	9
Thiamine (μg)	210	93
Riboflavin (μg)	105	138
Vitamin B6 (μg)	101	124
Vitamin B12 (μg)	0.42	0.17
Niacin (μg)	1680	1544
Folic Acid (μg)	30	10
Pantothenic Acid (μg)	421	620
Biotin (μg)	4.2	3.1
Choline (mg)	8	13
Inositol (mg)	5.1	23
Minerals		
Calcium (mg)	108	124
Phosphorus (mg)	81	93
Magnesium (μg)	8	12
Iron (mg)	1.8	1.85
Zinc (mg)	1.1	1.7
Manganese (μg)	93	90
Copper (μg)	126	124
Iodine (μg)	7	15
Sodium (mg)	45	37
Potassium (mg)	150	155
Chloride (mg)	60	77
Other Data		
Protein source	Free L- amino acids	Free L- amino acids
% Calories protein	15	12
Carbohydrate source	Corn syrup solids	Corn syrup solids
% Calories carbohydrate	43	47

Sources: Data collected from manufacturers of specified formulas.

Table 5–8 Standard Follow-up Formulas

	Similac 2 Advance per 100 kcals; Ross	*Enfamil Next Step Lipil per 100 kcals; Mead Johnson*	*Good Start 2 Essentials per 100 kcals; Nestle*	*Parents Choice 2 w/Lipids per 100 kcals; Wyeth-Ayerst*
Macronutrients				
Energy (kcals)	100	100	100	100
Protein (g)	2.07	2.6	2.6	2.6
Carbohydrate (g)	10.6	10.5	13.2	10
Fat (g)	5.49	5.3	4.1	5.4
Linoleic acid (mg)	1000	860	680	750
Vitamins				
Vitamin A (IU)	300	300	250	370
Vitamin D (IU)	60	60	60	65
Vitamin E (IU)	3	2	2	2
Vitamin K (IU)	8	8	8	9.9
Vitamin C (mg)	9	12	9	13
Thiamine (μg)	100	80	80	150
Riboflavin (μg)	150	140	140	220
Vitamin B6 (μg)	60	60	65	90
Vitamin B12 (μg)	0.25	0.3	0.25	0.29
Niacin (μg)	1050	1000	900	1020
Folic acid (μg)	15	16	15	15
Pantothenic acid (μg)	450	500	480	441
Biotin (μg)	4.4	3	2.2	2.9
Choline (mg)	16	12	12	15
Inositol (mg)	4.7	6	18	4
Minerals				
Calcium (mg)	118	195	120	120
Phosphorus (mg)	64	130	80	85
Magnesium (μg)	6	8	8	10
Iron (mg)	1.8	2	1.8	1.8
Zinc (mg)	0.75	1	0.8	0.88
Manganese (μg)	5	15	7	5.9
Copper (μg)	90	75	85	85
Iodine (μg)	6	10	10	10
Sodium (mg)	24	36	39	32
Potassium (mg)	105	130	135	125
Chloride (mg)	65	80	90	80
Other Data				
Protein source	Nonfat milk; Whey protein concentrate	Nonfat milk	Nonfat milk; Whey protein concentrate	Nonfat milk; Whey protein concentrate
% Calories protein	8	10.4	10.4	10.4
Carbohydrate source	Corn syrup solids; Sucrose	Corn syrup solids; Lactose		Corn syrup solids; Sucrose
% Calories carbohydrate	43	42	52.8	40

Sources: Data collected from manufacturers of specified formulas.

phosphorous. Vitamin A and D supplements are needed unless the evaporated milk is fortified. Additional vitamin C and iron[1] are needed unless the infant takes sufficient quantities of the appropriate solid foods. A supplemental fluoride is needed, after 6 months of age, unless the water used in formula preparation is fluoridated.[37–39] A vitamin A+D+C supplement drop is available on the market with or without iron and/or fluoride (see Table 5–9).

Management

Pediatric professionals should not assume that caregivers are familiar with how to purchase or prepare infant formulas. The Infant Formula Act requires packaging to provide instructions for preparation, including pictorials.[1] Bottle-feeding parents need assistance from their health care professionals on appropriate volumes required to meet nutrient needs and the addition of age appropriate solids.

Preparation of Infant Formulas

Infant formulas usually come packaged in three ways:

1. ready-to-feed
2. concentrated liquid
3. powder

Ready-to-feed formulas provide the convenience of offering sterile, accurately mixed formulas for those who do not have the capability of preparing formulas at the time of a feeding (e.g., while traveling). Concentrated liquid formulas are cheaper than ready-to-feed formulas, are readily available, mix easily, and can be the vehicle for fluoridated water. Powder is convenient if only a small amount of formula is desired and may be the cheapest form of formula. Powdered formula is popular among breastfeeding mothers who may have to supplement a feeding. Manufacturers recommend boiling water for 1–5 minutes and cooling it before mixing. In practice, some clinicians do not feel boiling water for formula preparation is necessary for healthy babies. The AAP recommends adding "potable water" that has been cooled after reaching a rolling boil for 1 minute.[1] Clinical judgement regarding the individual infant's immune system and water source should be made before deciding if boiling water is necessary or not.

Prepared formulas can be kept in the refrigerator for 24 to 48 hours; however, it is safest to consume formula within 24 hours. Open cans of powder have a 30-day shelf life. Clinical judgment should also be used to assess the need for sterilization of equipment. Sterilizing may be unnecessary if[41]

1. The formula source is a sterile, commercially prepared formula.
2. The water source is from a supervised city filtration plant.
3. Hands are washed during preparation and before feeding.
4. Equipment is washed well in warm, soapy water and rinsed thoroughly or washed in a dishwasher.
5. Formula is promptly refrigerated after preparation.[41]

There is currently no evidence that babies prefer warmed milk; however, most caregivers do not feed cold bottles from the refrigerator. Warming is best done quickly in a pan of hot water. Microwave heating is not advised because it is difficult to monitor the actual temperature of formula in the center of the bottle. In addition, steam building within the bottle can result in an explosion and spraying of hot liquid. Reports have associated facial and palatal burns of babies with the heating of bottles.[42,43]

Feeding Techniques and Schedules

Good bottle-feeding technique includes holding the infant so that face-to-face contact is maximized and tilting the bottle so that the nipple is filled with milk. Interaction between caregiver and infant can be just as intimate during bottle-feeding as with breastfeeding. Bottles should

Table 5–9 Products *Not* Recommended for Infant Feeding

Nutrient Distribution	*Ideal*[*]	*Goat's Milk*[†]	*Evaporated Milk*[‡]	*Whole Cow's Milk*[†]	*Skim Milk*	*Low-Fat Milk*[†]
kcal/100 mL	67	67	66	62	35	43
% Pro	7–16	20	16	21	38	31
% CHO	35–65	26	42	30	57	45
% Fat	30–55	54	45	49	5	24
Nutrient excesses		Protein	Butterfat	Protein	Protein	Protein
Nutrient deficiencies		Folic acid Iron	Vitamin C Iron	Vitamin C Iron	Vitamin C Iron Fat	Vitamin C Iron Fat
Daily supplementation required						
Vitamin C[‖]		+	+	+	+	+
Folic acid[¶]		+	–	–	–	–
Iron[¶]		+	+	+	+	+
Comments		High renal solute load with mineral composition similar to cow's milk[*#]	Cost is similar to powdered commercial infant formulas[*#]	High renal solute load; guaiac-positive stools may develop, precipitating iron deficiency anemia[#]	Unacceptable feeding alternative during infancy[#]	Unacceptable feeding alternative during infancy[#]

*Data from reference 110.
†Data from reference 104.
‡One can (13 oz) evaporated milk with 3 tbsp corn syrup and 19.5 oz water.
‖May be given as fruit juice (3.5 oz/d infant juice or 2 oz/d regular orange juice).
¶DRI.
#See text.

Source: Adapted with permission from R.J. Grand, J.L. Sutphen, and W.H. Dietz, *Pediatric Nutrition Theory and Practice,* p. 334, © 1987, Butterworth-Heinnemann, Newton, MA.

never be propped. This practice removes the socialization aspect of feeding and can lead to dental caries[44] and increased risk of ear infections.[45] There is also an increased risk of ear infections with feedings in the supine position with either breast- or bottle-feeding.[45] Infants should be fed in a semi-upright position.

The addition of sugar to the formula or sucrose-containing fluids in the bottle increases the risk of dental disease.[1] Adding solids, such as cereal to the bottle, also is not recommended. Many view this practice as a form of force-feeding and an indication that the infant may not be ready for spoon-feeding.

Most infants can finish a bottle in 15 to 20 minutes. If most feedings exceed this time frame, it is recommended that a pediatric feeding specialist evaluate the infant to rule out any severe oral or motor delay or dysfunction. Other possible reasons for slow feeding include a nipple with a hole that is too small or clogged or a collapsed nipple. Burping is usually done midway through the feeding and at the end of the feeding. Partially used bottles should be discarded after the feeding and not saved for the next feeding time. Table 5–10 gives a suggested bottle-feeding schedule for infants.

SUPPLEMENTATION

The human race has evolved over the centuries on an infant diet of human milk alone, raising the argument that no routine supplementation should be necessary. There are several nutrients, however, for which this may not be entirely true of the breast-fed infant. In addition, some vitamin and mineral supplements need to be discussed for the formula-fed infant. Table 5–11 summarizes the most up-to-date vitamin and mineral supplementation recommendations.[1] They include vitamin K, vitamin D, iron, and fluoride. Table 5–12 gives the composition of selected infant vitamin and mineral drops.

A one-time intramuscular dose of vitamin K at birth (0.5–1.0mg) is effective protection against hemorrhagic disease of the newborn.[1,46] This is recommended for both breast-fed and bottle-fed infants.

The need for supplemental vitamin D in exclusively breast-fed infants is somewhat controversial. However, breast-fed infants can and do develop rickets.[47] The AAP recommends supplementing all exclusively breast-fed infants with 200IU vitamin D within the first 2 months of life.[1] Infants particularly at risk[16] for vitamin D deficiency are those who

1. live in northern urban areas, especially during the winter
2. are dark skinned
3. are kept covered due to cultural practices or beliefs
4. have little exposure to sunlight
5. have mothers with inadequate intakes of vitamin D or little exposure to sunlight

Table 5–10 Suggested Number and Volume of Bottle Feedings for a Normal Infant

Age	*Number*	*Volume*
Birth–1 week	6–10	30–90 mL
1 week–1 month	7–8	60–120 mL
1 month–3 months	5–7	120–180 mL
3 months–6 months	4–5	180–210 mL
6 months–9 months	3–4	210–240 mL
10 months–12 months	3	210–240 mL

Source: Reprinted from *Manual of Pediatric Nutrition* (p. 38) by DG Kelts and EG Jones, 1984, Little, Brown, and Company, with permission from Lippincott Williams & Wilkins.

Term infants usually have adequate iron stores for the first 4 to 6 months of life regardless of route of nutrition.[1] Although the amount of iron in human milk is minimal, its bioavailability is quite high, approximately five times greater than bovine milk.[16] However, by 6 months of age, exclusively breast-fed infants require additional iron supplementation or introduction of soft-cooked red meat for delivery of higher concentration of heme iron in their diet.[48,49] The AAP now supports the use of iron-fortified formulas as the preferred alternative to feeding infants if breastfeeding is not chosen.[1] Several well-designed studies have shown that iron-fortified formulas are as well tolerated as low-iron formulas. Following these interventions with iron will decrease the risk of iron-deficiency anemia and its irreversible association with cognitive and motor impairments.[1,48,50]

The Committee on Nutrition of the AAP no longer recommends fluoride supplementation for any infants, breast-fed or formula-fed, from birth until 6 months of age. Commercial formulas do not contain fluoride, and if after 6 months they are mixed with fluoridated water, no supplement is needed. The AAP recommends daily supplements for those infants over 6 months of age living in areas where water supplies contain less than 0.3 ppm of fluoride or those exclusively breast-fed or given ready-to-feed formulas.[1,38] The current recommendation for any infant over 6 months of age, consuming nonfluoridated water (e.g., well water, bottled water) is a daily supplement of 0.25 mg fluoride.[1]

Diets of breastfeeding mothers should be assessed for adequacy of vitamin B12 if the mother is following an animal protein–restricted diet, especially those who comply with vegan guidelines.[16] When the mother takes a limited diet in any nutrient, supplementation is indicated for both the mother and infant (see Chapter 8 on vegetarianism in children).

WEANING AND FEEDING PROGRESSION

The introduction of solids into an infant's diet should balance nutrient needs with a variety of foods and textures while encouraging development of feeding skills. The goal of introducing complementary foods is the transition from liquid diet to a well-balanced table food diet. The latest pediatric nutrition handbook[1] by the American

Table 5–11 Suggested Vitamin and Mineral Supplementation for Full-Term Infants (0–12 Months)

	Infants Fed Human Milk	*Infants Fed Commercial Formula*
Vitamin K	Single dose at birth: IM 0.5–1.0 mg PO 2.0 mg 3 times in 1st month of life	Single dose at birth: IM 0.5–1.0 mg PO 2.0 mg
Vitamin D	200 IU/d Especially at-risk infants*	
Iron	1 mg/kg/d to maximum 15 mg/d by 4–6 months; iron drops are best source	1 mg/kg/d to maximum 15 mg/d by 4 months; iron-fortified formula is best source†
Fluoride	0.25 mg/d after 6 months if local H_2O has <0.3 ppm Fl	0.25 mg/d after 6 months if local H_2O has <0.3 ppm Fl or ready-to-feed formula is used

* See text for definition of at-risk infants.

†An iron-fortified formula (20 kcal/oz and 12 mg iron per quart) supplies approximately 2 mg/kg iron when fed at 120 kcal/kg.

Sources: Data from endnote references 1, 38, 39, 108, and 111–116.

Table 5–12 Composition of Selected Infant Vitamin and Mineral Drops

Product and Suggested Dose	*Vitamin D (IU)*	*Vitamin C (mg)*	*Vitamin A (IU)*	*Fe (mg)*	*Fl (mg)*
ADC drops 1.0 mL eg: Tri-Vi-Sol (Mead Johnson); Vi-Daylin ADC (Ross)	400	35	1500	—	—
ADC drops with iron 1.0 mL eg: Tri-Vi-Sol with iron (Mead Johnson); Vi-Daylin ADC plus iron (Ross)	400	35	1500	10	—
ADC drops with fluoride 1.0 mL* eg: Tri-Vi-Flor 0.25 mg (Mead Johnson); Vi-Daylin/F ADC (Ross)	400	35	1500	—	0.25
ADC drops with fluoride and iron* 1.0 mL eg: Tri-Vi-Flor 0.25 mg with iron (Mead Johnson); Vi-Daylin/F ADC plus iron (Ross)	400	35	1500	10	0.25
Iron drops: Fer-In-Sol (Mead Johnson) 0.6 mL	—	—	—	15	—
Fluoride drops Pediaflor (Ross)* eg: 0.5 mL	—	—	—	—	0.25

*Prescription required.

Sources: Data from product handbooks by Mead Johnson Nutritional Division and Ross Laboratories, 2003.

Academy of Pediatrics suggests considering the following factors when starting solids:

- energy requirements and growth of the infant
- iron, zinc, and vitamin D status of the infant and foods being introduced
- risk of infectious morbidity for the infant (especially in underdeveloped countries)
- risk of atopic disease
- long-term impact on neurocognitive development and behavior

Readiness generally occurs during the first 4 to 6 months of life, but observations of physical and psychologic developments are better determinants of readiness than age alone. When taking all these factors into account, the AAP and the World Health Organization (WHO) have stressed the benefits of exclusive breastfeeding for the first 6 months of life, but support, with limited contraindications, starting solids after 4 months of age if developmentally appropriate in "well-nourished infants".[1]

Nutrient Needs

In the absence of physical or developmental hindrance, a neonate can usually obtain the necessary calorie requirement from human milk or infant formula alone. As the infant reaches 4 to 6 months, nutrient needs become greater than human milk or formula can provide. Supplemental foods become necessary for adequate satiety. During infancy, distribution of calories is generally recommended to be 40% to 50% fat[51] and 7% to 11% protein, with the remaining calories from carbohydrates. The recommended water-to-energy ratio is 1.5 ml/kcal.[52] Adding supplemental foods to the diet may alter the distribution of nutrients. This is a significant factor when deciding on the type and amount of solids to add to the diet.

Vitamin and mineral intake is also affected by the introduction of solid foods, especially as the solids begin to replace the volume of milk taken daily by the infant. At this point in the changing infant's diet, the solids are relied upon to provide adequate vitamins and minerals. For this reason, any solids fed should be nutrient-dense items. Some studies have encouraged the introduction of meats between 4 to 6 months to help prevent deficiency of either iron or zinc.[1] It has been estimated that infants about 6 months old who are consuming age-appropriate solids still rely on about 80% of their energy intake from formula or breast milk and 20% from beikost. By 10 months of age, it is assumed that this infant will be able to take about 50% of energy intake from formula and 50% from other foods.[53]

Physical Readiness for Solids

Before 4 or 5 months of age, infants possess an extrusion reflex that enables them to swallow only liquid foods.[54] Around 4 to 6 months of age, an infant learns oral and gross motor skills that aid in accepting solid foods. Oral motor skills have evolved from the reflexive suck to the ability to swallow nonliquid foods and to transfer food from the front of the tongue to the back. Gross motor development includes sitting independently and maintaining balance while using hands to reach and grasp objects.[48] At this stage, the infant is ready to sit in a high chair and grasp pieces of food; however, the infant still lacks the hand-to-mouth coordination necessary to feed him- or herself.[55]

Psychologic Readiness for Solids

Independent eating behaviors are encouraged as the infant advances from reflexive and imitative behaviors to more independent and exploratory behaviors. This transitional milestone occurs sometime during the fourth month of life.[56] By 6 months, an infant is able to indicate a desire for food by opening his or her mouth, leaning forward to indicate hunger, and leaning back and turning away to show disinterest or satiety. Until an infant can express these feelings, feeding of solids will probably represent a type of forced feeding, potentially leading to overfeeding and obesity.

In addition to determining the quantity of feedings, the infant should be encouraged to develop more independence with feeding in the following ways:

- self-feeding of soft finger foods
- sipping from a cup by 6 to 8 months of age[56]
- holding the bottle or cup independently
- controlling the timing of feeds in an effort to promote self-regulation of hunger and satiety[57]

Later in infancy, a variety of foods are introduced into the diet. These introductions of unfamiliar foods are noteworthy as they allow the infant to gain experience with various tastes and textures, promoting successful weaning to the family diet. The importance of diversifying the diet at specific intervals during the infant's psychologic development can be observed in deprived environments in which the eating pattern is unvaried and monotonous, or where weaning is delayed. Both of these situations fail to stimulate interest in solid foods[57,58] or self-feeding.

First Foods

Around 4 to 6 months of age, infants are generally ready for the introduction of solids. Two indicators that an infant is ready for solids include the ability to hold the head up without support and disappearance of extrusion reflex. Commercial infant rice cereal thinned to a semiliquid consistency with breast milk or infant formula is generally recommended as an infant's first food, as it is an unlikely allergen.[48] The cereal is traditionally introduced on a small spoon. Resistance to the initial spoon-feeding is common as the infant is unaccustomed to the spoon as a dispenser of food. Holding the infant in one's arms, rather than sitting him or her in a high chair, may relieve some of the initial apprehension the infant may experience. A gag reflex of varying degrees is apparent until about the age of 7 to 9 months. At this time, most infants are beginning to chew and tolerate smooth to chunky foods, and normal gag is developing. Choking, however, indicates that, despite the infant's chronologic age, he or she is not ready for the transition to solid foods.

When initiating rice cereal as the first solid food in the infant's diet, it should be fed for 2 to 3 days while examining the infant for symptoms of intolerance, such as skin rashes, vomiting, diarrhea, or wheezing. In the absence of such symptoms, the quantity, frequency, and consistency of cereal feedings are increased, and a second food, such as oatmeal or barley cereal, is presented. Refer to Table 5–13 for further recommendations regarding the progression of solid foods.

Market Choices

Many commercial baby food products are available in markets today. Virtually all are prepared without added sodium and many without added sugar. Juices are generally enriched with vitamin C, and cereals are enriched with iron, thiamine, riboflavin, niacin, calcium, and phosphorus. Those advertised as "first foods" are single-ingredient foods, in contrast to "dinners," baked goods, desserts, "junior foods," and some cereals, which contain a combination of ingredients. Textures from strained to chunky are available, along with foods designed for teething.

Commercial baby foods are a time-efficient means of providing an infant with solids, and if chosen wisely, can supply a nutrient-dense diet. Certain items will provide more nutrients than seemingly comparable choices. For example, plain meats contain from 220% to 250% of the protein and up to 200% of the iron of "meat dinners." The nutrient contents of selected commercial baby foods are listed in Table 5–14.

Home Preparation of Baby Foods

Home-prepared baby foods are an alternative to commercially prepared foods. They are more economic and allow greater flexibility in altering food consistency, but preparation can be time consuming. Families should not be encouraged to prepare baby foods from their own meals if they lack variety in their diet, lack refrigeration and freezing, or have poor sanitation in their homes.[59] Home-grown foods should not be prepared for infants if the lead concentration of soil in residential areas is excessive.[60] These precautions are to ensure a varied diet and to prevent nutrient deficiencies, food-borne illness, and lead toxicity. Table 5–15 provides detailed instructions for the home preparation of baby foods.

DENTAL CARIES IN INFANCY

Baby bottle tooth decay (BBTD) is an oral health disorder characterized by rampant dental caries associated with inappropriate infant feeding practices (see Figure 5–1). The disorder affects the primary teeth of infants and young children, particularly those who are permitted to fall asleep with a bottle filled with juice or other fermentable liquid.[1] Nursing caries, similar to tooth decay caused by BBTD from formulas, can also occur with prolonged or inappropriate breastfeeding at naptime. Certain feeding practices can be altered to prevent BBTD.

Providing liquids concentrated in mono- and disaccharides, such as juice and sweetened beverages, is a leading cause of BBTD. While sleeping with a bottle in his or her mouth, an infant's swallowing and salivary flow decrease. This creates a pooling of liquid around the teeth. Sweet fluid contacting the teeth for a prolonged period of time provides plaque-forming bacteria, particularly Streptococcus mutans, with energy.[1,61] The outcome is otherwise known as dental plaque. Infants who refuse cold foods or grimace when chewing should be examined for BBTD. Those afflicted will have tooth discoloration varying from yellow to black. Preventive measures include the following:

- feeding only infant formula or water from a bottle
- cleaning the infant's teeth and gums with a damp washcloth or gauze pad after each feeding

Table 5–13 Guidelines for Progression of Solid Foods

Years in Months	*Feeding Skills*	*Oral Motor Skills*	*Types of Food*	*Suggested Activities*
Birth–4		Rooting reflex Sucking reflex Swallowing reflex Extrusion reflex	Breast milk Infant formula	Breastfeeding or bottle-feeding
5	Able to grasp objects voluntarily Learning to reach mouth with hands	Disappearance of extrusion reflex		Possible introduction of thinned cereal
6	Sits with balance while using hands Ready for high chair	Transfers food from front of tongue to back Closes lips around spoon	Infant cereal Strained fruit Strained vegetables	Prepare cereal with formula or breast milk to a semiliquid texture Use spoon Feed from a dish Advance to 1/3–1/2 cup cereal before adding fruits or vegetables
7	Improved grasp Drinks from cup with help	Mashes food with lateral movements of jaw	Infant cereal	Thicken cereal to lumpier texture
		Learns side-to-side or "rotary" chewing	Strained to junior texture of fruits, vegetables, and meats	Sit child in high chair with feet supported Introduce cup
8–10	Holds bottle without help Drinks from cup without spilling Decreases fluid intake and increases solids Coordinates hand-to-mouth movement	Swallows with closed mouth	Juices Soft, mashed, or minced table foods	Begin finger foods Do not add salt, sugar, or fats to food Present soft foods in chunks ready for finger feeding
10–12	Feeds self with fingers and spoon Holds cup without help	Tooth eruption Improved ability to bite and chew	Soft, chopped table foods	Provide meals in pattern similar to rest of family Use cup at meals

Sources: Data from endnote references 49, 70, and 117.

Table 5–14 Nutrient Composition of Selected Commercial Baby Food Products

Food	*Amount*	*Calories*	*Protein (g)*	*Carbohydrate (g)*	*Fat (g)*	*Sodium (mg)*	*Sugar (g)*	*Fiber (g)*
Infant cereal	15 g	60	1	12	0	10	1	0
Juice	4 oz	60	0	17	0	10	14	0
Stage 1 vegetables	2.5 oz	36	<1	8	0	15	4	1
Stage 1 fruit	2.5 oz	52	0	11	0	1	10	1
Stage 2 vegetables	4 oz	55	1	10	0	18	5	2
Stage 2 fruit	4 oz	78	0	18	0	10	15	1.5
Stage 2 dinner	4 oz	70	4.5	9	3	42	2	1.5
Stage 3 vegetables	6 oz	94	1	20	0	20	11	2.5
Stage 3 fruit	6 oz	111	0.5	27	0	8.5	20.5	2
Stage 3 dinner	6 oz	121	4.5	17.5	3.5	81	4	2

Note: Mean values derived from Gerber, Beech-Nut, and Del Monte/Heinz.

Sources: Mean values derived from Gerber, Beech-Nut, and Del Monte/Heinz labels.

Table 5–15 Steps in the Home Preparation of Baby Foods

1. Choosing appropriate foods.
   - Use fresh or unsalted frozen foods. Do not use canned foods because they may contribute excessive sodium to the infant diet.
   - Spinach, carrots, broccoli, and beets should not be pureed at home because they may contain sufficient nitrite to cause methemoglobinemia in young infants.
2. Preparing fruits and vegetables.
   - Thaw frozen vegetables; wash fresh produce.
   - Remove peels, cores, and seeds.
   - Steam or boil.
   - Puree in blender to desired consistency. Use liquid from cooking to preserve nutrients otherwise lost in cooking. Do not overblend because this may cause excessive oxidation of nutrients.
3. Preparing meats.
   - Bake, broil, or stew.
   - Remove all skins.
   - Chop into small pieces.
   - Puree in blender to desired consistency.
4. Storing prepared foods.
   - Keep refrigerated in a covered container. Use refrigerated foods within 48 hours.
   - Freeze in 2 tbsp portions by pouring pureed food into an ice cube tray. Thaw desired portions in refrigerator before using.

Sources: Data from endnote references 117–120.

- limiting juices and giving them with a cup rather than a bottle
- filling bedtime bottles with water if necessary

WHOLE COW'S MILK

The most recent recommendations by the AAP Committee on Nutrition suggest that, to maintain optimal nutrition status, infants should be provided breast milk for the first 12 months, with the only alternative being iron-fortified formulas.[1] According to R. Kleinman, "The use of infant formula or breastfeeding for the first year of life instead of feeding whole cow milk reduces the risk of malnutrition during this time."[1] Early introduction of whole cow's milk is associated with increased risks of milk protein allergy, gastrointestinal blood loss, poor iron delivery, and overall poor nutritional status of the infant.[1,62]

When the infant's diet is changed to cow's milk after the first year, it should be whole cow's milk, as opposed to 2% or skim milk to provide essential fat and calories. Incidence of cow's milk protein allergy is 1–2% during the first 2 years of life.[62,63] Very early exposure to cow's milk increases the risk of developing the allergy to milk protein and possibly to other foods as well. Resistance to allergy increases with gastrointestinal maturity,[1,64] so that at 6 months of age, cow's milk protein containing foods can be introduced into the infant's diet with a somewhat less risk of allergy. However, risks of iron deficiency anemia[50,64] and inadequate nutrient delivery are increased when cow's milk replaces breast milk or formula before 12 months of age.

Occult loss of blood from the gastrointestinal tract is associated with the introduction of cow's milk in both early and later infancy. Blood loss, along with the lower concentration and bioavailability of iron in cow's milk, predisposes the infant to iron-deficiency anemia.[50,65] When neonatal iron stores become depleted, around 4 to 6 months in term infants, iron-fortified infant cereal is traditionally introduced as an excellent source of iron. However, the bioavailability of the electrolytic iron powders presently fortifying the

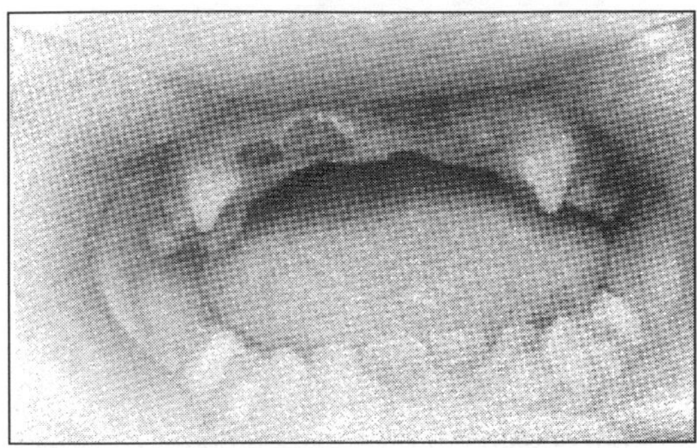

Figure 5–1 Baby Bottle Tooth Decay. *Source:* S.L. Groh and K. Antonelli, Normal Nutrition During Infancy, in *Handbook of Pediatic Nutrition*, P.M. Queen and C.E. Lang, eds., © 1993, Aspen Publishers, Inc. Gaithersburg, MD.

cereal is currently being scrutinized.[50,66–68] Heme-iron in meat is a reliable source of iron.[68] Until meat can be well tolerated in the diet, infants fed cow's milk or unfortified formula should be provided with an iron supplement. Cow's milk is also a poor source of vitamin C, vitamin E, and essential fatty acids (EFAs). When an infant is changed to cow's milk, high-vitamin-C foods such as fruits, fruit juices, and vegetables should be a regular part of the diet, or a supplement with vitamin C should be prescribed. The AAP recommends 2.7% of calories as EFAs in infancy.[69] Meeting this requirement and the RDAs for vitamin E may be difficult for the infant on cow's milk until a fairly wide variety of table foods are introduced into the diet.

Lastly, the additional protein and electrolytes in cow's milk increases the renal solute load and places the infant at risk for dehydration during periods of vomiting, diarrhea, or exposure to dry heat in winter or to the sun in the summer. For all of these reasons, it is best to delay the introduction of cow's milk until the infant is 1 year old.

JUICE CONSUMPTION DURING INFANCY

There is considerable controversy regarding the consumption of fruit juices during infancy. The debate revolves around the influence of fruit juice on inappropriate growth during infancy and malabsorption versus its role in relieving constipation.

The carbohydrate source in fruit juice is primarily from a combination of fructose, glucose, and sorbitol. See Table 5–16 for the carbohydrate sources in various fruit juices.[70] Studies summarized by Fomon suggest that infants have greater absorption and tolerance to juices containing fructose when found in combination with sucrose and glucose.[70,71] Fruit juices containing these sugars appear to have beneficial effects similar to those of fiber for infants suffering from constipation. Juices containing the greatest amounts of fructose and sorbitol include apple and pear juice.[72,73]

Consumption of fruit juices may displace the intake of nutrient-dense formulas essential for delivering the majority of an infant's nutritional needs. It is not uncommon to obtain a diet history from a caregiver of an infant with poor weight gain and to discover an excessive intake of fruit juice in the diet. Excessive fruit juice consumption for infants and toddlers is defined as an amount greater than 12 oz per day.[74] Some risks involved with overconsumption of juices include dental caries, failure to thrive, short stature, and obesity later in the preschool years.[74]

FEEDING PROBLEMS

Formula intolerance, constipation, acute diarrhea, and food refusal are common feeding problems encountered during infancy. These problems can usually be resolved through simple measures. If ignored, the problems may become exacerbated and cause detrimental effects to an infant's nutritional status.

Milk Allergy

Intolerance to lactose must not be confused with milk protein allergy. Lactose intolerance has an enzymatic etiology, whereas milk allergy is based on immunologic mechanisms. Gastrointestinal disturbance is common to both disorders. Diarrhea is frequently observed in both, but vomiting is exclusive to milk allergy. In addition to gastrointestinal symptoms, dermatologic, respiratory, and possibly systemic reactions, such as

Table 5–16 Carbohydrate Sources in Select Juices (g/100g of food) (mOsm/kg H_2O)

Juice	*Fructose*	*Glucose*	*Sucrose*	*Sorbitol*	*Osmolality*
Apple	6.0	2.4	2.5	0.5	638
Pear	6.6	2.0	3.7	2.2	764
White Grape	7.5	7.1	0.6		1030

Values may vary depending on the dilution of the juice and type of fruit used.

Sources: Data from endnote references 70, 72, and 121.

anaphylactic shock (although this is rare), may occur in milk allergy.[75]

The usual onset of milk allergy occurs in the first 4 months of infancy. This onset is due to the immaturity of both the gastrointestinal tract and the immune system. In early infancy, the gastrointestinal tract adapts to the extrauterine environment, protecting against the penetration of harmful substances such as bacteria, toxins, and antigens within the intestinal lumen.[76] Mechanisms act to control and maintain the epithelium as an impermeable barrier to the uptake of such antigens as β-lactoglobulin and α-lactalbumin found in cow's milk.

Treatment of milk allergy involves the elimination of suspected foods from the diet until 1 or 2 years of age, at which time a challenge with cow's milk is done to determine whether the allergy persists. Goat's milk has been used in the past for the treatment of cow's milk allergy. If the reaction to cow's milk is truly allergic, however, the infant will most likely react to goat's milk in the same way.[70] Unpasteurized, unfortified goat's milk also is not recommended because it contains inadequate folic acid, is excessive in protein and electrolytes, and is not reliably hypoallergenic. Canned goat's milk may be fortified but is still high in protein and not reliably hypoallergenic. Casein hydrolysate formulas are the feeding of choice in true cow's milk allergy.

Presence of milk protein allergy may correlate with allergies to other foods. Withholding the more allergenic foods from the diet for the first 6 to 12 months of life can be a prophylactic measure. Restricting these allergenic foods until the milk allergy has resolved may be indicated for more severe cases. The most common allergenic foods include: eggs, soy, nuts, peas, fish, chocolate, citrus fruit, corn products, wheat, chicken, and fish (see Chapter 9 on food sensitivities).

Constipation

There are many reasons an infant may experience constipation. The most common influencing factors include inappropriate fluid intake, excessive fluid losses, allergic etiology,[77] and medications. It is recommended that constipation be considered a symptom and not a diagnosis.[75] In simplest terms, it is defined as infrequent stooling as compared with usual number of bowel movements for that infant or as extremely dry, hard, or small stools. Normal stooling patterns vary from infant to infant and with differences in dietary intake. Constipation is rare in the breast-fed infant but more common in the bottle-fed infant.[54] Refer to Tables 5–17 and 5–18 for normal stooling patterns and colors in relation to type of infant formula or milk being consumed.

Treating nonanatomic constipation requires dietary intervention. Five measures can be taken in the following sequence:

1. Verify constipation through family interview.
2. Ensure the proper diet, including free fluid intake versus fluid losses.
3. Ensure accurate preparation of formula if infant is bottle-fed.
4. Feed two additional ounces of water after each feeding.
5. Provide two oz of pear or apple juice per day.

Table 5–17 Stool Characteristics

Protein Source	*Stool Characteristic*
Breast milk	Pasty, yellow, soft
Modified skim milk	Formed, greenish brown, very little free water
Whey, casein	Small volume, pasty yellow, some free water (similar to breast milk stool)
Whey, casein (with iron)	Soft, formed, yellowish green
Soy protein isolate	Soft, yellowish green
Casein hydrolysate	Green, some mucus, small volume
Sodium caseinate	Formed, greenish brown, little free water

Source: Reproduced with permission from *Pediatrics*, vol. 95, pages 50–54, 1995.

If there is no relief from these recommendations and the infant appears to be in pain or cramping, a physician should be notified.

Acute Diarrhea

Acute infantile diarrhea is defined as the sudden onset of increased stool frequency, volume, and water content.[78] The cause can be bacterial, viral, parasitic, or a result of large-dose antibiotics.[79,80] Diarrhea lasting more than 4 days or resulting in greater than 10% dehydration may require intravenous fluid therapy. However, bottle-fed infants suffering from mild to moderate diarrhea can be rehydrated with an oral rehydration solution for 4 to 6 hours (refer to Table 5–19).

The AAP recommends the reintroduction of age-appropriate foods and liquids after a brief rehydration period.[81] Studies revealed that this approach did not worsen stool output and helped with maintaining nutritional status.[82] Beverages such as juice, broth, carbonated beverages, or sport drinks should not be fed as their high osmolalities may induce osmotic diarrhea, exacerbating the initial problem.[83] Continued breastfeeding is beneficial, despite controversial concerns related to secondary lactose intolerance during acute diarrhea. Infants on formula should resume with their previous full-strength formulas.[82]

Stool Characteristics in Relation to Infant Formulas

It is not uncommon to obtain an infant's diet history and have a caregiver report various formula changes secondary to "formula intolerance." The frustration around this situation is that the perceived intolerance is usually nonspecific.

Table 5–18 Stool Frequency and Weight in Normal Infants

	1 Week	*8–28 Days*	*1–12 Months*	*13–24 Months*
No. stools/24 hr.	4	2.2	1.8	1.7
Weight (g)	4.3	11	17	35
Water content (%)	72	73	75	73.5

Source: Reprinted from *Gastrointestinal Problems in the Infant* by J Grybowski and WA Walker with permission of WB Saunders, © 1983.

A common complaint involves alterations in stool characteristics. Caregivers may fail to understand that different types of infant feedings are expected to produce variations in stool patterns. Infants being breast-fed or receiving hydrolyzed protein formulas typically experience between 1 and 12 bowel movements a day.[83] This can be at least twice as many stools as infants consuming cow's-milk-based or soy-based formulas.[84] The frequency of stools usually decreases considerably as infants reach their first birthday (see Table 5–18). Studies also suggest a variation in stool consistency in relation to type of formula. Infants fed soy-based formulas tend to have more stools, which are hard and firm.[84] Whether the perceived intolerance is valid or not, parents should be discouraged from "formula jumping." This only causes confusion for the infant and the professional attempting to distinguish between a "fussy" infant and a true allergic finding.

Gastroesophageal Reflux

Gastroesophageal reflux (GER), or chalasia, affects many infants. GER is otherwise referred to as regurgitation or spitting up. A clinical definition is the presence of gastric contents in the esophagus proximal to the stomach.[85] All infants experience some degree of GER. Most infants have no significant complications associated with it, whereas others may develop failure to thrive, anemia, or pulmonary aspiration with pneumonia. GER can potentially cause asthma or apnea.[85] Mild GER may be treated with modifications in feeding positions and dietary regimens. More severe GER may require pharmaceutical or surgical interventions.

An upright position during feeding may prevent GER. In this position, gravity may aid in gastric emptying. When an infant is placed in the semi-upright position of an infant seat, however, reduced truncal tone, common in early infancy, may result in slumping.[85] Slumping submerges the infant's posterior gastroesophageal junction into the stomach, increasing abdominal pressure and GER. A truly upright position is most reliable in preventing GER.[86] Studies indicate that infants maintained in an upright position for at least 15 minutes after a feeding have a lower incidence of ear infections. If this is not possible, a prone position with the head elevated to a 30° angle may also be effective.[87]

Thickening formula with cereal has been routine practice in preventing GER. There has been documentation of anecdotal responses to this treatment, including decreased emesis and crying time, and increased sleeping time in the postprandial period. Some believe a trial of a commercially prepared formula with added rice starch may be beneficial. However, there has been no proof of its efficacy in clinical studies,

Table 5–19 Nutrient Comparison of Clear Liquids and Rehydration Solutions

Product	*Na (mEq/L)*	*K (mEq/L)*	*Cl (mEq/L)*	*Sugar (g/L)*	*Starch (g/L)*	*Osmolality (mOsm/L)*
Cola	1.7	0.1–0.6	—	53–58.5	—	750
Apple juice	4.6	26	1.1	39.5	—	747
Gatorade	20–23	2.5–3	23	25–28	—	330–365
Chicken broth	250	8	—	—	—	500
Rehydralyte	75	20	65	25	—	305
Pedialyte	45	20	35	25	—	250
Ricelyte	50	25	45	—	30	200

Sources: Data from endnote references 122 and 123 and from product information provided by Ross Laboratories and Mead Johnson Nutritionals.

and it may even increase the frequency of asymptomatic reflux.[88–90] The clinician must also be aware that cereal increases the caloric concentration of formula, altering the protein:carbohydrate:fat ratio, interferes with breastfeeding, and may delay gastric emptying.

Food Refusal

Two important milestones during infancy are self-feeding and developing a positive relationship with food and eating. If these do not occur, a spiral effect of food refusal and poor nutrient intake can ensue. It is currently estimated that feeding problems may occur in up to 25–35% of infants and children.[91] Food refusal can occur in infancy because of physical or emotional stress and is more typically classified as organic, indicating a medical or functional etiology, referring to environmental influences. Illness and an unfavorable atmosphere for feeding are typical contributors to food refusal. The consequence of this problem is failure to thrive (see Chapter 18).

During illness, infants become irritable due to fever, congestion, or lack of sleep. At these times, food refusal is inevitable. The encouragement of oral fluids, and in severe cases administration of parenteral fluids, is necessary to prevent or treat dehydration. Although food refusal of this nature can still cause significant weight loss and deplete nutrient stores, if identified early, it is usually self-limited.

Food refusal originating from excessive or deficient stimulation is more difficult to discern. Commotion and overly aggressive or restrictive caregivers can cause development of negative associations with feeding. Routine negative interactions at mealtime can keep an infant from wanting to explore and advance with the normal self-feeding progression. As the stages of eating advance from complete liquid and dependence as a newborn to table foods as a toddler, the "balance of power" also shifts in the feeding relationship.[92] Similarly, a caregiver may restrict the infant's exploration of food and/or rush through a meal, disrupting the feeding pace. Under these circumstances, it is not uncommon for an infant to begin to refuse food entirely. Concerned that the infant is feeding poorly or losing weight, caregivers become tense. This tension only exacerbates the reluctance to feed.

The most effective means of treating feeding disorders after identification is to increase appropriate behavior and decrease maladaptive behavior between the infant and caregiver and between the infant and the feeding experience.[93] Most literature related to feeding disorders promotes a calm, interactive, and supportive environment and one that encourages the most positive relationship with infant feeding.

CONCLUSIONS

Issues related to breastfeeding, bottle-feeding, vitamin and mineral supplementation, the introduction and progression of solids, and common feeding problems have all been discussed in this chapter. Translating this scientific information into practical suggestions for parents is necessary, especially with the increasing prevalence of obesity and its relationship with pediatric nutrition. Pediatric patients at greatest risk for developing obesity include infants who were bottle-fed,[124] girls, Mexican-Americans (over non-Hispanic blacks and non-Hispanic whites),[125] those with obese parents,[126] and those from lower socioeconomic backgrounds.[127]

As early as infancy,[128,129] pediatric health care professions have a responsibility for identifying those at greatest risk of developing obesity and to provide appropriate education and intervention.

ACKNOWLEDGMENTS

We would like to extend a sincere thank you to Katie Dickman and Jennifer McKenna for their assistance with data collection and table development.

REFERENCES

1. Kleinman R. *Pediatric Nutrition Handbook,* 5th ed. American Academy of Pediatrics; 2004.
2. Lawrence RA, Lawrence RM. *Breastfeeding: A Guide for the Medical Profession,* 5th ed. St. Louis, MO: Mosby; 2003.

3. American Academy of Pediatrics. Breastfeeding and the use of human milk. *Pediatrics.* 1997;100:1035–1039.
4. Position of the American Dietetic Association. Promotion of breast-feeding. *J Am Diet Assoc.* 1997;97: 662.
5. Ryan A, Wenjun Z, Acosta A. Breastfeeding continues to increase into the new millennium. *Pediatrics.* 2002; 110:1103–1109.
6. Ross Products. *Mother's Survey.* Columbus, OH: Abbott Laboratories; 2002.
7. Ahluwalia I, Morrow B, Hsia J, Grummer-Strawn L. Who is breast-feeding? Recent trends from the pregnancy risk assessment and monitoring system. *J Pediatrics.* 2003; 142:486–491.
8. American Academy of Pediatrics, Committee on Practice and Ambulatory Medicine. Pediatrics' responsibility for infant nutrition. *Pediatrics.* 1997;99: 749–750.
9. Scott JA, Binns CW, Aroni RA. The influence of reported paternal attitudes on the decision to breast-feed. *J Pediatr Child Health.* 1997;33:305–307.
10. Heird W. The role of polyunsaturated fatty acids in term and preterm infants and breast-feeding mothers. *Pediatr Clin North Am.* 2001;48:173–188.
11. Scariati PD, Grummer-Strawn LM, Fein SB. A longitudinal analysis of infant morbidity and the extent of breast-feeding in the United States (Abstract). *Pediatrics.* 1997;99(6):5.
12. Dewey KG, Heinig MJ, Nommsen LA, et al. Breast-fed infants are leaner than formula-fed infants at 1 year of age: The DARLING Study. *Am J Clin Nutr.* 1993;57: 140–145.
13. Gdalevich M, Mimouni D, David M, Mimouni M. Breast-feeding and the onset of atopic dermatitis in childhood: A systemic review and meta-analysis of prospective studies. *J Am Acad Dermatol.* 2001;45: 520–527.
14. Gillman M. Breast-feeding and obesity. *J Pediatr.* 2002; 141:749–750.
15. American Academy of Pediatrics, Committee on Nutrition. Prevention of pediatric overweight and obesity. *Pediatr.* 2003;112:424–430.
16. Picciano MF. Representative values for constituents of human milk. *Pediatr Clin North Am.* 2001;48:263–264.
17. Karra MV, Udipi SA, Kirksey A, Roepke JLB. Changes in specific nutrients in breast milk during extended lactation. *Am J Clin Nutr.* 1986;43:495–503.
18. Lourdes B, Butte NF, Villalpando S, et al. Maternal energy balance and lactation performance of Mesoamerindians as a function of body mass index. *Am J Clin Nutr.* 1997;66:575–583.
19. Institute of Medicine. *Nutrition During Lactation.* Washington, DC: National Academy of Sciences; 1991.
20. Jensen RG. *Handbook of Milk Composition.* San Diego, CA: Academic Press; 1995.
21. American Academy of Pediatrics, Committee on Nutrition. Nutrition and lactation. *Pediatrics.* 1981;68:435–443.
22. Mellies MJ, Ishikawa TT, Gartside PS, et al. Effects of varying maternal dietary fatty acids in lactating women and their infants. *Am J Clin Nutr.* 1979;32:299–303.
23. Jakobsson I, Lindberg T. Cow's milk proteins cause infantile colic in breast-fed infants: A double-blind crossover study. *Pediatrics.* 1983;71:268–271.
24. Berlin CM, Denson HM, Daniel CH, Ward RM. Deposition of dietary caffeine in milk, saliva, and plasma of lactating women. *Pediatrics.* 1984;73:59–63.
25. Luck W, Nau H. Nicotine and cotinine concentrations in serum and urine of infants exposed via passive smoking or milk from smoking mothers. *J Pediatr.* 1985; 107:816–820.
26. Dewey KG, Peerson JM, Brown KH, et al. Growth of breast-fed infants deviates from current reference data: A pooled analysis of US, Canadian, and European data sets. *Pediatrics.* 1995;96(3):495–503.
27. Hamosh M. Breast feeding and the working mother. *Pediatrics.* 1996;97:492–498.
28. Life Science Research Office. LSRO report: Assessment of nutrient requirements for infant formulas. *J Nutr.* 1998;128:2059–2078.
29. Ziegler EE. Milk and formulas for older infants. *J Pediatr.* 1990;117:76.
30. American Academy of Pediatrics, Pediatric Nutrition Handbook. 4th ed. Evanston, IL: Am Acad of Pediatric, 1998;59.
31. Koo W, Hammami M, Margeson D. et al. Reduced bone mineralization in infants fed palm olein-containing formula: A randomize, double-blinded, prospective trial. *Pediatrics.* 2003;111:1017–1023.
32. American Academy of Pediatrics, Committee on Nutrition. Iron fortification of infant formulas. *Pediatrics.* 1999;104:119–123.
33. American Academy of Pediatrics, Committee on Nutrition. Soy protein-based formulas: Recommendations for use in infant feeding. *Pediatrics.* 1998;101: 148–153.
34. American Academy of Pediatrics, Committee on Nutrition. Hypoallergenic infant formulas. *Pediatrics.* 2000;106:346–349.
35. Zeiger RS, Sampson HA, Bock SA, et al. Soy allergy in infants and children with IgE-associated cow's milk allergy. *J Pediatr.* 1999;134:614–622.
36. American Academy of Pediatrics, Committee on Nutrition. Follow-up or weaning formulas. *Pediatrics.* 1989;83:1067–1068.
37. Fomon SJ, Filer LJ, Anderson TA, Ziegler EE. Recommendations for feeding normal infants. *Pediatrics.* 1979;63:52–59.

38. American Academy of Pediatrics, Committee on Nutrition. Fluoride supplementation for children: Interim policy recommendations. *Pediatrics.* 1995;95:777–778.
39. American Academy of Pediatrics, Committee on Nutrition. Vitamin and mineral supplement needs in normal children in the United States. *Pediatrics.* 1980;66: 1015–1021.
40. The American Dietetic Association. *Preparation of Infant Formulas: Guidelines for Health Care Facilities.* Chicago: ADA; 1991.
41. Gerber MA, Berliner BC, Karolus JJ. Sterilization of infant formulas. *Clin Pediatr.* 1983;22:344.
42. Hibbard RA, Blevins R. Palatal burn due to bottle warming in a microwave oven. *Pediatrics.* 1988;82: 382–384.
43. Puczynski M, Rademaker D, Gatson RL. Burn injury related to the improper use of a microwave oven. *Pediatrics.* 1983;72:714–715.
44. Shelton PG, Berkowitz RJ, Forrester DJ. Nursing bottle caries. *Pediatrics.* 1977;59:777–778.
45. Tully SB, Bar-Halm Y, Bradley RL. Abnormal tympanography after supine bottle-feeding. *J Pediatr.* 1995; 126:S105–S111.
46. American Academy of Pediatrics, Committee on Fetus and Newborn. Controversies concerning vitamin K and the newborn. *Pediatrics.* 2003;112:191–192.
47. Gartner L, Greer F, Section on Breastfeeding and Committee on Nutrition. Prevention of rickets and vitamin D deficiency: New guidelines for vitamin D intake. *Pediatrics.* 2003;111:908–910.
48. Fomon S. Feeding normal infants: Rationale for recommendations. *J Amer Diet Assoc.* 2001;101:1002–1005.
49. Butte N, Cobb K, Duyer J, Graney L, Heird W, Rickard K. The start healthy feeding guidelines for infants and toddlers. *J Amer Diet Assoc.* 2004;104:442–484.
50. Walter T, DeAndraca I, Chadud P, et al. Iron deficiency anemia: Adverse effects on infant psychomotor development. *Pediatrics.* 1989;84:7–17.
51. Fomon SJ. *Infant Nutrition,* 2nd ed. Philadelphia, PA: W.B. Saunders Company; 1974.
52. Hall B. Changing composition of human milk and early development of appetite control. *Lancet.* 1975;1:779.
53. Fomon SJ, Sanders KD, Ziegler EE. Formulas for older infants. *J Pediatr.* 1990;116:690–696.
54. Lipsitt L, Crook C, Booth C. The transitional infant: Behavioral development and feeding. *Am J Clin Nutr.* 1985;41:485–496.
55. Cloud H. Feeding problems of the child with special health care needs. In: Ekvall SW. *Pediatric Nutrition in Chronic Diseases and Developmental Disorders: Prevention, Assessment, and Treatment.* New York: Oxford University Press; 1993:203–218.
56. Chatoor I, Hirsch R, Persinger M. Facilitating internal regulation of eating: A treatment model of infantile anorexia. *Infants Young Child.* 1997;9(4):12–22.
57. Underwood B. Weaning practices in deprived environments: The weaning dilemma. *Pediatrics.* 1985;75 (suppl):194–198.
58. Pipes P, Trahms CM. *Nutrition in Infancy and Childhood,* 5th ed. St. Louis, MO: Mosby; 1993.
59. Oskarsson A. *Exposure of Infants and Children to Lead.* Rome, Italy: Food and Agriculture Organization of the United Nations; 1989.
60. Shils ME, Olson JA, Shike M. *Modern Nutrition in Health and Disease,* 8th ed. Philadelphia, PA: Lea & Febiger; 1994.
61. Nowak A. What pediatricians can do to promote oral health. *Contemp Pediatr.* 1993;10:90–106.
62. Foucard T. Development of food allergies with special reference to cow's milk allergy. *Pediatrics.* 1985;75 (suppl):177.
63. Committee on Nutrition, American Academy of *Pediatrics.* The use of whole cow's milk in infancy. *Pediatrics.* 1983;72:253–255.
64. Tunnessen WW, Oski FA. Consequences of starting whole cow milk at 6 months of age. *J Pediatr.* 1987; 111:813–816.
65. Ziegler EE, Fomon SJ, Nelson SE, et al. Cow milk feeding in infancy: Further observations on blood loss from the gastrointestinal tract. *J Pediatr.* 1990;116:11–18.
66. Fomon S. Bioavailability of supplemental iron in commercially prepared dry infant cereals. *J Pediatr.* 1987; 110:660–661.
67. Rios E, Hunter R, Cook J, et al. The absorption of iron as supplements in infant cereal and infant formulas. *Pediatrics.* 1975;55:686–693.
68. Monsen E. Iron nutrition and absorption: Dietary factors which impact iron bioavailability. J *Am Diet Assoc.* 1988;88:786–790.
69. Forbes GB, Woodruff CW, eds. *Pediatric Nutrition Handbook,* 2nd ed. Elk Grove Village, IL: American Academy of Pediatrics; 1985.
70. Fomon SJ. *Nutrition of Normal Infants.* St. Louis, MO: Mosby; 1993.
71. Hoeksttra JH, van Kempen AAMW, Kneepkens CMF. Apple juice malabsorption: Fructose or sorbitol? *J Pediatr Gastroenterol Nutr.* 1993;16:39–42.
72. Smith MM, Davis M, Chasalow FI, et al. Carbohydrate absorption from fruit juice in young children. *Pediatrics.* 1995;95:340–344.
73. Lifschitz CH. Fruit juice (Letter to the editor). *Pediatrics.* 1995;96:376.
74. Levine AA. Excessive fruit juice consumption: How can something that causes failure to thrive be associated with obesity? (Selected summary). *J Pediatr Gastroenterol Nutr.* 1997;25:554–555.
75. Wyllie R, Hyams JS. *Pediatric Gastrointestinal Diseases.* Philadelphia, PA: W.B. Saunders Company; 1993.

76. Walker A. Absorption of protein and protein fragments in the developing intestine: Role in immunologic/allergic reactions. *Pediatrics.* 1985;75(suppl):167.
77. Iacono G, Carroccio A, Cavataio F, et al. Chronic constipation as a symptom of cow milk allergy. *J Pediatr.* 1995;126:34–39.
78. Moffet H, Shulenburger BH, Burkholder BE. Epidemiology and etiology of severe infantile diarrhea. *J Pediatr.* 1968;72:1–14.
79. Snyder J. Oral rehydration therapy for acute diarrhea. *Semin Pediatr Gastroenterol Nutr.* 1990;1:8.
80. Provisional Committee on Quality Improvement, Subcommittee on Acute Gastroenteritis. Practice parameter: The management of acute gastroenteritis in young children. *Pediatrics.* 1996;97:424–436.
81. Duggan C, Nurleo S. "Feeding the gut:" The scientific basis for continued enteral nutrition during acute diarrhea. *J Pediatr.* 1997;131:801–808.
82. Moutos D. *Diarrhea: Building Blocks for Life.* Chicago: American Dietetic Association, Pediatric Nutrition Practice Group; 1996:20,3.
83. Hyams J, Treem WR, Etienne NL, et al. Effects of infant formula on stool characteristics of young infants. *Pediatrics.* 1995;95:50–54.
84. Hillemier C. Gastroesophageal reflux. *Pediatr Clin North Am.* 1996;43(1):197–212.
85. Herbst J. Gastroesophageal reflux. *J Pediatr.* 1981;98:859–870.
86. Orenstein S, Whitington P. Positioning for prevention of infant gastroesophageal reflux. *J Pediatr.* 1983;103:534–537.
87. Bailey D, Andres J, Danek G, Pineiro-Carrero V. Lack of efficacy of thickened feeding as treatment for gastroesophageal reflux. *J Pediatr.* 1987;110:187–189.
88. Orenstein S, Magill H, Brooks P. Thickening of infant feedings for therapy of gastroesophageal reflux. *J Pediatr.* 1987;110:181–186.
89. Ulshen M. Treatment of gastroesophageal reflux: Is nothing sacred? *J Pediatr.* 1987;110:254–255.
90. Benoit D. Phenomenology and treatment of failure to thrive. *Child Adolesc Psychiatr Clin North Am.* 1993;2:61–73.
91. Rudolph C, and Link D. Feeding disorders in infants and children. *Pediatr Clin N Am.* 2002;49:97–112.
92. Babbitt RL, Hoch TA, Coe DA, et al. Behavioral assessment and treatment of pediatric feeding disorders. *J Dev Behav Pediatr.* 1994;15:278–291.
93. Hollis BW, Ross BA, Draper HH, Lambert PW. Occurrence of vitamin D sulfate in human milk whey. *J Nutr.* 1981;111:384–390.
94. Jansson L, Akesson B, Holmberg L. Vitamin E and fatty acid composition of human milk. *Am J Clin Nutr.* 1981;34:8–13.
95. Haroon Y, Shearer MJ, Rahim S, Gunn WG, McEnergy G, Barkhan P. The content of phylloquinone (vitamin K1) in human milk, cow's milk and infant food determined by high-performance liquid chromatography. *J Nutr.* 1982;112:1105–1117.
96. Moran JR, Vaughan R, Stroop S, et al. Concentrations and total daily output of micronutrients in breast milk of mothers delivering preterm: A longitudinal study. *J Pediatr Gastroenterol Nutr.* 1983;2:629–634.
97. Ford JE, Zechalko A, Murphy J, Brooke OG. Comparison of the B vitamin composition of milk from mothers of preterm and term babies. *Arch Dis Child.* 1983;58:367–372.
98. Butte NF, Garza C, Smith EO, et al. Macro- and trace-mineral intakes of exclusively breast-fed infants. *Am J Clin Nutr.* 1987;45:42–48.
99. Lemons JA, Moye L, Hall D, Simmons M. Differences in composition of preterm and term human milk during early lactation. *Pediatr Res.* 1982;16:113.
100. Casey CE, Hambidge KM, Neville MC. Studies in human lactation: Zinc, copper, manganese and chromium in human milk in the first month of lactation. *Am J Clin Nutr.* 1985;41:1193–1200.
101. Smith AM, Picciano MF, Milner JA. Selenium intakes and status of human milk and formula fed infants. *Am J Clin Nutr.* 1982;35:521–526.
102. Ericsson Y, Hellstrom I, Hofander Y. Pilot studies on the fluoride metabolism in infants on different feedings. *Acta Paediatr Scand.* 1972;61:459–464.
103. Tomarelli RM. Osmolality, osmolarity, and renal solute load of infant formulas. *J Pediatr.* 1976;88:454.
104. United States Department of Agriculture. Composition of Foods: Dairy and Egg Products, Raw, Processed, Prepared. Handbook 8-1, Item No. 01-078. Washington, DC: Agricultural Research Service; 1976.
105. Casey CE, Hambidge KM. Nutritional aspects of human lactation. In: *Lactation: Physiology, Nutrition and Breastfeeding.* New York: Plenum Press; 1983.
106. Lammi-Keefe CJ, Jensen RG. Lipids in human milk: A review, II: Composition and fat-soluble vitamins. *J Pediatr Gastroenterol Nutr.* 1984;3:172–198.
107. Gebre-Medhin M, Vahlquist A, Hofvander Y, et al. Breast milk composition in Ethiopian and Swedish mothers, I: Vitamin A and B-carotene. *Am J Clin Nutr.* 1976;29:441–451.
108. Specker BL, Tsang RC, Hollis BW. Effect of race and diet on human-milk vitamin D and 25-hydroxyvitamin D. *Am J Dis Child.* 1985;139:1134–1137.
109. Greer FR, Tsang RC, Levin RS, et al. Increasing serum calcium and magnesium concentrations in breast-fed infants: Longitudinal studies of minerals in human milk and in sera of nursing mothers and their infants. *J Pediatr.* 1982;100:59–64.
110. American Academy of Pediatrics, Committee on Nutrition. Iron supplementation for infants. *Pediatrics.* 1976;58:765–768.

111. Fomon SJ. Reflections on infant feeding in the 1970s and 1980s. *Am J Clin Nutr.* 1987;46:171–182.

112. Food and Drug Administration. Rules and regulations. Nutrient requirements for infant formulas. *Fed Register.* 45106-8.21 CFR Sec 107. 1985;50:100.

113. Greer FR. Improving the vitamin K status of breast-feeding infants with maternal vitamin K supplements. *Pediatrics.* 1997;99:88–92.

114. Park MJ. Bone mineral content is not reduced despite low vitamin D status in breast milk-fed infants versus cow's milk based formula-fed infants. *J Pediatr*. 1998; 132:641–645.

115. Tsang R, Zlotkin SH, Nichols BL, et al. *Nutrition During Infancy, Principles and Practice,* 2nd ed. Cincinnati, OH: Digital Education Publishing; 1997.

116. Newman V. *Iron Needs of the Breastfed Infant. In Building Blocks for Life.* Chicago: American Dietetic Association, Pediatric Nutrition Practice Group: 1993; 17:3.

117. Hinton S, Kerwin D. *Maternal and Child Nutrition.* Chapel Hill, NC: Health Sciences Consortium Corporation; 1981.

118. American Academy of Pediatrics. *Pediatric Nutrition Handbook,* 4th ed. Evanston, IL: American Academy of Pediatrics; 1998;47.

119. American Academy of Pediatrics, Committee on Nutrition. Infant methemoglobinemia: The role of dietary nitrate. *Pediatrics.* 1970;46:475–478.

120. Kerr C, Reisinger K, Plankey F. Sodium concentration of homemade baby foods. *Pediatrics.* 1978;62:331–335.

121. Hyams JS, Etienne NL, Leichtner AM, et al. Carbohydrate malabsorption following fruit juice ingestion in young children. *Pediatrics.* 1988;82:64–68.

122. Snyder J. Oral rehydration therapy for acute diarrhea. *Semin Pediatr Gastroenterol and Nutr.* 1990;1:8.

123. Swedberg J, Steiner J. Oral rehydration therapy in diarrhea: Not just for Third World children. *Postgrad Med.* 1983;74:336.

124. Hediger ML, Overpeck MD, Ruan WJ, et al. Early infant feeding and growth status of US-born infants and children aged 4–71 mo: Analyses from the third National Health and Nutrition Examination Survey, 1988–1994. *Am J Clin Nutr.* 2000;72:159–167.

125. Ogden CL, Troiano RP, Briefel RR, et al. Prevalence of overweight among preschool children in the United State, 1971 through 1994. *Pediatrics.* 1997;99:1–7.

126. Whitaker RC, Wright JA, Pepe MS, et al. Predicting obesity in young adulthood from childhood and parental obesity. *N Engl J Med.* 1997;337:869–873.

127. Mei Z, Scanlon KS, Grummer LM, et al. Increasing prevalence of overweight among US low-income preschool children: The Centers for Disease Control and Prevention Pediatric Nutrition Surveillance, 1983 to 1995. *Pediatrics.* 1998;101:1–6.

128. Birch LL, Fischer JO. Development of eating behaviors among children and adolescents. *Pediatrics.* 1998;101: 539–549.

129. Christoffel KK. The epidemiology of overweight in children: Relevance for clinical care. *Pediatrics.* 1998: 101:103–104.

Chapter 6

Normal Nutrition from Infancy through Adolescence

Betty Lucas and Beth Ogata

Ages 1 year through adolescence incorporate most of the growing years. This includes physical, cognitive, and social-emotional growth. The 1-year-old toddler is taking his or her first steps into the bigger world, becoming more independent in self-help skills, and rapidly learning to communicate. At the other end of the spectrum, the 18-year-old is also taking steps into the wide world, becoming more independent and self-sufficient in many areas, and planning for the future. This chapter will focus on the nutritional needs and issues of normal, healthy children during these growing years.

PROGRESS IN GROWTH AND DEVELOPMENT

After the rapid growth of infancy, there is a considerable slowing in physical growth during the preschool and school years. The elementary school years are often referred to as the *latent period* prior to the pubertal growth spurt of adolescence. Children will have individual growth patterns, which may be erratic at times, with spurts in height and weight followed by periods of little or no growth. These patterns usually correspond to similar changes in appetite and food intake in healthy children and teenagers. Parents and other caregivers need to realize that these changes are normal so that they can avoid struggles over food and eating.

Developmental progress during the growing years influences many aspects of food and eating. The very young child prefers food that can be picked up or doesn't have to be chased across the plate. Food jags may be more an expression of independence than of actual likes and dislikes. In older children, the influence of peers and of the media will affect snack choices. Teenagers want foods that fit into their lifestyles, are quick and easy to fix, and are inexpensive. Understanding the developmental characteristics and milestones at any particular age will help parents and professionals to set realistic expectations, support eating behavior and food decisions that are developmentally appropriate, and avoid unnecessary conflicts. Satter[1] has described well the feeding relationship between parents and children of all ages, which incorporates these developmental aspects.

Nutrient Needs

A child's rate and stage of growth usually parallel nutrient needs and are primary factors in determining needs. Other factors include physical activity, body size, basal energy expenditure, and state of illness. There is a wide range of actual needs based on individual characteristics. The dietary reference intakes (DRIs), which include the recommended dietary allowances (RDAs) and adequate intake (AI), serve as a guide to prevent deficiency and/or to provide positive health benefits.[2] Many of the data for children and adolescents, however, are extrapolated values. Because these guidelines provide a margin of safety greater than the physiologic requirements for most children in the United States, they are not meant to be marker goals for individual children. Intakes less than these guidelines do not presume inadequacies or adverse effects (see Appendix I1 and I2).

Energy

Energy needs are the most variable, due to individual differences in basal metabolism, growth, physical activity, onset of puberty, and body size. The DRIs include equations for estimated energy requirements (EERs) for children who are not overweight and weight maintenance total energy expenditure (TEE) for children who are overweight. Unlike previous guidelines for energy intake, the DRIs incorporate direct measures of energy expenditure using doubly labeled water studies. EER equations through age 2 years include allowances for age and weight. EER and TEE equations for children 3 years and older include allowances for age, sex, weight, height, and level of physical activity.[3] These new references for energy intake in children and adolescents provide better tools to both assess energy intake and to develop nutrition care plans that incorporate the individual child's size, activity, and state of health.

Protein

Adequate protein intake is needed to provide for optimal growth in children and adolescents. National surveys have reported actual protein intakes to be in the range of 10–15% of energy for these ages.[4,5] This level assumes that enough energy is provided so that protein is spared for growth. Protein needs decrease as the growth rate slows after infancy, then increases again at puberty. Total protein intake increases steadily until about 12 years of age in girls and 16 years of age in boys.

In the United States, protein intakes usually exceed recommended allowances. Some children and adolescents, however, may be at risk for protein malnutrition; for example, those with inadequate energy intakes (extreme use of low-fat diets, limited access to food, dieting to lose weight, athletes in training who limit food), those who are strict vegetarians, and some with food allergies so that protein is used for energy. Dietary evaluation of protein intake should include the growth rate, energy intake, and quality of the protein sources.

Minerals and Vitamins

Although clinical signs of vitamin or mineral deficiency are rare in the United States, dietary intake studies have reported that the nutrients most likely to be low or deficient in the diets of children and adolescents are calcium, iron, vitamin A, folic acid, zinc, vitamin E, and vitamin B6.[5,6,7] Certain populations of children, such as low-income, Native American, and other groups with limited food and health resources (e.g., the homeless), are more at risk for poor diet and nutrient deficiencies.

Calcium

Primarily needed for bone mineralization, calcium needs are determined by growth velocity, rates of absorption, and other nutrients, such as phosphorus, vitamin D, and protein. Because of individual variability, a child receiving less than the recommended allowance of calcium is not necessarily at risk. Approximately 100 mg of calcium per day is retained as bone in the preschool years. This doubles or triples for adolescents during peak growth periods.[8] Adolescence is a critical period for optimal calcium retention to achieve peak bone mass, especially for females who are at risk for osteoporosis in later years. Calcium intake, however, often decreases during the teen years. Balance studies indicate that young adolescent girls (younger than 16 years of age) may need to consume as much as 1600 mg per day to achieve maximum calcium intake and calcium balance.[8] Even prepubertal children have demonstrated increased bone mineral density when their diets have been supplemented with calcium.[9] The Food and Nutrition Board recommends an AI of 1300 mg of calcium per day for ages 9 to 18 years to support optimal bone mineralization.[2]

Those who consume zero or only limited amounts of dairy products—the major source of calcium—are at risk for calcium deficiency. Some adolescents may also receive less calcium than needed because of rapid growth, dieting practices, and substituting carbonated beverages for milk. In assessing calcium status, vitamin D intake should be considered because of its major role in calcium metabolism. For children with limited sunshine exposure, dietary intake is critical. Vitamin D–fortified milk is the primary food source of this nutrient; other dairy products are not usually made with fortified milk. A child may be receiving adequate calcium from cheese and yogurt but taking very little fluid milk and, thus, receiving minimal dietary vitamin D. Table 6–1 contains a list of calcium food sources. Levels of physical activity also affect an individual's calcium needs for optimal bone development.[10]

Iron

Requirements for iron are determined by the rate of growth, iron stores, increasing blood volumes, and rate of absorption from food sources. Menstrual losses, as well as rapid growth, increase the need in adolescent females. To reach adulthood with an adequate storage of iron, recommended daily intakes are 7 mg for children ages 1 to 3 years, 10 mg for 4 to 8-year olds, 11 mg for pubertal males, and 15 mg for pubertal females.[11] (See the iron deficiency anemia discussion later in this chapter.)

Vitamins

Vitamins function in numerous metabolic processes. Vitamin needs are often dependent on energy intake or other nutrient levels. Most of the recommended allowances for children and adolescents have been extrapolated from studies on infants and adults.

Table 6–1 Calcium Equivalents

1 cup whole milk =	1 cup skim milk*	
	1 cup 1% or 2% milk	
	1 cup buttermilk	= 300 mg
	1 cup (8 oz) yogurt	calcium
	1 cup calcium-fortified orange juice	(approximately)
	1 cup calcium-fortified soy milk**	
3/4 cup milk =	1 oz cheddar, jack, or Swiss cheese	
2/3 cup milk =	1 oz mozzarella or American cheese	
	2 oz canned sardines (with bones)	
1/2 cup milk =	2 oz canned salmon (with bones)	
	1/2 cup custard or milk pudding	
	1 cup cooked greens (mustard, collards, kale)	
1/4 cup milk =	1/2 cup cottage cheese	
	1/2 cup ice cream	
	3/4 cup dried beans, cooked or canned	

*Some low-fat or skim milks and some low-fat yogurts have additional nonfat dry milk (NFDM) solids added. Some labels will read "fortified." Such products will contain more calcium than indicated here.

**Amount of calcium varies; not all soy milks are fortified with calcium and/or vitamin D.

Source: US Department of Agriculture, Agriculture Research Service, USDA Nutrient Data Laboratory. 2004. *USDA National Nutrient Database for Standard Reference,* Release 17. Retrieved August 19, 2004, from www.nal.usda.gov/fnic/foodcomp.

Vitamin-Mineral Supplements

After infancy, the use of supplements decreases but is still a common practice in the United States. About 54% of preschool children take supplements, typically a multivitamin mineral preparation with iron.[12] The use of supplements is generally less in older children and adolescents. Children taking supplements do not necessarily represent those who need them most. Higher rates of use are found in families with more education and income. However, the supplements may not be providing the marginal or deficient nutrients either; for example, a child may be taking a children's vitamin but may actually need extra calcium, not always provided in a supplement.

Except for fluoride supplementation in nonfluoridated areas, the American Academy of Pediatrics does not support routine supplementation for normal, healthy children.[13] It does, however, identify six groups at nutritional risk who might benefit from supplementation. These include children and adolescents

1. with anorexia, poor appetites, or who consume fad diets
2. with chronic disease, e.g., cystic fibrosis, inflammatory bowel disease
3. from deprived families, especially those who are abused or neglected
4. using diets to manage obesity
5. who do not consume adequate amounts of dairy products
6. who do not get regular sunlight exposure or do not take vitamin D–fortified milk.

Both the American Medical Association and the American Dietetic Association have also recommended that nutrients for healthy children should come from food, not supplements.[14,15]

Dietary evaluation will determine the need for supplements. Children with food allergies, those who omit entire food groups, and those with limited food acceptances will be likely candidates for supplementation. No risk is involved if parents wish to give their children a standard pediatric multivitamin. Megadose levels of nutrients should be discouraged and parents counseled regarding the dangers of toxicity, especially of fat-soluble vitamins. The DRIs include tolerable upper intake levels (UL), which can be used to determine excessive levels of vitamins and minerals from supplemental sources.[2] Because many children's vitamins look and taste like candy, parents should be educated to keep them out of reach of children.

Use of other dietary supplements, including herbal preparations, is becoming more widespread. While many supplements are harmless and may be beneficial, others may be dangerous and/or affect nutritional status. Evaluation of dietary intake should include questions about the use of supplements.[16] This topic is covered in Chapter 26.

FOOD INTAKE PATTERNS AND GUIDELINES

Because appetite usually follows the rate of growth, food intake is not always smooth and consistent. After observing a good appetite in infancy, parents frequently describe their preschool children as having fair to poor appetites, a response to a slower growth rate. There is a wide variability in nutrient intake in healthy children. Daily energy intake of preschool children is surprisingly constant, despite a high variability from meal to meal. One classic longitudinal study found that the maximum intake of energy, carbohydrate, fat, and protein was two to three times the minimum intake. For ascorbic acid and carotene, the maximum/minimum ratios were 10:1 and 20:1, all in healthy children.[17] With such variability (especially in micronutrient intake) being the norm for children, nutrition professionals need to use dietary assessment tools that include intake over time.

Just as there are changing trends of dietary patterns in the general public, similar patterns are seen in children. National dietary studies have shown decreased intake of whole milk and eggs, greater use of low-fat and nonfat milk, more snacking, and more eating away from home among children and adolescents.[5] These shifts in intake, however, still do not meet national recommendations such as the United States Dietary Guidelines or the USDA Food Guide (see Appendix J1). Using national data, one study reported an average of 35% of energy intake from fat, and only about one third of the group met recommendations for fruit, vegetable, grain, and meat intake.[18]

FACTORS INFLUENCING FOOD INTAKE

Food intake and habits are determined by numerous factors. Major influences for children include the family, peers, media, and body image.

Family

Family food choices and eating-related behaviors influence the types of foods children will accept.[19] Eating habits and food likes and dislikes are formed in the early years and often continue into adulthood. Parents and siblings are primary models for young children to imitate behavior. Mealtime atmosphere, both positive and negative, can influence how a child approaches and handles family meals. As children move into adolescence, they eat fewer meals at home.[20]

With more women employed outside the home, there may be less time available for food preparation and more use of fast food, prepared foods, and restaurant meals. Mothers' employment, however, is not associated with poorer dietary intakes for their children.[21] There is also a larger percentage of single-parent families, usually headed by women. This usually translates into lower income, with less money available for food.

Quality of dietary intake has been linked to family meals. School-aged children and adolescents who ate dinner with their families most often had higher consumptions of fruits and vegetables and nutrients including fiber, folate, calcium, iron, vitamins B6, B12, C, and E. Intakes of saturated fat, soda, and fried foods were lower among individuals who ate with their families more often than among children with less frequent family meals.[22]

Media

Television is the primary media influence on children of all ages. It has been estimated that by the time the average American child graduates from high school, he or she will have watched about 15,000 hours of television, compared with spending 11,000 hours in the classroom. The average child views more than 500 food references per week on television.[23] In addition, food products are marketed through cross-promotions with programs and characters and through fast-food restaurant promotions. The food items generally advertised to young audiences are sweetened cereals, fast food, snack foods, and candy; foods high in sugar, fat, and salt.[24]

The commercial messages are not based on nutrition but on an emotional/psychological appeal; fun, gives you energy, yummy taste. Younger children generally cannot discriminate between the regular program and commercial messages, frequently giving more attention to the latter because of their fast, attention-getting pace. Television viewing has been suggested as a factor in the rising rate of obesity among American children and teenagers, and television viewing has been inversely associated with fruit and vegetable intake.[25,26] In addition to encouraging inactivity, there is the steady presentation of food and eating cues.

Peers

As children move into the world, others influence their food choices. In preschool, the group snack time may encourage a child to try a new food. During school years, friends rather than the menu may decide participation in the school lunch program. Peer influence is particularly strong in adolescence as teenagers strive for more independence and eating becomes a more social activity outside the home. A chronic illness or disorder that requires diet modification, such as diabetes, phenylketonuria, or food allergies, can be a problem for children and teenagers when they want to be part of the group. These individuals need education regarding diet rationale appropriate to their developmental level, as well as avoid problem-solving methods to explain it to their peers.

Body Image

Puberty is the period of greatest awareness of body image. It is normal for teens to be uncomfortable and dissatisfied with their changing bodies. The media and popular idols offer a standard that adolescents compare themselves with, no matter how unrealistic it may be (e.g., store mannequins are usually size 7 or 8, and magazine models weigh about 23% less than the average female). Even prepubertal school-age girls have been increasingly preoccupied with body image and "dieting." To change their body image, they may try restrictive diets, purchase weight loss products, or in the case of males, try supplements or diets in the hope of increasing their muscles. Some of these dietary measures may put them at risk for poor nutritional status. The increasing prevalence of childhood overweight has also impacted the positive body image of growing children and adolescents.

Feeding the Toddler and Preschool Child

Parents often become concerned when their toddler refuses some favorite foods and appears to be disinterested in eating. These periods (food jags) vary in intensity from child to child and may last a few days or years. At the same time, the child is practicing self-feeding skills, with frequent spills, and is often resorting to the use of fingers. These changes and behaviors during the preschool years are a normal part of the development and maturation of young children. When parents understand this, they are more likely to avoid struggles, issues of control, and negative feedback around food and eating.

Portion sizes for young children are small by adult standards. Table 6–2 provides a guide for foods and portion sizes. A long-standing rule of thumb is to initially offer 1 tablespoon of each food for every year of age for preschool children, with more provided according to appetite.

Because of smaller capacities and fluctuating appetites, most children eat four to six times a day. Snacks contribute significantly to the total day's nutrient intake and should be planned accordingly. Foods that make nutritious snacks are listed in Table 6–3. Foods chosen for snacks should be those least likely to promote dental caries.

Parents of young children frequently become concerned about the adequacy of their children's intakes; plain meats are often refused because they are more difficult to chew, very little or too much milk may be consumed, cooked vegetables are pushed away. Table 6–4 offers nutrition solutions to these common, normal variations in eating behaviors.

Just as important as providing adequate nutrients to young children is supporting a positive feeding environment—both physically and emotionally—so that, as they grow, they acquire skills, develop positive attitudes, and have control over food decisions as appropriate for their developmental level. General guidance in this area is listed in Table 6–5.

Children under age 4 are at greatest risk for choking on food. In some cases, this can lead to death from asphyxiation.[27] Foods most likely to cause choking are those that are round, hard, and do not readily dissolve in saliva, such as hot dogs, grapes, raw vegetables, popcorn, peanut butter, nuts, and hard candy. Other foods can also cause choking problems if too much is stuffed into the mouth, if the child is running while eating, or if the child is unsupervised. Choking episodes can be prevented by common-sense management of foods and the eating environment. Table 6–6 outlines the preventive approaches.

Fruit juice, especially apple, has become a common beverage for young children, usually replacing water and frequently replacing milk. Excessive fruit juice consumption has been linked to chronic diarrhea and failure to thrive.[28,29] Both conditions improved when juice intake was limited. One report of preschool children found an association between short stature or obesity and the consumption of more than 12 oz of juice daily,[30] but other studies have not shown associations between fruit juice intake and growth parameters.[31,32] It is understandable that frequent juice intake could dull the appetite

Table 6–2 Feeding Guide for Children

This is a guide to a basic diet. Fats, sauces, desserts, and snack foods will provide additional energy to meet the growing child's needs. Foods can be selected from this pattern for both meals and snacks.

Food	2- to 3-Year-Olds Portion Size	Servings	4- to 6-Year-Olds Portion Size	Servings	7- to 12-Year-Olds Portion Size	Servings	Comments
Milk and dairy products	1/2 cup (4 oz.)	4–5	1/2–3/4 cup (4–6 oz.)	3–4	1/2–1 cup (4–8 oz.)	3–4	The following may be substituted for 1/2 cup liquid milk: 1/2–3/4 oz. cheese, 1/2 cup yogurt, 2 1/2 Tbsp. nonfat dry milk.
Meat, fish, poultry, or equivalent	1–2 oz.	2	1–2 oz.	2	2 oz.	3–4	The following may be substituted for 1 oz. meat, fish or poultry: 1 egg, 2 Tbsp. peanut butter, 4–5 Tbsp. cooked legumes.
Fruits and vegetables							
Vegetables		4–5		4–5		4–5	Include one green leafy or yellow vegetable for vitamin A, such as carrots, spinach, broccoli, or winter squash.
Cooked	2–3 Tbsp.		3–4 Tbsp.		1/4–1/2 cup		
Raw*	Few pieces		Few pieces		Several pieces		
Fruit							Include one vitamin C–rich fruit, vegetable or juice, such as citrus juices, orange, grapefruit, strawberries, melon, tomato, broccoli.
Raw	1/2–1 small		1/2–1 small		1 medium		
Canned	2–4 Tbsp.		4–6 Tbsp.		1/4–1/2 cup		
Juice	3–4 oz.		4 oz.		4 oz.		

continues

Table 6–2 continued

Food	2- to 3-Year-Olds	4- to 6-Year-Olds	7- to 12-Year-Olds	Comments
	Portion Size/Servings	*Portion Size/Servings*	*Portion Size/Servings*	
Bread and grain products	3–4	3–4	4–5	The following may be substituted for 1 slice of bread: 1/2 cup spaghetti, macaroni, noodles, or rice; 5 saltines; 1/2 English muffin or bagel; 1 tortilla
Whole-grain or enriched bread	1/2–1 slice	1 slice	1 slice	
Cooked cereal	1/4–1/2 cup	1/2 cup	1/2–1 cup	
Dry cereal	1/2–1 cup	1 cup	1 cup	

*Do not give to young children until they can chew well.

Source: Adapted from Lowenberg ME, Development of food patterns in young children. In: PL Pipes ed., *Nutrition Infancy and Childhood,* 4th ed. (pp. 146–147) Times Mirror/Mosby College Publishing; 1989 ©. With permission of W.B. Saunders Company.

Table 6–3 Foods that Make Nutritious Snacks

Protein Foods	*Fruits***
Natural cheese	Apple wedges*
Milk	Bananas
Plain yogurt	Pears
Cooked turkey or beef	Berries
Unsalted nuts and seeds*	Melon
Peanut butter*	Oranges and other citrus fruits
Hard-cooked eggs	Grapes*
Cottage cheese	Unsweetened canned fruit
Tuna	Unsweetened fruit juices
Breads and Cereals*	***Vegetables***
Whole-grain breads	Carrot sticks*
Whole-grain, low-fat crackers	Celery*
Rice crackers	Green pepper strips*
English muffins	Cucumber slices*
Bagels	Cabbage wedges*
Tortillas	Tomatoes
Pita bread	Jicama*
Popcorn*	Vegetable juices
	Cooked green beans
	Broccoli and cauliflower flowerettes

*Foods that are hard, round, and do not easily dissolve can cause choking. Do not give to children under 3 years of age. (Peanut butter is more dangerous when eaten in chunks or spread thickly rather than thinly spread on crackers or bread.)

**Fruits, juices, and most cereal/bread products contain fermentable carbohydrate, which is a factor in the development of dental caries. Try to limit these foods to one serving in a snack.

enough to result in less food consumed at regular meals, or, for some children, the energy from juice (instead of water) in addition to other foods could cause excess weight gain. The American Academy of Pediatrics (AAP) suggests that fruit juice intake be limited to 4 to 6 oz per day for children 1 to 6 years of age and 8 to 12 oz for children 7 to 18 years old. The AAP recommends that fruit juice provide up to half of the suggested servings of fruit, and the consumption of whole fruit should be encouraged to provide dietary fiber.[33]

Feeding the School-Age Child

The years from 6 to 12 are a period of slow but steady growth, with increases in food intake as a result of appetite (see Table 6–2). Most food behavior problems from early childhood have been resolved except for extreme cases, but food dislikes may persist, especially if attention is given to them.

Because children are in school, they may eat fewer times in the day, but after-school snacks usually are a routine. Skipping breakfast may begin in these years, with contributing factors such as time constraints, children left to get themselves off to school, and early school starts. With participation in organized sports, music lessons, and other activities, sitting down to a family meal may be less frequent.

An emerging trend in the United States is the increased responsibility of children not yet in their teens to do family shopping and cooking. Some children are frequently responsible for

Table 6–4 Common Feeding Concerns in Young Children

Common Concerns	*Possible Solutions*
Refuses meats	• Offer small, bite-size pieces of moist, tender meat or poultry. • Incorporate into meat loaf, spaghetti sauce, stews, casseroles, burritos, pizza. • Include legumes, eggs, cheese. • Offer boneless fish (including canned tuna and salmon).
Drinks too little milk	• Offer cheeses and yogurt, including cheese in cooking, eg., macaroni and cheese, cheese sauce, pizza. Use milk to cook hot cereals; offer cream soups, milk-based puddings and custards. • Allow child to pour milk from a pitcher and use a straw. • Include powdered milk in cooking and baking; eg., biscuits, muffins, pancakes, meat loaf, casseroles.
Drinks too much milk	• Offer water if thirsty between meals. • Limit milk to one serving with meals or offer at end of meal; offer water for seconds. • If bottle is still used, wean to cup.
Refuses vegetables and fruits	• If child refuses vegetables, offer more fruits and vice versa. • Prepare vegetables that are tender but not overcooked. • Steam vegetable strips (or offer raw if appropriate) and allow child to eat with fingers. • Offer sauces and dips; eg., cheese sauce for cooked vegetables, dip for raw vegetables, yogurt to dip fruit. • Include vegetables in soups and casseroles. • Add fresh or dried fruit to cereals. • Prepare fruit in a variety of ways, eg., fresh, cooked, juice, in gelatin, as a salad. • Continue to offer a variety of fruits and vegetables.
Eats too many sweets	• Limit purchase and preparation of sweet foods in the home. • Avoid using as a bribe or reward. • Incorporate into meals instead of snacks for better dental health. • Reduce sugar by half in recipes for cookies, muffins, quick breads, etc. • Work with staff of day care, preschools, etc., to reduce use of sweets.

their own breakfasts, lunches, snacks, and even the dinner meal. They also do food shopping on a regular basis and influence the family food purchases. Several factors contribute to this trend, including working parents, increased use of microwave ovens, more money available to spend on convenience and prepared foods, and less emphasis on family meals. Along with this trend, increasingly sophisticated advertising is being aimed at these children.

Children usually participate in the school lunch program or bring a packed lunch from home. The National School Lunch Program is administered by the U.S. Department of Agriculture (USDA) and supported by means of reimbursements and supplemental commodity foods. Federal guidelines are established for food groups and portion sizes so that the lunch provides approximately one third of the RDAs or AIs for students. About 70% of schools also participate in the School Breakfast

Table 6–5 Tips for a Happy Mealtime

Physical Setting

- Schedule meals at regular times.
- Avoid having a child get too hungry or too tired before mealtime.
- Snacks should be at least 1½ to 2 hours before meals.
- Child should be able to sit up to the table comfortably without reaching.
- Provide support for the legs and feet, such as a booster seat, stool, etc.
- Use nonbreakable, sturdy dishes with sides to push food against.
- Spoons and forks should be blunt with broad, short handles.
- Use cups that are nonbreakable, broad based, and small.

Social-Emotional

- Serve a new food with familiar ones—don't be surprised by an initial rejection.
- Offer at least one food at a meal that you know your child will eat, but do not cater to his or her likes and dislikes.
- Avoid coaxing, nagging, bribing, or any other pressure to get your child to eat.
- Serve dessert (if any) with the meal—it becomes less important and cannot be used as a reward.
- Let children determine when they are full; amounts eaten will vary from child to child and day to day.
- Use the child's developmental stage to determine expectations for neatness and manners, but set limits on inappropriate behaviors; eg., throwing food, playing.
- Attempt to have family meals be as pleasant as possible; avoid arguments and criticism.
- Allow children to help set the table or do part of the meal preparation.

Program. Free and reduced-price meals are available for low-income children. Problems with the school lunch program have included plate waste, poor menu acceptance by students, competition from vending machines, and concerns regarding the amount of fat, sugar, and salt in the food. These problems have been addressed by including the students in menu planning, offering popular items more frequently (e.g., pizza, tacos, hamburgers, salad bars), and allowing students to refuse one or two items from the menu. Incorporating the U.S. Dietary Guidelines into child nutrition programs has also encouraged menus with a lower fat content, more fresh fruits, vegetables, and whole-grain products.[34] A sack lunch prepared at home will likely provide fewer nutrients than will the school lunch meal.[35] The same favorite foods tend to be packed with less variety, and foods are limited to those that don't require heating or refrigeration.

Vending machines, especially those that sell soft drinks, are becoming increasingly available to children during the school day. This issue becomes complex as educators and health care providers weigh the health risks associated with excessive intake of these foods and beverages with the funding that is often provided by vending machine profits and pouring rights. Problems associated with increased consumption include risk of obesity, deficits in bone mass (because of decreased intake of calcium and other nutrients when soft drinks replace milk), and increased dental caries. The AAP encourages health care providers to work to eliminate sweetened drinks in schools.[36] Other approaches to promoting better choices from vending machines include price reductions on lower fat options. In one study, this approach did not affect profits.[37]

Feeding the Adolescent

Adolescents in their rapid-growth period seem to eat all the time. Their appetites usually guide their intakes. As teenagers achieve more independence and spend a greater amount of time away from home, they have additional variable intakes and irregular eating patterns. Skipping meals is greatest in this age group, particularly for breakfast and lunch. On the other hand, snacking

Table 6–6 Guidelines for Feeding Safety—Preschool Children

1. Insist that children eat sitting down. It lets them concentrate on chewing and swallowing.
2. An adult should supervise children while they eat.
3. Food on which preschoolers often choke, such as hot dogs, peanut butter, hard pieces of fruit and vegetables, should be avoided for children under 3 years of age.
4. Well-cooked foods, modified so that the child can chew and swallow without difficulty, should be offered.
5. Eating in the car should be avoided. If the child starts choking, it is hard to get to the side of the road safely.
6. Rub-on teething medications can cause problems with chewing and swallowing because the muscles in the throat may also become numb. Children who receive such medications should be carefully observed during feeding.

Source: Reprinted from Pipes, PL ed. *Nutrition in Infancy and Childhood,* 4th ed. (p 126) Times Mirror/Mosby College Publishing; 1989 ©. With permission from W.B. Saunders Company.

tends to be a common practice. Whether they are called snacks or meals, adolescents who eat less than three times a day have poorer diets than do those eating more often.

Although fast foods are popular with all segments of the population, they appeal most to teenagers. The food is inexpensive, well-accepted, and can be eaten informally without utensils or plates. Fast food restaurants are also socially acceptable and a common employer of adolescents. Generally, the menu items tend to be energy-dense, high in fat (some items provide more than 50% of energy as fat), high in sodium, and low in fiber, vitamin A, ascorbic acid, calcium, and folate. Although these establishments now offer more salads and lower-fat sandwiches, these foods are not necessarily chosen by teens. Any negative impact of fast foods on the diets of adolescents will depend on how frequently they are eaten and the choices made.

Other Nutrition Issues

As children grow and develop, various nutrition-related issues or problems arise. These are not uncommon in otherwise healthy children, and they can be prevented or managed with minimal intervention. Other specific problems—obesity, allergies, and chronic diseases—are discussed in other chapters.

DIET AND ORAL HEALTH

Despite successful efforts in the past few decades, dental caries remain a common oral health disease in the pediatric population. National Health and Nutrition Examination Survey III (NHANES III) data reveal that 45% of children and adolescents have caries.[38] The rate changes with age; 62% of children ages 2 to 9 were caries-free, while only 33% of adolescents ages 12 to 17 were caries-free.

Nutrition and oral health are closely related. Inadequate intake of energy and protein can delay tooth eruption, affect tooth size, and cause salivary gland dysfunction. Micronutrients (e.g., calcium and vitamin D for mineralization and fluoride for enamel formation) are also critical to the development and maintenance of oral structures.[39,40]

Poor oral health can negatively affect a child's nutritional status and has implications for overall health as well. Missing or decayed teeth may increase risk of nutrient deficiency by preventing a child from eating certain foods. Pain or malformed teeth can contribute to problems with speech and communication, interfere with sleep, and negatively affect an individual's self image, psychological status, and overall social function.

Dental caries develops in the presence of carbohydrate, bacteria, and a susceptible tooth. The process of decay begins with the interaction of bacteria (*Streptococcus mutans*) and fermentable carbohydrate on the tooth surface. When the bacteria within the dental plaque (the gelatinous substance on the tooth surface) metabolize the carbohydrate, organic acids are produced. When the acid reduces the pH to 5.5 or less, demineralization of the tooth enamel occurs.[41] Some individuals seem to be more susceptible to caries than others, suggesting a hereditary influence. About 80% of the caries in 5–17 year olds is found in only 25% of the children and adolescents.[38] Individual salivary counts of *S. mutans* that are high appear to be a risk for caries.[42]

Sucrose is the most common carbohydrate recognized in the caries process. Although starch is considered less cariogenic than sucrose, it can easily be broken down into fermentable carbohydrate by salivary amylase. Also, many foods high in starch often contain sucrose or other sugars, which may make the food more cariogenic than sugar alone because starch is retained longer in the mouth. Honey is just as cariogenic as sucrose.

The cariogenicity of specific foods depends not only on the type and amount of fermentable carbohydrate but also on the retentiveness of foods to the tooth surface and the frequency of eating. Dental researchers believe that all of these factors influence the length of time the teeth are exposed to an acidic environment, which leads to tooth decay.[41]

Some protein foods (e.g., nuts, hard cheeses, eggs, and meats) do not decrease plaque pH and are thought to have a protective effect against caries.[43] Eating these foods at the same time as high-sugar foods prevents a reduction in plaque pH. Why these foods are protective is not known, but theories include the presence of protein and lipids in these foods, the presence of calcium and phosphorus, and the stimulation of alkaline saliva. Chewing gum sweetened with xylitol or sorbitol after a sugar-containing snack may also counteract the decrease in pH and reduce caries.[44]

Prevention of Caries

Because children of all ages eat frequently, snacks should emphasize foods that are low in sucrose, are not sticky, and stimulate saliva flow, thereby limiting acid production in the mouth (Table 6–3). Including protein foods such as cheese and nuts may provide nutritional as well as dental benefits. Desserts, when consumed, should be eaten with meals. School-age children and adolescents may benefit from chewing sugarless gum after snacks containing fermentable carbohydrate.

Good oral hygiene complements dietary efforts. In infancy, parents can clean the gums and teeth with a clean cloth. The toothbrush should be introduced in the toddler period. The key is to incorporate brushing and flossing as a regular, consistent routine, with parental supervision in the early years. If the water supply is not fluoridated, a fluoride supplement is recommended into the teen years. See Table 6–7 for recommended fluoride dosages. Topical fluoride applications are used in many communities. Varnishes, rinses, gels, and foams are also available to prevent caries and are often incorporated into local public health activities (e.g., partnership with the public health department, schools, and early intervention program).

The AAP and American Academy of Pediatric Dentistry (AAPD) suggest regular dental visits beginning in early childhood; AAPD recommends a visit by 12 months of age or 6 months after the first tooth erupts.[45,46]

The U.S. Surgeon General's Report on Oral Health identifies assessment and action by nondental providers as critical to improving oral health. Screening (and appropriate referral) and anticipatory guidance are included in these actions.[47]

Early Childhood Caries

Children under 3 years of age are most likely to have early childhood caries (ECC). ECC is also known as baby bottle tooth decay, nursing caries, and nursing bottle caries. ECC has been estimated to affect 10% of 2 year olds.[48] In some nonfluoridated communities, the prevalence is about 20%; in Native American and Native Alaskan preschool children, the rate is more than 50%.[49] Rampant caries develops on the primary upper front teeth (incisors) and often on the cheek surface of primary upper first molars. Children from poor families are at highest risk

Table 6–7 Recommended Dietary Fluoride Supplement* Schedule

	*Fluoride concentration in community drinking water***		
Age	*Less than 0.3 ppm*	*0.6–0.6 ppm*	*Greater than 0.6 ppm*
0–6 months	None	None	None
6 months–3 years	0.25 mg/d	None	None
3–6 years	0.50 mg/d	0.25 mg/d	None
6–16 years	1.0 mg/d	0.50 mg/d	None

*Sodium fluoride (2/2 mg sodium fluoride contains 1 mg fluoride ion)
**(1.0 parts per million (ppm) = 1 mg/L)

Source: Centers for Disease Control and Prevention. Recommendations for using fluoride to prevent and control dental caries in the United States. *MMWR.* 2001;50(No.RR-14):8.

for ECC. A history of ECC seems to increase the risk for future caries in permanent teeth.[48]

The primary cause of ECC is prolonged exposure of the teeth to a sweetened liquid (formula, milk, juice, soda pop, sweetened drinks). This occurs most often when the child is routinely given a nursing bottle at bedtime or during naps. During sleep, the liquid pools around the teeth, saliva flow decreases, and the child may continue to suck liquid over an extended period of time. Although ECC has been documented in ad libitum breastfeeding, the occurrence is believed to be less than with bottle-feeding.[49] Toddlers who hold their own bottles and have access to bottles or sippy cups with sweetened liquids anytime throughout the day are also at high risk. Dental treatment of ECC is expensive, often requires a general anesthetic, and may be traumatic for the child and family.

Education is the primary strategy to prevent ECC. Parents should be counseled about the disorder early in infancy and encouraged to avoid putting a baby to sleep with a bottle, as previously addressed in Chapter 5. Juices and liquids other than milk or formula should be offered in a cup. In typically developing infants, weaning from the bottle should begin at about 1 year of age. Day care providers and other caregivers should also be informed of the threat to oral health posed by use of the nursing bottle as a pacifier. For this educational approach to be successful, families often need help with positive parenting strategies and behavioral counseling.

Iron Deficiency Anemia

Iron deficiency anemia is most common in children between 1 and 3 years of age with a prevalence of about 9%.[50] Other high-risk groups are young adolescent males and females of childbearing age. Over the past two decades, there has been an overall decrease in the prevalence of iron deficiency anemia, both in low-income and middle-class pediatric populations. Factors influencing this positive trend include increased and prolonged use of iron-fortified infant formulas, more breastfeeding, increased iron intake from other food sources, and the Women, Infants, and Children (WIC) food program. Despite the encouraging trends, some young children, especially those in low-income households, are at high risk for iron deficiency. Although the relationship between iron deficiency and cognitive/behavioral function has been debated for a long time, poorer cognitive performance and delayed psychomotor development have been reported in infants and preschool children with iron deficiency, compared with children without iron deficiency.[51] Iron deficiency in infancy may have long-term consequences, as demonstrated by poorer performance on developmental tests in late childhood and early adolescence.[52] Children who are iron deficient are also at risk for increased lead absorption when exposed to sources of lead.

Dietary factors, as well as growth and physiologic needs, play a role in development of anemia. Some toddlers consume a large volume of milk to the exclusion of solids; plain meats are often not well-accepted by preschool children because they require more chewing. For many of these children, most dietary iron comes from nonheme sources such as vegetables, grains, and cereals. Because the typical American mixed diet contains approximately 6 mg iron per 1000 calories, adolescents dieting to lose weight will have minimal iron intake, especially if animal protein is limited.

Absorption of iron from food depends on several factors. One is the iron status of the individual; those with low iron stores will have a higher absorption rate. There is a higher rate of absorption from heme-iron (in meat, fish, and poultry) than from nonheme-iron (in vegetables and grains). Absorption of nonheme-iron can be increased by two enhancing factors: (1) ascorbic acid and (2) meat, fish, or poultry (MFP).[53] The presence of an ascorbic acid–rich food and/or MFP in a meal will increase the rate of nonheme iron absorption. Other food or compounds inhibit iron absorption. Table 6–8 identifies good iron sources as well as absorption enhancers and inhibitors. Simple but conscientious menu planning can help improve iron availability to children and teenagers.

Hemoglobin and hematocrit are the main biochemical screening tests for iron deficiency anemia. The AAP recommends either universal or selective screening for infants between 9 and 12 months of age, with a second screening 6 months later.[54] Universal screening for children up to 2 years of age is recommended for communities and populations with significant levels of iron deficiency anemia or for infants whose diets put them at risk. Selective screening would be based on individual risk factors such as prematurity, low-birth-weight infants, and dietary intake. Routine screening is not recommended after age 2 except for risk factors; poor diet, poverty/limited access to food, and special health care needs. Guidelines for treatment and follow-up of iron deficiency anemia have been developed.[54]

EFFECT OF DIET ON LEARNING AND BEHAVIOR

What impact does a child's diet have on his or her school performance and behavior? For decades people have debated whether skipping breakfast affects classroom learning. Food additives, sugar, and allergies have been suggested as causes of hyperactivity in children. Although these are controversial issues, some scientific studies have examined them.

Diet and Learning Behavior

Although severe malnutrition early in life is known to negatively affect intellectual development, the impact of marginal malnutrition, skipping meals, or hunger has been more difficult to document. Experimental studies have used standardized tests to measure cognitive functions (e.g., problem solving, attention, and memory) in healthy school-age children who were given either breakfast or no breakfast. The "fasted" children had slower memory recall, increased errors, and slower stimulus discrimination.[55] Similar studies comparing healthy children to those stunted, those who suffered severe malnutrition early in life, and those currently wasted (low weight for height) showed even poorer results for the malnourished/undernourished children when they missed breakfast.[55,56]

In a community study, standardized achievement test scores were compared before and after implementation of the School Breakfast Program in six schools in a predominantly low-income community.[57] Children participating in the breakfast program demonstrated improved academic performance compared with those qualified but not participating. The findings also noted decreased tardiness and absenteeism among the children in the breakfast program. These results and results of other similar studies indicate that

Table 6–8 Food Sources of Iron

	Iron (mg)
Meat, Fish, and Poultry* (1 oz)	
Chicken liver	3.8
Beef liver	1.7
Turkey, roasted	0.7
Beef pot roast	0.7
Hamburger	0.7
Fresh pork, roasted	0.4
Ham	0.3
Chicken	0.5
Tuna, canned	0.4
Hot dog	0.3
Salmon	0.3
Fish stick	0.2
Cereals, Grains, Vegetables, Fruits**	
Cooked cereals (1/2 cup)	0.2–1.2
Ready-to-eat cereals (3/4 cup)	1.3–13.0
Whole-wheat bread, enriched bread (1 slice)	0.6–0.8
Legumes, cooked (1/2 cup)	1.2–1.8
Greens (spinach, mustard, beet), cooked (1/2 cup)	0.3–1.4
Green peas, cooked (1/2 cup)	1.2
Dried fruit (1/4 cup)	0.2–0.8
Nuts (2 tbsp)	0.5–1.4
Wheat germ (1 tbsp)	0.5
Molasses, light (1 tbsp)	0.9

Dietary Enhancers of Nonheme Iron Absorption	*Dietary Inhibitors of Nonheme Iron Absorption*
Meat, fish, poultry	Tea (tannic acid)
Ascorbic acid	Sequestering additives (such as EDTA used in fats and soft drinks to clarify and prevent rancidity)
Antacids	

*Heme iron sources (approximately 40% of the iron in these foods); well-absorbed.

**Nonheme sources; lower level of absorption; enhancers eaten at the same time will increase absorption.

Source: US Dept. of Agriculture, Agriculture Research Service, USDA Nutrient Data Laboratory. 2004. *USDA National Nutrient Database for Standard Reference, Release 17.* Retrieved August 19, 2004, from www.nal.usda.gov/fnic/foodcomp.

efforts of nutrition education and feeding programs should be targeted to children at risk so that they might be better able to achieve in school.[58]

The impact of diet and nutrition on a child's behavior has been a controversial topic for some time. Although malnourished children and those experiencing iron deficiency anemia often demonstrate decreased attention and responsiveness, less interest in their environment, and reduced problem-solving ability, the effects of periodic hunger or "food insecurity" is less clear. A report of families from a large Community

Childhood Hunger Identification Project (CCHIP) found that the "hungry" children were three times more likely than "at-risk for hunger" children, and seven times more likely than "not hungry" children, to have scores indicating irritability, anxiety, aggression, and oppositional behavior.[59] Data from NHANES III showed negative academic and psychosocial outcomes associated with food insufficiency. Children who were classified as food-insufficient had lower math scores and were more likely to have repeated a grade, seen a psychologist, and have difficulty getting along with other children. Adolescents with food insufficiency also more likely have been suspended from school.[60] Although other unstudied factors could also be related to these negative behaviors, they could be tied to the family's food insecurity. With federal welfare reform legislation and state budget limitations, more low-income families are likely to be at risk for limited food resources. Without broad policies to ensure children their basic needs, these children may suffer worsening behavioral and academic functioning.

Attention Deficit Hyperactivity Disorder

Commonly known as hyperactivity, attention deficit hyperactivity disorder (ADHD) is a developmental disorder with specific criteria; inattention, impulsivity, hyperactivity, onset before 7 years of age, and duration of at least 6 months. The etiology of ADHD is not clear, however, some dietary factors have been proposed as causes, including food additives, sugar, and food allergies. Although treatment usually includes behavioral management, medication, and/or special education, various dietary treatments have been proposed.

The Feingold diet, popularized in the 1970s, theorized that artificial colorings and flavorings in the food supply caused hyperactivity. Treatment was to remove from the child's diet those substances, natural salicylates (found mostly in fruits), and some preservatives (BHA, BHT). Controlled double-blind challenge studies have not supported the Feingold hypothesis,[61] although it is generally accepted that a small percentage (no more than 5–10%) of children with ADHD (usually preschoolers) may benefit from the diet. Another report, using the Feingold diet plus elimination of foods that the family thought were bothersome to their child, (e.g., chocolate, sugar, or caffeine) found that almost 50% of the preschool hyperactive boys showed some improvement in behavior, using accepted rating scales.[62] The modified Feingold diet, including fruits, has been evaluated favorably according to nutrient content and thus poses little risk for the child.[63] Families using the diet should receive nutritional counseling and should not disregard other helpful treatment for their child's ADHD.

Sugar (sucrose) is popularly believed to cause hyperactivity in children or behavior problems and delinquency in adolescents. Controlled challenge studies, however, have failed to show any negative behavioral effects from sucrose.[64] In one study, children receiving the sugar were less active and quieter afterward than were those receiving the placebo.[65] A double-blind challenge study with juvenile delinquents did not show impaired behavioral performance after a sucrose load.[66] There are many good reasons for reducing sugar consumption, including improved oral health and diets that are more nutrient dense. This can be reinforced with families, while helping them remain objective about a sugar-behavior relationship. There is always the rare possibility that a child may have an individual intolerance to sugar.

Stimulant medications, such as methylphenidate (e.g., Ritalin, Concerta, Metadate, and Focalin), dextroamphetamine (e.g., Dexedrine or Dextrostate), and mixed salts of a single entity amphetamine (e.g., Adderall), are commonly used to treat ADHD.[67] These medications are available in short- and long-acting preparations. They usually result in improvement of motor restlessness, short attention span, and irritability. Anorexia is a side effect that has been shown to cause suppression of physical growth. Over time, there seems to be more tolerance for a medication's negative effect on growth, but the response is individual. Data suggests that there is a direct relationship between dosage of the medication and the degree of reduced growth.[68] The effects of stimulant medications on height gain, however, seem to be temporary, with no differences in heights-for-age by late adolescence.[68] Nonstimulant medications, including atomoxetine (Strattera), are sometimes prescribed for ADHD.

Although the mechanisms involved are not clear, decreased energy intake is a factor. Children receiving these medications should have regular monitoring of growth, and the efficacy of the drug effect should be reassessed routinely. Because the effect of the medication will be noted about half an hour after being ingested, food should be offered to take advantage of the child's optimal appetite; in other words, the medication should be given with or after meals and healthy snacks offered when the effects of the short-action preparations are wearing off. The long-acting preparations appear to suppress appetite less dramatically, but more continuously throughout the day.

Megavitamin therapy has been promoted for many disorders, including ADHD and behavior problems. Of the controlled studies done, none have supported the use of megavitamins, and there is the potential for vitamin toxicity or other negative effects.[69] The use of fatty acid supplements, specifically polyunsaturated fatty acids such as docosahexaenoic acid (DHA) and evening primrose oil, has been suggested because of observed differences in plasma and erythrocyte phospholipid levels in children with ADHD. One double-blind, placebo-controlled study indicated no significant clinical improvements with DHA supplementation after 4 months. The authors suggest future supplementation studies with different doses and other fatty acids.[70]

Food allergies as a factor in ADHD or behavioral difficulties in children are unclear. Many reports are subjective and the validity and interpretation of allergy tests can be controversial. It is certainly possible that children with allergies may manifest behaviors (irritability, poor attention) seen in children with ADHD, but whether or not elimination diets alleviate these symptoms is not clear. Children suspected of having food allergies should be seen by an allergist for diagnosis. Periodic nutrition evaluations are warranted for any child using an atypical dietary regimen.

ADOLESCENT PREGNANCY

Although pregnancy is a normal physiologic state, there are more risks and complications for pregnant teens compared to any other age group. They have higher rates of low-birth-weight infants, especially among those younger than 15 years old. Birth rates among adolescents have been declining during the 1990s; there were 43 births per 1000 females 15 to 19 years of age in 2002.[71] The biggest decline was in adolescent black females ages 15 to 17. The nutritional status of the pregnant adolescent is influenced by both physiologic and environmental/social factors. There is evidence that young pregnant teenage girls are still growing, creating a maternal-fetal competition for nutrients, and thus indicating increased nutrient needs in addition to pregnancy.[72] Other risk factors include a low prepregnancy weight and minimal nutrient stores at the time of conception. Many social factors can also affect the health and nutritional status of the teen, including late or no prenatal care, little financial support, limited food resources, poor eating habits, family difficulties, and various other emotional stresses.

For a positive outcome of pregnancy, weight gain for the pregnant adolescent may need to be more than the usual 25 to 35 pounds. The Committee on Nutritional Status During Pregnancy and Lactation of the Food and Nutrition Board recommends that pregnant teens gain at the upper end of the recommended range for their prepregnancy weight[73] (see Appendix I). The pattern of weight gain is important, with weight gain in the first and early second trimesters being related to improved birth weights.[74] Studies, however, document that weight gain in adolescent pregnancy results in a reduced birth weight infant and greater maternal stores than would be expected in the pregnant adult.[75]

Dietary guides for pregnant teens have usually added the pregnancy DRIs to the DRIs for 15 to

18-year-old females (see Appendix I-1 and I-2). Energy needs can vary greatly, depending on pubertal maturation and physical activity. An adequate weight gain is the best indicator of an appropriate energy intake. The pregnancy RDA for protein is 0.88 grams protein per kilogram body weight per day, which is slightly more than the RDA for 14- to 18-year old females.[3] Higher protein intakes may be needed, depending on body build and growth needs. A sufficient energy intake will protect the protein to be used for growth. Individualized nutrition assessments will help identify the nutrition and diet concerns to be prioritized for ongoing nutrition counseling and education. An iron supplement is routinely recommended for the second and third trimesters, and vitamins B6, C, folate, and calcium may be indicated in the presence of dietary and social-environmental risk factors.[76] Recommendations for folate during pregnancy suggest a daily intake of 600 μg. Because this is greater than the amount usually consumed through diet (including enriched cereals and breads), a supplement is often necessary.[77]

Education and counseling are needed for the teen to accept the needed weight gain, plus the likelihood of a higher postpartum weight as part of a healthy pregnancy. An interdisciplinary health care team can best help pregnant teenagers to deal with their multiple health, psychosocial, and economic issues. This is most effective when provided as accessible prenatal care targeted to the teenage population in their own communities.[78] Because most of them keep their babies, education and resource referrals are needed regarding infant care and feeding, continued schooling of the mother, parenting, and financial services (see also Chapter 3).

SUBSTANCE ABUSE

Alcohol, tobacco, and marijuana are the most widely used substances among teenagers. During the 1990s, there was an increase in the percentages of 8th, 10th, and 12th graders who smoked daily, drank heavily, or used illegal drugs.[79] Alcoholism in adolescence is a significant public health problem. More than 90% of teenagers have had some experience with alcohol by the 12th grade, with many having their first exposure as early as 12 years of age.[80] Any negative effect on nutritional status will depend on the frequency and amount of drinking as well as usual food habits. A survey of teenage males who were alcohol and marijuana abusers did not show significant differences in biochemical measures, but decreased intakes of milk, fruits, and vegetables were reported, as well as more snack food consumption and more symptoms of poor nutrition (tiredness, bleeding gums, muscle weakness).[81] For the female who consumes alcohol and becomes pregnant, there is risk of fetal alcohol syndrome in her infant.

Despite a decrease in cigarette smoking among adults in recent years, smoking remains relatively popular among teenagers. There may be increased need for some nutrients such as ascorbic acid, and smoking during pregnancy can reduce infant birth weight. Smokeless (chewing) tobacco has become popular with both school-age children and adolescents.[82] Not a benign substance, regular use is related to periodontal disease, oral cancer, dependence, and hypertension.

The negative nutritional consequences of a substance user's habit will depend on factors such as lifestyle, available food, and money to buy food. During a nutrition evaluation, the areas of alcohol consumption, tobacco use, and illegal drug use should be considered. Information will most likely be shared if a matter-of-fact, nonthreatening approach is used. Depending on the individual's situation, nutrition education and counseling can focus on improving health and nutrition. Other teenagers will need comprehensive treatment programs, which include a nutrition component.

HEALTH PROMOTION

Americans have been gradually altering their eating habits as a result of increased interest in their health and their concern about preventing heart disease, cancer, obesity, and hypertension. The federal government and nonprofit organizations have provided recommendations, such as the dietary guidelines, to promote healthy eating. To what degree, if any, should this advice be applied to growing children and adolescents?

The federally sponsored National Cholesterol Education Program (NCEP) recommends that everyone over 2 years of age follow a diet that includes no more than 30% of energy as fat (10% or less from saturated fat, up to 10% from unsaturated fat, 10–15% from monounsaturated fat) and no more than 300 mg cholesterol per day.[83] The panel also recommends cholesterol screening for children at risk: those with parents or grandparents diagnosed with coronary heart disease or a cardiac event before age 55 and those with one or both parents having a serum cholesterol of 240 mg or more. Although controversy exists regarding universal versus selective cholesterol screening,[84] screening in childhood appears to be a sensitive predictor of adult lipid levels.[85]

For children identified by screening, the NCEP intervention is dependent on low-density lipoprotein (LDL) cholesterol categories.[83] For those with an acceptable level (less than 110 mg/dL), the recommended dietary pattern (step-one diet) is suggested, with a repeat lipoprotein analysis in 5 years. Children with a borderline level of LDL cholesterol (110–129 mg/dL) would be provided with a step-one diet prescribed and individualized for them and a reevaluation in 1 year. Those with high LDL cholesterol levels (greater than 130 mg/dL) would initially be given the step-one diet, and if necessary the step-two diet (further reduction to less than 7% saturated fat and less than 200 mg cholesterol per day).

Some experts believe that these recommendations are not appropriate, especially for the young child.[86] Growth failure has been seen in some infants and toddlers whose parents, well intentioned but misguided, restricted their children's diet to prevent atherosclerosis, obesity, and poor eating habits[87] (See Chapter 18). Although there is little evidence that dietary intervention in the growing years will decrease serum cholesterol levels or modify other risk factors later in life,[88] young children appear to be able to consume low-fat diets (less than 30% of energy as fat) without negatively influencing the level of energy or micronutrients consumed or affecting growth.[89,90] It seems appropriate to recommend a gradual transition to a diet meeting the NCEP guidelines for children over 2 years of age.

A 10-year study of 2379 girls showed that a significant number of adolescents are exceeding NCEP recommendations for total and saturated fat and cholesterol intakes. A higher percentage of black girls than white girls are not meeting recommendations.[91] Another large national study indicated that children in low-income families with food insufficiency had higher cholesterol intakes than their peers from higher income, food-sufficient households. They were more likely to be overweight, consumed less fruit, and watched more television than peers from low-income, food-sufficient families.[92]

Prevention of osteoporosis begins with optimal calcium intake and maximal bone density in the growing years. However, many young people, especially adolescents, do not receive the recommended AI of 1,300 mg calcium. Those who consume limited amounts of dairy products are at risk for calcium deficiency. Some adolescents may also receive less calcium than needed because of rapid growth, dieting practices, and substituting carbonated beverages for milk. Nutrition education public media campaigns are being used to improve these diet trends.

National diet intake data have shown that children and adolescents consume a less-than-desirable intake of fiber and whole-grain foods, similar to the adult population.[93] An AI for fiber has been established as part of the DRIs. This new recommendation is significantly higher for children and adolescents than previous guidelines[3] (see Appendix I-1 and I-2). Increasing dietary fiber can help prevent constipation, protect against coronary heart disease, and often results in greater intake of fruits and vegetables.

For overall health promotion, moderation and common sense continue to be the best policy. Although prevention of obesity and other chronic conditions are worthy goals, there is no conclusive data to support a massive change in the diets of growing children. For healthy, growing children, the use of low-fat dairy products and fewer high-fat foods is appropriate for those over 2 years of age. Limiting the intake of fermentable carbohydrate will enhance dental health. Increasing the intake of fruits, vegetables, whole-grain products, and legumes above the usual reported levels can have several benefits: reducing the percentage of fat in the diet, increasing the fiber content, increasing the amount of beta-carotene and other dietary factors that may help prevent cancer, and making the total diet more nutrient dense. The more varied the diet, the more likely that the child's nutrient needs will be met.

NUTRITION EDUCATION

Children first learn about food and nutrition from their families in their own homes. This begins in an informal manner, with parental attitudes, foods commonly served (e.g., potatoes or tortillas may be served daily; okra or bok choy may never be served), and family opinions about what foods are good nutritionally. Later, more formal nutrition education occurs in preschools, Head Start programs, day care, schools, and clubs such as 4-H. Information is also assimilated from the media, advertising, written materials, the Internet, and peers.

A child's developmental level should be taken into account when teaching nutrition concepts. For example, Piaget's learning theory can be used to correlate developmental periods and cognitive characteristics with progress in feeding and nutrition.[94] Younger children definitely do best with hands-on personal experience with food, not abstract nutrition concepts. A personal approach works well with children and adolescents, such as the use of computer software to examine their own dietary profiles. Using theoretical concepts to design nutrition education programs and evaluating the effectiveness of these programs is necessary to have an impact on the target population.[95,96] The use of an ecological model has been suggested to increase understanding of eating behaviors, especially among adolescents. The ecological model examines the influences of individual (e.g., biologic), social environmental (e.g., peers), physical environmental (e.g., school), and macrosystem or societal (e.g., marketing) factors on behaviors.[97] Lastly, nutrition education efforts for children should not overlook parents and the family as a whole (see Chapter 7).

REFERENCES

1. Satter E. *How to Get Your Kid to Eat...But Not Too Much*. Palo Alto, CA: Bull Publishing Co; 1987.
2. Food and Nutrition Board, Institute of Medicine, National Academy of Sciences. *Dietary Reference Intakes: Calcium, Phosphorus, Magnesium, Vitamin D and Fluoride*. Washington, DC: National Academy Press; 1997.
3. Food and Nutrition Board, Institute of Medicine, National Academy of Sciences. *Dietary Reference Intakes for Energy, Carbohydrate, Fiber, Fat, Fatty Acids, Cholesterol, Protein, and Amino Acids*. Washington, DC: National Academy Press; 2002.
4. Bialostosky K, et al. *Dietary Intake of Macronutrients, Micronutrients, and Other Dietary Constituents. United States. 1988–94*. National Center for Health Statistics, Vital Health Stat. 11(245); 2002.
5. US Department of Agriculture, Agricultural Research Service. *Food and Nutrient Intakes by Children 1994–96, 1998*. ARS Food Surveys Research Group. Available on the "Products" page, retrieved February 10, 2004, from www.barc.usda.gov/bhnrc/foodsurvey/home.htm.
6. Alaimo K, McDowell MA, Briefel RR, et al. Dietary intake of vitamins, minerals, and fiber of persons ages 2 months and over in the United States: Third National Health and Nutrition Examination Survey, Phase I, 1988–1991. *Advance Data from Vital Statistics*. 1994; No. 258 (PHS) 95–1250 Hyattsville, MD: National Center for Health Statistics.
7. Suitor CW, Gleason PM. Using dietary reference intake–based methods to estimate the prevalence of inadequate nutrient intake among school-aged children. *J Am Diet Assoc*. 2002;102(4):530–536.
8. Matkovic V, Fontana D, Tominac C. Factors that influence peak bone mass formation: A study of calcium balance and the inheritance of bone mass in adolescent females. *Am J Clin Nutr*. 1990;52:878–888.
9. Johnston CC, Miller JZ, Slemenda CW, et al. Calcium supplementation and increases in bone mineral density in children. *N Engl J Med*. 1992;327:82–87.
10. Anderson JJ. Calcium requirements during adolescence to maximize bone health. *Pediatrics*. 2001;20(2 Suppl): 186S–191S.
11. Food and Nutrition Board, Institute of Medicine, National Academy of Sciences. *Dietary Reference Intakes: Vitamin A, Vitamin K, Arsenic, Boron, Chro-*

mium, Copper, Iodine, Iron, Manganese, Molybdenum, Nickel, Silicon, Vanadium, and Zinc. Washington, DC: National Academy Press; 2001.

12. Yu SM, Kogan MD, Gergen P. Vitamin-mineral supplement use among preschool children in the United States. *Pediatrics*. 1997;100(5):E4.
13. Feeding the child. In: American Academy of Pediatrics, Committee on Nutrition. *Pediatric Nutrition Handbook*, 5th ed. Elk Grove Village, IL: The American Academy of Pediatrics; 2004:125–126.
14. American Dietetic Association. Position of the American Dietetic Association: Food fortification and dietary supplements. *J Am Diet Assoc*. 2001;101:115–125.
15. American Medical Association, Council on Scientific Affairs. Vitamin preparations as dietary supplements and as therapeutic agents. *JAMA*. 1987;257:1929.
16. Lanski SL, Greenwald M, Perkins A, Simon HK. Herbal therapy use in a pediatric emergency department population: Expect the unexpected. *Pediatrics*. 2003;111(5): 981–985.
17. Beal VA. Dietary intake of individuals followed through infancy and childhood. *Am J Public Health*. 1961;51: 1107–1117.
18. Munoz KA, Krebs-Smith SM, Ballard-Barbash R, et al. Food intakes of U.S. children and adolescents compared with recommendations. *Pediatrics*. 1997;100:323–329.
19. Galloway AT, Lee Y, Birch LL. Predictors and consequences of food neophobia and pickiness in young girls. *J Am Diet Assoc*. 2003;103(6):692–698.
20. Nielsen SJ, Siega-Riz AM, Popkin BM. Trends in food locations and sources among adolescents and young adults. *Prev Med*. 2002;35(2):107–113.
21. Johnson RK, Crouter AC, Smiciklas-Wright H. Effects of maternal employment on family food consumption patterns and children's diets. *J Nutr Educ*. 1993;25:130–133.
22. Gillman MW, Rifas-Shiman SL, Frazier AL, et al. Family dinner and diet quality among older children and adolescents. *Arch Fam Med*. 2000;9:235–240.
23. Borzekowski D. Watching what they eat: A content analysis of televised food references reaching preschool children. Unpublished Manuscript. 2001 [as cited in Kaiser Family Foundation. *The Role of Media in Childhood Obesity*. 2004].
24. American Public Health Association. Policy Statement 2003-17. *Food Marketing and Advertising Directed at Children and Adolescents: Implications for Overweight*. Retrieved February 13, 2004, from www.apha.org/legislative/policy/2003/2003-017.pdf.
25. Kohl HW, Hobbs, KE. Development of physical activity behaviors among children and adolescents. In: Hill JO, Trowbridge FL. The causes and health consequences of obesity in children and adolescents. *Pediatrics*. 1998;101 (suppl):549–554.
26. Boynton-Jarrett R, Thomas TN, Peterson KE, et al. Impact of television viewing patterns on fruit and vegetable consumption among adolescents. *Pediatrics*. 2003;112(6 Pt1):1321–1326.
27. Harris CS, Baker SP, Smith GA. Childhood asphyxiation by food: A national analysis and overlook. *JAMA*. 1984;251:2231–2235.
28. Smith MM, Davis M, Chasalow FI, et al. Carbohydrate absorption from fruit juice in young children. *Pediatrics*. 1995;95:340–344.
29. Smith MM, Lifshitz F. Excess fruit juice consumption as a contributing factor in nonorganic failure to thrive. *Pediatrics*. 1994;93:438–443.
30. Dennison BA, Rockwell HL, Baker SL. Fruit juice consumption by preschool-aged children is associated with short stature and obesity. *Pediatrics*. 1997;99:15–22.
31. Skinner JD, Carruth BR, Moran J, et al. Fruit juice intake is not related to children's growth. *Pediatrics*. 1999;103(1):58–64.
32. Alexy U, Sicher-Hellert W, Kersting M, et al. Fruit juice consumption and the prevalence of obesity and short stature in German preschool children: Results of the DONALD Study. *J Pediatric Gastroenterology and Nutrition*. 1999;29(3):343–349.
33. Committee on Nutrition. American Academy of Pediatrics. The use and misuse of fruit juice in pediatrics. *Pediatrics*. 2001;107(5):1210–1213.
34. U.S. Department of Agriculture. Child Nutrition Programs: School meal initiatives for healthy children. *Fed Reg*, 7CFR, Part 220, Food and Consumer Service, USDA; 1995.
35. Ho CS, Gould RA, Jensen LN, et al. Evaluation of the nutrient content of school, sack and vending lunch of junior high students. *Sch Food Serv Res Rev*. 1991;15:85–90.
36. Committee on Nutrition, American Academy of Pediatrics. Soft drinks in schools. *Pediatrics*. 2004;113(1): 152–154.
37. French SA, Jeffery RW, Story M, et al. Pricing and promotion effects on low-fat vending snack purchases: The CHIPS study. *Am J Public Health*. 2001;91(1):112–117.
38. Kaste LM, Selwitz RH, Oldakowski RJ, et al. Coronal caries in the primary and permanent dentition of children and adolescents 1–17 years of age: United States, 1988–1991. *J Dent Res*. 1996;75:631–641.
39. Faine MP. Nutrition and oral health. In: Proceedings of *Promoting Oral Health of Children with Neurodevelopmental Disabilities and Other Special Health Care Needs*. May 4–5, 2001. Seattle, WA. Retrieved February 10, 2004, from www.depts.washington.edu/ccohr/resource/LEND_2001.pdf.
40. Palmer CA. *Diet and Nutrition in Oral Health*. Upper Saddle River, NJ: Prentice Hall; 2003.
41. White-Graves MV, Schiller MR. History of foods in the caries process. *J Am Diet Assoc*. 1986;86:241–245.

42. Garcia-Closas R, Garcia-Closas M, Sera-Majem L. A cross-sectional study of dental caries, intake of confectionery and foods rich in starch and sugars, and salivary counts of Steptococcus mutans in children in Spain. *Am J Clin Nutr*. 1997;66:1257–1263.

43. Navia JM. Carbohydrates and dental health. *Am J Clin Nutr*. 1994;59(suppl):719S–727S.

44. Makinen KK, Hujoel PP, Bennett CA, et al. A descriptive report of the effects of a 16-month xylitol chewing-gum programme subsequent to a 40-month sucrose gum programme. *Caries Res*. 1998;32:107–112.

45. American Academy of Pediatric Dentistry. *Policy on Early Childhood Caries (ECC): Classifications, Consequences, and Preventive Strategies*. 2003. Retrieved November 13, 2003, from www.aapd.org/members/referencemanual/pdfs/02-03/Policy_ECCClass.pdf.

46. American Academy of Pediatrics, Section on Pediatric Dentistry. Oral health risk assessment timing and establishment of the dental home. *Pediatrics*. 2003;111(5): 1113–1116.

47. US Department of Health and Human Services. *Oral Health in America: A Report of the Surgeon General—Executive Summary*. Rockville, MD: US Department of Health and Human Services, National Institute of Dental and Craniofacial Research, National Institutes of Health; 2000. Retrieved November 13, 2003, from www.nidcr.nih.gov/sgr/sgr.htm.

48. Faine MP. The role of dietetics professionals in preventing early childhood caries. *Building Block for Life*. 2001; 25(1).

49. Johnsen D, Nowjack-Raymer R. Baby bottle tooth decay (BBTD): Issues, assessment, and an opportunity for the nutritionist. *J Am Diet Assoc*. 1989;89:112–116.

50. Looker AC, Dallman PR, Carroll MD, et al. Prevalence of iron deficiency in the United States. *JAMA*. 1997; 277:973–976.

51. Walter T, De Andraca I, Chadud P, et al. Iron deficiency anemia: Adverse effects on infant psychomotor development. *Pediatrics*. 1989;84:7–17.

52. Lozoff B, Jimenez E, Hagen J, Mollen E, Wolf AW. Poorer behavioral and developmental outcome more than 10 years after treatment for iron deficiency in infancy. *Pediatrics*. 2000;105(4):e51.

53. Monsen ER, Hallberg L, Layrisse M, et al. Estimation of available dietary iron. *Am J Clin Nutr*. 1978;31:134–141.

54. Iron deficiency. In: American Academy of Pediatrics, Committee on Nutrition. *Pediatric Nutrition Handbook*, 5th ed. Elk Grove Village, IL: The American Academy of Pediatrics; 2004.

55. Pollit E, Cueto S, Jacoby ER. Fasting and cognition in well- and undernourished school children: A review of three experimental studies. *Am J Clin Nutr*. 1998; 67(suppl):779S–784S.

56. Simeon DT, Grantham-McGregor S. Effects of missing breakfast on the cognitive functions of school children of differing nutritional status. *Am J Clin Nutr*. 1989;49: 646–653.

57. Meyers AF, Sampson A, Weitzman M, et al. School breakfast program and school performance. *Am J Dis Child*. 1989;143:1234–1239.

58. Powell CA, Walker SP, Chang SM, Grantham-McGregor SM. Nutrition and education: A randomized trial of the effects of breakfast in rural primary school children. *Am J Clin Nutr*. 1998;68:873–879.

59. Kleinman RE, Murphy J, Little M, et al. Hunger in children in the United States: Potential behavioral and emotional correlates. *Pediatrics*. 1998;101:e3.

60. Alaimo K, Olsom CM, Frongillo EA. Food insufficiency and American school-aged children's cognitive, academic, and psychosocial development. *Pediatrics*. 2001; 108(1):44–51.

61. Lipton MA, Mayo JP. Diet and hyperkinesis: An update. *J Am Diet Assoc*. 1983;83:132–134.

62. Kaplan BJ, McNicol J, Conte RA, et al. Dietary replacement in preschool-aged hyperactive boys. *Pediatrics*. 1989;83:7–17.

63. Harper PH, Goyette CH, Conners CK. Nutrient intakes of children on the hyperkinesis diet. *J Am Diet Assoc*. 1978;73:515–519.

64. Wolraich ML, Wilson DB, White JW. The effect of sugar on behavior or cognition in children: A metaanalysis. *JAMA*. 1995;274:1617–1621.

65. Behar D, Rapoport JL, Adams AJ, et al. Sugar challenge testing with children considered behaviorally sugar reactive. *Nutr Behav*. 1984;1:277–288.

66. Bachorowski J, Newman JP, Nichols SL, et al. Sucrose and delinquency: Behavioral assessment. *Pediatrics*. 1990;86:244–253.

67. American Academy of Pediatrics Subcommittee on Attention-Deficit/Hyperactivity Disorder. Clinical practice guideline: Treatment of the school-aged child with attention-deficit/hyperactivity disorder. *Pediatrics*. 2001;108(4):1033–1044.

68. Spencer T, Biederman J, Wilens T. Growth deficits in children with attention deficit hyperactivity disorder. *Pediatrics*. 1998;102:501–506.

69. Haslam RHA, Dalby JT, Rademaker AW. Effects of megavitamin therapy on children with attention deficit disorders. *Pediatrics*. 1984;74:103–111.

70. Voigt RG, Llorente AM, Jensen CL, et al. A randomized, double-blind, placebo-controlled trial of docosahexaenoic acid supplementation in children with attention-deficit/hyperactivity disorder. *J Pediatr*. 2001;139: 189–196.

71. US Department of Health and Human Services. *US Birth Rate Reaches Record Low*. 2003. Centers for Disease

Control and Prevention, National Center for Health Statistics. Retrieved February 10, 2004, from www.cdc.gov/nchs/releases/03news/lowbirth.htm.

72. Hediger ML, Scholl TO, Schall JI. Implications of the Camden study of adolescent pregnancy: Interactions among maternal growth, nutritional status, and body composition. *Ann NY Acad Sci.* 1997;817:281–291.
73. National Academy of Sciences. *Nutrition During Pregnancy*. Washington, DC: National Academy Press; 1990.
74. Hediger ML, Scholl TO, Belsky DH, Ances IG, Salmon RW. Patterns of weight gain in adolescent pregnancy: Effect on birth weight and preterm delivery. *Obstet Gynecol.* 1989;74:6–12.
75. Scholl TO, Hediger ML, Schall JI. Maternal growth and fetal growth: Pregnancy course and outcome in the Camden study. *Ann NY Acad Sci.* 1997;817:292–301.
76. American Dietetic Association. Nutrition care for pregnant adolescents. *J Am Diet Assoc.* 1994;94:449–450.
77. Food and Nutrition Board, Institute of Medicine, National Academy of Sciences. *Dietary Reference Intakes: Thiamin, Riboflavin, Niacin, Vitamin B6, Folate, Vitamin B12, Pantothenic Acid, Biotin, and Choline*. Washington, DC: National Academy Press; 1998.
78. Story M. Promoting healthy eating and ensuring adequate weight gain in pregnant adolescents: Issues and strategies. *Ann NY Acad Sci.* 1997;817:321–333.
79. Federal Interagency Forum on Child and Family Statistics. *America's Children: Key National Indicators of Well-Being*. Washington, DC: US Government Printing Office, Pub no. 065-000-01162-0; 1998.
80. Johnston LD, O'Malley PM, Bachman JG. *National Survey Results on Drug Use from the Monitoring the Future Study, 1975–1995.* Rockville, MD: US Department of Health and Human Services, Public Health Services; 1996.
81. Farrow JA, Rees JM, Worthington-Roberts B. Health, developmental and nutritional status of adolescent alcohol and marijuana abusers. *Pediatrics.* 1987;79:218–223.
82. Centers for Disease Control and Prevention. Tobacco use among middle and high school students—United States, 2002. *Morb Mortal Wkly Rep.* 2003;52(45):1096–1098.
83. National Heart, Lung, and Blood Institute, National Cholesterol Education Program. *Report of the Expert Panel on Blood Cholesterol Levels in Children and Adolescents*. Bethesda, MD: National Heart, Lung, and Blood Institute; 1991.
84. Steiner NJ, Neinstein LS, Pennbridge J. Hypercholesterolemia in adolescents: Effectiveness of screening strategies based on selected risk factors. *Pediatrics.* 1991;88:269–275.
85. Stuhldreher WL, Orchard TJ, Donahue RP, et al. Cholesterol screening in childhood: Sixteen-year Beaver County Lipid Study experience. *J Pediatr.* 1991;119:551–556.
86. Olson RE. The folly of restricting fat in the diet of children. *Nutr Today.* 1995;30(6):234–245.
87. Pugliese MT, Weyman-Daum M, Moses N, et al. Parental health beliefs as a cause of nonorganic failure to thrive. *Pediatrics.* 1987;80:175–182.
88. Luepker RV, Perry CL, McKinlay SM, et al. Outcomes of a field trial to improve children's dietary patterns and physical activity. The Child and Adolescent Trial for Cardiovascular Health (CATCH). *JAMA.* 1996;275:768–776.
89. Dixon LB, McKenzie J, Shannon BM, et al. The effect of changes in dietary fat on the food group and nutrient intake of 4- to 10-year-old children. *Pediatrics.* 1997;100:863–872.
90. Obarzanek E, Kimm SYS, Barton BA, et al. Long-term safety and efficacy of a cholesterol-lowering diet in children with elevated low-density lipoprotein cholesterol: Seven-year results of the Dietary Intervention Study in Children (DISC). *Pediatrics.* 2001;107(2):256–264.
91. Kronsberg SS, Obarzanek E, Affenito SG, et al. Macronutrient intake of black and white adolescent girls over 10 years: The NHLBI Growth and Health Study. *J Am Diet Assoc.* 2003;103(7):852–860.
92. Casey PH, Szeto K, Lansing S, et al. Children in food-insufficient, low-income families: Prevalence, health, and nutrition status. *Arch Pediatr Adolesc Med.* 2001;155(4):508–514.
93. Harnack L, Walters SH, Jacobs DR. Dietary intake and food sources of whole grains among US children and adolescents: Data from the 1994–1996 Continuing Survey of Food Intakes by Individuals. *J Am Diet Assoc.* 2003;103(8):1015–1019.
94. Lucas B. Nutrition in childhood. In: Mahan LK, Escott Stump S, eds. *Krause's Food, Nutrition, & Diet Therapy*, 11th ed. Philadelphia: W.B. Saunders Company; 2004:269.
95. Contento I, Balch GI, Bronner YL, et al. The effectiveness of nutrition education and implications for nutrition education and policy, programs, and research: A review of research. *J Nutr Educ.* 1995;27:298–311.
96. Sigman-Grant M. Strategies for counseling adolescents. *J Am Diet Assoc.* 2002;102(3 Suppl):S32–S39.
97. Story M, Neumark-Sztainer D, French S. Individual and environmental influences on adolescent eating behaviors. *J Am Diet Assoc.* 2002;102(3 Suppl):S40–S51.

CHAPTER 7

Nutrition Counseling

Bridget Klawitter

COUNSELING CHILDREN: WHAT IS THE DIFFERENCE?

Historically, the dietetic practitioner received little training to differentiate between nutrition counseling and nutrition education. Often, even less was learned about the distinction between how to counsel children and adults. Children learn naturally through experience and play. Adults often are able to identify their concerns and express them to the nutrition counselor. Children are more likely to express their concerns and feelings, either indirectly through play or directly through behavior. This chapter attempts to distinguish for the reader some of the differences the nutrition counselor may encounter with various age and developmental levels in the pediatric population.[1]

HOW CHILDREN LEARN

Information is processed through attention, perception, memory, thinking, and problem solving.[2] Gullo[3] has provided a discussion of how young children process information using these stages. An expansion of this to the field of nutrition counseling is warranted.

Attention

Before children can respond to something, they must recognize it. For the infant, recognition of a parent, and the smile and giggling it elicits, is an early example. Pellegrini and Smith[4] suggest that forms of physical activity and play serve a developmental function and have labeled this dimension of activity in infants as rhythmic stereotypes that serve to improve control of specific motor patterns.

Perception

As the child grows older, attention to objects and events in the environment elicit more specific responses. Once an element in the environment has the child's attention, the child must be able to make sense of it. For example, the infant and toddler soon learn to associate elements of their environment to foods. The sight of the breast or bottle for the infant or the bright colors on the cereal box for the toddler usually attract attention and elicit a response based on the meaning associated with the item. Counseling strategies aimed at the toddler should focus on attracting attention. For example, brightly colored food models or brightly colored pictures can gain the attention of the toddler who is being asked to identify foods.

Memory

The retention of information over time is one of the primary goals of nutrition counseling. Jackson and associates[5] outlined four ways to facilitate memory in young children:

1. Make it familiar, meaningful, and containing similar characteristics (such as pictures of fruits).

2. Have the child actively involved with the information (such as playing with food models).
3. Give the child repeated exposure to the information (parents reinforce food groups at home).
4. Make sure the information is of interest, fun, and holds the child's attention (fruits are cut in different shapes and/or the child is involved in food preparation).

Thinking

This aspect appears to become more evident in the older preschool and school-aged group and is often illustrated by the decision-making process that children demonstrate. One strategy that uses this skill is having children plan a meal using the USDA Food Guide (see Appendix J1) or food models. Challenging them to include a food from each group can facilitate the thinking and decision-making processes.

Problem Solving

Through experience, children learn the consequences of their actions and decisions. Skills in problem solving will increase with exposure to various situations in the environment. For the older child and adolescent, the nutrition counselor may be able to present scenarios and ask them what actions they would take.

DEVELOPMENTAL STAGES

Children perceive, discern, and react to elements in their environment based on their experiences and level of development. Understandably, their reactions change over time as their base of experience and developmental stage changes. A brief discussion of each age group and the typical developmental stages the counselor may encounter can assist in developing counseling strategies appropriate for the age and developmental stage of the children seen.

Infant and Toddler

Biologic, cognitive, and psychosocial development begin and advance quite rapidly during the infant and toddler years. For infants, the parent or caretaker should become the focus of the nutrition counseling session. Two primary reasons that the nutrition counselor should ask parents to bring the infant or toddler to the counseling session are to assess the child's developmental level and to evaluate the parent-child or caretaker-child interaction.[6]

Observation and appropriate interview probes can provide the nutrition counselor with valuable information about the infant or toddler. The nutrition counselor should be familiar with the normal course of child development and should be able to determine any deviations from the norm that may influence feeding ability. An evaluation of parenting skills and interactions is invaluable, due to the infant or toddler's total dependence on the parent for nutritional well-being.

For many new parents, learning the normal developmental stages of the infant and the range of individual differences can be quite overwhelming. The infant's growth and development pattern is the most suitable guide to introducing semisolid foods. The feeding of semisolid foods should be delayed until the consumption of food is no longer a reflexive process and the infant has the fine, gross, and oral motor skills to appropriately consume nonliquid foods safely. Infants need appropriate stimulation to thrive; thus, they usually love colors, talking, music, and being physically held. The attention span of infants is short, but they enjoy sharing pictures, songs, or nursery rhymes, which can encourage cognitive development. The nutrition counselor has a prime opportunity to assist parents during this learning stage to understand the importance of stimulation for their infant as well as the consistency in meeting the infant's needs. The skilled nutrition counselor adapts the parent-learning experience to include issues that cause stress related to the care of the infant and food.

The toddler stage is a time of rapid development and increasing autonomy. Temper tantrums and negative behaviors are common but usually become tempered as the toddler starts to learn socialization skills. As language skills develop, toddlers gradually start to recall past events and to anticipate the consequences of their actions. By 2 or 3 years of age, the toddler can problem solve through physical and mental experimentation, differentiate space and colors, and identify symbols. Although the attention span of the toddler is limited, play that involves the toddler can be beneficial. Although the parent will be the primary recipient of nutrition and feeding information, children in the toddler stage are capable of understanding some basic nutrition concepts, especially if they are fun. During the toddler phase, parents must continue to be supported, and the nutrition counselor should provide reinforcement for positive changes. The use of small utensils and dishes that are easily manipulated until motor skills are better developed should be encouraged. The nutrition counselor should emphasize the importance of continued parental stimulation and a good parent-child relationship during this period.

Cognitive Behavioral Play Therapy (CBPT) is a technique that may be useful to help young children express their feelings and to understand basic nutrition facts.[7] Play is one of the most powerful ways young children learn, and it provides an important base for cognitive, language, and social development. Play is a natural medium for self-expression; open-ended play encourages children to think and to reflect about their environment. As challenges naturally arise in the course of play, the child seeks meaningful solutions. Play is a voluntary activity, and the child is in control.

Through play, children feel control over situations because they can decide what to play and how long to play. Pretend play allows children to create an imaginary world that they can master. In the early years, children think primarily in concrete terms and have no concept of the abstract. The toddler is unable to reason, and, instead, takes words literally. As vocabulary increases, so does the child's ability to express thoughts, needs, and desires. Play therapy is one method that permits children to express their needs and to discover solutions in a safe, therapeutic environment.

Preschool Children

As the toddler matures, the need for social experiences increases. The preschooler can understand his or her physical needs, such as hunger and tiredness, but usually has a poor perception of time. Preschoolers may be able to express their fears and frustrations but may often use play to express these feelings. As the child enters the preschool years, gross motor skills improve dramatically; fine motor skills remain limited.[8] Social interaction increases as the child more actively participates in play, both real and imaginary. Children begin to interact with one another, as well as to communicate with imaginary playmates. Preschool children continue to develop their own identities and to expand their world through outside social contacts. Social skills start to develop as the child attempts to model observed behaviors. The preschooler's maturing cognitive skills produce endless curiosity, as evidenced by the now-constant question "Why?" Explanations must be kept simple and to the point. The counselor should take this opportunity to involve the child, using language and tools appropriate to the child's developmental level. Opportunities to observe the child at play can provide insight into neuromuscular and cognitive development. At this stage, it is also important for the nutrition counselor to develop a rapport with the child to promote behavior change.

Parents should be provided guidance and encouragement in making appropriate nutrition changes. The nutrition counselor should assess parental nutrition knowledge and attitudes toward food during this period, because the influence of the parent on the child's behavior is tremendous. It is during this time that "food jags" and the parent's response may become a challenge of control. The nutrition counselor becomes a support for parents in understanding usual developmental behavior and effective parental responses.

School-Aged Children

School-aged children rapidly build on motor and social skills as they spend more time away from home and enter the formal education environment. Although the attention span of the school-aged child is longer, the nutrition counselor must be attuned to the length of time the child remains attentive during a counseling session. School-aged children will begin to establish self-concept and values through interaction with others in their environment. At this stage, children start to realize cause-and-effect relationships and gradually logical reasoning develops. The school-aged child enjoys learning new words and science principles in simple terms. Children in this age group enjoy play that involves winning: Stickers, stars, or "points" may provide an incentive for learning and compliance. By age 10 to 12 years, the child begins to choose friends more selectively, and the influence of peers becomes more predominant. The nutrition counselor should strive to promote more one-on-one interaction with the child during the counseling session and to have parents reinforce the concepts at home. Parents should be encouraged to foster the child's sense of independence and to praise accomplishments within the nutrition care plan.

It is also during this period that the environment becomes more structured and routine; consequently, physical activity levels may decline, and the incidence of obesity increases. Much research has been done on the growing problem of childhood obesity.[9–11] The nutrition counselor can play a major role in assisting parents to understand the important relationship between diet and physical activity, and the potential negative long-term effects of dieting to promote weight loss. It is also a period during which the nutrition counselor can aid the child in learning self-management skills with parental support.

Adolescents

The nutrition counselor may use group therapy or one-to-one interaction with adolescents. Children at this stage are usually able to give facts accurately and are becoming more autonomous in their actions and decisions. Adolescents are usually able to understand abstract ideas and concepts and will sometimes verbalize disagreement with nutrition concepts. The adolescent may readily absorb medical terminology but often needs clarification of definitions. Improving self-esteem may make adolescents more compliant because peer relationships are important as the adolescent strives to "fit in." Adolescents also have difficulty imagining themselves vulnerable to illness or disease, and this may impact compliance with the nutrition plan of care. Thus, it is important to emphasize the importance of nutrition and physical activity in relationship to the adolescent's current lifestyle—not for the prevention of disease.

The limits of confidentiality should be established early.[6] Two types of information that nutrition counselors may need to pass on to caregivers include their opinion on the nutritional status of the adolescent and what information the adolescent has revealed either verbally or nonverbally that impacts the nutrition plan of care. Being honest and frank with the adolescent aids in establishing trust and can facilitate the interview process. Studies noted by Hayes[12] have found caregivers are usually receptive to the issue of confidentiality and to recognize its importance in building relationships with a child. In many instances, adolescents will give permission to the counselor to share the details of the session with their parents, and this makes the counseling experience more open. Respecting the individuality of the adolescent can go a long way in establishing the trust needed for a productive nutrition counseling experience.

A strong preoccupation with body image may also accompany this group and interfere with comprehension of healthy lifestyle practices. Growing evidence[13] suggests that body image is just as important to young boys as it is to girls. The primary difference is that boys worry more about not having enough size. Society views being big and powerful as being "manly," as evidenced by messages sent in films, on television, by rock groups, and in video games. Men in athletics, taller men, or those involved in physical activity are also valued by society in general. Approximately 90% of individuals treated for eating disorders are female; however, the number of males appears to be increasing.[14] The same factors—decreased self-esteem, feeling the need to be "perfect," and the desire to feel in control of the environment—accompany eating disorders in both males and females.

Adolescents are capable of abstract thinking and logical reasoning, and these should become the major focus of the counseling session. Adolescents may rebel against authority as they struggle to establish their own identities. Establishing rapport with the adolescent and facilitating the relationship between the child and the family in following recommendations is perhaps the most challenging aspect of counseling this age group. Parents should be encouraged to set realistic limits for adolescents while fostering independence.

CREATING A LEARNING ENVIRONMENT

Interviewing Techniques

Some general techniques for interviewing children using the five-stage model[15] are provided in Exhibit 7–1. Interviewing the child or adolescent can present many unique challenges to the nutrition counselor.[6] Interviewing is quite different from counseling the adult and the younger the client, the greater will be the difference. The nutrition counselor will find that children and adolescents will vary in their cognitive and language skills—at times independent of chronological age. Others often bring children and adolescents (either willing or unwilling) to the counseling experience. Occasionally, an older adolescent will come on his or her own initiative. Children and adolescents may often perceive the nutrition counseling experience as a reflection of misdeeds; that is, "eating wrong" or having an "imperfect body." This perception can lead to barriers that the nutrition counselor must recognize and overcome for the counseling to be effective. Finally, nutrition counseling sessions may involve children or adolescents who have difficulty with communication, either voluntary or involuntary. The skilled nutrition counselor will possess a variety of counseling methodologies to assist the child to participate actively in the learning experience as much as possible.

Establishing rapport is key to the success of the counseling experience. The counselor must be warm, empathetic, and genuine and should develop a warm and friendly relationship with the child. At the first visit, the primary focus should be the establishment of rapport, rather than simply determining facts about the child. With very

Exhibit 7–1 Interviewing Children Using the Five-Stage Model

Stage 1 Establish a rapport.
Establish a rapport in your own way: Use facial expressions (i.e., smile, laugh), play activities, or draw.

Stage 2 Gather data emphasizing strengths.
Paraphrase, reflect the child's feelings, summarize frequently. Keep questions and concepts concrete and avoid abstract talk. Identify positive aspects.

Stage 3 Determine goals.
Ask what the child wants to happen. Accept a child's goals but focus on concrete, short-term goals. Allow the child to explore his or her ideal world and discover their fantasies and desires.

Stage 4 Generate alternative solutions and actions.
Utilize creative brainstorming techniques. Try small groups with children having similar problems. Imagine the future and explore various alternatives.

Stage 5 Allow time to try new behaviors and ideas.
Maintain concrete goals day to day. Homework assignments are useful. Observe behavior and interactions with others.

Source: Adapted with permission from Ivey AE, Ivey MB, and Simek-Morgan L. *Counseling and Psychotherapy: A Multicultural Perspective,* 4th ed.

young children, it is especially important to explore their world with them before introducing change. Nutrition counselors should take the time to show interest in the child and should genuinely care about who the child is.

It is important for the nutrition counselor to have a flexible approach to counseling children. This includes being aware of feedback that the child may provide, either verbal or nonverbal. The nutrition counselor should be alert to the feelings of the child and should be able to reflect those feelings back to the child in a manner that the child understands. It is usually possible—through skillful probing—to determine whether a child is ready to learn a particular nutrition concept. The nutrition counselor should respect the child's ability to solve problems when given the opportunity to do so. As with adults, the responsibility to make choices and to make change rests with the child.

THE COUNSELING EXPERIENCE

Role of the Child

The role of the child is to be him- or herself. It is important for the nutrition counselor to realize that the ultimate decision to change rests with the child and that the counseling approach, as well as strategies used, must take this into consideration to be successful.

Role of the Parent

The role of the parent in the counseling experience changes as the child matures. For the infant, the parent's primary role is to engage in social interaction with the child and counselor and to attend to the needs of the infant on cue. As the child enters the toddler stage, the parental role is to provide opportunities for the child to explore and experiment with his or her environment. Children love mastering new skills and the preschooler relishes completing tasks for the parent. The preschooler also enjoys reenacting experiences through imaginary play, and the parental role is to provide props and to acknowledge the child's progress and accomplishments. As the child enters school and takes charge of a greater number of activities, the parent becomes a mentor offering information and assistance. Adolescence is the child's final push for independence as the child, now a youth, "practices" adulthood; the parental role gradually decreases to offering objective, succinct information for the adolescent's decision-making process.

Parents appear to respond best to information that focuses on their specific needs and problems.[16] Verbal suggestions can be effective for conveying brief, concrete nutrition concepts, but clearly written information should be provided for both reinforcement and more complex, detailed information. Modeling or role playing may be a useful technique for parents who need visual examples or when the issue involves problematic parent or child behavior. The counselor may ask, "What could you do differently in that circumstance?" These various techniques, if applied wisely and appropriately, can facilitate nutrition and activity behavior changes.

Exercising together as a family should be promoted as an excuse to have fun. Families should find various activities that can be accomplished at different skill levels and enjoyed on a regular basis. The benefits of an active lifestyle to children include improved motor skills, increased self-confidence, and maximized time together as a family unit. Inactivity is often accompanied by poor eating habits during childhood and can contribute to a lifetime of health problems. General guidelines issued by the American Heart Association for healthy physical activity can aid families in increasing physical activity in their children.[17] Some key points to suggest to parents include:

- Encourage regular walking, bicycling, and outdoor play; use of playgrounds and gyms; and interaction with other children.
- Limit watching television or videotapes and video games to less than 2 hours per day.
- Encourage weekly participation in age-appropriate organized sports, lessons, or team activities.
- Seek out daily school or day care physical

activity that includes at least 20 minutes of coordinated large muscle exercise.
- Plan regular family outings that involve walking, cycling, swimming, or other recreational activities.
- Be a positive role model for a physically active lifestyle and look for other caregivers and school personnel who do the same.

Role of the Counselor

A counselor can help guide the child through a developmentally and age-appropriate play experience to learn basic health concepts and can assist parents or caregivers to discover the correct balance of independence for a child. Certain limits required by family structure and therapeutic diet modifications may also need to be communicated.

Counseling Environment

The nutrition counselor must provide a physical environment that will facilitate the counseling experience for both the parent and the child. Using concepts outlined by Barker,[6] the nutrition interview should be conducted in counseling rooms or playrooms designed for younger children.

Key elements include:

- comfortable chairs and tables of sizes suitable for the age of the child being seen
- book shelves with a selection of age-appropriate books, especially those illustrating nutrition and physical fitness concepts
- paper and drawing materials
- child-centered and age-appropriate surroundings
- culturally sensitive toys
- well-designed cupboards and other readily accessible storage space
- cleaning solution to sanitize items between sessions, especially toys and food models

Arrangement of the room, perhaps by age category or developmental level, can assist in directing a child's attention to items that are likely of interest and age appropriate. Older adolescents are usually comfortable in an adult environment. Elements key to an environment conducive to counseling adults may include such factors as[18,19]:

- Adults want to be treated as adults and as individuals.
- Most adults prefer objectivity and a business-like approach.
- Adults want counseling to address their perceived needs.
- Adults need positive reinforcement and feedback.
- Adults want to be active participants in the counseling experience.
- Adults prefer a counseling location that is clean, safe, private, and furnished with the adult client in mind.

PROVIDING DEVELOPMENTALLY APPROPRIATE EXPERIENCES

Biologic Experiences

As the infant grows and develops, important biologic experiences occur that can influence food habits later on. The process of introducing solid foods is a primary learning ground for food tastes and textures. Caregivers should be prepared for initial refusal of new textures and flavors and counseled on how to encourage an infant without force-feeding. Negative food experiences during this time can often develop into food aversions. Trying foods too early or in a certain order may influence a child's food preferences and acceptance. The role of the nutrition counselor involved during this early period is to assist parents in identifying when their infant is developmentally ready to advance food types and textures and to assist parents in recognizing cues their infant gives in regard to acceptance of the food.

Physical Experiences

Infants prefer exploring objects with all their senses. Many parents comment: "Everything goes in the mouth!" Mobiles, musical toys, and bright colors and shapes all stimulate the infant's senses. As mobility increases, the child's ability to explore tends to increase, and toys should have a variety of colors, shapes, and sizes to stimulate interest. Safety is an important feature during this stage as children explore their environment.

Role playing is evident as the maturing child "pretends" during play. The preschooler often will be found modeling the behavior of the waitress at the restaurant and taking orders for food from stuffed animals. Pretending allows children to recall events in their environment and to translate those into play experiences. The nutrition counselor may want to consider role-playing activities to teach and evaluate basic nutrition concepts.

Pictures, puzzles, and games can challenge children as they develop cognitive and motor skills. For very young children, coloring a picture of the USDA Food Guide or drawing a picture of a favorite food in each group can foster both motor and cognitive skill building. Use of the food pyramid and food models to plan a special meal or to go on a trip to the grocery store can be an exciting activity. School-aged children can often incorporate math and reading skills into food activities by planning the number of servings per day of a food or measuring the ingredients for baking. Cutting out magazine pictures of food and arranging them in a collage or mobile by food group can spur interest in food variety.

Children learn important nutrition concepts through daily food experiences. Cooking can be an enjoyable activity for many children; however, many parents may be reluctant to use this activity, anticipating chaos and inedible results. The nutrition counselor should encourage parents to use this activity and to plan ahead, taking time to help children prepare simple recipes. Cooking helps develop important skills in a number of areas, including language, science, nutrition, art, sensory-motor development, socioemotional development, social studies, and mathematics.[20]

Social Experiences

Family mealtime can provide high-quality, positive social interactions that facilitate a child's cognitive abilities, enhance the nurturing process, promote family values, and affirm a sense of identity and security. Unfortunately, many families find it difficult to eat together regularly. The role of the nutrition counselor is to encourage parents to provide at least one family mealtime daily, where the child can experience the companionship of family members and a positive feeding environment. To assist families to "reconnect," meals can be planned outside in the yard, at a park, or at a restaurant with as many family members present as possible.

ROLE OF THE PARENT

Developmental Stage of the Parent

The nutrition counselor must assess not only the developmental level of the child, but also that of the parent. Providing complex information that the parent is unable to understand or apply will serve only to stress the family environment and to decrease compliance. In general, the nutrition counselor may want to consider having all initial materials provided to parents to be written at a 6th-grade reading level to facilitate learning and to provide quick access for review at a later time. More complex information can always be provided as the situation demands.

Cultural Influences

In today's multicultural society, sensitivity to the ethnic and religious facets of a child's environment is critical to long-term compliance with the nutrition plan of care. Incorporating ethnic foods into the meal plan can facilitate the entire family unit supporting the diet interventions versus expectations that the child must eat "differently." Knowledge of cultural and religious traditions and how these can be integrated into day-to-day meals and activity is also an important asset for the nutrition counselor to possess.[21]

At times, it may be difficult to ascertain if a child and/or caregiver with cultural considerations understands the information relayed. Asking directly, or through an interpreter, for the client to describe, demonstrate, or apply key concepts will assist in assessing counseling efforts. Before providing written materials, determine the client's reading ability. Written information resources may be obtained from local health departments or health care facilities who utilize translators. Curriculum development specialists in local school districts may be useful to identify cross-cultural materials or resources targeted at child nutrition. State or federal health programs may often be an additional resource on non-English materials.

Feeding Relationship

The ability to observe the feeding relationship between child and parent can provide tremendous insight into potential barriers to adequate nutrition. For children with feeding difficulties enrolled in rehabilitation programs, observation of a feeding session with a speech therapist can provide valuable information on the parent-child relationship. Asking parents to record a food diary for 2 to 3 days, including the time of feedings and where the feedings took place, provides information on the structure of the family lifestyle. For older children, input from caregivers or school personnel, where available, can be helpful as well. In addition, in-depth probing on the parent's feelings toward food and the child's particular feeding issues can assist in developing a successful nutrition care plan.

Psychosocial Relationship with Child

Parents will sometimes comment on the difficulty they have in getting a child to eat or to comply with a modified diet. Careful attention to the feelings of the parent in regard to the child's actions can aid the nutrition counselor in assessing the parent-child psychosocial relationship when it comes to food. Food can become a power struggle; one that usually neither side wins without outside intervention. It is also important to assess the relationship between parents. One parent sabotaging the other's efforts will often be picked up on quickly by the child, making compliance with the nutrition plan difficult and challenging.

Model Behavior

Children look to their parents as role models. The nutrition counselor must help parents to understand that the family must help the child adapt to any needed diet modifications, but in many cases, the nutrition plan of care can be used by all members of the family to promote health. For the child who is battling a weight problem, having the entire family become more active and follow a low-fat, balanced diet will facilitate compliance and improve the health status of the entire family. In some cases, the nutrition counselor may, in fact, become a role model for the child if the family situation lacks the support and follow-through.

COUNSELING THE CHILD WITH SPECIAL NEEDS

The nutrition counselor who sees children with special needs must be attuned to the developmental stages and cues previously discussed. Chronological age often does not correlate with the abilities of the child, and the level of parental involvement can vary significantly. The etiology of the disability and its physiologic and psychosocial implications on nutrition status must be determined. The medical nutrition therapy protocols (such as for failure to thrive[22,23]) can provide the nutrition counselor with clinical and functional outcomes to be monitored, as well as with potential interventions that may be considered.

The first step that the nutrition counselor should consider is accommodations required by the population served to make services as accessible as possible. Laurel Hayes[24] outlines many of the general considerations that the counselor should take into account. Specific to the field of nutrition counseling, scales and other equipment should be calibrated to accommodate the non-ambulatory client. Reference materials specific to special populations (such as growth grids and activity conversion factors) should be readily available. The nutrition counselor should also have a good working knowledge of the disabilities most frequently encountered and the impact on the family unit as a whole. Play therapy allows many children with special needs to discover what strengths they have in relation to their disabilities. The involvement of parents and/or caregivers becomes key in this population and may also entail coordination of efforts with other health care professionals.

SUMMARY

Developmental considerations are important in determining the interview approach to be used. Flexibility and the establishment of rapport are key to a successful nutrition interview. Key tips for parents to facilitate nutrition learning experiences include:

- establish routines for the feeding experience
- talk to children about how they feel about foods and any necessary diet modifications prescribed by the health care provider
- help children tie their self-worth to actions regarding food selections instead of body image
- model appropriate behavior, including diet selections and physical activity behavior
- re-direct a child's attention or activity by using neutral or positive language (such as "Potato chips are fine for an occasional snack, but here is some fresh fruit that would be a better snack.")
- acknowledge positive behavior (such as "You helped me plan a very healthy meal for dinner tonight.")
- do not make food and diet selections a power struggle
- do not use food as a reward or a punishment
- recognize that each child is an individual and is unique

Evers[25] summarizes the most successful approach to pediatric nutrition counseling with what she calls the FIB (fun, integrated, behavior change) approach to nutrition education. First, the nutrition counseling experience should be fun for the parent, child, and nutrition counselor. Creating engaging methods to illustrate basic nutrition concepts can be a challenge but an enjoyable one. Secondly, nutrition should be integrated wherever possible. The effective nutrition counselor finds ways for parents and children to integrate the basic nutrition concepts into their daily lifestyle. Change may be gradual but gradual change may be more permanent. Last, but not least, behavior change is key. Possessing the knowledge is one thing; making the necessary lifestyle changes is another. The nutrition counselor must assist the parents in making healthy choices as a family unit, not expecting the change to affect just the child. Changes isolated only to the child foster noncompliance and can potentially influence the child's self-image negatively in the long term. Involving the whole family in making wise food and activity choices can promote a more permanently healthy lifestyle for all involved.

REFERENCES

1. Klawitter B. Counseling: Child, adolescent, and family. In: King K, Klawitter B, eds. *Nutrition Therapy: Advanced Counseling Skills,* 2nd ed. Lake Dallas, TX: Helm Publishing; 2003:19–29.
2. Yusson SR, Santrock JW. *Child Development: An Introduction.* Dubuque, IA: WC Brown Co; 1982.
3. Gullo DF. *Developmentally Appropriate Teaching in Early Childhood.* Washington, DC: National Education Association; 1992.
4. Pellegrini AD, Smith PK. Physical activity play: The nature and function of a neglected aspect of play. *Child Dev.* 1998;69:577–598.
5. Jackson NE, Robinson HB, Dale PS. *Cognitive Development in Young Children.* Washington, DC: National Institute of Education; 1976.
6. Barker P. *Clinical Interviews with Children and Adolescents.* New York: WW Norton and Company; 1990.
7. Knell SM. Cognitive-behavioral play therapy. *J Clin Child Psych.* 1998;27(1):28–33.
8. Anderson JR. *Cognitive Psychology and Its Implications,* 3rd ed. New York: WH Freeman; 1990.
9. Committee on Nutrition. Prevention of pediatric overweight and obesity. *Pediatrics.* 2003;112(2);424–430.

10. Arluk SL, Branch JD, Swain DP, Dowling FA. Childhood obesity's relationship to time spent in sedentary behavior. *Mil Med.* 2003;168(7):583–586.
11. Barlow SE, Dietz WH. Management of child and adolescent obesity: Summary and recommendations based on reports from pediatricians, pediatric nurse practitioners, and registered dietitians. *Pediatrics.* 2002;110(1 Part 2):236–238.
12. Hayes LL. Counseling resistant teens. *CTOnline.* 1997;40:1–3.
13. Andersen AE. Eating disorders in males. In: Brownell K, Fairburn CG, eds. *Eating Disorders and Obesity. A Comprehensive Handbook.* New York: Guilford Press; 1995:177–182.
14. Holbrook TL, Weltzin TE. Eating disorders in males: A neglected problem revisited. *Treatment Today.* 1998;10.
15. Ivey AE, Ivey MB, Simek-Morgan L. *Counseling and Psychotherapy: A Multicultural Perspective,* 3rd ed. Boston, MA: Allyn & Bacon; 1993.
16. Glascoe FP, Oberklaid F, Dworkin PH, Trimm F. Brief approaches to educating patients and parents in primary care. *Pediatrics.* 1998;101:E10.
17. American Heart Association. *Exercise (Physical Activity) and Children.* AHA Scientific Position. Chicago, IL: 1998.
18. Klawitter B. Counseling: The adult learner. In: King K, Klawitter B, eds. *Nutrition Therapy: Advanced Counseling Skills,* 2nd ed. Lake Dallas, TX: Helm Publishing; 2003:31–45.
19. King K. Successful business skills. In: King K, Klawitter B, eds. *Nutrition Therapy: Advanced Counseling Skills,* 2nd ed. Lake Dallas, TX: Helm Publishing; 2003: 261–269.
20. Vaughn S. *Cooking and Learning Together.* Resource Sheet #22. Ontario, Canada: Canadian Child Care Federation; 1996.
21. Gonzales R, Klawitter B. Cultural competency in counseling. In: King K, Klawitter B, eds. *Nutrition Therapy: Advanced Counseling Skills,* 2nd ed. Lake Dallas, TX: Helm Publishing; 2003:57–74.
22. American Dietetic Association and Morrison Healthcare, Inc. *Medical Nutrition Therapy Across the Continuum of Care: Supplement 1.* Chicago, IL: American Dietetic Association; 1997.
23. Dietitians Independent Practice Association. *The Handbook of Medical Nutrition Therapy: Practice Guidelines, Protocols, Codes, and Outcomes.* Lake Dallas, TX: Helm Publishing; 1998.
24. Hayes LL. Counseling individuals with disabilities. *CTOnline.* 1997;40:2–5.
25. Evers CL. *How to Teach Nutrition to Kids*. Tigard, OR: Carrot Press; 2003.

Chapter 8

Vegetarian Diets for Children

Virginia Messina

Appropriately planned lacto-ovo vegetarian and vegan diets can meet nutrient needs during all stages of the lifecycle. These diets have been associated with reduced risk for chronic disease in adulthood and have also been shown to reduce risk factors for future heart disease in children.[1] All parents face challenges in helping children choose healthful foods regardless of the type of diet the family follows. Normal variations in growth patterns and psychosociological development throughout childhood affect children's food preferences and behaviors. For parents of vegetarian children, particular attention should be given to those nutrients that are traditionally supplied by animal foods in American diets. When parents follow appropriate guidelines, plant-based diets are adequate and sometimes superior nutrition throughout childhood.

This chapter provides an overview of the nutrients that deserve special attention in vegetarian diets followed by discussions of growth and development of vegetarian infants, children, and adolescents. Guidelines for meal planning and recommendations for addressing special situations for vegetarian children and teens are offered.

TYPES OF VEGETARIAN DIETS

Although the concept of vegetarianism appears in writings from as early as the 6th century BCE, the term was not coined until the mid-1800s when national vegetarian societies were formed in both England and the United States. Vegetarian diets were associated with some Christian church denominations in the 19th century and with the health reform movement of the Victorian era.

Today, a diverse group of individuals choose vegetarian diets for different reasons, most citing ethical (animal welfare), environmental, spiritual, or health reasons. An important influence has been the Seventh-day Adventist church, a Christian denomination that encourages a healthful lifestyle, including exercise, abstinence from smoking and alcohol, and vegetarian diet. It is believed that approximately 50% of church members are vegetarian. Large-scale epidemiologic studies conducted by Adventist-affiliated institutions have provided a wealth of information about health status of vegetarians.

The number of self-described vegetarians in the United States was approximately 12 million people in 1992 according to a Gallup poll, but the number of people who actually adhere to a meatless diet is probably much smaller.[2] According to a Harris poll conducted for the Vegetarian Resource Group in 2003, and which surveyed actual eating habits, there were approximately 5.7 million adult vegetarians in the United States, or 2.8% of the population.[3]

Most vegetarians consume either a lacto-ovo vegetarian or vegan diet. Vegans consume no meat, fish, poultry, eggs, or dairy products. Lacto-ovo vegetarians consume no meat, fish, or poultry but do consume eggs and dairy products. Although the widely held perception has been that most vegetarians consume a lacto-ovo vegetarian diet, this appears to be true only when the population of self-described vegetarians is considered. Polls of actual eating habits suggest that one third to one half of actual vegetarians are vegan.[3,4] A Roper poll conducted in 2000 suggested that 2% of American children (ages 8 to 17) are vegetarian and approximately 25% of these children consume a vegan diet.[5]

NUTRITIONAL CONSIDERATIONS IN VEGETARIAN DIETS FOR CHILDREN

Protein

Concerns about protein in vegetarian diets have focused largely on the fact that plant proteins have lower concentrations of certain limiting amino acids and are less well digested. However, the Institute of Medicine, in establishing protein RDAs for Americans concluded that protein recommendations are no higher for vegetarians than omnivores, provided vegetarians consume a complementary mixture of plant proteins.[6] In the past, it was believed that vegetarians needed to consume complementary proteins at the same time. It is now recognized that consuming a variety of foods throughout the day and meeting energy needs will ensure adequate protein intake for vegetarians.[7]

Although protein combining at meals is not necessary for adults, it may be helpful in meeting protein needs of infants and young children. One study in children showed that the supplementary effect of beans added to a corn-based diet was less when beans were eaten more than 6 hours after corn was eaten.[7] Because children eat frequently throughout the day, however, their meals are likely to be timed closely enough to provide the benefits of complementary amino acid profiles.

Some nutritionists have suggested that vegan children may have slightly higher protein requirements to compensate for digestibility and amino acid composition.[8] For young children, this might translate to just 1 to 9 additional grams of protein per day and needs are easily met when children include small amounts of legumes, nuts, and soyfoods in their diet.

Fat

Like vegetarian adults, children on vegetarian diets consume a smaller percentage of their calories from fat.[9,10] Studies in nonvegetarian children suggest that reduced fat intakes do not compromise growth in childhood when fat intake is between 21% and 38% of calories.[11] However, in some vegetarian families, an emphasis on very low fat intakes may translate to restrictions of healthful foods such as nuts, seeds, and soy products. These foods can be important in helping young children meet nutrient needs and their inclusion in vegetarian diets should be encouraged. The judicious use of added fats can also help to support adequate energy intake in vegetarian, and particularly vegan, children.

Vegetarian diets for children should include good sources of the essential omega-3 fatty acid, linolenic acid. These include ground flaxseed, canola oil, walnuts, and soy products. Both linoleic acid and trans fatty acids can interfere with conversion of alpha linolenic acid to the long chain omega-3 fatty acids.[12,13] Therefore, limiting solid vegetable fats like margarine and vegetable shortening and vegetable oils that are rich in linoleic acid such as safflower and sunflower oils, can help maximize conversion of alpha-linolenic acid to the long chain omega-3 fatty acids.[12,13]

Calcium

Vegan children who do not consume fortified foods are at risk for not meeting calcium requirements. One factor affecting calcium intake in vegan families may be the belief held by some vegans that calcium requirements are lower on plant-based diets compared to omnivore diets. This is based on research linking lower intakes of animal proteins to better calcium retention and reduced risk of fracture. Ecological studies support such a relationship, but epidemiologic studies within populations generally do not. For example, higher calcium intakes (342 vs. 1056 mg/d) in Gambian children on near-vegan diets were shown to improve bone mineral status.[14] Chinese children with very low calcium intakes also had improved bone density after 18 months of calcium supplementation.[15] Both genetics and a variety of lifestyle factors affect bone density and possibly calcium requirements. Vegan parents should be encouraged to provide diets for their children that meet calcium recommendations established by the Institute of Medicine. At this time, there is no reason to believe that Western vegan children have lower calcium needs than their omnivore peers.

An important consideration is bioavailability of calcium from plant foods. Calcium is poorly absorbed from some beans, unhulled sesame seeds, and high-oxalate vegetables such as spinach and beet greens. It is well-absorbed from soy products, fortified juices, and low-oxalate vegetables such as kale, collards, mustard greens, turnip greens, and broccoli.[16] Although unfortified plant foods are generally lower in calcium than cow's milk, the high absorption rates from some of these foods, such as the low-oxalate vegetables, makes them good sources of this nutrient overall.

Plant sources of calcium often provide other compounds that may contribute to bone health such as isoflavones in soyfoods[17] and vitamin K in vegetables.[18] Both lacto-ovo vegetarian and vegan children should be encouraged to consume a variety of calcium-rich plant foods. See Exhibit 8–1 for food sources of selected nutrients.

Vitamin D

For light-skinned children in sunny climates, exposing the hands and face to the sun two or three times a week for about 20 to 30 minutes per time has been shown to be adequate exposure for synthesis of vitamin D.[19] However, a number of factors interfere with vitamin D synthesis. These include use of sunscreen, smog, low sunlight levels at northern latitudes (in the Northern Hemisphere), and darker skin pigmentation. A regular source of dietary vitamin D is recommended for children who are otherwise at risk for vitamin D deficiency.

Vitamin D is poorly supplied by foods with fish and egg yolks being among the few natural sources. Therefore, for both vegetarian and nonvegetarian children, fortification is nearly always depended upon for vitamin D. Lacto-ovo vegetarian children can obtain adequate vitamin D from cow's milk, which is fortified in the United States. A number of vegan products are vitamin D fortified, including various brands of soymilk or rice milk and many commercial cereals.

Vitamin B12

Vitamin B12 occurs naturally only in animal foods or in foods contaminated with B12-produc-

Exhibit 8–1 Food Sources of Selected Nutrients for Vegetarians

Protein	Soyfoods and soymilk, legumes, nuts, seeds, cow's milk
Calcium	Almond butter, tahini, figs, textured soy protein, soynuts, kale, broccoli, collards, mustard greens, turnip greens, corn tortillas (processed with lime), vegetarian baked beans, black beans, blackstrap molasses, fortified soymilk, fortified rice milk, fortified almond milk, fortified fruit juices, calcium-set tofu, cow's milk, cheese
Iron	Bran flakes, instant oatmeal, whole-wheat bread, enriched white bread, nuts, nut butters, potatoes (with skin), dried fruits, legumes, enriched cereals, whole grain cereals
Zinc	Whole grains, nuts, seeds, legumes, fortified breakfast cereals, cow's milk, cheese
Vitamin B12	Fortified meat analogues, fortified breakfast cereals, fortified soymilk, nutritional yeast (Red Star Vegetarian Support Formula), cow's milk, cheese, and yogurt
Vitamin D	Fortified soymilk, fortified cow's milk, and fortified breakfast cereals
Linolenic acid	Flaxseed, flaxseed oil, canola oil, walnuts, soyfoods, eggs (if chickens are fed omega-3 fatty acid-rich diet)

ing microbes. Throughout the world, people on plant-based diets may obtain adequate vitamin B12 due to bacterial contamination, but in the more hygienic environments of the United States, it is risky to depend on these sources. Sea vegetables and cultured soy products such as miso and tempeh, once believed to be sources of vitamin B12, have been shown to be poor sources of the active vitamin.[20] The presence of B12 analogues in these foods could increase the likelihood of deficiency because they interfere with absorption of the active vitamin. All vegetarians should be counseled on the need to identify and regularly consume dietary sources of vitamin B12. These can be dairy products for lacto-ovo vegetarians, fortified foods such as many brands of soymilk, meat analogues, and breakfast cereals, or a vitamin supplement pill. Nutritional yeast that is grown on a vitamin B12-rich medium is a popular source of vitamin B12 for vegans. Parents should be advised that neither brewer's yeast nor active baking yeast are sources of this nutrient and that nutritional yeast is a good source only if the growing medium contains vitamin B12. A reliable source is Red Star brand Vegetarian Support Formula nutritional yeast.

Iron

Vegetarian diets are typically higher in iron than diets that contain meat, with vegan intakes being higher than lacto-ovo.[21,22] However, the nonheme iron found in plant foods has lower bioavailability than heme iron in meats, and vegetarians have been shown to have smaller body stores of iron.[2,23] Therefore, the Institute of Medicine has specified higher iron RDAs for vegetarians.[24] The actual requirement for iron, however, depends on inhibitors and enhancers of iron absorption in the diet and some vegetarians probably have needs that are lower than those recommended by the Institute of Medicine.

Despite smaller iron stores, vegetarians are no more likely to be diagnosed with iron deficiency anemia than omnivores.[25,26] However, because iron deficiency anemia is the most common childhood nutritional problem in all dietary populations with risk highest for toddlers and teenage girls, it is very important to counsel vegetarians about sources of iron and ways to maximize absorption.

The main inhibitor of iron in vegetarian diets is phytate found in whole grains and legumes. Leavening of grains with yeast hydrolyzes phytate and makes iron more available so that breads are better sources of available iron than grains and crackers.[27]

Vitamin C enhances the absorption of nonheme iron in the diet when these nutrients are consumed at the same meal.[28] Other organic acids in fruits and vegetables may also improve iron absorption.[29]

Excessive consumption (more than 3 cups daily after age 1 year) of milk and other dairy products can raise the risk for iron deficiency because cow's milk is devoid of iron and can displace iron-rich foods in the diet.[30] Both milk and calcium are also potent inhibitors of iron absorption,[31,32] and milk can cause iron loss through intestinal bleeding in infants.[33] Lacto-ovo vegetarians should be counseled to use dairy foods in moderation and calcium supplements should be taken between meals.

Zinc

Vegetarians may require up to 50% more zinc than the RDA depending on the composition of their diet, because both fiber and phytate interfere with zinc absorption.[24] In developing countries, overt zinc deficiency has been seen in children with diets high in unleavened whole grain breads and who have other predisposing factors for zinc deficiency such as parasitic infections. This does not predict zinc status in Western vegetarians, however, where zinc absorption is likely to be considerably better. Dairy products are good sources of zinc for lacto-ovo vegetarian children. Parents of young vegans should be encouraged to regularly include legumes and nuts in children's diets because these foods are rich in both protein and zinc, and protein enhances zinc absorption.[34] Zinc is also well-absorbed from yeast-leavened breads and fermented soy products such like tempeh and miso. Although zinc absorption is lower from whole grains, the total amount of zinc absorbed is greater than from refined grains, which are very low in this nutrient.[35] Soaking dried beans and discarding the soaking water prior to cooking can reduce phytate content and improve zinc absorption. If a vegan child's diet is based on high-phytate cereals and legumes, zinc supplementation should be considered.

VEGETARIAN INFANTS

Children can safely be raised on vegetarian diets from birth. All infants are, or should be, essentially vegetarian during the first 7 to 8 months of life because meats are generally not included in diets until that time. First solid foods, ideally introduced between 4 and 6 months of age, are usually infant cereals, followed by vegetables and fruits. Vegetable proteins (legumes or tofu) can be substituted for strained meats in the diets of older infants.

Growth in Vegetarian Infants

With the exception of some macrobiotic populations, infants born to vegetarian mothers have birth weights similar to norms and to those of infants born to nonvegetarian women.[36,37] Vegetarian infants who receive adequate breast milk or formula, including soy infant formula, and whose diets include adequate sources of iron, vitamin B12, and vitamin D, grow well.[1] Vegetarian mothers are more likely to breastfeed, which may explain the slightly slower rate of growth seen in vegetarian infants.[38,39]

Nutritional deficiencies and poor growth have been seen in some populations that follow unusually restrictive diets that do not conform to appropriate guidelines for feeding infants.[40–42] These findings are not appropriate arguments against the suitability of well-planned vegetarian diets for infants. When vegetarian families have access to good information about diet and have regular access to a qualified health care provider, diets are far more likely to be adequate.

Guidelines for Feeding Vegetarian and Vegan Infants

For the first 4 months of life, vegetarian infants, like all infants, require only breast milk or commercial infant formula. Vegan women need to supplement their diet with vitamin B12 if their infant does not receive a B12 supplement because vitamin B12 from a woman's stores may not be available in her milk.[43]

Infants in vegan families should receive 0.4 μg/day of vitamin B12 starting at birth if the mother's diet is not supplemented. Like all infants, vegetarian infants should receive vitamin D supplements beginning in the first 2 months and sources of iron (iron-fortified cereal, supplemental drops, or iron-fortified formula) beginning at age 4 months. Where water is not fluoridated, fluoride supplements are usually prescribed at approximately 6 months of age. Some experts recommend zinc supplements during the time when solid foods are being introduced to the infant's diet if these foods are low in zinc or zinc bioavailability.[44] Although this may be of particular importance for some vegetarian infants, zinc supplements are not routinely recommended for all vegetarian infants because zinc deficiency is rarely seen in these infants.[45] If zinc supplements are used for older infants, total zinc intake should not exceed 5 mg/day.

Solid foods should be introduced by age 6 months, with developmental signs of readiness rather than age serving as a guide (see Chapter 5). Exhibit 8–2 shows a flexible set of guidelines for introduction of solid foods to a vegetarian infant. Vegetarian parents should be encouraged to prepare their own infant foods in order to expand choices. If local soil is high in lead, however, parents should be cautioned against making these foods from home-grown vegetables.

Soy Formulas

Infant soy formulas are based on soy protein that has been fortified with methionine, carnitine, and taurine. All soy formulas are fortified with iron, zinc, and calcium, and are lactose free. The calcium, phosphorus, and protein contents of these formulas are higher than in cow's milk formula to compensate for lower bioavailability of these nutrients. Soy formula supports normal growth and development in full-term infants.[46] Soy formulas are not recommended for preterm

Exhibit 8–2 Introduction of Solid Foods in the Diets of Vegetarian Infants

4–6 months	• Introduce iron-fortified rice cereal, according to the guidelines in Chapter 5, followed by oat and barley cereals. • When infants are consuming 1/3 to 1/2 cup of cereal per day over several feedings, mashed fruits and vegetables can be introduced. Good choices include smooth applesauce; pureed peaches and pears canned in their own juice; strained potatoes, carrots, sweet potatoes, and green beans; and mashed bananas and avocados.
7–9 months	• Most infants will begin to drink from a cup, allowing introduction of juices such as apple juice. • Higher protein foods are typically introduced at this age. Choices for first protein-rich foods for vegetarian infants include thoroughly cooked and pureed legumes or mashed tofu. In lacto-ovo vegetarian families, infants may also have pureed cottage cheese, yogurt, and egg yolks. • Stronger tasting vegetables may be introduced at this time. Blending vegetables such as kale and collards with blander foods like avocado, applesauce, tofu, or cottage cheese, can temper the flavor and make them more acceptable to infants.
10–12 months	• Older vegetarian infants can begin to eat finger foods such as tofu chunks, crackers, and bread.
12 months	• Infants can begin to consume the smooth nut and seed butters that are popular in many vegetarian families such as tahini and almond butter. As for all infants, peanut butter should not be fed to vegetarians before 18 months of age because of concerns about allergic reactions.

infants and therefore, there is currently no vegan formula available for preterm infants.[47]

Estimates are that between 50% and 85% of infants with cow's milk allergy will not develop allergies to soy protein.[48] Therefore, soy formula can be a viable option for many infants with a milk allergy. Soy formula used in the place of cow's milk formula has also been shown to reduce colic symptoms.[49]

Recently, questions have arisen about the effects of soy isoflavones (phytoestrogens) in infants, because these compounds have a variety of hormonal and nonhormonal effects.[50] Soy formulas contain significant levels of soy isoflavones ranging from 155.1 to 281.4 μg/g and infants who consume soy infant formula have elevated plasma isoflavone levels.[51] However, a study of close to 250 adults who had received soy formula as infants found no effect of soy formula on fertility, miscarriage rate, birth defects in offspring, and maturation.[52]

It is important that parents understand the difference between soy infant formula and commercial soy beverages. Although small amounts used in food preparation are acceptable, commercial soy beverages should not be used in place of breast milk or soy infant formula for the same reasons that cow's milk is not an appropriate substitute for cow's milk formula.

PRESCHOOL AND SCHOOL-AGE CHILDREN

Growth of Vegetarian Children

Although stature is widely perceived as an important measure of health among populations, optimal health is not related to height. In fact, taller individuals appear to be at increased risk for both cancer[53] and hip fracture.[54] Lower body mass index in childhood may be associated with a reduction in cardiovascular mortality in adulthood and risk for obesity.[55,56] Nevertheless, a normal growth pattern is an important indicator of health and comparison of growth of vegetarian children to omnivore children is commonly used to assess adequacy of vegetarian diets.

Studies suggest that when diets are adequately planned, lacto-ovo vegetarian children have similar growth patterns to omnivore children.[57,58] Growth rates of Seventh-day Adventist children, a large percentage of whom are lacto-ovo vegetarian, equal or exceed those of omnivore children.[59,60] One exception is seen in Seventh-day Adventist preadolescent girls who are slightly shorter than omnivore controls. This may be due to a later growth spurt among Adventist girls[61] and may be associated with a reduced risk for breast cancer in adulthood.[62]

Older studies of growth in vegan children have been somewhat problematic because they included children following macrobiotic diets. These diets can be considerably different from more usual vegan eating patterns with many more food restrictions and are generally not useful in assessing growth in vegan children today.[63]

A study of 404 nonmacrobiotic vegan children aged 4 months to 10 years who lived in a vegan community in Tennessee, showed that although they were slightly shorter than controls at ages 1 through 5, they were comparable in height by age 10.[37] British vegan children aged 1 to 18 years also exhibited normal growth.[39]

Diets of Vegetarian Children

Children following lacto-ovo, vegan, and macrobiotic diets have average protein intakes that meet or exceed recommendations.[9,58,63,64] Fat and cholesterol intakes of vegetarian children come closer to meeting recommendations of the National Cholesterol Education Program and vegetarian children have been shown to have lower blood cholesterol levels than omnivore children.[65,66]

Although data are limited, calcium intakes of lacto-ovo vegetarian children generally exceed calcium recommendations,[10] while limited data suggest that the calcium content of vegan children's diets is lower than recommendations.[38]

Like vegetarian adults, children consuming plant-based diets have higher iron intakes than omnivore children.[38,67] Although vegetarian children have been shown to have lower iron stores compared to omnivores, they are no more likely to suffer from iron deficiency anemia.[68,69] Zinc supplementation may be indicated in young children following a vegan diet based on high-phytate cereal and legumes, but experts do not advocate supplementation of this nutrient other than on an individual basis.

Meeting Dietary Needs of Young Vegetarian Children

Tables 8–1 and 8–2 show guidelines for feeding vegetarian toddlers and children. Although milk is not essential in diets of children, vegetarian children may meet nutrient needs more easily if some type of fortified milk is consumed. Lacto-ovo vegetarian children may consume vitamin D–fortified whole cows' milk beginning at the first birthday and this should be changed to a low-fat milk at age 2. Both lacto-ovo and vegan children may use a full-fat soymilk (which has a fat content similar to 2% cow's milk) that is fortified with calcium, vitamin D, and vitamin B12. Rice and almond milks are lower in protein and calories than soymilk and are generally not recommended as a primary milk for young children. When they are chosen, due to preference or allergies, it is important to choose fortified brands and to emphasize other protein-rich foods in the diet. Breast milk is also an option, and many children may consume breast milk well into their second year.

It is important that parents of vegan children identify a regular source of vitamin B12 to be included in the diet. This might be a fortified soymilk, nutritional yeast, fortified breakfast cereals, fortified meat analogues, or a vitamin supplement. Children should have two servings of these foods per day.

Toddlers typically experience a decrease in appetite and this, along with increasing independence, can manifest in picky eating habits. Both vegetarian and omnivore families face challenges in providing adequate nutrition to children at this time. While most children enjoy grains,

Table 8–1 Meal Planning Guidelines for Children, 1–3 years

Food	*Servings per day*
Grains A serving is 1/2 to 1 slice bread; 1/4 to 1/2 cup cooked cereal, grain, or pasta; 1/2 to 1 cup ready-to-eat cereal.	6+
Legumes, nuts, and other protein-rich foods A serving is 1/4 to 1/2 cup cooked beans, tofu, tempeh, or textured vegetable protein; 1 oz meat analogue; 1–2 tbsp nuts seeds, or nut or seed butter; 1 egg; 3/4 oz cheese; 1/2 cup yogurt.	2+ (vegan children should include at least 1 serving per day of nuts or seeds or 1 full-fat soy product)
Vegetables A serving is 1/4 to 1/2 cup cooked; 1/2 to 1 cup raw.	2+
Fruits A serving is 1/4 to 1/2 cup canned; 1/2 cup juice; 1/2 medium piece of fruit.	3+
Fats A serving is 1 tsp margarine or oil.	3–4 (include one serving daily of a source of omega-3 fatty acids)
Fortified soymilk, cow's milk, or breast milk A serving is 1 cup.	3

Source: Reprinted with permission from Mangels AR, Messina VK, Messina MJ. *The Dietitian's Guide to Vegetarian Diets: Issues and Applications.* Sudbury, MA: Jones and Bartlett; 2004.

fruits, and nuts, they may be reluctant to try new vegetables and legumes.

Familiarity is an important dimension of food preference for young children and they may need to be presented with a new food as many as 10 times before they will try it.[70] New foods may be more acceptable to children if they are offered in small amounts along with familiar, well-liked foods. Children prefer foods that are easy to eat such as strips of vegetables or mashed beans served with crackers or chips for dipping. Raw vegetables may be more acceptable than cooked ones. Flavors of strong-tasting vegetables such as kale, collards, or other greens can be tempered by blending them with bland-tasting foods, such as tofu, avocado, or ricotta cheese. To increase a child's intake of vegetables, these foods can be shredded or chopped finely and mixed into soups, spaghetti sauce, or veggie burgers.

The high fiber content of vegetarian meals can fill a child up quickly. Including some refined foods in a young child's diet can help ensure adequate energy intake. Nutritious choices include hot cereals such as farina or Cream of Rice, many ready-to-eat cereals, muffins made with 1/2 white flour and 1/2 whole-wheat flour, applesauce, fruit juice, and white rice. Other ways to increase the energy content of a child's diet are to include higher-calorie foods such as bean spreads, nut butters, avocado as a sandwich spread or in small chunks, soymilk shakes with fruits, and dried fruit spreads. Small amounts of added fats, such as mayonnaise (eggless mayonnaise is available for vegans) on sandwiches, a small amount of margarine on vegetables or bread, or foods sautéed in oil, can also help boost a child's calorie intake.

The use of supplemental foods can also make a significant contribution to a child's nutrient intake. Nutritional yeast that is reliably rich in vitamin B12 can be added to homemade veggie burgers and loaves, scrambled tofu, bread dough, white sauce to create a cheese-like sauce, or

Table 8–2 Diet-Planning Guidelines for School-Aged Children and Adolescents

Food Groups	*Ages (number of servings/day)*			
	Calcium-rich choices	*4–8 yrs*	*9–13 yrs*	*14–18 yrs*
Grains				
A serving is 1/2 cup cooked cereal, pasta, rice, or other grain; 1 oz ready-to-eat cereal; 1 slice bread.	1 oz calcium-fortified cereal	8	10	10
Legumes, Nuts, and Soyfoods				
A serving is 1/2 cup cooked beans, tofu, tempeh, fortified soymilk; 1/4 cup nuts; 1 oz meat analogue; 2 tbsp nut or seed butter.	Fortified soymilk, tempeh, calcium-set tofu, almonds, almond butter, tahini, soybeans, and soynuts	5	6	6
Vegetables				
A serving is 1/2 cup cooked vegetables, 1 cup raw vegetables, 1/2 cup vegetable juice.	Bok choy, broccoli, collards, Chinese cabbage, kale, mustard greens, turnip greens okra, fortified tomato juice	4	4	4
Fruits				
A serving is 1 medium fresh fruit, 1/2 cup cooked or cut-up fruit, 1/2 cup fruit juice, 1/4 cup dried fruit.	Calcium-fortified fruit juice; dried figs	2	2	3
Fats				
A serving is 1 tsp mayonnaise, soft margarine, or oil.		2	3	3

Food choices should include

- 6 servings from calcium-rich choices for 4–8 year olds and 10 choices for children 9–18.
- 2 servings per day of foods rich in omega-3 fatty acids (1 tsp faxseed oil, 1 tbsp ground flaxseed, 1 tbsp canola oil; 1/4 cup walnuts)
- 3 servings per day of foods rich in vitamin B12 (1 tbsp nutritional yeast, 1/2 cup cow's milk or fortified soymilk, 1/2 cup yogurt, 1 egg).
- A vitamin D supplement or fortified foods if children don't have regular exposure to sunshine.

Source: Adapted with permission from Mangels AR, Messina VK, Messina MJ. *The Dietitian's Guide to Vegetarian Diets: Issues and Applications.* Sudbury, MA: Jones and Bartlett; 2004.

sprinkled over popcorn. Blackstrap molasses is an excellent source of both calcium and iron. It can be added to baked beans or vegetable stew, used in muffin, cake, or cookie batter, mixed into milkshakes, or blended with nut butters. Exhibit 8–3 shows snack ideas.

Special Issues for Vegetarian School-Age Children

Peer pressure is an important influence on school-age children and some young vegetarians may be uncomfortable with their family's eating habits. Nutrition education in school may also be at variance with the family's eating practices. Vegetarian diets have an increasingly attractive image among young people, however. Parents can help by providing foods that appear more "mainstream" such as sandwiches made with meat analogues and soy cheese.

Some foods that are important parts of many vegetarian diets are not allowable items in the National School Lunch Program. For example, fortified soymilk cannot be served as a milk substitute. The US Department of Agriculture has recently ruled that there is no limit on the amount of vegetable protein products (soy, peanuts, tree nuts, or seeds) that can be used in the school lunch program and removal of this restriction may allow more vegetarian options to be served.[71]

Schools can choose from among four approaches to meal planning. The Nutrient Standard Menu Planning Approach and the Assisted Nutrient Standard Menu Planning Approach are computer-based systems that allow meals that meet a specific nutrient standard. These approaches can allow use of a greater number of vegetarian menu items than the more traditional approaches. For example, although tofu is not considered a vegetable protein product under the traditional menu planning approaches, it could easily be included in the School Lunch Program under the Nutrient Standard Menu Planning Approaches.

Lunches brought from home provide a better alternative to school lunches for many vegetarian children. Planning nutritious lunches around a child's food preferences increases the likelihood that lunches will be consumed. For vegan children, lunch brought from home is the only practical option in most school systems. Exhibit 8–4 offers ideas for bag lunches for vegetarian children.

Exhibit 8–3 Snacks for Vegetarian Children

Research indicates that children who eat more than six times per day are more likely to have higher intakes of calories, calcium, and vitamin C than average, whereas those who eat less than four times a day have lower than average intakes of iron and protein. Good snack ideas for vegetarian children include:

- muffins
- fruit-flavored milkshakes or smoothies using cow's or vegetable milk
- vegetable soup with crackers
- crackers spread thinly with nut butter
- trail mix (for older children)
- oatmeal cookies or graham crackers with juice
- frozen bananas
- frozen juice bars
- dried fruits
- fresh fruit
- yogurt with fruit
- bagel or English muffin half with fruit spread
- cold cereal with or without milk
- vegetables with dip (salsa or blended and flavored tofu, for example)

VEGETARIAN DIETS FOR ADOLESCENTS

Nutrition is often a low priority for teens, and poor eating habits can be typical of teenagers no matter what type of diet they choose. Omnivore teens often have diets that are low in zinc, folate, calcium, iron, vitamin A, and magnesium.[72]

Growth of Vegetarian Adolescents

Studies suggest there is little difference in growth between vegetarian and nonvegetarian teens.[73–75] In a study of 1,800 lacto-ovo vegetarians between the ages of 7 and 18 years, vegetarians were slightly taller than omnivores.[60] The exception was 11- and 12-year-old girls who were slightly shorter than omnivore peers, a finding that may be related to later age of menarche in vegetarians that has been seen in some[76] but not all[75] vegetarian girls.

Diets of Vegetarian Adolescents

Some research suggests that vegetarian adolescents have more healthful diets than their omnivore peers. Female vegetarian adolescents

Exhibit 8–4 Bag Lunch Ideas for Vegetarian Children

Sandwiches:

- Hummus spread with sliced tomatoes and lettuce
- Almond or peanut butter with shredded carrots
- Peanut butter blended with pureed tofu, ricotta cheese, or dried fruits
- "Missing egg" salad (egg salad with chopped tofu in place of the eggs and vegan mayonnaise)
- Avocado blended with chopped or shredded raw vegetables
- Peanut butter mixed with crushed pineapple and raisins
- "No tuna" salad (chopped chickpeas flavored with kelp powder and lemon in place of tuna)
- Submarine sandwich with cheese (soy or dairy), lettuce, tomatoes, and other sliced vegetables
- Veggie deli slices with sliced tomatoes
- Bean loaves or burgers with catsup or salsa
- Tofu burgers with catsup, mustard, pickle relish, lettuce, and tomatoes on a bun
- Cheese with sliced apples
- Mashed kidney beans and salsa in a whole-wheat tortilla

Lunch box stuffers:

- Fresh fruit
- Raw carrots, celery, or zucchini rounds or strips
- Trail mix
- Dried fruit
- Rice cakes
- Muffins
- Pasta salad
- Yogurt, dairy or soy
- Oatmeal cookies or other homemade cookies
- Graham crackers
- Granola bars
- Pretzels
- Individual containers of soy, rice, or almond milk
- Juice
- Water

were found to consume 40% more fiber and 20% more vitamin C than omnivores.[73] Vegetarian adolescents have also been found to be twice as likely as omnivores to consume fruits or vegetables, one third as likely to consume sweets, and one fourth as likely to eat salty snack foods more than once a day.[77] Vegetarian adolescents in Canada consumed more legumes, nuts, and vegetables than omnivores.[74] Diets of vegetarian teens are lower in total fat, saturated fat, and fast food and higher in vegetables, fiber, vitamin A, iron, and folate than their nonvegetarian peers.[78] Protein intake has been shown to be above requirements and similar to nonvegetarians.[74]

Omnivore teenagers, particularly girls, often do not meet the calcium RDA, and some data indicate lacto-ovo vegetarian adolescents also have diets that fall short in this nutrient.[68,75] Vegetarian girls have also been reported to have later menarche, which may raise the risk for osteoporosis, possibly due to shorter exposure to estrogen.

In a study of Canadian female teenagers, twice as many vegetarians as omnivores had ferritin levels indicative of depleted iron stores, although fewer vegetarians had two or more abnormal indices of iron status.[73,74] As for all teenage girls, there is a great need to emphasize good sources of iron in the diets of vegetarians.

Vegetarian teens had lower vitamin B12 intakes than nonvegetarian teens in one study, but average vitamin B12 intake of both groups was above current recommendations.[78]

Zinc is needed for growth and sexual maturation in adolescence. Zinc intake among vegetarian adolescents has been shown to be below the RDA,[25,58] although at least one study found higher zinc intake in vegetarian teens compared to omnivores.[79]

Meal Planning for Vegetarian Adolescents

Table 8–2 (see page 151) illustrates meal-planning guidelines for vegetarian teens. Particular attention should be given to iron, zinc, and calcium sources and a regular source of vitamin B12 should be identified in the diet of every vegetarian teen. When these nutrient needs are not being met, a supplement is warranted.

In planning menus for this age group, it is important to consider factors that impact food choices such as convenience and time. Teenagers consume many of their calories as snacks and consume many meals away from home. Parents can help to ensure better food choices by stocking the kitchen with healthful foods that can serve as quick snacks, portable meals, and even breakfasts that can be consumed en route to school.

Food choices can be a point of intense conflict in families, especially where teenagers choose a diet that is different from that of the rest of the family. When vegetarian teens live in an omnivore household, it is important to elicit support for, and interest in, the teen's diet from the parents. Some adolescents may experience difficulty in planning appropriate vegetarian diets if parents do not willingly cooperate by purchasing "special" foods such as soymilk, beans, and meat analogues.

Introducing more vegetarian meals that the whole family enjoys, such as spaghetti with tomato sauce or bean burritos, can be a unifying approach. Meals that can be served with or without meat, such as stir-fried dishes, are also helpful.

Eating Disorders

One survey has shown that vegetarian teenagers were more likely to have disordered eating behaviors including frequent dieting, binge eating, self-induced vomiting, and laxative use for weight control, than nonvegetarians.[77] Another study found that teens who described themselves as vegetarian were more weight conscious and more likely to have been told they had an eating disorder.[78] However, fully half of the self-described vegetarians in this study actually consumed meat. Limited data suggest that vegetarian diets are sometimes selected as a way to hide a pre-existing eating disorder,[79] with vegetarianism being chosen before the onset of anorexia nervosa in only 6% of cases examined in one study.[80] Eating disorders are multifaceted and have a complex etiology. There is no evidence that vegetarian diets increase risk for developing disordered eating behavior.[81,82]

Risk of Amenorrhea in Female Vegetarians and Female Vegetarian Athletes

Secondary amenorrhea, defined as the absence of three or more consecutive menstrual periods after menarche has been seen in some athletes and some vegetarians and appears to be due to a dysfunction of the hypothalamus. Amenorrhea associated with low estrogen levels in young women has been linked to decreased bone mineral density and increased risk for osteoporosis.[83]

Studies on menstrual cycle disturbances in vegetarians yield conflicting results. In a 6-month prospective study of 23 vegetarians and 22 nonvegetarian women who were not athletes, the vegetarians actually had a higher proportion of normal ovulatory cycles than nonvegetarians (76.7% versus 61.9%).[84] In a study of girls with a mean age of 16.2 years, there was no difference between lacto-ovo vegetarians and omnivores in the percentage of girls with normal ovulatory cycles.[85]

However, several cross-sectional studies have found menstrual cycle disturbances to be more common in vegetarians.[86–88] A study at The Pennsylvania State University found that 26.5% of vegetarian women experienced menstrual irregularities compared to just 4.9% of omnivore women.[87] However, in this study the nonvegetarians had used birth control pills longer than the vegetarians, which may have affected menstrual cycle regularity.

Vegetarians have been reported to have lower blood levels of estrogen and higher levels of the sex hormone–binding globulin, which would effectively lower the amount of biologically active estrogen in the circulation.[89] These effects may be due to the high-fiber and low-fat intake of vegetarians.[90,91] Other dietary factors that differ between vegetarians and nonvegetarians and that may affect menstrual cycle include fiber, fat, and meat intake. It has also been found that high blood levels of carotene may increase risk for irregular menstrual cycles.[92,93] This may help to explain why adoption of a mixed diet by sedentary amenorrheic vegetarian and semivegetarian women resulted in ovulation.[92] Some factors that affect menstrual cycle such as low-energy availability and excessive exercise may be at work in women who adopt vegetarian diets for weight loss.

Among athletes, several studies have reported a higher incidence of amenorrhea in vegetarians and semivegetarians compared to omnivores.[94,95] Other research has found rates of amenorrhea to be no higher among vegetarian athletes than nonvegetarians.[95]

Because of the many confounding variables in studies of amenorrhea, it has not been possible to establish vegetarianism as a clear risk factor. Low intakes of fat and energy and higher intakes of fiber may be factors. For these reasons, and pending further research, it is important to help vegetarian girls and young women choose diets that are adequate in fat and calories.

Macrobiotics Diets for Children

Macrobiotic philosophy is linked to the Chinese principles of yin and yang and foods central to this diet reflect Asian influences. The diet makes extensive use of brown rice, sea vegetables, Asian condiments such as tamari, miso, umeboshi plum, and root vegetables like daikon. Although there is wide variation in practice, traditionally, grains make up about 50% to 60% of the diet. Vegetables and miso soup play a central role and beans are also important parts of meals. Fruits, nuts, and seeds are used in moderation. Foods typically avoided are nightshade vegetables, like potatoes or eggplant, and tropical fruits, dairy foods, and processed sweeteners. Although some macrobiotic followers include fish in their diets, many consume a vegan diet.

Several studies of macrobiotics in the United States and the Netherlands have revealed nutritional deficiencies in macrobiotic infants.[41,42] Smaller size in macrobiotic children has been attributed to inadequate calories, calcium, vitamin B12, riboflavin, and zinc.[9,40,67,96,97]

Breastfeeding is common among macrobiotics, and mothers tend to breastfeed for longer than is typical in the general population.[98] However, in some cases, infants and toddlers may be weaned onto a homemade grain-based milk that is low in protein, calories, iron, and calcium and devoid of vitamin B12 and vitamin D. Tofu, legumes, and vegetables, including sea vegetables, may be added several months after weaning.

Deficiencies may occur on macrobiotic diets when tofu, legumes, and vegetables are the sole sources of calcium. If fat is restricted, the diet can be too low in energy. If the use of fortified foods is prohibited, macrobiotic children may suffer deficiencies of vitamin B12 and vitamin D.

Macrobiotic diets should not be confused with nonmacrobiotic vegan diets. Macrobiotic diets are generally more restrictive and often do not include fortified foods. However, because diets vary greatly among followers of macrobiotics, it cannot be assumed that these diets are deficient. Many infants and children in macrobiotic families are well-nourished. Those who counsel macrobiotic families should be prepared to work to the extent possible within the guidelines of macrobiotic principles. Diets for macrobiotic children can be planned using the guidelines in Tables 8–1 and 8–2 (see pages 150–151). It may be advisable to limit intake of sea vegetables in the diets of macrobiotic children whose intake of vitamin B12 is low. Although these foods may contain some active B12, they can also contain analogues that may interfere with the absorption of active vitamin B12. As for all vegetarian children, macrobiotic children must consume a reliable source of vitamin B12. Frequent sun exposure should be encouraged to ensure adequate vitamin D synthesis. However, because macrobiotics is popular in some northern areas of the United States and Europe, a supplemental form of vitamin D will almost always be advisable.

CONCLUSION

Studies of growth and development of vegetarian children produce expected results. When vegetarian children are fed well-balanced diets that follow appropriate guidelines, they grow well. Often, their diets come closer to recommendations by nutrition experts. Health parameters in well-nourished vegetarian children may be closer to optimal than children following more standard American patterns. However, when children are fed inappropriately restrictive diets that do not follow accepted guidelines for vegetarian meal planning, they are at great risk for nutrient deficiency and for compromised growth and health.

Parents of vegetarian children face many of the same challenges as their omnivore peers in providing healthful foods to their families. Additional obstacles can be encountered because some foods that play important roles in vegetarian diets are unpopular with many children. Those who counsel vegetarian families need to be prepared to provide suggestions on incorporating legumes, soyfoods, and a variety of vegetables into children's diets.

All parents should be aware of the importance of identifying good sources of calcium, iron, zinc, omega-3 fatty acids, vitamin B12, and vitamin D in their child's diet. In the case of vitamin B12, fortified foods or supplements are essential for vegan children. The same may be true regarding vitamin D for some children. When children consume a variety of plant foods and attention is given to these nutrients, vegetarian diets are appropriate choices for all stages of childhood.

REFERENCES

1. Position of the American Dietetic Association and Dietitians of Canada. Vegetarian diets. *J Am Diet Assoc.* 2003;103:748–765.
2. Yankelovich, Skelly, White/Clancy, Shulman, Inc. The American vegetarian: Coming of age in the 90s (A study of the vegetarian marketplace conducted by *Vegetarian Times, Inc.*). Oak Park, IL; 1992.
3. Vegetarian Resource Group. *How Many Vegetarians Are There?* Harris Poll 2003. Retrieved from www.vrg.org/journal/vj2003issue3/vj2003issue3poll.htm.
4. Vegetarian Resource Group. *How Many Vegetarians Are There?* Zogby Poll 2000. Retrieved from www.vrg.org/nutshell/poll2000.htm.
5. Vegetarian Resource Group. *How Many Teens Are Vegetarian? How Many Kids Don't Eat Meat?* Roper Poll 2000. Retrieved from www.vrg.org/journal/vj2001jan/2001janteen.htm.
6. Institute of Medicine, Food and Nutrition Board. *Dietary Reference Intakes for Energy, Carbohydrate, Fiber, Fat, Fatty Acids, Cholesterol, Protein, and Amino Acids.* Washington, DC: National Academy Press; 2002.
7. Young VR, Pellett PL. Plant proteins in relation to human protein and amino acid nutrition. *Am J Clin Nutr.* 1994; 59(suppl):1203S–1212S.
8. Messina V, Mangels AR. Considerations in planning vegan diets. II. Children. *J Am Diet Assoc.* 2001;101: 661–669.
9. van Staveren WA, Dhuyvetter JHM, Bons A, Zeelen M, Hautvast JGAG. Food consumption and height/weight status of Dutch preschool children on alternative diets. *J Am Diet Assoc.* 1985;85:1579–1584.
10. Tayter M, Stanek KL. Anthropometric and dietary assessment of omnivore and lacto-ovo-vegetarian children. *J Am Diet Assoc.* 1989;89:1661–1663.
11. Lagstrom H, Seppanen R, Jokinen E, et al. Influence of dietary fat on the nutrient intake and growth of children from 1 to 5 years of age: The Special Turku Coronary Risk Factor Intervention Project. *Am J Clin Nutr.* 1999; 69:516–523.
12. Bremer RR, Peluffo RO. Regulation of unsaturated fatty acid biosynthesis. *Biochem Biophys Acta.* 1969:176: 471–479.
13. Koletzko B. Trans fatty acids may impair biosynthesis of long-chain polyunsaturates and growth in man. *Acta Paediatr.* 1992;81:302–306.
14. Dibba B, Prentice A, Ceesay M. Effect of calcium supplementation on bone mineral accretion in Gambian children accustomed to a low-calcium diet. *Am J Clin Nutr.* 2000;71:544–549.
15. Lee WTK, Leung SSF, Wang S-H, et al. Double-blind, controlled calcium supplementation and bone mineral accretion in children accustomed to a low-calcium diet. *Am J Clin Nutr.* 1994;60:744–750.
16. Weaver CM, Proulx WR, Heaney R. Choices for achieving adequate dietary calcium with a vegetarian diet. *Am J Clin Nutr.* 1999;70(3 Suppl):543S–548S.

17. Arjmandi BH, Smith BJ. Soy isoflavones' osteoprotective role in postmenopausal women: Mechanism of action. *J Nutr Biochem.* 2002;13:130–137.
18. Feskanich D, Weber P, Willett WC, Rockett H, Booth SL, Colditz GA. Vitamin K intake and hip fractures in women: A prospective study. *Am J Clin Nutr.* 1999;69:74–79.
19. Specker BL, Valanis B, Hertzberg V, et al. Sunshine exposure and serum 25-hydroxyvitamin D concentrations in exclusively breast-fed infants. *J Pediatr.* 1985;107: 372–376.
20. Donaldson MS. Metabolic vitamin B12 status on a mostly raw vegan diet with follow-up using tablets, nutritional yeast, or probiotic supplements. *Ann Nutr Metab.* 2000;44:229–234.
21. Haddad EH, Berk LS, Kettering JD, Hubbard RW, Peters WR. Dietary intake and biochemical, hematologic, and immune status of vegans compared with nonvegetarians. *Am J Clin Nutr.* 1999;70(suppl):586S–593S.
22. Alexander D, Ball MJ, Mann J. Nutrient intake and haematological status of vegetarians and age-sex matched omnivores. *Eur J Clin Nutr.* 1994;48:538–546.
23. Hua NW, Stoohs RA, Facchini FS. Low iron status and enhanced insulin sensitivity in lacto-ovo vegetarians. *Br J Nutr.* 2001;86:515–519.
24. Institute of Medicine, Food and Nutrition Board. *Dietary Reference Intakes for Vitamin A, Vitamin K, Arsenic, Boron, Chromium, Copper, Iodine, Iron, Manganese, Molybdenum, Nickel, Silicon, Vanadium, and Zinc.* Washington, DC: National Academy Press; 2001.
25. Larsson C, Johansson G. Dietary intake and nutritional status of young vegans and omnivores in Sweden. *Am J Clin Nutr.* 2002;76:100–106.
26. Ball MJ, Bartlett MA. Dietary intake and iron status of Australian vegetarian women. *Am J Clin Nutr.* 1999;70: 353–358.
27. Sandberg AS, Brune M, Carlsson NG, Hallberg L, Skoglund E, Rossander-Hulthen L. Inositol phosphates with different numbers of phosphate groups influence iron absorption in humans. *Am J Clin Nutr.* 1999;70: 240–246.
28. Monsen ER, Balintfy JL. Calculating dietary iron bioavailability: Refinement and computerization. *J Am Diet Assoc.* 1982;80:307–311.
29. Gillooly M, Bothwell TH, Torrance JD, MacPhail AP, Derman DP, Bezwoda WR, Mills W, Charlton RW. The effects of organic acids, phytates, and polyphenols on the absorption of iron from vegetables. *Br J Nutr.* 1983;49: 331–342.
30. Centers for Disease Control and Prevention. Recommendations to prevent and control iron deficiency in the United States. *MMWR.* 1998;47(No. RR-3):1–29.
31. Hallberg L, Rossander-Hultén L, Brune M, Gleerup A. Calcium and iron absorption: Mechanism of action and nutritional importance. *Eur J Clin Nutr.* 1991;46:317–327.
32. Gleerup A, Rossander-Hultén L, Gramatkovski E, Hallberg L. Iron absorption from the whole diet: Comparison of the effect of two different distributions of daily calcium intake. *Am J Clin Nutr.* 1995;61:97–104.
33. Ziegler EE, Foman SJ, Nelson SE, et al. Cow milk feeding in infancy: Further observations on blood loss from the gastrointestinal tract. *J Pediatr.* 1990;16:11–18.
34. Gibson RS, Yeudall F, Drost N, et al. Dietary interventions to prevent zinc deficiency. *Am J Clin Nutr.* 1998; 68(suppl):484S–487S
35. Sandstrom B, Arvidsson B, Cederblad A, Bjorn-Rasmussen E. Zinc absorption from composite meals I. The significance of wheat extraction rate, zinc, calcium, and protein content in meals based on bread. *Am J Clin Nutr.* 1980;33:739–745.
36. Drake R, Reddy S, Davies J. Nutrient intake during pregnancy and pregnancy outcome of lacto-ovo-vegetarians, fish-eaters and non-vegetarians. *Veg Nutr.* 1998;2:45–52.
37. O'Connell JM, Dibley MJ, Sierra J, Wallace B, Marks JS, Yip R. Growth of vegetarian children: The Farm study. *Pediatrics.* 1989;84:475–481.
38. Sanders TAB. Growth and development of British vegan children. *Am J Clin Nutr.* 1988;48:822–825.
39. Dewey KG, Heinig MJ, Nommsen LA, et al. Growth of breast-fed and formula-fed infants from 0 to 18 months: The DARLING study. *Pediatrics.* 1992;89:1035–1041.
40. Dagnelie PC, van Staveren WA, Vergote FJVRA, et al. Nutritional status of infants aged 4 to 18 months on macrobiotic diets and matched omnivorous control infants: A population-based mixed-longitudinal study. II. Growth and psychomotor development. *Eur J Clin Nutr.* 1989; 43:325–338.
41. Dagnelie PC, van Staveren WA. Macrobiotic nutrition and child health: Results of a population-based, mixed-longitudinal cohort study in the Netherlands. *Am J Clin Nutr.* 1994;59(suppl):1187S–1196S.
42. Dagnelie PC, Vergot F, van Staveren WA, van den Berg H, Kingjan PG, Hautvast J. High prevalence of rickets in infants on macrobiotic diets. *Am J Clin Nutr.* 1990;51: 202–208.
43. Specker BL, Black A, Allen L, Morrow F. Vitamin B12: Low milk concentrations are related to low serum concentrations in vegetarian women and to methylmalonic aciduria in their infants. *Am J Clin Nutr.* 1990;52: 1073–1076.
44. Allen LH. Zinc and micronutrient supplements for children. *Am J Clin Nutr.* 1998;68(suppl):495S–498S.
45. American Academy of Pediatrics, Committee on Nutrition. *Pediatric Nutrition Handbook,* 4th ed. Elk Grove Village, IL: AAP; 1998.
46. Lasekan JB, Ostrom KM, Jacobs JR, et al. Growth of newborn, term infants fed soy formulas for 1 year. *Clin Pediatr.* 1999;38:563–571.

47. American Academy of Pediatrics, Committee on Nutrition. Soy protein-based formulas: Recommendations for use in infant feeding. *Pediatrics.* 1998;101: 148–153.

48. Businco L, Bruno G, Giampietro PG. Soy protein for the prevention and treatment of children with cow-milk allergy. *Am J Clin Nutr.* 1998;68(suppl):1466S–1473S.

49. Campbell JP. Dietary treatment of infant colic: A double-blind study. *J R Coll Gen Pract.* 1989;39:11–14.

50. Irvine C, Fitzpatrick M, Robertson I, Woodhams D. The potential adverse effects of soybean phytoestrogens in infant feeding. *N Z Med J.* 1995;108:208–209.

51. Setchell KDR, Zimmer-Nechemias L, Cai J, Heubi J. Exposure of infants to phytoestrogens from soy infant formulas. *Lancet.* 1997;350:23–27.

52. Strom BL, Schinnar R, Ziegler EE, et al. Exposure to soy-based formula in infancy and endocrinological and reproductive outcomes in young adulthood. *JAMA.* 2001;286:807–814.

53. Albanes D, Taylor PR. International differences in body height and weight and their relationship to cancer incidence. *Nutr Cancer.* 1990;14:69–77.

54. Hemenway D, Azruel DR, Rimm EB, Feskanich D, Willett WC. Risk factors for hip fracture in US men aged 40 through 75 years. *Am J Public Health.* 1994;84: 1843–1845.

55. Gunnell DJ, Frankel SJ, Nanchahal K, et al. Childhood obesity and adult cardiovascular mortality: A 57-y follow-up study based on the Boyd Orr cohort. *Am J Clin Nutr.* 1998;67:1111–1118.

56. Guo SS, Wu W, Chumlea WC, et al. Predicting overweight and obesity in adulthood from body mass index values in childhood and adolescence. *Am J Clin Nutr.* 2002;76:653–658.

57. Nathan I, Hackett AF, Kirby S. A longitudinal study of the growth of matched pairs of vegetarian and omnivorous children, aged 7–11 years, in the north-west of England. *Eur J Clin Nutr.* 1997;51:20–25.

58. Leung SSF, Lee R, Sung S, et al. Growth and nutrition of Chinese vegetarian children in Hong Kong. *J Paediatr Child Health.* 2001;37:247–253.

59. Sabaté J, Linsted KD, Harris RD, Johnston PK. Anthropometric parameters of schoolchildren with different life-styles. *Am J Dis Child.* 1990;144:1159–1163.

60. Sabaté J, Linsted KD, Harris RD, Sanchez A. Attained height of lacto-ovo vegetarian children and adolescents. *Eur J Clin Nutr.* 1991;45:51–58.

61. Sabaté J, Llorca C, Sanchez A. Lower height of lacto-ovovegetarian girls at preadolescence: An indicator of physical maturation today? *J Am Diet Assoc.* 1992;92: 1263–1264.

62. Peeters PHM, Verbeek ALM, Krol A, Matthyssen MMM, de Waard F. Age of menarche and breast cancer risk in nulliparous women. *Breast Cancer Res Treat.* 1994;33: 55–61.

63. Sanders TAB, Manning J. The growth and development of vegan children. *J Hum Nutr Diet.* 1992;5:11–21.

64. Dwyer JT, Dietz WH Jr, Andrews EM, Suskind RM. Nutritional status of vegetarian children. *Am J Clin Nutr.* 1982;35:204–216.

65. Ruys J, Hickie JB. Serum cholesterol and triglyceride levels in Australian adolescent vegetarians. *Br Med J.* 1976;2:87.

66. Sanders TAB, Purves R. An anthropometric and dietary assessment of the nutritional status of vegan preschool children. *J Hum Nutr.* 1981;35:349–357.

67. Thane CW, Bates CJ. Dietary intakes and nutrient status of vegetarian preschool children from a British national survey. *J Hum Nutr Dietet.* 2000;13:149–162.

68. Nathan I, Hackett AF, Kirby S. The dietary intake of a group of vegetarian children aged 7–11 years compared with matched omnivores. *Br J Nutr.* 1996;75:533–544.

69. Sanders TAB. Vegetarian diets and children. *Pediatr Clin N Am.* 1995;42:955–965.

70. Hammer LD. The development of eating behavior in childhood. *Pediatr Clin North Am.* 1992;39:379–394.

71. *Modification of the "Vegetable Protein Products" Requirements for the National School Lunch Program,* School Breakfast Program, Summer Food Service Program and Child and Adult Care Food Program (7 CFR 210, 215, 220, 225, 226). *Fed Reg.* March 9, 2000;65: 12429–12442.

72. ARS/USDA. *Continuing Survey of Food Intakes of Individuals,* 1994–96, 1998. Table Set 17: Food and Nutrient Intakes by Children, 1994–96, 1998. Retrieved from www.barc.usda.gov/bhnrc/foodsurvey/pdf/scs_all.pdf.

73. Donovan UM, Gibson RS. Iron and zinc status of young women aged 14–19 years consuming vegetarian and omnivorous diets. *J Am Coll Nutr.* 1995;14:463–472.

74. Donovan UM, Gibson RS. Dietary intakes of adolescent females consuming vegetarian, semi-vegetarian, and omnivorous diets. *J Adolesc Health.* 1996;18:292–300.

75. Hebbelinck M, Clarys P, De Malsche A. Growth, development, and physical fitness of Flemish vegetarian children, adolescents, and young adults. *Am J Clin Nutr.* 1999;70(suppl):579S–585S.

76. Sanchez A, Kissinger DG, Phillips RL. A hypothesis on the etiological role of diet on age of menarche. *Med Hypothesis.* 1981;7:1339–1345.

77. Neumark-Sztainer D, Story M, Resnick MD, Blum RW. Adolescent vegetarians: A behavioural profile of a school-based population in Minnesota. *Arch Pediatr Adolesc Med.* 1997;151:833–838.

78. Perry CL, McGuire MT, Neumark-Sztainer D, et al. Characteristics of vegetarian adolescents in a multiethnic urban population. *J Adol Health.* 2001;29:406–416.

79. Martins Y, Pliner P, O'Connor R. Restrained eating among vegetarians: Does a vegetarian eating style mask concerns about weight? *Appetite.* 1999;32:145–154.

80. O'Connor AM, Touyz WS, Dunn SM, Beumont PJ. Vegetarianism in anorexia nervosa? A review of 116 consecutive cases. *Med J Aust.* 1987;147:540–542.

81. Janelle KC, Barr SI. Nutrient intakes and eating behavior scores of vegetarian and nonvegetarian women. *J Am Diet Assoc.* 1995;95:180–186, 189.

82. Barr SI. Vegetarianism and menstrual cycle disturbances: Is there an association? *Am J Clin Nutr.* 1999;70(suppl): 549S–554S.

83. Emans SJ, Grace E, Hoffer FA, et al. Estrogen deficiency in adolescents and young adults: Impact on bone mineral content and effects of estrogen replacement therapy. *Obstet Gynecol.* 1990;76:585–592.

84. Barr SI, Janelle KC, Prior JC. Vegetarian vs. nonvegetarian diets, dietary restraint, and sub-clinical ovulatory disturbances: Prospective 6-mo study. *Am J Clin Nutr.* 1994;60:887–894.

85. Persky VW, Chatterton RT, Van Horn LV, Grant MD, Langenberg P, Marvin J. Hormone levels in vegetarian and nonvegetarian teenage girls: Potential implications for breast cancer risk. *Cancer Res.* 1992;50:578–583.

86. Pirke KM, Schweiger U, Laessle R, et al. Dieting influences the menstrual cycle. Vegetarian versus nonvegetarian diet. *Fertil Steril.* 1986;46:1083–1088.

87. Pedersen AB, Bartholomew MJ, Dolence LA, et al. Menstrual differences due to vegetarian and nonvegetarian diets. *Am J Clin Nutr.* 1991;53:879–885.

88. Lloyd T, Schaeffer JM, Walker MA, Demers LM. Urinary hormonal concentrations and spinal bone densities of premenopausal vegetarian and nonvegetarian women. *Am J Clin Nutr.* 1991;54:1005–1010.

89. Barbosa JC, Shultz TD, Filley SJ, Nieman DC. The relationship among adiposity, diet, and hormone concentrations in vegetarian and nonvegetarian postmenopausal women. *Am J Clin Nutr.* 1990;51:798–803.

90. Rose DP, Boyar AP, Cohen C, Strong LE. Effect of a low-fat diet on hormone levels in women with cystic breast disease. I. serum steroids and gonadotropins. *J Natl Cancer Inst.* 1987;78:623–626.

91. Rose DP, Goldman M, Connolly JM, Strong LE. High-fiber diet reduces serum estrogen concentrations in postmenopausal women. *Am J Clin Nutr.* 1991;54:520–525.

92. Kemmann E, Pasquale SA, Skaf R. Amenorrhea associated with carotenemia. *JAMA.* 1983;249:926–928.

93. Martin-Du Pan RC, Hermann W, Chardon F. Hypercarotenemia, amenorrhea and vegetarian diet. *J Gynaecol Obstet Bio Reprod.* 1990;19:290–294.

94. Brooks SM, Sanborn CR, Albrecht BH, et al. Diet in athletic amenorrhea. *Lancet.* 1984;1:559–560.

95. Slavin J, Lutter J, Cushman S. Amenorrhea in vegetarian athletes. *Lancet.* 1984;1;1974–1975.

96. Dwyer JT, Andrew EM, Berkey C, Valadian I, Reed RB. Growth in "new" vegetarian preschool children using the Jenss-Bayley curve fitting technique. *Am J Clin Nutr.* 1983;37:815–827.

97. Dwyer JT, Dietz WH Jr, Andrews EM, Suskind RM. Nutritional status of vegetarian children. *Am J Clin Nutr.* 1982;35:204–216.

98. Dagnelie PC, van Staveren WA, Verschuren SAJM, Hautvast JGAJ. Nutritional status of infants aged 4 to 18 months on macrobiotic diets and matched omnivorous control infants: A population-based mixed-longitudinal study. I. Weaning pattern, energy, and nutrient intake. *Eur J Clin Nutr.* 1989;43:311–323.

CHAPTER 9

Food Hypersensitivities

Lynn Christie

Identifying health problems associated with foods, the mechanisms of the problems, and appropriate treatments have plagued medicine for centuries. Hippocrates was one of the first to report an adverse food reaction to milk over 2000 years ago.[1] The National Institutes of Allergy and Infectious Diseases and the American Academy of Allergy, Asthma, and Immunology established a common language describing adverse food reactions. An adverse food reaction is a clinically abnormal response to an ingested food or food additive. Adverse food reactions (food sensitivities) are categorized either as hypersensitivities (food allergy) or as intolerances. Food hypersensitivity is caused by an immunologic reaction resulting from the ingestion of a food or food additive. Food intolerance is an abnormal physiological response to an ingested food or food additive that has not been proven to be immunologic in nature.

Food hypersensitivity is an immunoglobulin E (IgE), mast cell dependent reaction (Type I). After ingestion of a specific food, an IgE-mediated reaction typically occurs within 1 hour and can be followed by late-phase reaction. Additional immune mechanisms (non-IgE), such as protein-induced malabsorption syndromes and gluten-sensitive enteropathy, are suspected to play a role in food sensitivities. Food hypersensitivities are further described in Table 9–1 by their clinical manifestations and whether the disorder is IgE mediated.

Food intolerances, that are proven not to be immunologic in nature, are secondary to factors that include toxic contaminants, pharmacological properties of foods, metabolic disorders, and idiosyncratic responses. Table 9–2 provides a differential diagnosis for adverse food reactions.

The prevalence of immediate food hypersensitivity reactions is up to 8% in children less than 3 years of age and 1–2% in older children and adults.[2,3] Milk, egg, peanut, soybean, and wheat are the primary foods responsible for hypersensitivity reactions in children. Fish, shellfish, tree nuts, and peanuts are the main culprits of food hypersensitivities in older children and adults. Eggs, milk, peanuts, soybeans, wheat, tree nuts, and fish account for approximately 90% of positive food challenges in children in the United States.[4,5] Table 9–3 lists common label ingredients that indicate the presence of food allergens in 5 categories.

One prospective survey[6] demonstrated the prevalence of adverse food reactions to ingested foods in a pediatric practice of 480 children followed from birth to 3 years of age. Physicians or family suspected that 133 (28%) of the children had adverse food reactions. When food challenges were performed, 75 (15%) of the children experienced skin rashes and diarrhea following the ingestion of fruits and fruit juices (food intolerance). Excluding those reactions, only 37 (8%) of the 480 children had reproducible reactions to foods, usually milk, egg, soy, peanut, and wheat (food hypersensitivity).

Pathophysiology

The allergic immune response begins with sensitization to a particular antigen. Therefore,

Table 9–1 Food Hypersensitivity Disorders

Gastrointestinal
- **IgE mediated**
  - Oral allergy syndrome (oral and perioral pruritis and angioedema, throat tightness)
  - Gastrointestinal anaphylaxis (nausea, cramping, emesis, diarrhea)
  - Infantile colic (~15% of infants with colic)
- **Mixed** (may involve both IgE-mediated and cell-mediated mechanisms)
  - Allergic eosinophilic esophagitis (subset)
  - Allergic eosinophilic gastroenteritis (postprandial nausea, emesis, weight loss)
- **Non-IgE mediated**
  - Food-induced enterocolitis (1 to 3 hr postingestion: emesis, diarrhea, failure to thrive, and rarely, hypotension)
  - Food-induced proctocolitis (2 to12 hr postingestion; blood in stools)
  - Food-induced malabsorption syndrome ("celiac-like"; nausea, steatorrhea, weight loss)
  - Celiac disease

Cutaneous
- **IgE mediated**
  - Acute (common) and chronic (rare) urticaria
  - Generalized flushing
- **Mixed**
  - Atopic dermatitis (pruritic morbilliform rash leading to eczematous lesion)
- **Non-IgE mediated**
  - Dermatitis herpetiformis
  - Contact hypersensitivity
  - Contact irritation (especially with acid fruits and vegetables)

Respiratory
- **IgE mediated**
  - Rhinoconjunctivitis
  - Laryngeal edema
- **Mixed**
  - Asthma (both acute wheezing and increased bronchial hyper-reactivity)
- **Non-IgE mediated**
  - Heiner's syndrome (rare form of pulmonary hemosiderosis)

Other: Mechanism Unknown
- Migraine (rare)

Source: Adapted with permission from Sampson HA. Diagnosing food allergies in children, In: Lichtenstein LM, Busse WW, Raif SG. *Current Therapy in Allergy, Immunology, and Rheumatology*, 6th ed. St. Louis, MO: Mosby; 2004:147–153.

---

the susceptible individual must come in contact with a food before becoming allergic. The B cells begin producing IgE to a particular food antigen. The food specific IgE becomes bound to mast cells and basophils, then recurrent antigen exposure leads to a cross-linking of the food-specific IgE molecules activating the mast cells and basophils. This activation causes the release of histamine, leukotrienes, and other mediators. These mediators produce the vasodilation, smooth muscle contraction, and mucous secretion resulting in the clinical symptoms detected in the skin,

Table 9–2 Differential Diagnosis for Adverse Food Reactions

- I. Food additives
  - A. Food colors: Azo dye F, D, & C, yellow no. 5 (tartrazine)
  - B. Preservatives
    - 1. Sulfiting agents
    - 2. Nitrate/nitrite
    - 3. BHA/BHT
  - C. Flavor enhancers: l-monosodium glutamate (MSG)
  - D. Sweeteners: aspartame, sorbitol, sucrose
  - E. Miscellaneous: antibiotics (penicillin)
- II. Unintentional food contaminants
  - A. Plant toxins
    - 1. Cyanogenic compounds: glycosides in fruit pits and cassava
    - 2. Oxalates: spinach
    - 3. Solanine alkaloids: potatoes
  - B. Microbial toxins
    - 1. Bacterial
      - a. *Staphylococcus aureus, Clostridium botulinum,* etc.
      - b. Scromboid poisoning: tuna, mackerel
    - 2. Fungal (mycotoxins): aflatoxins, ergot
    - 3. Algal (dinoflagellates)
      - a. Ciguatera poisoning: grouper, snapper, barracuda
      - b. Saxitoxin: shellfish
  - C. Food-borne infectious agents
    - 1. Bacterial: salmonellosis, *Campylobacter jejuni, Clostridium perfringens*, etc.
    - 2. Parasitic: *Giardia lambia, Trichinella spiralis*, flukes, etc.
    - 3. Viral: hepatitis
- III. Naturally occurring pharmacologic agents
  - A. Methylxanthines: caffeine, theobromine
  - B. Biologically active amines: tyramine, phenylethylamine, serotonin, histamine
- IV. Gastrointestinal diseases
  - A. Structural abnormalities
    - 1. Gastroesophageal reflux
    - 2. Hiatal hernia
    - 3. Pyloric stenosis
    - 4. Intestinal obstruction
  - B. Carbohydrate intolerance
    - 1. Congenital carbohydrate deficiency: lactase, sucrase, isomaltase, galactose-4-epimerase
    - 2. Acquired carbohydrate intolerance: lactase, sucrase, isomaltase
  - C. Malignancy
  - D. Other Conditions
    - 1. Gastroenteritis
    - 2. Gastric/duodenal ulcer disease
    - 3. Cholelithiasis
    - 4. Pancreatic insufficiency
    - 5. Irritable bowel syndrome
    - 6. Inflammatory bowel disease
    - 7. Mucosal damage secondary to drug therapy
- V. Other conditions
  - A. Malnutrition
  - B. Endocrine disorders: hypothyroidism, hyperthyroidism
  - C. Eating disorders

Source: Adapted with permission from Olejer V. Food hypersensitivities. In: Queen PM, Lang CE, eds., *Handbook of Pediatric Nutrition*, Aspen Publishers, Inc. 1993:206–231.

Table 9–3 Label Ingredients that Indicate the Presence of Food Allergens

Milk		
artificial butter flavor	custard	sour cream
butter	half & half	whey
buttermilk	ghee	yogurt
casein (rennet casein)	lactoglobulin	milk solids (dry)
caseinate (all forms)	lactoferrin	
cheese	lactulose	
cream	milk (all forms dry, goats, malted, powder, solids)	
cottage cheese	nougat yogurt	
curds	pudding	
Label Ingredients that MAY indicate the Presence of Milk Protein		
chocolate	high-protein flour	
flavorings (caramel or natural)	lactose	
margarine	non-dairy products	
Egg		
albumin	egg including white, yolk, dried, powdered, solids	
eggnog	lysozyme	
mayonnaise	meringue	
surimi		
Label Ingredients that MAY indicate the Presence of Egg		
flavoring (including natural and artifical)		egg substitutes
lecithin	macaroni	nougnut
marzipan	marshmallows	pasta
Soybean		
Edamame	miso	
Natti	shoyu sauce	
soy sauce (Tamari)		
textured vegetable protein (TVP)		
tempeh	tofu (soybean curd)	
soy flour, soy grits, soy milk, soy nuts, soy sprouts		
soy protein concentrate, soy protein isolate, hydrolyzed soy protein		
Label Ingredients that MAY Indicate the Presence of Soy Protein		
flavorings	hydrolyzed vegetable protein	
hydrolyzed plant protein	natural flavoring	
vegetable broth, vegetable gum, vegetable starch		
Wheat		
bran	bread crumbs	bulgur
couscous	cracker meal	durum flour
gluten	kamut	matzoh, matzoh meal
pasta	seitan	semolina
spelt	vital gluten	whole-wheat berries
wheat (bran, germ, gluten, malt, starch)		
flour (all-purpose, cake, enriched, graham, high-protein, self-rising, whole-wheat)		

continues

Table 9–3 continued

Label Ingredients that MAY Indicate the Presence of Wheat Protein		
gelatinized starch hydrolyzed	vegetable protein	flavorings (natural and artificial)
modified food starch	modified starch	soy sauce
starch	surimi	
Peanuts		
artificial nuts	beer nuts	goobers
ground nuts	mandelonas	mixed nuts
monkey nuts	nutmeat	peanut
peanut flour	peanut butter	
cold pressed, expressed, or expelled peanut oil		
Foods that MAY Indicate the Presence of Peanut Protein		
African, Asian, Chinese, and Thai dishes	enchilada sauce	
	flavoring (natural and artificial)	
baked goods (pasties, cookies, etc.)	marzipan	
candy	nougat	
chili	egg rolls	
chocolate (candy, candy bars)		

Source: Adapted with permission. *How to Read Label Cards.* © 1990–2004, The Food Allergy and Anaphylaxis Network.

respiratory system, and gastrointestinal system. The immediate allergic reaction can occur within seconds and up to 2 hours after contact with the food allergen. This cross-linking can lead to the synthesis of proinflammatory cytokines and chemokines that are responsible for a late-phase reaction that might occur within 2 to 24 hours after the initial exposure. A chronic inflammatory response that is seen primarily with the skin and respiratory systems is thought to be due to the repetitive ingestion of a food allergen.[7]

CLINICAL MANIFESTATIONS

IgE-Mediated Food Hypersensitivities

The organ systems generally related to IgE-mediated allergic reactions are the skin, gastrointestinal (GI) tract, and respiratory tract. Once foods are ingested, there may be immediate oral symptoms such as itching and swelling of the lips, palate, tongue, or throat. In the gastrointestinal tract, nausea, cramping, gas, distention, vomiting, abdominal pain, or diarrhea may be experienced. Once the antigen spreads through the blood stream and lymphatics, degranulation of mast cells may occur in the skin, causing urticaria, angioedema, pruritis, or an erythematous macular rash. Respiratory symptoms include coughing, wheezing, profuse nasal rhinorrhea, sneezing, or laryngeal edema. The eyes may experience edema, tearing, excess mucus, itching, or burning. The relationship of food hypersensitivities to migraine headaches, epilepsy, rheumatoid arthritis, enuresis, or attention deficit hyperactivity remains controversial.[8]

Systemic anaphylaxis is an acute and potentially fatal reaction. Anaphylaxis can begin with any of the symptoms just mentioned plus cardiovascular symptoms including chest tightness, tachycardia, hypotension, and shock. A fatal reaction may begin with mild symptoms and progress to cardiorespiratory arrest and shock rapidly within 1 to 3 hours. The most severe reactions are usually associated with the ingestion of peanuts, tree nuts, fish, and shellfish. Milk, egg, and soy are less likely to produce fatal reactions in children. *Risk factors for fatal or near-fatal hypersensitivity reactions include children with asthma, allergies to peanut, tree nuts, fish, and/or shellfish, individuals who do not receive epinephrine immediately after the reaction begins, and patients who had a previous allergic reaction to a food.*[9]

Exercise-induced anaphylaxis is associated with the ingestion of a specific food prior to exercise. Then, during or shortly after exercise the individual experiences allergic symptoms that may progress to anaphylaxis.[10] The individual can usually exercise without any reaction as long as the specific food has not been ingested within the past 8 to 12 hours. Individuals with exercise-induced anaphylaxis typically have a positive prick skin test to foods that provoke symptoms. Management requires identifying the food through a challenge with an exercise challenge after food ingestion and avoiding the food at least 8 to 12 hours prior to any expected exercise.

Oral Allergy Syndrome (OAS) is another form of IgE-mediated food allergy.[11] OAS occurs mainly in patients allergic to pollens (seasonal allergic rhinitis). The pollens that cause allergic rhinitis are similar to the allergens in foods causing cross reactivity. The reaction is limited to the lips, tongue, palate, and throat, followed by a rapid resolution of symptoms. People allergic to birch tree pollen may have symptoms when they eat carrots, celery, apples, pears, cherries, apricots and kiwis. Those allergic to ragweed may react when they eat watermelon, cantaloupe, honeydew, and bananas. Generally, cooked foods are less likely than raw foods to cause OAS symptoms.

To diagnose the OAS, a skin prick test is recommended with the prick + prick technique. This involves pricking the fresh food first and then the patient's skin with the same lancet.[12] This induces a minor reaction which does not require a challenge to confirm. It is important to distinguish the OAS from oropharyngeal symptoms that may precede systemic symptoms, including urticaria, gastrointestinal (GI) symptoms, rhinitis, and anaphylactic shock.

Infants with cow's milk allergy have a high rate (44%)[13] of colic that improves with hypoallergenic formulas that are not cow's milk or soybean based. All causes of colic need to be considered, but if there are additional symptoms of cow's milk allergy or a poor response to other measures (for example, medicines), a trial elimination diet may be reasonable.

Non-IgE–Mediated Food Hypersensitivity

Dietary protein enterocolitis, dietary protein enteropathy, dietary protein colitis, and celiac disease (gluten-sensitive enteropathy) are immunologically mediated food hypersensitivity disorders, but are not IgE mediated.[14] Dietary protein enterocolitis, enteropathy, and protocolitis tend to be outgrown by 12 to 36 months of age. Treatment is dietary elimination of the offending foods.

Allergic eosinophilic esophagitis or gastroenteritis may have an IgE component. If dietary proteins do play a role in this disease, there is an IgE reaction upon testing. If a food allergy is diagnosed, elimination of the food is indicated, otherwise, treatment is with corticosteroids.

Dietary protein enterocolitis usually presents by 6 months of age. Symptoms appear 2 to 6 hours following ingestion of the food. Symptoms include projectile emesis, diarrhea, dehydration, and/or a "septic" appearance. Diagnosis is confirmed with a food challenge using 0.6 g protein of the suspected food per kg body weight. Cow's milk, soybeans, grains, vegetables, and/or poultry are often the offending foods.[15]

Dietary protein enteropathy is seen in those with a history of atopy. The onset of symptoms mimics acute enteritis with transient emesis, anorexia, and protracted diarrhea that leads to failure to thrive. Diagnosis through biopsy reveals patchy, subtotal villus injury. The foods commonly associated with food-sensitive enteropathy are cow's milk, soy, chicken, egg, rice, and/or fish.

Dietary protein proctocolitis presents with rectal bleeding within the first few months of life in well-nourished infants. Biopsy of the large intestine reveals eosinophils in the lamina propria. Cow's milk and soy proteins are the usual offending foods.

Celiac disease is an intolerance to gliadin, which is found in wheat, spelt, kamut, rye, and barley. Oats do not contain gliadin and are safe for those with celiac disease. However, oats are contaminated during processing with other grains that do contain gliadin.[16] Diagnosis is made by obtaining a biopsy prior to starting dietary treatment and an follow-up biopsy showing mucosal recovery after a gluten-restricted, gliadin-free diet. Refer to Chapter 16 on gastrointestinal disorders for more information on celiac disease.

DIAGNOSING FOOD HYPERSENSITIVITY

History

The evaluation of a suspected adverse food reaction requires a thorough medical history, physical examination, possibly a diet diary and various laboratory studies. If a food hypersensitivity is suspected, an elimination diet is indicated and food challenges may need to be performed. Incomplete food hypersensitivity work-ups and unorthodox procedures can label one with erroneous food allergies, resulting in incorrect diagnoses, nutrient deficiencies (e.g., calcium or vitamin D), and delay in treating treatable disease.[17–20]

The medical history is useful in diagnosing food allergy in acute events (e.g., systemic anaphylaxis following the ingestion of peanuts). Historically reported adverse food reactions have been confirmed less than 50% of the time using double-blind, placebo-controlled, food challenge (DBPCFC).[21,22] The history may be helpful in distinguishing IgE-mediated type food reactions from other forms of adverse food reactions. The history should include:

- the food suspected to have provoked the reaction
- the quantity of the food ingested
- the length of the time between ingestion and development of symptoms
- a description of the symptoms provoked
- what similar symptoms developed on other occasions when the food was eaten
- if other factors (e.g., exercise) are necessary
- the length of time since the last reaction

If reactions occur within minutes to hours of ingesting a specific food and the symptoms are consistent with those previously mentioned, one should suspect a food hypersensitivity.

Adverse food reactions and disorders that mimic food allergic reactions are listed in Table 9–2. Lactose intolerance produces symptoms similar to cow's milk allergy. Lactose intolerance is frequently seen after a bacterial or viral gastroenteritis. Toddler's diarrhea or chronic nonspecific diarrhea is aggravated by consumption of simple sugars, especially, sorbitol found in fruits (e.g., apple and pear juice), some sugar-free candies, and chewing gums. Unintentional consumption of food contaminants (infectious organisms and toxins) may result in symptoms similar to an allergic reaction.

Physical Exam

No specific features of the physical examination will suggest IgE-mediated food hypersensitivity. The physical exam can identify atopic diseases such as allergic rhinitis, atopic dermatitis (eczema), and asthma which increases the chance that the symptoms are related to a food hypersensitivity. Thirty-five percent of young children with atopic dermatitis have food allergies as a trigger for the condition.[4] Anthropometrics, assessment of growth and development, and nutritional status should be performed (refer to Chapter 2). Abnormal physical findings and a patient's behavior may suggest a diagnosis other than adverse reactions to foods.

Skin Testing and In Vitro Assays

If an IgE-mediated food sensitivity is suspected, prick (puncture) skin testing (PST) with food extracts will help screen for the responsible food allergens. Glycerated food extracts, positive (histamine) and negative (saline) controls are applied by a prick (or puncture) technique.[23] After 15 to 20 minutes, the diameter of the wheal is measured. If the wheal (not including erythema) is at least 3mm greater than the negative control, it is considered positive; anything else is considered negative. A positive PST indicates the presence of specific IgE to that food, not necessarily that the child will have a clinical reaction to the food. Individuals may or may not be hypersensitive to a specific food because the positive predictive accuracy of a PST is less than 50%. A good history is critical when evaluating PST results. A negative PST confirms the absence of an IgE-mediated reaction. The negative predictive value is greater than 95%. Intradermal skin tests are not recommended because of the increased risk of inducing a systemic reaction.[23]

There are a few exceptions to the clinical findings to consider when interpreting the PST results. A child less than 1 year of age may have an IgE-mediated food allergy without a positive PST because of the lower concentration of IgE present in the skin; a child less than 2 years of age may have smaller wheals when tested by the PST method.[24] Therefore, do not discount histories of strongly suspected foods for which the PST is negative. Patients may have positive PST long after they have outgrown the food allergy. As mentioned with OAS, IgE-mediated sensitivity to several fruits and vegetables are detected with fresh extracts, not commercial food extracts.[25] Another exception is when a PST is positive to a food; if that food had been ingested in isolation causing a serious systemic anaphylactic reaction, this scenario is considered diagnostic. A PST is not indicated in patients with extensive skin disease, dermatographism, those who cannot be taken off antihistamines, or if prior exposure to minute amounts resulted in near-fatal anaphylaxis. In vitro tests for specific IgE would be indicated in these patients.

Radioallergosorbent tests (RAST) are the most commonly used in vitro assays that detect and quantitate serum-specific IgE antibodies. The CAP fluorescent enzyme immunoassay (FEIA); Pharmacia-Upjohn Diagnostics, Uppland, Sweden RAST (CAP RAST) system has been validated with double-blind, placebo-controlled food challenges to show that there are specific levels of IgE for individual foods that indicate a less-than 95% probability of a reaction if that individual undergoes a food challenge to a specific food.[26] This information confirms the presence of a food hypersensitivity and that no food challenge is needed if a CAP RAST is (in kilounits of antibody/liter):

egg $\geq$ 7 kU_A/L
milk $\geq$ 15 kU_A/L
peanut $\geq$ 14 kU_A/L
tree nuts $\geq$ 15 kU_A/L
fish $\geq$ 20 kU_A/L

If a child is less than 2 years of age with an egg CAP RAST $\geq$ 2 kU_A/L or a child less than 1 year of age has a milk CAP RAST $\geq$ 5 kU_A/L, both indicate that a positive reaction is highly probable.[27,28] The CAP RAST is helpful in quantifying the amount of food-specific IgE for other foods but it has not been validated to predict reactivity to those foods. Like PST, the false positive rate is less than 50% for CAP RAST test to other foods.

Cross-reactivity is when an individual is allergic to more than one food in a food family. Positive PST and CAP RAST for specific IgE suggest that there is a significant amount of cross-reactivity. Clinical reactivity to more than one member of an animal species or botanical family is rare. SPT and CAP RAST cannot determine the clinical relevance of cross-reactivity between foods. It should be assumed that there is no cross-reactivity unless proven with a food challenge. Otherwise, the patient and family will be unnecessarily avoiding foods. The exception to this is with hypersensitivity to fish,[29,30] shellfish, and OAS as mentioned previously.[31]

Diet Diary

A diet diary may be helpful in identifying a relationship between the foods ingested and the symptoms experienced. Families are asked to keep a timed, chronological record of the amount of formula and/or food (including condiments) ingested for each meal or snack over a specified period of time. Brand names (with ingredient labels), methods of preparation, and recipes are important. The families and other caregivers should record any prescription or over-the-counter medications, including vitamin and mineral supplements or herbal preparations, along with the duration and severity of any symptoms experienced during this time. This experience helps the family pay greater attention to what the child is actually eating. The registered dietitian can evaluate the diet for nutritional adequacy. If a food intolerance is responsible for the symptoms, minor dietary changes may be adequate as opposed to elimination diets.

Elimination Diets

Food elimination followed by selected food challenges is important to determine whether a food is responsible for the reported symptoms. The food(s) to be eliminated and tested by oral food challenge are based on patient history, food diary, skin prick test, and/or CAP RAST results. The elimination diet used in diagnosing a food allergy may be the same as one needed in treatment of the diagnosed food hypersensitivity.

If an infant is breast-fed, the mother will need to eliminate the food(s) in question from her diet.[32,33] Formula-fed infants will need to be on an extensively hydrolyzed protein formula, such as Nutramigen, Pregestimil, or Alimentum. A child with gastrointestinal problems suggesting a non-IgE hypersensitivity may need an amino acid formula, such as Neocate or Elecare if a protein hydrolysate is not tolerated. In older children, two to three foods may need to be eliminated from the diet 2 to 3 weeks before oral food challenges are started.

A strict allergen elimination diet is needed when the history and laboratory test fail to identify the potential food allergens, but should be used with caution because it can lead to iatrogenic malnutrition. A strict allergen elimination diet should be followed for less than 6 weeks unless the necessity is confirmed by a DBPCFC. The following strict allergen elimination diet is recommended by Barnes-Koerner and Sampson.[34] Each step builds upon the previous step as the infant/child gets older.

- Infants under 4 months: casein hydrolysate infant formula (Nutramigen, or Alimentum) or amino acid formula (e.g., Neocate or Elecare)
- 4–8 months: infant diet + rice cereal (nonflavored) + pears
- 9–24 months: 4–8 months diet + rice + squash + lamb
- over 24 months: 9–24 months diet + fresh lettuce + potato + safflower oil + tea + sugar or amino acid formula (e.g., Neocate One)

For older children not drinking formula, an elimination diet using fortified rice milk and the foods mentioned are permitted. In addition, the fruit and fruit juice of apricots, cranberries, peaches, grapes, and apples are allowed. Beets, carrots, corn, sweet potatoes, tapioca, white vinegar, olive oil, honey, cane sugar, and salt are also allowed. The purpose of the strict allergen elimination diet is to provide a clean baseline. Food challenges then would begin with the patient's favorite and nutrient-dense foods.

Resolution of symptoms during the elimination phase suggest that the symptoms were triggered by one or more of the eliminated foods. A food challenge is recommended to re-introduce foods that are not responsible for the clinical reactions. In order to diagnose the allergy or intolerance appropriately, the symptoms must be documented after oral ingestion of the suspected food. If improvement of symptoms is not detected within 2 weeks on the elimination diet either:

- a food sensitivity is not responsible for the symptoms
- there is poor dietary compliance
- the unrecognized offending food continues to be present in the diet
- other chronic conditions cause flair of symptoms (i.e., asthma, atopic dermatitis)

Food Challenges

Food challenges (FC) determine if an individual is, in fact, reactive to a food. There are three types of FC: (1) open, (2) single-blinded, and (3) double-blinded, placebo-controlled. The double-blind, placebo-controlled food challenge (DBPCFC) is considered the "gold standard" for accurately diagnosing food allergies and for examining a wide variety of food related complaints.[35,36,37] Open or single-blinded food challenges are useful in the medical practice setting to determine whether symptoms can be reproduced when the food is ingested. Challenges are labor intensive, requiring equipment to treat an anaphylactic reaction, if necessary.

Open Food Challenge

During open FC, the patient eats a serving of the food in its traditional form (cup of milk, egg scrambled). Examples of good candidates are patients who have had negative skin tests and doubtful histories and/or patients who have been "avoiding the food" yet ingests foods that contain the allergen (example: eats pancakes that contain milk and eggs). Open challenges are also performed following a single-blinded or double-blinded FC. An open challenge will convince the individual that the food is not responsible for the symptom.

Single-Blinded Food Challenge

A single-blinded FC is where the patient and parent do not know what food is being challenged; therefore, it eliminates the bias of the subject and family. It is easily performed in an office setting to confirm objective symptoms. This challenge would be performed under the same conditions as a double-blind, placebo-controlled food challenge (outlined later) except the nurse, dietitian, or doctor performing the challenge would know which food is being challenged. Any challenge should be supervised by personnel appropriately trained to recognize and manage any severe food reaction.[38,39] Multiple positive challenges should be confirmed by a DBPCFC.

Double-Blinded, Placebo-Controlled Food Challenge

The DBPCFC has the patient, parent, and medical personnel performing the challenge "blinded" to what substance is being administered, placebo versus the food being tested. The DBPCFC is the most objective test and provides the most accurate information. For the DBPCFC or other food challenges to be accurate, suspected foods should be totally eliminated for at least 10 to 14 days or up to 12 weeks in some gastrointestinal disorders prior to the challenge. The subject should be symptom free during the elimination diet. It might be assumed that once symptoms resolve and the skin tests are positive, a diagnosis could be made. However, less than 50% of histories will be confirmed by DBPCFC.[22] Certain medications (e.g., antihistamines and oral or injected steroids) may inhibit food hypersensitivity reactions. Recommended avoidance of medication prior to food challenge may range from 36 hours to 1 month.[5] Children with atopic dermatitis may require aggressive skin care prior to food challenges. *Note of caution:* If there is a clear history of severe anaphylaxis following an isolated ingestion of a specific food and there is a positive skin test, this patient should *not* be challenged.

Foods to be used in challenges can usually be found locally. Powdered milk, individually packed flours, and baby foods are found in regular and health food stores. Dried whole eggs can be found through bakery suppliers. A challenge substance and placebo material is well mixed in a vehicle. The vehicle should mask the smell, flavor, and texture of the food to be tested. Vehicles to use in food challenges are fruit juices, elemental formulas with or without flavor packets, baby fruits, hot cereals, and ground chicken or beef patty. Placebos can be safe foods not under suspicion, such as dextrose, cornstarch, another grain, or baby food meat.

The DBPCFC is administered in the fasting state, starting with a dose unlikely to cause symptoms (125 to 500 mg of dry powder food, 1/20 of the total amount to be consumed). The dose is doubled every 10 to 60 minutes, depending on the type of reaction that might occur based on the history. Clinical reactivity is generally ruled out once the patient has tolerated 10 grams of the dried food or 60 to 100 grams of the wet food (blinded) without symptoms. Following completion of the challenge, the individual should be observed for 1 to 2 hours for food allergic reactions and 4 to 8 hours for food intolerances, based on history. If the immediate onset of symptoms is suspected, the DBPCFC can be performed in a day. One series of challenges (active or placebo) is given over 1 to 2 hours in the morning. In the afternoon, a second series of challenges (opposite of earlier challenge) is performed. If the blinded challenge is negative, the food *must* be given openly in usual quantities, under observation, to rule out a rare false-negative challenge. Overall, this method works well except for delayed or late onset reactions. The Food Allergy and Anaphylaxis Network has recently published a book titled *A Health Professional's Guide to Food Challenges* that is more detailed for those interested in performing food challenges.[40]

Correctly diagnosing a food hypersensitivity can be a long and tedious process. Controversial diagnostic techniques that are not found to be effective in the diagnosing of food allergies are abundant. These include cytotoxic testing, sublingual or subcutaneous provocative challenge, ELISA/ACT, IgG or IgG4 antibody food test, lymphocyte activation, food antigen-antibody complexes, and electrodiagnostic devices.

Summation of Food Challenges

In summary, the medical history identifies possible food hypersensitivity reactions. If IgE-mediated food hypersensitivity is suspected, perform prick skin tests for suspected and common food allergens (milk, egg, wheat, soy, peanut, fish). If positive, perform CAP RAST to those foods. If negative, either stop or consider other possible non-IgE immunological disorders (see Tables 9–1 and 9–2 on pages 162 and 163). If the tests are positive and there is a convincing history of anaphylaxis, restrict the food(s) and stop the work-up. Otherwise, place the child on an elimination diet for the suspected food allergens for 2 to 4 weeks. If there is no improvement, food hypersensitivity may not be the cause. If there is improvement and considering the CAP RAST results, begin the food-challenge process. If one suspects food protein–induced enteropathy, do not challenge the patient. If a food intolerance is suspected, eliminate the suspected offending food(s) from the diet. If symptoms persist, add the foods back and look for other causes. If symptoms improve, add the food(s) back to the diet after food challenges.

THERAPY

Education

Once a diagnosis has been made, strict avoidance of the offending allergen(s) is the only proven therapy for food hypersensitivities. Education is the cornerstone for good compliance and a nutritionally adequate diet. This requires extensive education for the patient and family regarding all forms of the food to be avoided, how to read food labels, where the food may be hidden, and alternative food sources for the nutrients that may be affected. This is overwhelming to the family and impacts most aspects of their life. Accidental ingestions do occur in spite of the best avoidance efforts and the family will need to be educated on how to manage an allergic reaction. Cooking from scratch is one of the best ways to avoid accidental ingestions. Follow-up for newly diagnosed individuals needs to be 1 to 2 months after diagnosis to reinforce education and address issues that have come up with the family. If a child is allergic to a single food, such as peanuts or fish, the nutritional adequacy of the diet may not be compromised, however, the elimination of milk, eggs, soybeans, or wheat can have a major impact on the quality of a diet. These foods are found in the food supply in many forms, making complete elimination difficult. Milk, soy, wheat, and egg food hypersensitivities traditionally can be outgrown. Therefore, long-term follow-up involves repeated testing to determine if a child is still hypersensitive to a food and to prevent unnecessary food avoidance.

In a recently published study,[41] children with two or more food hypersensitivities were shorter in length and height stature than those with only one food hypersensitivity. Twenty-five percent of the children with food hypersensitivities consumed inadequate amounts of calcium, vitamin D, and vitamin E. Children with two or more food hypersensitivities and those hypersensitive to milk were at greatest risk. A nutritional assessment (refer to Chapter 2), including a 3-day diet record, should be collected a least once a year. When evaluating a 3-day diet record, inadequate intake is considered to be less than two thirds of the RDAs and AIs of a nutrient. Counseling on alternative sources of the nutrient(s) will be needed.

Labels

Label reading is critical to successfully avoid a food allergen. The patient and family should read all labels every time they shop because ingredients change without warning. This is the only way food manufacturers communicate that the ingredients have changed. One brand may be allergen free but another brand of the same food may not. Patients and families may be deceived by labels. For example, nondairy creamers contain caseinates (milk protein). This is why the patient and family need a good command of the terms used by the food industry to detect the presence of a specific food allergen. Other household products, including pet food, cosmetics, bath products, lotions, sunscreens, and so forth are known to contain food allergens and their ingredient labels also need to be reviewed.

Specific ingredients on food labels identify foods that contain a particular food allergen. Patients and families should look for these terms when reading food labels so that they can appropriately avoid the offending foods. Table 9–3 on pages 164 and 165 contains terms used on labels that indicates the presence of food allergens for milk, egg, soybean, wheat, and peanuts. There are diet manuals and books[34,42] available that also have appropriate information regarding the scientific and technical names for foods. The diet manuals traditionally provide lists of foods to avoid and foods that are safe. The Food Allergy and Anaphylaxis Network is another valuable resource that provides booklets on guidelines for food allergies, how to work with the schools, cook books, newsletters, and wallet-size cards that contains the terms used on labels for the common individual food allergens. Additional resources for the professional and families are listed at the end of this chapter.

There are obscure terms on food labels that suggest the presence of a food allergen. Modified food starch, modified starch, vegetable starch, or food starch could be from corn, tapioca, wheat, soy, potato, or rice. Vegetable gums may be from corn, wheat, soy, or guar. Hydrolyzed plant or vegetable protein may indicate the presence of wheat or soy protein. Caramel is usually from browned sugar, but could be made with corn syrup or contain milk protein. Contacting the individual food companies is the only way to clarify whether a food is safe. If there is any doubt about a food or there is no ingredient list, it is best to avoid that food.

Kosher dietary laws prohibit eating dairy products together with meat or fowl. If the word "Parve" or rabbinical agency symbols (such as a "K" in a star or triangle or a "U" in a circle) are on the label, the product is identified by a rabbinical agency as one that does not contain dairy. However, under Jewish law, a food product can contain a small amount of milk and meet specifications for "parve." Therefore, these foods may not be safe for those with milk hypersensitivity. A "D" (dairy) or "DE" (dairy equipment) indicates the possible presence of milk protein, which may or may not be found in the ingredient statement.

Cross-contact

Another major source of hidden allergens is cross-contact. Food proteins mix when one food comes in contact with another food. Cross-contact can occur during food preparation and presentation of the food at the manufacturing plant, grocery store, restaurants, and at home. Packaged and processed foods are at risk because related products are made on shared equipment. Failure to clean the equipment satisfactorily between processing different products can leave allergenic food residues. This may occur with any food; for example, egg-containing and egg-free pastas and breakfast cereals and rice cakes with or without nuts. Industry utilizes leftovers by adding what is left over to the next batch. This is called re-work. For example, ingredients such as nuts may be filtered out of the re-work, but nut residues remain and are added to a new batch of nut-free ice cream. Some manufacturers are adding precautionary labeling, such as "may contain," to the label because of potential cross-contact. Other mistakes are packaging a different, yet similar food, in the wrong package or a formulation error.

At the grocery store, cross-contact can occur in the deli where meats and cheese are sliced on the same equipment, pastries are side by side, and bulk foods are accidentally mixed. In the food service industry, cooking utensils, serving utensils, and containers may be shared. Not washing hands after handling allergen-containing foods can contaminate allergen-free foods. Frying oils may be used for all deep-fat fried foods (e.g., potatoes, fish, foods dipped in egg or milk and battered). The same grill can be used to grill seafood and steaks. Creative or ethnic recipes may contain unexpected ingredients, such as tree nuts and peanuts.

ELIMINATION DIETS

All forms of a food to be eliminated must be completely removed from an individual's diet once diagnosed with a food hypersensitivity. Labels must be read to identify words that are terms for the offending foods (see Table 9–3, pages 164 and 165).

Milk Hypersensitivity

If milk-protein hypersensitivity is suspected in infancy, an extensively hydrolyzed protein-based formula (Alimentum, Nutramigen, or Pregestimil) rather than a soy-based formula is recommended until the child is 1 year of age or has had a negative test to soy. Partially hydrolyzed milk-based formulas, such as Good Start, contain whole cow's milk allergens and will continue to cause allergic reactions in the milk-allergic child. In children with IgE-associated hypersensitivity to milk, 14% cannot tolerate soy formulas[43] where 30–50% of the non-IgE–mediated enterocolitis and enteropathy syndromes are reactive to soy protein. If an infant or toddler fails to tolerate a protein-hydrolysate formula, then an amino acid–based formula (Neocate, Neocate One +, Elecare) will be required.[44,45,46] Other amino acid–based formulas are available but are not appropriate for infants. Health professionals also need to contact these companies to ensure the product is free of milk or soy contamination. As infants become toddlers and are beginning to trust their food, rarely will they want to change their "safe formula." Goat's milk is not an alternative to cow's milk because of the potential cross-reactivity with the beta-lactoglobulins in cow's milk.[47] The vitamin- and mineral-fortified infant casein hydrolysate formulas will provide the calcium, phosphorus, vitamin D, vitamin B12, riboflavin, and pantothenic acid that would be provided by the milk products. Encourage parents to continue milk-free formulas as long as the milk-hypersensitive child will consume it; age not being a factor. If the child refuses formula, a calcium- and vitamin D–fortified soy beverage is an alternative, but lacks the methionine fortification found in infant and toddler soy formulas. Calcium- and vitamin D–fortified rice beverages lack protein; therefore, stress the need for amounts of high biological proteins during counseling. A calcium and vitamin D supplement may be needed. Some ready-to-eat cereals, breads, and fruit juices are calcium fortified but may not be fortified with vitamin D. When cooking from scratch at home, fruit juice, water, rice milk, or soy milk are appropriate substitutes for milk in recipes. Whole grains, legumes, meats, and nuts can provide alternative sources of other nutrients like phosphorus, riboflavin, and pantothenic acid that are found in milk.

Egg Hypersensitivity

Nutrients in eggs are easily replaced by other high-protein foods and whole grains. However, eggs are incorporated into breads, pastas, baking mixes, breaded or processed meats, custards, fat substitutes, salad dressings, sauces, and other commercially prepared foods. It is the elimination of all of these other foods containing egg that cause problems in providing a nutritionally balanced diet. For instance, eggs are used for a shiny glaze on products in bakeries. Beware of fried foods because eggs are frequently used in batters and consequently the oil may be contaminated with egg protein.

Families can be taught how to modify recipes at home providing substitutes for the binding and leavening properties of eggs. Not all egg substitutes are alike; egg whites are commonly used in most egg substitutes, for example, Egg Beaters, Ener-g Foods, Inc., has an egg-free powder called Egg Replacer. For other substitutes for eggs in a recipe, try one of the following for each egg:[34,48]

- 1 tsp of baking powder + 1 Tbsp of water + 1 Tbsp of vinegar (add vinegar separately at end)
- 1 tsp baking soda + 1 Tbsp oil + 2 Tbsp baking powder + 1 Tbsp vinegar (add vinegar separately at end)
- 1 tsp of yeast dissolved in 1/4 cup of warm water
- 1 1/2 Tbsp of water + 1 1/2 Tbsp of oil + 1 tsp of baking powder
- 1 Tbsp of apricot puree (binder)
- 1 packet of plain gelatin mixed with 1 cup boiling water (binder). Substitute 3 Tbsp of this liquid for each egg. Refrigerate remainder for 1 week, microwave to liquefy.

Soybean Hypersensitivity

Soybean flour and soybean protein are major ingredients used by food manufacturers. Soy can be found in processed grains (crackers, cereals, baked goods), processed meats, frozen dinners, salad dressings, sauces, Asian foods, and soups. A balanced diet may be a challenge in this population and cooking from scratch with basic ingredients may be a necessity. Soybean oil and soy lecithin are considered safe for most soy allergic individuals because the processing of the oil removes the protein portion.[49]

Wheat Hypersensitivity

Wheat and wheat products are the foundation of the American diet and are difficult to eliminate from the diet. They are found in baked products, pastas, cereals, snacks, sauces, soups, and breaded and processed meats. Products made with the flours of amaranth, arrowroot, barley, buckwheat, corn, oats, potato, quinoa, rice, rye, soybean, and tapioca are suitable wheat alternatives. These foods and grains can be found in grocery stores, health food stores, and mail-order companies. Gluten-free products used by individuals with celiac disease may be good alternatives but often contain milk or egg products. Wheat flours are fortified with niacin, riboflavin, thiamin, and iron. A child's diet composed of very few grain products may be deficient in these and many other nutrients. Children with a wheat allergy should have their intake evaluated at least annually to ensure overall nutritional adequacy.

Peanut Hypersensitivity

Peanuts are legumes, but an allergy to peanuts does not automatically make one allergic to other legumes (soybeans, peas, beans, green beans, and lentils). However, there is a strong possibility of cross reaction between peanuts and lupine.[50] Individuals allergic to peanuts are advised to avoid tree nuts (such as pecans, almonds, and walnuts) for several reasons. One, however, is that roughly a third of the people who are allergic to peanuts are also allergic to one other type of tree nut.[51] Peanuts are often substituted for tree nuts or flavored as tree nuts. Tree nuts are commonly processed on equipment shared with peanuts. Peanuts, especially peanut flour, are found in pastries, candies, fruit nut breads, salads, sauces, cereals, crackers, soups, and ethnic foods, particularly those of Africa, China, and Thailand. Peanut oil is considered safe for most individuals with peanut allergies[52] *except* crude peanut oil that has been cold pressed, expressed, or expelled. Nutrients such as vitamin E, niacin, magnesium, manganese, and chromium found in peanuts can also be found in legumes, whole grains, meats, and vegetable oils.

Tree Nut Hypersensitivity

Tree nut hypersensitivity is more common in adults than children and has a reputation of causing anaphylactic reactions. When a child is diagnosed with any food allergy, the physician may also recommend that the child avoid peanuts, tree nuts, fish, and shellfish until the child is 3 or 5 years old to avoid developing these life-long food allergies. Tree nuts are used in cereals, crackers, ice cream, and sauces, making avoidance more difficult. Nut paste and nut butters are often made on shared equipment. Pure tree nut extracts, such as almond, walnut, may contain allergens.

Individuals hypersensitive to any tree nut are advised to avoid all tree nuts because of potential cross-reactivity.[51] The nuts are frequently processed on the same equipment and substituted for each other in recipes.

Fish and Shellfish Hypersensitivity

An individual may be hypersensitive to one fish and tolerate others[29] but in the marketplace, substituting one fish for another is a common occurrence and is dangerous for the fish-allergic individual. In addition, there is a 50% rate of cross-reactivity with fish allergies.[31] Cross-contamination occurs in restaurants because of shared equipment (frying oil, grill, spatula). Those allergic to fish but not shellfish need to be aware of Surimi, an imitation shellfish made with fish. Common foods that contain fish include Caesar salad dressing and Worcestershire sauce. Nutrients in fish such as vitamin B6, vitamin B12, vitamin E, niacin, phosphorus, and selenium are also found in meats, grains, and oils.

If one is allergic to shellfish, all shellfish, such as shrimp, crabs, lobster, and crawfish, need to be avoided. If allergic to mollusks, then all clams, oysters, and scallops are to be avoided. The risk of cross-reactivity is 75% with shellfish.[31] Shellfish are traditionally not hidden in foods but beware of cross-contamination in seafood restaurants. Asian dishes use a number of fish and shellfish and should also be avoided. Imitation seafood may not be safe because the flavoring used may be made from shellfish.

OTHER PRINCIPLES OF MANAGEMENT AND TREATMENT

The registered dietitian can play a critical role in working with children with food hypersensitivities and their families. The key is avoiding all forms of the known allergens all of the time. The Food Guide Pyramid for Young Children[53] is a wonderful tool to explain what the child can eat: fruits, vegetables, meats, grains, and milk. Alternative foods based on the allergens to avoid can be worked into the pyramid to demonstrate a balanced diet. Families need to be educated about new cooking techniques, eating out, social events, dealing with other family members, and schools. Cooking from scratch is an excellent way to protect the allergic child from accidental ingestions, however, families may need to be educated on cooking basics. Cooking lessons with recipes can alleviate anxiety and help with the time management of cooking. Ideally, everyone in the family follows the allergen-free diet at home. If this is not possible, the allergen-free meal should be prepared first and protected from cross-contact before mealtime.

When eating out, the parent needs to review the menu to determine if there is something the child can eat before they go or they can bring their child's safe foods (easy with older infants). Different restaurants may prepare the same dish with different ingredients. Always ask the manager or chef, not the wait staff, questions about ingredients and preparation methods. Order single ingredient foods, such as broiled meats or baked potatoes. Avoid sauces, desserts, fried foods, and combination foods such as stews.[54] If there is a restaurant that the family prefers, get to know the manager or owner so your child's special requests can be met. Avoid the restaurant's busiest time.

Social events can be stressful because there is food "everywhere" and the parent has no idea how most of the foods were prepared. Other individuals may try to feed the allergic child without knowing of the child's food hypersensitivity. Children need to be taught not to accept any food or candy from anyone without their parent's approval. Eating before events may help curb the child's hunger. Grandparents and other close friends need to be educated on a child's food hypersensitivity. The parent must be firm about avoiding allergens with those who do not understand that even a little can hurt the child.

Schools and day cares need aggressive education for those caring for children with peanut and other food allergies. Contact with peanut butter and jelly sandwiches or projects using peanut butter (as part of a bird feeder) can trigger a severe allergic reaction. Thanks to Public Law 93-112, The Rehabilitation Act of 1973, Section 504, and the U.S. Department of Agriculture's 7 CFR 15b, schools are required to modify their health services, which include making available menu information, providing substitutions for the foods to be omitted (identified by a doctor's signed statement) and administering medications at school. The Food Allergy and Anaphylaxis Network[55] developed a program to assist in managing food allergy at school and day cares.

As stated previously, accidental ingestions do occur and the patient, family members, and caregivers should be educated regarding signs and symptoms of anaphylaxis and appropriate treatment. Most accidental ingestions that lead to severe systemic anaphylaxis occur when foods are eaten away from home and are disguised. Examples include sandwiches at a restaurant or hors d'oeuvres at a party. If the allergic reaction is mild (only urticaria or rhinitis), the treatment may be an antihistamine. Antihistamines, however, are never a substitute for epinephrine when severe reactions occur. Individuals with moderate to severe food hypersensitivities must be taught how to self-inject epinephrine once an allergic reaction is recognized. Epinephrine is available for emergency use in premeasured doses, available by prescription. These include EpiPen Jr. and the EpiPen (Center Laboratories; Port Washington, New York) and Ana-Kit and the Ana-Guard (Miles Inc.; Allergy Products, West Haven, Connecticut). Because accidental ingestions commonly occur away from the home, it should be stressed to carry emergency medicine at all times. Epinephrine provides valuable time for transport to the hospital emergency room for observation. Once epinephrine is used, the individual must go to a hospital emergency room. The medically supervised observation period is critical for immediate treatment of an unexpected late phase reaction. No one can predict how a reaction will progress; guidelines are available on medical treatment.[56] Emergency medical identification systems (MedicAlert; Turlock, California) may also be indicated.

Preventive therapies using drugs such as antihistamines, corticosteroids, ketotifin, and oral cromolyn sodium, may modify symptoms but have minimal efficacy.[5] At this time, the only proven treatment is strict elimination of the offending allergen. Rotation diets (where the offending food is eliminated and rotated back into the diet every few days) are not recommended for children. Strict elimination is needed to "outgrow" some food allergies and a rotation diet is thought to keep the individual sensitized, prolonging this process. The effectiveness of subcutaneous neutralization, provocation, or oral, desensitization has not been demonstrated. Untested herbal remedies and nutrition supplements do not affect the outcome of a food hypersensitive reaction. Atopic individuals should be warned of rare but potential adverse reactions after ingesting some nutrition supplements. Case reports have documented anaphylaxis to bee pollen,[57,58] royal jelly,[59,60] and echinacea.[61]

Research efforts are directed at identifying the molecular and immunologic mechanisms involved in food allergen-receptor recognition and the cascade of events that lead to allergic reactions through anti-IgE, probiotics, and vaccines. Immunotherapy[62] methods are under investigation and appear to help prevent serious food allergic reactions in the future.

NATURAL HISTORY AND PREVENTION

The general understanding is that most children "outgrow" food hypersensitivities by school age.[6,63] The allergens responsible for the sensitivities and the compliance with allergen elimination diets will affect whether one will "outgrow" the allergic response. Children with peanut, tree nut, fish, or shellfish hypersensitivity will rarely lose their clinical reactivity. The exception is that roughly 20% of children with peanut hypersensitivity do lose their clinical reactivity.[64,65] If the child has not had a clinical reaction to peanut for 1 to 2 years and the peanut CAP RAST is low (under 2),[66] this child may have lost clinical reactivity; consider a food challenge to peanut. Infants with non-IgE–mediated food hypersensitivities also appear to outgrow their food reactivity by 3 years of age.[67] Celiac disease is an exception, where gliaden must be avoided for life.

The American Academy of Pediatrics (AAP) has published guidelines for the primary prevention of food allergy in high-risk children.[68] AAP defines a high-risk infant as one with both parents or a parent plus a sibling with atopic diseases (environmental and/or food hypersensitivities, atopic dermatitis, allergic rhinitis, or asthma). A pregnant woman does not need to avoid food allergens in her diet with the possible exception of peanuts. It is recommended that she exclusively breastfeed the high-risk infant, if possible, for the first 6 months. Breastfeeding mothers who have high-risk infants ought to consider the elimination of allergens in her diet; this should be discussed with her physician. If a formula is needed for a high-risk infant, extensively hydrolyzed protein formulas (Nutramigen, Alimentum) should be used instead of partially hydrolyzed, milk, or soy-based formulas.

If an infant is diagnosed with food hypersensitivity and is breast-fed, the mother will need to completely remove the allergen from her diet.[32,33] This may place the lactating mother at nutritional risk. She will need to be counseled on alternative sources of the nutrients loss through the avoidance diet. This can be difficult, may impact her nutritional status, and can have an impact on the infant's growth.[69] If the mother cannot follow a strict avoidance diet, an extensively hydrolyzed formula is appropriate.

The AAP recommends delaying the introduction of any solids for the high-risk infant until 6 months of age and to delay the introduction of allergenic foods. Single ingredient foods should be conservatively introduced one at a time, weekly or biweekly. This allows for the identification of any problems. Delay the introduction of milk or soy until after 1 year of age; eggs until 2 years of age; and peanuts, tree nuts, fish, and shellfish until after 3 years of age. Baby food labels always need to be read because they can contain allergens that are to be avoided. Families need to be reminded to offer foods with textures so that developmental milestones are not missed. Postponing the introduction of food allergens does not prevent this disorder, but does delay the development of food hypersensitivity and other atopic diseases in high-risk infants.[70,71]

In summary, it is important to make an accurate diagnosis of food hypersensitivity. Nutrition assessment and education for avoidance diets is complex. Without appropriate education, the child is at risk of accidental reactions, persistent food allergies, growth problems, and social stigmas. Education may also prevent the development of additional food hypersensitivities.

REFERENCES

1. Anderson JA, Song DD, eds. American Academy Allergy & Immunol/NIAID: Adverse reactions to foods. *NIH Publ.* #84-2442;1984:1–6.
2. Sampson HA. Immediate reactions to foods in infants and children. In: Metcalfe DD, Sampson HA, Dimon RA, eds. *Food Allergy: Adverse Reactions to Foods and Food Additives,* 2nd ed. Malden, MA: Blackwell Science, Inc.;1997: 169–182.
3. Wood RA. The natural history of food allergy. *Pediatrics.* 2003;111:1631–1637.
4. Burks AW, James JM, Heigel A, et al. Atopic dermatitis and food hypersensitivity reactions. *J Pediatr.* 1998;132: 132–136.
5. Sampson HA. Food allergy. Part 2. Diagnosis and management. *J Allergy Clin Immunol.* 1999;103:981–999.
6. Bock SA. Prospective appraisal of complaints of adverse reactions to foods in children during the first 3 years of life. *Pediatrics.* 1987;79:683–688.
7. Bischoff SC, Sellge G. Immune mechanisms in food-induced disease. In: Metcalfe DD, Sampson HA, Simon RA. *Food Allergy: Adverse Reactions to Foods and Food Additives,* 3rd ed. Malden, MA: Blackwell Science, Inc.; 2003:14–37.
8. Metcalfe DD, Sampson HA, Simon RA. *Food Allergy: Adverse Reactions to Foods and Food Additives,* 3rd ed. Malden, MA: Blackwell Science, Inc.; 2003.
9. Burks WA, Sampson HA. Anaphalaxis and food allergy. In: Metcalfe DD, Sampson HA, Simon RA. *Food Allergy: Adverse Reactions to Foods and Food Additives,* 3rd ed. Malden, MA: Blackwell Science, Inc.; 2003;192–205.
10. Tilles S, Schocket A, Milgrom H. Exercise-induced anaphylaxis related to specific foods. *J Pediatr.* 1995;127: 587–589.
11. Pasterello EA, Incorvaia C, Ortolani C. Mouth and pharynx. *Allergy.* 1995;50:41–44.
12. Dreborg S, Foucard T. Allergy to apple, carrot, and potato in children with birch pollen allergy. *Allergy.* 1983;36: 167–170.

13. Sicherer SH. Clinical aspects of gastrointestinal food allergy in childhood. *Pediatrics.* 2003;111:1609–1616.
14. James JM, Burks AW. Food-associated gastrointestinal disease. *Curr Opin Pediatr.* 1996;8:471–475.
15. Norwak-Wegrzyn A, Sampson HA, Wood RA, et al. Food protein-induced entercolitis syndrome caused by solid food proteins. *Pediatrics.* 2003;111:829–835.
16. Janetuinen EK, Kemppainen TA, Julkunen RJ, et al. No harm from five-year ingestion of oats in celiac disease. *Gut.* 2002;50:332–335.
17. Lloyd-Still JD. Chronic diarrhea of childhood and the misuse of elimination diets. *J Pediatr.* 1979;95:10–13.
18. Libib M, Gama R, Wright J, Marks V, et al. Dietary maladvice as a cause of hypothyroidism and short stature. *Br Med J.* 1989;298:232–233.
19. Robertson DAF, Ayres RCS, Smith CL, Wright R. Adverse consequences arising from misdiagnosis of food allergy. *Br Med Jr.* 1988;297:719–720.
20. Roesler TA, Barry PC, Bock SA. Factitious food allergy and failure to thrive. *Arch Pediatr Adolesc Med.* 1994; 148:1150–1155.
21. Bock SA, Lee WY, Remigio LK, et al. Studies of hypersensitivity reactions to foods in infants and children. *J Allergy Clin Immunol.* 1978;62:327–334.
22. Sampson HA, Albergo R. Comparison of results of skin test, RAST and double-blind, placebo-controlled food challenge in children with atopic dermatitis. *J Allergy Clin Immunol.* 1984;74:26–33.
23. Bock SA, Buckley J, Houst A, May CD. Proper use of skin test with food extracts in diagnosis of food hypersensitivity. *Clin Allergy.* 1978;8:559–564.
24. Menurdo JL, Bousquet J, Rodiere M, et al. Skin test reactivity in infancy. *J Allergy Clin Immunol.* 1985;74: 646–651.
25. Ortoloni C, Ispano M, Partorella EA, et al. Comparison of results of skin prick test (with fresh foods and commercial food extracts) and RAST in 100 patients with oral allergy syndrome. *J Allergy Clin Immunol.* 1989;83:683–689.
26. Sampson HA. Utility of food specific IgE concentration in predicting symptomatic food allergy. *J Allergy Clin Immunol.* 2001;107:891–896.
27. Garcia-Ara C, Boyano-Martinez T, Diaz-Pena JM, et al. Specific IgE levels in the diagnosis of immediate hypersensitivity of cows' milk protein in the infant. *J Allergy Clin Immunol.* 2001;107:185–190.
28. Boyano-Martinez T, Garcia-Ara C, Diaz-Pena JM, et al. Validity of specific IgE antibodies in children with egg allergy. *Clin Exp Allergy.* 2001;31:1464–1469.
29. Bernhisel-Broadbent J, Scanlon SM, Sampson HA. Fish hypersensitivity. I. In vitro and oral challenge results in fish allergic patients. *J Allergy Clin Immunol.* 1992;89: 730–737.
30. Bernhisel-Broadbent J, Strause D, Sampson HA. Fish hypersensitivity. II. Clinical relevance of altered fish allergenicity caused by various preparation methods. *J Allergy Clin Immunol.* 1992;90:622–629.
31. Sicherer SH. Clinical implications of cross-reactive food allergens. *J Allergy Clin Immunol.* 2001;108:881–890.
32. Jarvinen KM, Makinen-Kiljunen S, Suomalainen H. Cow's milk challenge through human milk evokes immune responses in infants with cow's milk allergy. *J Pediatr.* 1999;135:506–512.
33. Vadas P, Wai Y, Burks AW, et al. Detection of peanut allergens in breast milk of lactating women. *JAMA.* 2001;106:346–349.
34. Barnes-Koerner C, Sampson HA. Diets and nutrition. In: Metcalfe DD, Sampson HA, Simon RA. *Food Allergy: Adverse Reactions to Foods and Food Additives,* 3rd ed. Malden, MA: Blackwell Science, Inc.; 2003;438–460.
35. Sampson HA, McCaskill CM. Food hypersensitivity and atopic dermatitis: Evaluation of 113 patients. *J Pediatr.* 1985;107:669–675.
36. Sicherer SH, Morrow EH, Sampson HA. Dose response in double blind placebo controlled oral food challenges in children with atopic dermatitis. *J Allergy Clin Immunol.* 2001;105:582–586.
37. Sicherer SH. Food allergy: When and how to perform oral food challenges. *Pediatr Allergy Immunol.* 1999;10: 226–234.
38. Reibel S, Rohr C, Zeigert M, et al. What safety measures need to be taken in oral food challenges in children? *Allergy.* 2000;55:940–944.
39. Executive committee of the Academy of Allergy and reactions caused by immunotherapy with allergic extracts (position statement). *J Allergy Clin Immunol.* 1986;77: 271–273.
40. Mofidi S, Bock SA. A health professional's guide to food challenges. Fairfax, VA: The Food Allergy & Anaphylaxis Network, 2004.
41. Christie L, Hine RJ, Parker JG, et al. Food allergies in children affect nutrient intake and growth. *J Am Diet Assoc.* 2002;102:1648–1651.
42. Nevin-Folino NL, ed. *Pediatric Manual of Clinical Dietetics,* 2nd ed. Chicago, IL. American Dietetic Association; 2003:259–281.
43. Zeiger RS, Sampson HA, Bock SA, et al. Soy allergy in infants and children with IgE-associated cow's milk allergy. *J Pediatr.* 1999;134:614–622.
44. Sampson HA, James JM, Berhisel-Broadbent J. Safety of an amino acid–derived infant formula in children allergic to cow milk. *Pediatrics.* 1992;40:463–465.
45. Niggerman B, Christaine B, Dupont C, et al. Prospective, controlled, multi-center study on the effect of an amino acid based formula in infants with cow's milk allergy/ intolerance and atopic dermatitis. *Pediatr Allergy Immunol.* 2001;12:78–82.

46. Sicherer SH, Noone SA, Koerner CB, et al. Hypoallergenicity and efficacy of an amino acid–based formula in children with cow's milk and multiple food hypersensitivities. *J Pediatr.* 2001;138:688–693.
47. Bellioni-Businco B, Paganelli R, Lucenti P, et al. Allergenicity of goat's milk in children with cow's milk allergy. *J Allergy Clin Immunol.* 1999;103:1191–1194
48. Muñoz-Furlong A. *Food Allergy News Cookbook.* Minneapolis, MN. Chronimed Publishing; 1998.
49. Bush RK, Taylor CL, Nordlee JA, Busse WW. Soybean oil in not allergenic to soybean-sensitive individuals. *J Allergy Clin Immunol.* 1985:76:242–245.
50. Moneret-Vuatrin DA, Guerin L, Kanny G, et al. Cross-allergenicity of peanut and lupine: The risk of lupine allergy in patients allergic to peanuts. *J Allergy Clin Immunol.* 1999;104:883–888.
51. Sicherer S, Burks AW, Sampson H. Clinical features of acute allergic reactions to peanut and tree nuts in children. *Pediatrics*. 1998;102:6.
52. Taylor SL, Busse WW, Sachs MI, Parker JL, et al. Peanut oil is not allergenic to peanut-sensitive individuals. *J Allergy Clin Immunol.* 1981;68:372–375.
53. US Department of Agriculture, Center for Nutrition Policy and Promotion. *Food Guide Pyramid for Young Children 2 to 6 Years of Age.* Washington, DC: US Department of Agriculture, Center for Nutrition Policy and Promotion; 1999.
54. Sicherer SH, DeSimone J, Furlong TJ. Peanut and tree nut allergic reactions in restaurants and food establishments. *J Allergy Clin Immunol.* 2001;107:S231.
55. Muñoz-Furlong A. *The School Food Allergy Program.* Fairfax, VA: The Food Allergy and Anaphylaxis Network; 1995.
56. Sampson HA. Anaphylaxis and emergency treatment. *Pediatrics.* 2003;111:1601–1608.
57. Mansfield LE, Goldstein GB. Anaphylactic reaction after ingestion of local bee pollen. *Annals of Allergy.* 1981;47: 154–156.
58. Cohen SH, Yunginger JW, Rosenberg N, Fink JN. Acute allergic reaction after composite pollen ingestion. *J Allergy Clin Immunol.* 1979;64:270–274.
59. Leung R, Ho A, Chan J, Choy D, et al. Royal jelly consumption and hypersensitivity in the community. *Clin Exp Allergy.* 1997;27:333–336.
60. Thien FC, Leung R, Baldo BA, Weiner JA, et al. Asthma and anaphylaxis induced by royal jelly. *Clin Exp Allergy.* 1996;26:216–222.
61. Mullins RJ. Echinacea-associated anaphylaxis. *Med J Australia.* 1998;168:170–171.
62. Leung DY, Sampson HA, Yunginger JW, et al. Effect of anti-IgE therapy in patients with peanut allergy. *N England J Med.* 2003;348:986–993.
63. Host A, Halken S. A prospective study of cow milk allergy in Danish infants during the first 3 years of life. Clinical course in relation to clinical and immunological type of hypersensitivity reaction. *Allergy.* 1990;45: 587–596.
64. Hourihane JO, Roberts SA, Warner JO. Resolution of peanut allergy: Case-control study. *BMJ.* 1998;316: 1271–1275.
65. Skolnick HS, Conover-Walter MK, Barnes-Koerner C, et al. The natural history of peanut allergy. *J Allergy Clin Immunol.* 2001;107:265–274.
66. Fleischer DM, Conover-Walker MK, Christie L, et al. The natural progression of peanut allergy: Resolution and the possibility of recurrence. *J Allergy Clin Immunol.* 2003;112:183–189.
67. Host A, Halken S, Jacobsen HP, et al. The natural course of cow's milk allergy in Danish infants during the first 3 years of life. Clinical course in relation to clinical and immunological type of hypersensitivity reaction. *Allergy.* 1990;45:587–596.
68. American Academy of Pediatrics, Committee on Nutrition. Hypoallergenic infant formulas. *Pediatrics.* 2000; 106:346–349.
69. Isolauri E, Tahvanainen A, Peltola T, et al. Breast-feeding of allergic infants. *J Pediatr*. 1999;134:27–32.
70. Kjellman MIM. Atopic disease in seven-year-old children. Incidence in relation to family history. *Acta Paediatr Scand.* 1977;66:465–471.
71. Zeiger RS, Heller S. The development and prediction of atopy in high-risk children: Follow-up at age 7 years in a prospective randomized study of combined maternal and infant food allergen avoidance. *J Allergy Clin Immunol.* 1995;95:1179–1190.

RESOURCES FOR FOOD HYPERSENSITIVITIES

Allergy and Asthma Network/Mothers of Asthmatics, Inc.
3554 Chain Bridge Road, Suite 200
Fairfax, Virginia 22030
(800)878-4403
Web site: www.aanma.org

To locate a board-certified allergist, contact:
American Academy of Allergy, Asthma, & Immunology
611 East Wells Street
Milwaukee, Wisconsin 53202
(800)822-2762
Web site: www.aaai.org

Asthma and Allergy Foundation of America
1233 20th Street, Suite 402
Washington, DC 20036
(800)7-ASTHMA
Web site: www.aafa.org/

The American Dietetic Association
216 West Jackson Boulevard
Chicago, Illinois 60606-6995
Web site: www.eatright.org

National Eczema Association for Science and Education
6600 SW 92nd Avenue, Suite 230
Portland, Oregon 97223-0704
(800)818-7546
Web site: www.nationaleczema.org

The Food Allergy Network
10400 Eaton Place, Suite 107
Fairfax, Virginia 22030-2208
(800)929-4040
(703)691-2713
Web site: www.foodallergy.org

Ener-G Foods, Inc.
5960 1st Avenue, South
P.O. Box 84487
Seattle, Washington 98124-5787
(206)767-6660
Web site: www.ener-g.com

Miss Roben's
P.O. Box 1149
Frederick, Maryland 21702
(800)891-0083
Web site: www.missroben.com

The Gluten-Free Pantry
P.O. Box 840
Glastonbury, Connecticut 06033
(800)291-8386
Web site: www.glutenfree.com

Mead Johnson Nutritionals
Bristol-Myers Squibb Company
2400 West Lloyd Expressway
Evansville, Indiana 47721
(800)BABY-123
Web site: www.meadjohnson.com

Abbott Laboratories/Ross Products Division
625 Cleveland Avenue
Columbus, Ohio 43216
(800)227-5767
Web site: www.ross.com

Novartis Nutrition
5100 Gamble Drive
St. Louis Park, Minnesota 55416
(800)999-9978
Web site: www.novartis.com

Scientific Hospital Supplies
P.O. Box 117
Gaithersburg, Maryland 20884
(800)365-7354
Web site: www.allegromedical.com/scientific_hospital.html

MedicAlert Foundation
P.O. Box 1009
Turlock, California 95381
(800)344-3226
Web site: www.medicalert.org

Chapter 10

Weight Management: Obesity to Eating Disorders

Bonnie Spear

Obesity has been declared an epidemic in the United States. With dramatic increases between 1987 and 2000, there are now an estimated 45 million overweight or obese US adults—nearly 65% of the population. The number of overweight and obese youth also continues to rise despite efforts by government officials, academic researchers, weight loss industry, and the media. The percentage of children and adolescents who are overweight also has more than doubled since the early 1970s. The Centers for Disease Control and Prevention (CDC) reports that African-American and Hispanic children and youth are disproportionately affected by this problem. Current medical and scientific evidence suggests that overweight and obesity result from the interaction of a variety of factors including personal behaviors, biological issues related to weight regulation, genetic predisposition, excessive dietary fat intake, low levels of physical activity, as well as sociocultural and environmental influences.

In a culture that glorifies being thin, many youth become overly preoccupied with their physical appearance and in an effort to achieve or maintain a thin body, begin to diet obsessively. A minority of these youth eventually develops an eating disorder such as anorexia nervosa, bulimia nervosa, or eating disorders not otherwise specified. Between 0.5% and 1% of all females between the ages of 12 to 18 years have anorexia nervosa and 1% to 5% have bulimia nervosa, with perhaps 20% engaging in unhealthy dieting behaviors. Symptoms of eating disorders usually first become evident early in adolescence. Factors that appear to place girls at increased risk include low self-esteem, poor coping skills, and perfectionism. Additionally, daughters of women with eating disorders are at particular risk for developing an eating disorder themselves.

Adults and health professions should take it seriously when children or adolescents express concern about their body weight. Health professionals can help children and their parents understand the importance of physical activity and appropriate nutrition for maintaining health. In doing so, it is important to keep in mind a family's resources and its cultural background, which may influence a child's ability to make change.

OVERWEIGHT/OBESITY

Introduction

Childhood obesity has become the most prevalent pediatric nutritional problem in the United States.[1,2] It affects as many as 15% to 30% of grade school children and adolescents.[3,4] The prevalence rate has been rising steadily since 1965, with a relative increase of 20% in children aged 6–11 years and 18% in adolescents from 1976 to 1991.[1] There are variations in the prevalence of obesity among different ethnic groups. Among school-aged children, there is a higher occurrence of obesity in black, Native American, Puerto Rican, Mexican, and Native Hawaiians.[5] Children are also becoming obese at younger ages. This increased prevalence is problematic because obesity that occurs early in life and persists throughout childhood is more difficult to treat. If obesity continues into adolescence, it is unlikely that he or she will outgrow it.[6,7]

Prevalence and Trends

The words *pandemic* and *epidemic* have been used to describe the recent dramatic upward trends in childhood overweight/obesity. The most recent NHANES (NHANES IV) data shows a continuing increase in overweight status. As shown in Table 10–1, the increase in overweight from NHANES III (1988–1994) to NHANES IV (1999–2000) has been significant.[8] Data from the CDC[9] shows that African-American and Hispanic children and youth are disproportionately affected by this problem, with 21.5% and 21.8% respectively classified as overweight compared to 12.3% of non-Hispanic white children.

Concerns for children and adolescents experiencing rapid weight gain are seen in the research indicating that children are likely to carry obesity into adulthood and thus experience health problems related to obesity. Several studies[10,11] have documented the persistence of obesity from childhood into adolescence and on into adulthood. The probability that overweight school age children will become obese adults is estimated at 50%, while the likelihood that obese adolescents will become obese adults is between 70–80%.

Medical Complications in Children/Adolescents

Obesity is associated with significant health problems in the pediatric age group and is an important early risk factor for much of adult morbidity and mortality. Medical problems are common in obese children and adolescents and can affect cardiovascular health (hypercholesterolemia, dyslipidemia, hypertension), the pulmonary system, musculoskeletal system, the endocrine system (hyperinsulinism, insulin resistance, impaired glucose tolerance, type 2 diabetes mellitus, menstrual irregularity), and mental health status (depression, low self-esteem).[12]

Cardiovascular

With overweight children, cardiovascular risk factors tend to cluster. Data from the Bogalusa Heart Study[13] showed that children who were overweight (above the 95th percentile for BMI) had a greater risk for cardiovascular risk factors. The cardiovascular risk factor increased from 27% (nonoverweight) to 61% (overweight). Overweight children also had increased risks for elevated cholesterol (2.4% increased risk), elevated triglycerides (7.1% increased risk), and low HDL-C (3.4% increased risk). This data also showed that overweight children had a 2.5 to 4.5% increased risk for elevated blood pressure.

Pulmonary

Childhood obesity is related to increases in childhood pulmonary complications, such as sleep apnea, exercise intolerance, and asthma. Gennuso

Table 10–1 Prevalence/Trend of Overweight in Children (defined as ≥ 95th percentile BMI for age and gender)

Age	*NHANES III, 1988–1994 (in %)*	*NHANES IV, 1999–2000 (in %)*	*Change in %*
2–5 year olds	7.2	10.4	3.2
6–11 year olds	11.3	15.3	4.0
12–19 year olds	10.5	15.5	5.0

Source: NHANES III, NHANES IV.

and associates[14] showed that there were significantly more children with asthma (30.6%) who were overweight (above the 95th BMI percentile) compared with only 11.6% of the nonoverweight. The difference in asthma between obese and nonobese was significant for both sexes and across all age groups, although the severity of asthma was not related to obesity.

Musculoskeletal

Overweight is associated with an increased incidence of slipped capital femoral epiphysis (SCFE), the most common hip disorder among young teenagers. SCFE happens when the cartilage plate (epiphysis) at the top of the thighbone (femur) slips out of place. This only happens during growth before the epiphysis plates fuse.[15]

Endocrine

In 1988, Reaven first described the metabolic syndrome in adults, also called dysmetabolic syndrome or Syndrome X.[16] It is defined as a link between insulin resistance and hypertension, dyslipidemia, type 2 diabetes, and other metabolic abnormities associated with an increase risk of atherosclerotic cardiovascular disease in adults. The large variety of symptoms and signs associated with the metabolic syndrome has made it difficult to define the clinical syndrome with precision.[17] The World Health Organization[18] and the National Cholesterol Education Program (NCEP)[19] have provided diagnostic criteria for adults.

Obesity is the most common cause of insulin resistance in children and is associated with dyslipidemia, type 2 diabetes, and long–term vascular complications. The NHANES III (1988–1994) showed a prevalence of metabolic syndrome was 6.8% among overweight adolescents and 28.7% among obese adolescents. However, these rates may underestimate the current extent of the problem because both the magnitudes and the prevalence of childhood obesity have increased in the past decade.[20] Weiss and colleagues[20] modified the adult criteria to apply to children and adolescents. Because body proportions normally change during pubertal development and may vary among persons of different races and ethnic groups, waist-to-hip ratios (used as criteria in adults) are difficult to interpret and not appropriate to use in children.[20]

In the study by Weiss and associates, children and adolescents were classified as having metabolic syndrome if they met 3 or more of the following criteria:[20]

1. BMI above the 97th percentile
2. A triglyceride level above the 95th percentile
3. An HDL cholesterol level below the 5th percentile
4. Systolic or diastolic blood pressure above the 95th percentile (for age, gender, and height)
5. Impaired glucose tolerance

Results of this study suggested that the metabolic syndrome was more common among children and adolescent than previously reported and that its prevalence increased directly with the degree of obesity. Insulin resistance in obese children is strongly associated with specific adverse metabolic factors. C-reactive protein and interleukin-6 levels, which are putative biomarkers of inflammations and potential predictors of adverse cardiovascular outcomes, rose with the degree of obesity.[20]

Preliminary follow-up of the subjects suggested that the metabolic syndrome persists over time and tends to progress clinically. Many of the children diagnosed with metabolic syndrome developed type 2 diabetes in a very short period of time. The authors felt that the incidence of type 2 diabetes may represent only the tip of the iceberg and may indicate the emergence of an epidemic of advancing cardiovascular disease.[20]

The American Diabetes Association reports that type 2 diabetes now accounts for 8% to 45% of newly diagnosed cases of diabetes in children and adolescents, especially minority youth.[21] This increase in adolescent diabetes is almost completely attributable to childhood obesity. Family history is strongly associated with type 2 diabetes in children. The frequency of a history of type 2 diabetes is a first- or second-degree relative has a range from 74–100%. There is also a concern that with the relatively recent recognition of type 2 diabetes in children, many may be misdiagnosed as having type 1 diabetes.[21]

PolyCystic Ovary Syndrome (PCOS), also referred to as Stein-Leventhal syndrome, is characterized by a group of symptoms plus physical and laboratory findings that *may* present in young women as overweight (but not always), menstrual cycle disturbance often starting at puberty that may lead to infertility, insulin resistance, a propensity to develop diabetes, elevated blood pressure, elevated lipids, acne, and male-pattern hair growth: balding and excessive body hair.[22–24] PCOS experts usually agree that the two consistent components of PCOS are hyperandrogenism (increased male hormones) and chronic lack of ovulation.[22] PCOS patients have more androgen production because they have enlarged sclerocystic ovaries containing many small cysts that form from arrested follicular development; the cysts produce a relatively large amount of androgens.[22–24]

PCOS is a diagnosis of exclusion because so many things must be checked and ruled out before PCOS is considered the cause of the symptoms. The early signs of PCOS may be passed over, and although this may not alter fertility or long-term health, self-image and quality of life can be affected. Laboratory tests needed to make diagnosis usually include basic endocrine tests: estradiol, thyroid-stimulating hormone, possibly DHEAS and testosterone. Ninety percent of PCOS patients can be diagnosed with a pelvic ultrasound.[22]

Therapy for PCOS may consist of hormone therapy, a pharmaceutical agent for insulin resistance/type 2 diabetes (like Metformin), and if overweight is an issue, use of a lower calorie diet and increased physical activity. Infertility may be treated with fertility drugs.[24] Because patients' symptoms vary so greatly, medical treatment and physicians' experience with the condition vary greatly. There are support groups worldwide for women, young and old, with PCOS; most can be found through search engines on the Internet.

Assessment and Diagnosis

The assessment of the obese child is critical in the treatment of childhood obesity. Persistence of the condition is based on a wide variety of factors, including age, sex, family, history of obesity, developmental stage, ethnicity, and social environment. Each of these factors will influence the treatment goal, the selection of type of treatment, and the course of therapy. Obesity is a complex disease, and even with excellent adherence to treatment recommendations, progress may be slow. Because of the extended time that children may need to be in treatment, the assessment must include a careful review of family lifestyle patterns and the child's social environment. The first step, however, is the physical assessment. This will establish whether the obesity is accompanied by any other disorder and whether the child has any physical limitations that will be affected by an exercise program.

Growth Assessment

In children and teens, the body mass index is used to assess underweight, overweight, and the risk for overweight. Children's body fatness changes over the years as they grow. Also, girls and boys differ in their body fatness as they mature. This is why BMI for children, also referred to as BMI-for-age, is gender and age specific.[25,26] The following identifies how to interpret BMI for assessing overweight/obesity.

BMI	*Interpretation*
≥ 85th but < 95th percentile	At risk for overweight
≥ 95th percentile	Overweight

BMI Rebound

BMI changes substantially with age. After about 1 year of age, BMI-for-age begins to decline and it continues falling during the preschool years until it reaches a minimum around 4 to 6 years of age. After that age, BMI-for-age begins a gradual increase through adolescence and most of adulthood. The rebound or increase in BMI that occurs after it reaches its lowest point is referred to as BMI rebound.[27–28] This is a normal pattern of growth that occurs in all children. Recent research has shown that the age when the BMI rebound occurs may be a critical period in childhood for the development of obesity as an adult.[28] An early BMI rebound, occurring before ages 4 to 6, is associated with obesity in adulthood. However, studies have yet to determine whether the higher BMI in childhood is truly adipose tissue versus lean body mass or bone. Additional research is needed to further understand the impact of early BMI rebound on adult obesity.

Screening

The first step in screening is to assess and interpret BMI. Figure 10–1 shows recommended overweight screening procedures.[29] For children who have BMIs less than 85th percentile, recommendations are to provide nutrition and physical activity anticipatory guidance and evaluate in 1 year. For children between the 85th and 95th percentile, recommendations are for a second-level assessment/screening.

The following five items should be screened. If any are positive, then the patient should be referred for an in-depth medical assessment and behavioral management. The second-level screening includes:

1. Family history—A positive family history includes history of early cardiovascular disease, parental hypercholesterolemia, unknown family history, parental obesity, first- or second-generation relative with type 2 diabetes.

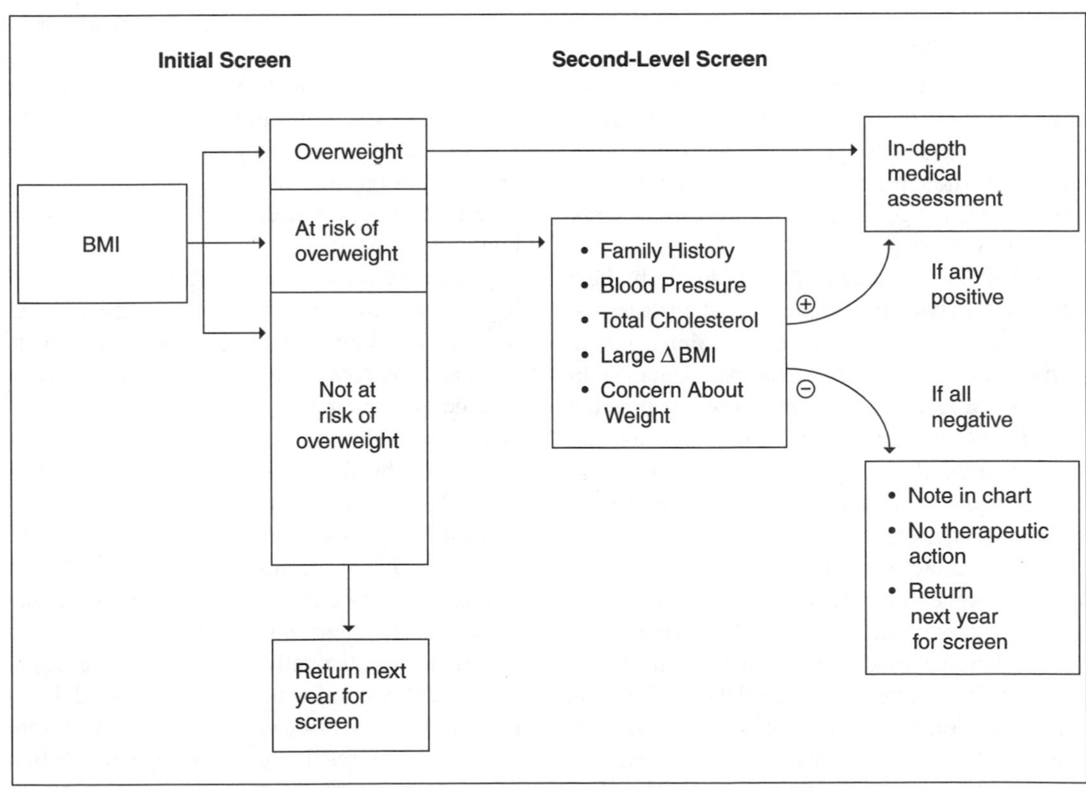

Figure 10–1 Screening for Obesity. *Source:* Himes J, Dietz W. Guidelines for overweight in adolescents preventative services. *Am J Clin Nutr.* 1994;59:307–316.

2. Blood pressure—Children/adolescents' blood pressure evaluation should be based on age, gender, and height. Blood pressures greater than the 90th percentile for age/gender/height is considered at risk and blood pressure over the 95th percentile for age/gender/height is considered high.
3. Total cholesterol—Fasting blood cholesterol levels 200 mg/dl or greater are considered a positive finding.
4. Large change in BMI—An increase of more than two or three points in BMI in 1 year is considered a positive finding.
5. Concern about weight—If the child/adolescent or family has concerns over the child/adolescents' weight, then this is considered a positive finding.

Factors Contributing to Obesity

Nutritional Intakes

It is estimated that 40% of the calories in children's diets come from added fats and sugars.[30] In fact, intakes of fruits, vegetables, dairy products, and whole grains are very low and in some cases, decreasing, while intakes of higher energy dense food have gone up.

Soft drinks represent the 6th single highest contribution of energy to the diets of adolescents. Between 12–16% of the daily caloric intake comes from soft drinks alone. Data from Ludwing and associates[31] has shown that as the number of servings of soft drinks increase, so does the risk of obesity. Unfortunately, much of the increase in soft drinks is at the expense of milk and other dairy products.

Studies show a role for calcium and dairy in obesity prevention/intervention in modulating body fat. Zemel[32] demonstrated that increased dietary calcium inhibited adipocyte intracellular calcium resulting in increased stimulation of lipolysis and inhibition of lipogenesis during energy restriction. NHANES III data showed an inverse relationship between calcium and BMI. This data indicates that individuals with higher calcium intake had lower BMIs. More recently Skinner and associates[33] showed the same effect in children. In examining children 9 to 14 years, she found that those who consume more calcium tend to weigh less and have lower body fat than those with low calcium consumption. In this study, the intake of calcium accounted for 4.5–9.0% of the variance in body fat. Skinner suggested that children could reduce their body fat if they increased their calcium intake with one glass of skim milk or 8 oz of yogurt per day. Even the slightest decrease in body fat could help in preventing comorbidities associated with overweight/obesity.

Physical Activity

Along with diet, physical activity is the other key factor in the maintenance of energy balance. Physical activity provides numerous mental and physical benefits to health including reduction in the risk of cardiovascular disease, hypertension, diabetes, depression, and cancer. According to the U.S. surgeon general's report,[34] the greatest benefits of physical activity are gained from regular participation for at least 30 minutes per day, at least four to five times per week. Unfortunately, the trend is for children to spend less and less time engaging in physical activity with U.S. children spending approximately 75% of their waking hours being inactive.

The decrease in the number of children walking to and from school, the increased use of technology by children (computers, TV in bedrooms, etc.), and the concern about after-school play in safe neighborhoods have all contributed to increased sedentary time.

A study by the Kaiser Family Foundation[35] showed that children watch an average of 2.5 hours of TV per day with one in five kids watching TV for 5 hours or more every day. Robinson[36] implemented a controlled study to promote the reduction of TV viewing. The intervention group experienced statistically significant decreases in BMI, waist circumference, triceps skinfold thickness, and self-reported decrease in eating in front of the TV. The results of this study showed that TV viewing contributes to increased body fatness and that reducing TV time improves BMI as well as body fatness.

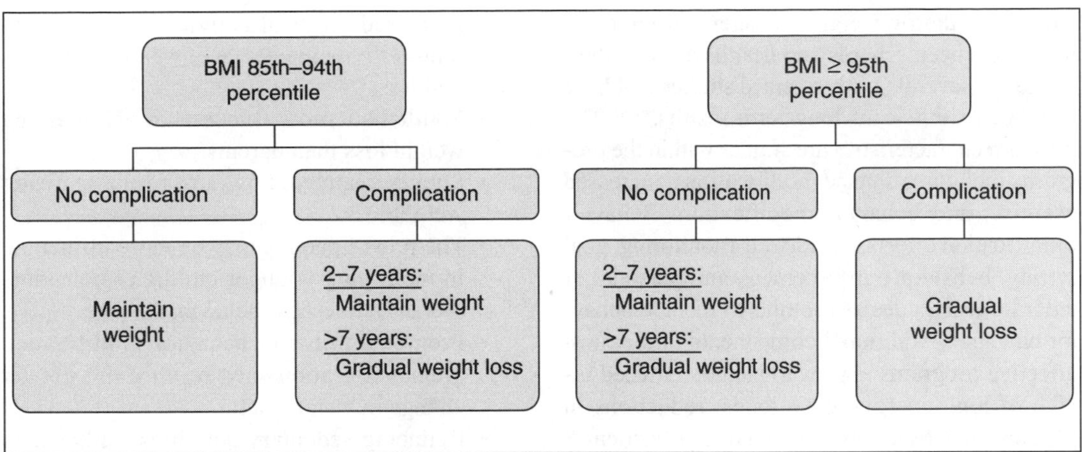

Figure 10–2 Weight Goals for Overweight Children. *Source:* Barlow SE, Dietz WH. *Pediatrics.* 1998; 102:e29. Available at www.pediatrics.org/cgi/content/full/102/3/e29.

Treatment

An expert committee was convened by the Maternal and Child Health Bureau to develop recommendations for treatment for childhood overweight.[37] The expert committee recommendations provided guidelines for treatment based on the BMI percentile (Figure 10–2). The committee recommends that for children from 2 to 7 years of age with a BMI between the 85th and 94th percentile to work on weight maintenance. For 2- to 7-year-olds with a BMI in the 95th or more percentile but without complications, the treatment should also be weight maintenance. However, for the 2- to 7-year-old whose BMI is in the 95th percentile or greater with complications, treatment should include gradual weight loss. For children over 7 years of age with a BMI between the 85th and 94th percentile without complications, treatment should be weight maintenance. However, for children over 7 years of age with a BMI between the 85th and 94th percentile with complications or with a BMI of 95th percentile or more, treatment should also include gradual weight loss. The primary goals of treatment should be related to eating and physical activity behaviors in addition to resolving any comorbidities. Interventions should not be focused only on weight loss but on healthy dietary changes, increasing physical activity, and behavior modification. Practitioners who advocate the nondiet or Health At Every Size (HAES) tenets, also believe in improving self-esteem, normalizing a person's relationship with food, finding enjoyment in activities, and learning to eat according to the person's appetite, not emotions. Goal weight is wherever it lands with healthy habits.

Intervention, Programs, and Resources

Childhood obesity treatment recommendations from the expert committee suggest that the degree of obesity and the existence of obesity-related complications determine the type of intervention to be utilized.[37] In a review of literature, Glenny and associates[38] determined that family intervention and lifestyle modification seem to be effective in the prevention and treatment of childhood but not necessarily adult obesity. Furthermore, research indicates that obese children are better able to maintain weight loss over a long-term period than adults.[39]

A variety of programs have been implemented to address childhood overweight. The primary sites for pediatric weight management interventions have been schools and health care facilities. There are several youth-oriented studies that have produced significant long-term results.[40–41] The program characteristics are similar within the programs including dietary modifications, increased exercise, and behavior modification. Behavior modification efforts include self-monitoring, goal setting, behavior reinforcement, and personal or environmental cues as prompts to include behavior change.[42] Additional components of the most effective programs appear to include reduced intake of high-energy-dense foods, reductions in physical inactivity, and parental involvement.[43] The most successful interventions also use a team of health experts.[44]

Health Care Setting (Individual and Family-Based Treatment)

The use of formal weight loss programs in health care settings has increased in recent years. Several academic institutions in conjunction with their associated medical school or health systems have implemented and evaluated child and adolescent weight-management programs. The advantages of clinical weight loss interventions delivered in the health care setting is the ability to utilize a "team" of experts from the different areas for the treatment programs and the ability of researchers to follow patients over an extended period of time. Disadvantages have tended to be associated with higher costs and dropout rates.

Much of the current understanding of individual/family treatment of pediatric overweight comes from four long-term family-based studies conducted by Epstein.[45] Epstein's studies targeted children between 6 and 12 years of age. Common program features included counseling sessions for parents and children (treatment varied from 8 to 26 weeks), the "stoplight diet" where no foods are forbidden, physical activity, and behavior modification. Key findings from Epstein's 10-year follow-up on treatment of overweight[46–48] and other long-term studies[49–52] indicate that:

- Child outcomes were improved when both parents and children were targeted for behavior change.
- Increased physical activity was critical to long-term maintenance of weight control in children.
- Youth had more success in maintaining weight loss than parents.
- Longer treatment programs result in greater weight loss.
- The role of parents may be more influential in modifying younger children's behaviors (versus adolescent behavior).
- Programs utilizing behavior modification (versus education only) resulted in a greater change in weight status.
- Reducing sedentary activities (rather than increasing structured physical activity) achieved better long-term physical activity levels.
- The caloric intake in most childhood treatment programs ranged from 900 to 1500 kilocalories/day depending on the severity and the presence of medical complications.

Through his interventions, Epstein[53] also developed a multiple-stage model for the treatment of obesity. This model shifts the responsibility for habit change from the parent to the child based on the child's developmental capabilities. Although these can be used as a guide, the interventionist must evaluate the child's cognitive ability and tailor the program to meet the family/individual's needs. These guidelines include:

1. Age 1 to 5 years: The program must focus on parent management, because parents are the major influences on child eating and activity. Children of this age are probably not motivated to lose weight.
2. Age 5 to 8 years: A program in this age group must focus on parent management, but the child must be trained to handle any social situation in which food is offered. The child can learn to solicit parental cooperation so that reciprocal reinforcement occurs with the parent or significant adult.
3. Age 8 to 12 years: Although children are still responsive to parent management methods, they can take greater responsibility for

weight loss. Reading and writing skills are more advanced and children are capable of self-monitoring and goal setting. Children at this age are more motivated to lose weight to improve athletic performance, look better, and avoid criticism from peers.

4. Age 13 and older: Children at this age possess the motivation and capability of managing their program with appropriate support from their parents. Behavior management programs for adolescents must be carefully planned because conflict can arise when parents are involved as the adolescent is struggling for independence.

Many programs are available for individual/family interventions. Unfortunately, many do not have long-term outcomes. The following is a list of programs that are nationally available and have long-term outcomes.

KidShape is designed for children K-8 to increase healthy eating and physical activity participation while building self-esteem for entire families. Results showed 87% of participants lost weight and 80% kept if off for at least 2 years. Two programs are available: Kidshape and KinderShape (designed for day care parents and workers). See http://kidshape.com.

Shapedown is a family-based intervention for children and teens (ages 6 to 18) that has been shown effective at 10-year follow-up. Goals are to enhance self-esteem, improve peer relationships, adopt healthier habits, and begin to normalize weight. See www.Shapedown.com.

Committed to Kids is an individualized approach to weight management conducted in an outpatient, group setting for children and teens ages 6 to 18 years of age. Significant decreases in body weight, BMI, and body fat have been observed short-term as well as long-term. See www.committed-to-kids.com/home.html.

SUNY–Buffalo Childhood Weight Control Program is a 6-month program designed to decrease the intake of energy-dense foods in younger children and includes individual counseling as well as group education sessions that focus on behavioral choice theory. At the 10-year follow-up, 34% of participants had maintained a decreased weight of more than 20%. For information, contact ckk@buffalo.edu.

Health Works! is a program for ages 5 to 18 and utilized a team-based treatment team to provide intervention in overweight kids through diet modification, lifestyle physical activity promotion, behavioral intervention, parental involvement, and comprehensive medical evaluations. Long-term results showed decreases in BMI. See www.cicinnatichildrens.org/svc/prog/healthworks/default.htm.

L.E.S.T.E.R. (Let's Eat Smart Then Exercise Right) is an 8-week program focused on a balance diet, increasing physical activity, and addressing emotional relationships within the family. There were significant decreases in BMI upon completion of the program and continued improvement of BMIs at the 4-year follow-up. Contact Susan.Teske@chsys.org for further information.

On Target is an intervention program for families of overweight teens. The program is designed to provide lifetime skills for weight management including nutrition, physical activity, and behavioral management. Long-term results showed improvement in BMI but greater improvement in males than females. Improvements were also shown in lipid levels. Contact the Schneider Children's Hospital in New York City.

School Settings

The school environment provides an ideal setting in which to intervene and improve children's nutrition and physical activity habits. Much has been written in the media and scientific literature about the need for modification of the school environment, including policy changes to promote healthier dietary intake and more opportunities for physical activity.[54–55] Past research has demonstrated the link between a child's health and his or her ability to learn but few studies have examined the combination of a healthful diet and activity behaviors on academic performance.[55]

The school environment is recognized as having a powerful influence on student's eating behaviors. Reimbursable school meals offered through the USDA School Lunch and Breakfast Programs must meet federally managed nutrition guidelines, but "competitive foods" such as those sold a la carte or in vending machines have no federal guidelines.

A 2003 study by Kubik and colleagues[56] demonstrated a negative and adverse association between physical factors in the school food environments such as a la carte programs, snack vending machines, and fried potatoes being served daily to students and these students' consumption of fruits, vegetables, and dietary fat. Interestingly, they found that beverage vending machines were not a significant correlate of any of the dietary behaviors studied. They concluded that the school food environment and its influence on dietary behavior extended beyond the school lunchroom. Students are exposed to foods throughout the school day and this repeated exposure, especially to less-healthful foods, is likely to influence food selection outside the school as well.

The School Health Policies and Programs Study (SHPPS) is a national survey periodically conducted to assess school health policies and programs at the state, district, school, and classroom levels. In the 2000 SHPSS data,[57] nationwide 95% of the high schools had access to soft drinks and vending machines; 80% offered high-fat cookies or cakes; 76% offered pizza, burgers, or sandwiches; and 62% offered French fries in the a la carte areas on a daily basis; while 13% of schools actually offered name-brand fast foods. Most of the items included in the vending were foods high in fat, sugar, and sodium as well as energy-dense foods.

French and associates[59,60] examined the effects of pricing strategies on sales of fruits and vegetables in a high school setting. Prices on fruit, carrots, and salads were reduced by 50% and sales were monitored; the prices were returned to the original price and sales continued to be monitored. With the less-expensive prices, fruit sales increased from 14% to 63%, carrot sales increase from 35.6% to 77.6%, and there was no significant difference in the percent of salad sales. Their results showed that lower pricing for fruits and vegetables with minimal promotion increased sales of these items among high school students.

French and colleagues[61] also researched the effect of pricing in vending machines. First, they identified the low-fat foods (less than 3g fat/package) by an orange dot. After 4 weeks, prices were reduced by 50%. During the price intervention, sale of low-fat foods increased by 80% from 25.7% to 45.8% of total sales. However, purchases returned to baseline when prices were returned to normal. Results of this study showed that without affecting overall sales volume, sales of low-fat snacks from vending machines increased significantly when prices were lowered and in the absence of a concurrent nutrition education intervention.

Concerns about the financial feasibility and long-term sustainability of the price reduction strategy have prevented it from being widely adopted as a way to promote healthful food choices. Schools are concerned with providing healthful food choices, yet as a business operation, revenues remain a primary concern. A pricing strategy that simultaneously raises prices on higher fat foods and lowers prices on lower volume, low-fat foods could address the issue of long-term financial sustainability. Increased revenues from the small increase in price on popular higher fat foods could offset lower revenues from lower priced low-fat foods. Students are an important consumer group, and a la carte and vending sales to students generate an important revenue stream for schools. Alternative funding sources need to be identified to replace potential revenue reduction that might come from policies that ensure a healthy school food environment.

School Interventions

Most school-based overweight treatment interventions have resulted in positive, though modest, and short-term effects.[62] Based on a review of literature, Story[62] identified 12 controlled school-based treatment studies of overweight children. Of these, four involved children 5 to 10 years old; six involved adolescents aged 12 to 15 years. Interventions aimed at younger children were generally more successful than interventions targeting adolescents. Interventions ranged from 9 weeks to 6 months and included nutrition education, physical activity, and behavioral modification. In all but one of the studies, the intervention group had significantly greater weight loss than the control group. Unfortunately, only two of these studies included long-term follow-up and in only one was weight loss maintained at 6 months post-interventions.

However, few school-based studies specifically targeted overweight children have been published since 1984.[63] It is speculated that the reason for this may be increased sensitivity to the stigma associated with participation in such programs at school. More recent programs have provided for school-wide interventions addressing healthy eating, increasing physical activity, and behavior change. Many have also focused on changing the school environment.

A number of evaluated school intervention programs are available addressing the topics of childhood obesity, prevention, physical activity, and nutrition behaviors. These may provide nutrition professionals the opportunity to reach out to local schools to serve as partners in education to promote a healthy school environment. A selected few school and government programs are reviewed here. A more comprehensive list of programs can be found at www.ILSI.org under documents: Physical Activity and Nutrition Programs.

Pathways is a multi-center school-based intervention to reduce obesity in American Indian children in grades 3 through 5. The overall goals are to implement a culturally appropriate school-based intervention to promote healthy eating, increase physical activity, and decrease obesity in this population. For more information, see http://hsc.unm.edu/pathways. Modules are available from the Web.

GEMS (Girls Health Enrichment Multi-site Program) is a school-based program designed for 8- to 10-year-old African-American females with the goals to reduce risk for obesity using a family-based behavioral intervention program. For more information, see www.bsc.gwu.edu/gems/.

Planet Health is a school-based program designed for adolescents in 6th and 7th grades with the goals of obesity reduction through decrease TV viewing, increased fruit and vegetable intake, and increased physical activity. See www.humankinetics.com.

Health Hearts is a Web-based interdisciplinary instructional model for 5th and 6th grade children focusing on cardiovascular disease risk factors including physical activity, nutrition and tobacco. It is designed to be used by classroom teachers. For more information, see www.healthyhearts4kids.org.

CATCH (Coordinated Approach to Child Health), originally called the Child and Adolescent Trial for Cardiovascular Health, was develop to produce school environmental changes in food service and physical activity. The program also included classroom and family education. The intervention was targeted for grades K-5. See www.flaghouse.com or www.CATCHTEXAS.org.

TEENS (Teens Eating for Energy and Nutrition at School) is a school-based program designed for 7th grade students to improve fruit and vegetable consumption, and reduce fat intake. For more information, see www.learningzoneexpress.com.

Take 10! is an elementary school–based curriculum developed by the International Life Science Institutes' Center for Health Promotion. It is designed to integrate at least 10 minutes of moderate-to-vigorous physical activity with grade-specific academic learning objectives to reinforce required concepts and skills. See www.take10.net.

Healthy Start was funded by the NIH to develop an elementary school–based intervention in changing nutrition patterns in school centers. It focuses on nutrition education and food service intervention. This is one of the few programs that has long-term intervention outcomes. See www.health-start.com for more information.

The SPARK Programs (Sports, Play and Active Recreation in Kids) is designed for pre-K through 8th grade to increase physical activity during physical education classes and outside of school. See www.sparkpe.org.

Bienestar (Spanish for "Well-being") is an intervention program designed for grades 3rd through 5th. It includes bilingual instruction materials to decrease dietary saturated fat intake, increase dietary fiber, increase fitness levels, and decrease obesity rates. Contact srhct@msn.com for more information.

CANFit is an intervention for children 10 to 14 years of age designed to improve nutritional status and physical fitness of California's low-income African-American, Latino, and Pacific Islander youth. For more information, see www.canfit.org.

Prevention

Intervention programs are few and their costs may prevent them from being integrated into school curriculums. As society continues to intervene with already-at-risk children and adolescents, it also needs to increase our preventive measures. Prevention is the responsibility of the provider, the family, the child, the school, and the community as well as the insurer and government agencies. The following provides an overview of prevention activities for each level.

Primary Care Provider

1. Early recognition of overweight/obesity: Plot BMI routinely. If it is increasing, address this prior to being higher than 95% BMI.
2. Identify those at risk:
   - Parents are overweight.
   - Sibling is overweight.
   - Family has lower socioeconomic status.
   - Children have less cognitive stimulation.
3. Provide anticipatory guidance in nutrition and physical activity.
4. Promote water and milk consumption over juice and soda.
5. Suggest eating as a family.
6. Encourage nonsedentary family activities.
7. Do not use food as a reward.
8. Limit TV/computer/video games to 1 to 2 hours per day.
9. Do not eat in front of the TV.
10. Do not put a TV in the child's room.

Parents

Act as a role model for nutrition and physical activity

Limit eating out

Encourage family meals

Set "Special times" that do not have to involve food or sedentary activities

School

Promotes physical activity

Provides nutritious meals

Has recess prior to lunch when possible

Controls vending machines/ healthy vending

Has nutrition and activity education integrated into school curriculum

Encourages children to walk or bike to school when safe

Community

Has safe playgrounds

Provides safe places for bike riding and walking

Promotes physical activity

Insurance and Government

Acknowledge obesity as a medical condition for which one can be reimbursed

Provide reimbursement for anticipatory guidance for nutrition and physical activity

Additional Web-Based Resources

www.apha.org/ppp/obesity_toolkit—A collection of tools and information regarding obesity in children (American Public Health Association).

www.brightfutures.com/nutritionfamfact—Bright Futures Nutrition Fact Sheets; materials also available in Spanish.

www.nutrition.gov—Information on nutrition for infants and children.
www.kidnetic.com—Interactive Web site for middle school children to learn about nutrition and physical activity. Includes games, contests, and puzzles.
www.4girls.gov—Nutrition and fitness information of 7- to 18-year-old females and their parents.
http://nature.berkeley.edu/cwh—The Center for Weight and Healthy at the University of California, Berkeley; provides information on nutrition and health as well as links to other sources.
www.fns.usda.gov/TN/Resources/index—Nutrition resources for schools and school-aged children; some material available in Spanish.
www.bam.gov—Provides information for teachers, providing them with interactive activities to support their health and science curriculums.
www.nat.uiuc.edu/energy—Provides a free Web-based program that allows anyone to determine the amount of physical activity needed to lose weight as well as resource information on physical activity.

EATING DISORDERS

Introduction

Eating disorders are complex illnesses that are affecting children and adolescents with increasing frequency.[64–65] Although considered to be psychiatric disorders, they are remarkable for their nutrition and medical-related problems, some of which can be life threatening. As a general rule, eating disorders are characterized by abnormal eating patterns and cognitive distortions related to food and weight, which in turn result in adverse effects on nutrition status, medical complications, and impaired health status and mental function.[66–70] The major characteristic of eating disorders are the disturbed body image in which one's body is perceived as being fat (even at normal or low weight), an intense fear of weight gain or becoming fat, and a relentless obsession to become thinner.[71,72]

Diagnosis Criteria

Diagnostic criteria for anorexia nervosa, bulimia nervosa, and eating disorders—not otherwise specified (EDNOS) are identified in the fourth edition of the *Diagnostic and Statistical Manual of Mental Disorders* (DSM-IV)[73] (see Table 10–2). These clinical diagnoses are based on psychological, behavioral, and physiological characteristics. It is important to note that patients cannot be diagnosed with both anorexia nervosa (AN) and bulimia nervosa (BN) at the same time. Patients with EDNOS do not fall into the diagnostic criterion for either AN or BN, but account for about 50% of the population with eating disorders and up to 70% of children and adolescents. Binge eating disorder is currently classified within the EDNOS grouping.

In a medical setting, often the psychiatric diagnoses of AN and BN are *not* used because medical providers are not trained in psychiatric diagnosis. Because physicians are treating the medical problems, the diagnoses are related to medical problems/symptoms such as severe malnutrition, bradycardia, hypotension, amenorrhea, vomiting, and esophageal pain.

Because of the complex biopsychosocial aspects of eating disorders, the optimal assessment and ongoing management of these conditions appear to be under the direction of an interdisciplinary team consisting of professionals from medical, nursing, nutrition, and mental health disciplines.[64,65] Medical nutrition therapy (MNT) provided by a registered dietitian trained in the area of eating disorders and pediatrics is an integral component of treatment and management of children and adolescents with eating disorders.

Children and Adolescents

Eating disorders rank as the third most common chronic illness in adolescent females, with an incidence of up to 5%. The prevalence has increased

Table 10–2 Diagnostic Criteria for Eating Disorders

Anorexia Nervosa (Diagnostic Code 307.10)

A. Refusal to maintain body weight at or above a minimally normal weight for age and height, e.g., weight loss leading to maintenance of body weight less than 85% of that expected; or failure to make expected weight gain during period of growth, leading to body weight less than 85% of that expected.
B. Intense fear of gaining weight or becoming fat, even though underweight.
C. Disturbance in the way in which one's body weight, size, or shape is experienced; undue influence of body weight or shape on self-evaluation; or denial of the seriousness of the current low body weight.
D. In postmenarcheal females, amenorrhea, i.e., the absence of at least three consecutive menstrual cycles. (A woman is considered to have amenorrhea if her periods occur only following hormone, e.g., estrogen, administration.)

Specify Type:
Restricting Type: During the current episode of Anorexia Nervosa, the person has not regularly engaged in binge eating or purging behavior (i.e., self-induced vomiting or the misuse of laxatives, diuretics, or enemas).

Binge Eating/Purging Type: During the current episode of Anorexia Nervosa, the person has regularly engaged in binge eating or purging behavior (i.e., self-induced vomiting or the misuse of laxatives, diuretics, or enemas).

Bulimia Nervosa (Diagnostic Code 307.51)

A. Recurrent episodes of binge eating. An episode of binge eating is characterized by both of the following:
   (1) eating, in a discrete period of time (e.g., within any 2-hour period), an amount of food that is definitely larger than most people would eat in a similar period of time under similar circumstances.
   (2) a sense of lack of control over eating during the episode (e.g., a feeling that one cannot stop eating or control what or how much one is eating).
B. Recurrent inappropriate compensatory behavior in order to prevent weight gain, such as self-induced vomiting; misuse of laxatives diuretics, enemas, or other medications; fasting or excessive exercise.
C. The binge eating and inappropriate compensatory behaviors both occur, on averge, at least twice a week for 3 months.
D. Self-evaluation is unduly influenced by body shape and weight.
E. The disturbance does not occur exclusively during episodes of Anorexia Nervosa.

Specific Type:
Purging Type: During the current episode of Bulimia Nervosa, the person has regularly engaged in self-induced vomiting or the misuse of laxatives, diuretic or enemas.

Nonpurging Type: During the current episode of Bulimia Nervosa, the persona has used other inappropriate compensatory behaviors, such as fasting or exessive exercise, but has not regularly engaged in self-induced vomiting or the muses of laxative, diuretic, or enemas.

Eating Disorders Not Otherwise Specified (EDNOS) (Diagnostic Code 307.5)

The Eating Disorder Not Otherwise Specified category is for disorders of eating that do not meet the criteria for any specific eating disorders. Examples include:

1. For females, all of the criteria for Anorexia Nervosa are met except that the individual has regular menses.

continues

Table 10–2 continued

2. All of the criteria for Anorexia Nervosa are met except that despite significant weight loss, the individual's current weight is in the normal range.
3. All of the criteria for Bulimia Nervosa are met except that the binge eating and inappropriate compensatory mechanism occurs at a frequency of less than twice a week or for a duration of less than 3 months.
4. The regular use of inappropriate compensatory behavior by an individual of normal body weight after eating small amounts of food (e.g., self-induced vomiting after the consumption of two cookies).
5. Repeatedly chewing and spitting out, but not swallowing large amounts of food.
6. Binge-eating disorder: recurrent episodes of binge eating in the absence of the regular use of inappropriate compensatory behaviors characteristic of Bulimia Nervosa.

Binge-Eating Disorder (Research Criteria of EDNOS)

A. Recurrent episodes of binge eating (rapid consumption of a large amount of food in a discrete period of time).
   (1) eating, in a discrete period of time* (e.g., within any 2-hour period), an amount of food that is definitely larger than most people would eat in a similar period of time under similar circumstances.
   (2) a sense of lack of control over eating during the episode (e.g., a feeling that one cannot stop eating or control what or how much one is eating).
B. The binge-eating episodes are associated with three (or more) of following:
   (1) eating much more rapidly than normal
   (2) eating until feeling uncomfortably full
   (3) eating large amounts of food when not feeling physically hungry
   (4) eating alone because of being embarrassed by how much one is eating
   (5) feeling disgusted with oneself, depressed, or very guilty after overeating
C. Marked distress regarding binge eating is present.
D. The binge eating occurs, on average, at least 2 days a week for 6 months.
E. The binge eating is not associated with the regular use of inappropriate compensatory behaviors (e.g., purging, fasting, excessive exercise) and does not occur exclusively during the course of Anorexia Nervosa or Bulimia Nervosa.

Source: Reprinted with permission from the American Psychiatric Association. *Diagnostic and Statistical Manual of Mental Disorders,* 4th ed. text revised, Washington, DC: American Psychiatric Association; 2000 (10).

*The method of determining frequency differs from that used for Bulimia Nervosa; future research should address whether the preferred method of setting a frequency threshold is counting the number of days on which binges occur on counting the number of episodes of binge eating.

dramatically over the past three decades.[69,72,74] Large numbers of adolescents who have disordered eating do not meet the strict DSM-IV criteria for either AN or BN but can be classified as EDNOS. Diagnostic criteria for eating disorders such as DSM-IV may not be entirely applicable to children and adolescents. The wide variability in the rate, timing, and magnitude of both height and weight gain during normal puberty, the absence of menstrual periods in early puberty along with the unpredictability of menses soon after menarche, and the lack of abstract concepts, limit the application of diagnostic criteria to adolescents.[68,75]

Because of the potentially irreversible effects of an eating disorder on physical and emotional growth and development in adolescents, the onset and intensity of the intervention in adolescents should be more aggressive than with adults.

Medical complications in adolescents that are potentially irreversible include (1) growth retardation if the disorder occurs before closure of the epiphyses, pubertal delay, or arrest; (2) impaired acquisition of peak bone mass during the second decade of life, increasing the risk of osteoporosis in adulthood; and (3) structural brain changes.[70,76]

Health Care Team

Adolescents with eating disorders require evaluation and treatment focused on biological, psychological, family, and social features of these complex, chronic health conditions. The expertise and dedication of the members of a treatment team who work specifically with adolescents and their families are more important than the particular treatment setting. In fact, traditional settings such as a general psychiatric ward/clinic may be less appropriate than an adolescent medical clinic/unit. Smooth transition from inpatient to outpatient care can be facilitated by an interdisciplinary team that provides continuity of care in a comprehensive, coordinated, developmentally oriented manner. The health care team needs to be familiar with working not only with the patient, but also with the family, school, coaches, and other agencies or individuals who are important influences on healthy adolescent development.[64,65,72] Many patients with eating disorders have a fear of eating in front of others. Often it can be difficult for the patient to achieve adequate intake from meals at school. Because school is a major element in the life of adolescents, team members need to be able to help adolescents and their families work within the system to achieve a healthy and varied nutrition intake. In working with the family of an adolescent, it is important to remember that the adolescent is the patient and that all nutritional therapy should be planned on an individual basis. It is often helpful to have the dietitian meet with adolescent patients and their parents to provide nutrition education and to clarify and answer questions. Parents are often frightened and want a quick fix. Educating the parents regarding the stages of the nutrition plan may be helpful.

Prognosis

There is limited research in the long-term outcomes of adolescents with eating disorders. There appears to be limited prognostic indicators to predict outcome.[67,69,74,77] Generally, poor prognosis has been reported when adolescent patients have been treated almost exclusively by mental health care professionals.[67,69] Data from treatment programs based in adolescent medicine show more favorable outcomes. Reviews by Kreipe and associates[67,69,71,78] showed a 71% to 86% satisfactory outcome when treated in adolescent-based programs. Strober and associates[77] conducted a long-term prospective follow-up of severe AN patients admitted to the hospital. At follow-up, results showed that nearly 76% of the cohort met criteria for full recovery. In this study, approximately 30% of patients had relapses following hospital discharge. The authors also noted that the time to recovery ranged from 57 to 79 months.

Adolescents who recover medically and are able to maintain a healthy weight, usually have no long-term medical side effects of the malnutrition. The only exception may be that total peak bone density may not reach the genetic potential. This is especially critical to individuals who suffer the malnutrition during the peak growth phases. Bone density may be in the normal range, but may not be as high as it would have been without the eating disorder.

Nutrition Assessment

The initial interview/visit provides the dietitian with the first opportunity to develop a therapeutic alliance with the patient while gathering information critical to the assessment. Developing an alliance with the patient is important in building a trusting relationship. Ensuring an atmosphere of acceptance during the interview allows the patient to feel comfortable and to share openly. Table 10–3 lists the topics to cover during the initial interview. In addition to the information gathered from the initial interview, a nutrition assessment should include data listed in Table

Table 10–3 Important Topics for Initial Interviews

1. Background information
   - Diagnosis
   - Age and age of onset
   - Treatment history: treaters, time in treatment
   - Weight: premorbid and current
   - Height
   - Menstruation history: last menstrual period, typical cycle
2. Food/dieting
   - "Usual" intake prior to diagnosis
   - Typical day's intake or food frequency or 24-hour recall
   - Safe and forbidden foods
   - Food likes and dislikes
   - Weight-loss techniques employed
3. Exercise history
   - Exercise and activity level: current and premorbid
     Including
       Type of exercise (e.g., running, weight training, riding bike)
       Intensity (e.g., how long to run 1 mile, how many miles)
       Setting (alone in room, at gym, etc.)
4. Weight history
   - History of weight conflicts
   - Weight high/low
   - Patient's goal weight
   - Total weight loss
5. Binge/purge activity
   - Frequency of binges
   - Method of purging
   - Frequency of purging
   - Subjective report on severity of bingeing/purging
6. Family history
   - Family members at home
   - Food/dieting/exercise/weight conflicts among other members
   - Heights and weights of family members
   - History of psychiatric illness, especially affective illness
   - Mother or sibling with eating disorder
7. Social history
   - School and grade
   - Overall school performance: current and premorbid
   - Peer interactions: current and premorbid
8. Physical status
   - General observations: hair loss; dry, flaking skin; swollen parotid glands; calluses on knuckles (Russell Sign)
   - Reported clinical effects of starvation: decreased tolerance to cold, poor sleep habits, light-headedness, dizziness, symptoms of hypoglycemia, increased moodiness
9. Medication and substance use
   - Prescription medication
   - Over-the-counter medication, including laxatives, diuretics, and vomiting agents, such as ipecac
   - Alcohol use
   - Other substance use

Table 10–4 Additional Data Needed for the Initial Assessment

1. Growth data
   - Height
   - Weight
   - BMI percentile
   - Expected weight range for height (using Hamwi method)
   - Percent ideal body weight for height
2. Energy
   - Basal energy expenditure (BEE) for ideal body weight for height
   - Requirement for weight gain (BEE × 1.5)
3. Body composition data (if appropriate)
   - Skinfolds: tricep, bicep, subscapular, suprailliac
   - Calculate percent body fat
4. Physical assessment
   - Subjective muscle wasting (e.g. gluitial wasting)
   - Symptoms of GER or H pylori
   - Symptoms of hypoglycemia (lightheadedness, dizziness)
   - Callus on knuckles
   - Dental erosions
5. Biochemical data (labs are based on symptoms; not all will be needed)
   - CBC
   - Electrolytes
   - Glucose
   - Bone density (only recommended if more than 6 months amenorrheic)
   - Lipid status (cholesterol level)
   - Phosphorus status
   - Urine specific gravity
   - Amylase
   - Stool Antigen for H pylori
   - T4, TSH

10–4. These topics will be covered in more detail in the following sections.

Medical Consequences and Intervention in Eating Disorders

Nutritional factors and dieting behaviors may influence the development and course of eating disorders.[65,67,70,79,80] Higher prevalence rates among specific groups, such as athletes and patients with diabetes mellitus,[81] support the concept that increased risk occurs with conditions in which dietary restraint or control of body weight assumes great importance. However, only a small proportion of individuals who diet or restrict intake develop an eating disorder. In many cases, psychological and cultural pressures must exist along with physical, emotional, and societal pressures for an individual to develop an eating disorder.

Anorexia Nervosa

Medical Symptoms

Essential to the diagnosis of AN is that patients weigh less than 85% of that expected (Table 10–2). There are several ways to determine the less than 85th percentile. For post-menarchal adolescents and young adults, the Hamwi method[82] can be used to determine expected weight for height. This method allows 100 pounds for 5 feet of height plus 5 lb for each inch over 5 ft tall, the

10% or greater to determine 90% to 110% expected weight for height, which is a normal healthy range. The 85th percentile of expected weight for height can be diagnostic of AN.[69,70,83,84] Additionally, for children and younger adolescents, the percent of expected weight-for-height can be calculated by using CDC growth charts or the CDC body mass index charts (see Appendix B).[85] Individuals with BMI's less than the 10th percentile are considered at risk for underweight and BMIs less than 5th percentile are at risk for AN.[67,69–71] In all cases, the patient's body build, weight history, and stage of sexual development should be considered.

Physical characteristics include lanugo hair on face and trunk, brittle listless hair, cyanosis of hands and feet, and dry skin. Cardiovascular changes include bradycardia (HR <60 beats/min), hypotension (systolic <90 mm HG), and orthostatic changes in pulse and blood pressure.[66,67,70] Many patients, as well as some health providers, attribute the low heart rate and low blood pressure to their physical fitness and exercise regimen. However, Nudel and colleagues[86] showed these lower vital signs actually altered cardiovascular responses to exercise in patients with AN. A reduced heart mass has also been associated with the reduced blood pressure and pulse rate.[87–92] Cardiovascular complications have been associated with death in AN patients.

Anorexia nervosa can also significantly affect the gastrointestinal tract and brain mass of these individuals. Self-induced starvation can lead to delayed gastric emptying, decreased gut motility, and severe constipation. There is also evidence of structural brain abnormalities (tissue loss) with prolonged starvation, which appears early in the disease process and may be of substantial magnitude. Although it is clear that some reversibility of brain changes occurs with weight recovery, it is uncertain whether complete reversibility is possible. To minimize the potential long-term physical complication of AN, early recognition and aggressive treatment is essential for young people who develop this illness.[76,93–96]

Amenorrhea is a primary characteristic of AN. Amenorrhea is associated with a combination of hypothalamic dysfunction, weight loss, decreased body fat, stress, and excessive exercise. The amenorrhea appears to be caused by an alteration in the regulation of gonadotropin-releasing hormone. In AN, gonadotropins revert to prepubertal levels and patterns of secretion.[67,70,97]

Osteopenia and osteoporosis, like brain changes, are serious and possibly irreversible medical complications of anorexia nervosa. This may be serious enough to result in vertebra compression and stress fractures.[98–99] Results indicate that some recovery of bone may be possible with weight restoration and recovery, but compromised bone density has been evident 11 years after weight restoration and recovery.[100,101] In younger adolescents, more bone recovery may be possible. Providing exogenous estrogen (e.g., oral contraceptives) has not been shown to preserve or restore bone mass in the anorexia nervosa patient.[102] Calcium supplementation alone (1500mg/d) or in combination with estrogen have not been observed to promote increased bone density.[66] However, adequate calcium intake may help to lessen bone loss.[70] Only, weight restoration to greater than 90% of expected weight/height has been shown to increase bone density.

Laboratory values in patients with AN usually remain in normal ranges until the illness is far advanced, although true laboratory values may be masked by chronic dehydration. Some of the earliest lab abnormalities include bone marrow hypoplasia including varying degrees of leukopenia and thrombocytopenia.[103–105] Despite low-fat and low-cholesterol diets, patients with AN often have elevated cholesterol and abnormal lipid profiles. Reasons for this include mild hepatic dysfunction, decreased bile acid secretion, and abnormal eating patterns.[106] Additionally, serum glucose tends to be low, secondary to a deficit of precursors for gluconeogenesis and glucose production.[71] Patients with AN may have repeated episodes of hypoglycemia.

Despite dietary inadequacies, vitamin and mineral deficiencies are rarely seen in AN. This has been attributed to a decreased metabolic need for micronutrients in a catabolic state. Additionally, many patients take vitamin and mineral supplements, which may mask true deficiencies. Despite low iron intakes, iron deficiency anemia is rare. This may be due to decreased needs due to amenorrhea, decreased needs in a catabolic state, and altered states of hydration.[107] Prolonged malnutrition, however, may lead to low levels of zinc, vitamin B12, and folate. Any low nutrient levels should be treated appropriately with food and supplements as needed.

Medical and Nutritional Management

Treatment for anorexia nervosa may be inpatient or outpatient based, depending upon the severity and chronicity of both the medical and behavioral components of the disorder. No single professional or professional discipline is able to provide the necessary broad medical, nutritional, and psychiatric care necessary for patients to recover. This teamwork is necessary whether the individual is undergoing inpatient or outpatient treatment.

Out-Patient

In AN, the goals of outpatient treatment are to focus on nutritional rehabilitation, weight restoration, cessation of weight reduction behaviors, improvement in eating behaviors, and improvement in psychological and emotional state. Clearly weight restoration alone does not indicate recovery, and forcing weight gain without psychological support and counseling is contraindicated. Typically, the patient is terrified of weight gain and may be struggling with hunger and urges to binge, but the foods he or she allows him- or herself are too limited to enable sufficient energy intake.[67,108] Individualized guidance and a meal plan that provides a framework for meals, snacks, and food choices (but not a rigid diet) are helpful for most patients.

The registered dietitian determines the individual caloric needs and with the patient develops a nutrition plan that allows the patient to meet these nutrition needs. In the early treatment of AN, this may be done on a gradual basis, increasing the caloric prescription in increments to reach the necessary caloric intake. The dietitian helps the patient to select acceptable food, thereby starting the process of relearning how to eat normally. A critical balance exists between allowing gradual, small changes in a patient with very restricted eating patterns and ensuring adequate nutrition and weight gain. Reminding the patient that the treatment team does not want the patient's weight gain to be out of control but reflective of physiologic changes may soothe fears about adding new foods and increasing the amount of calories consumed. Guidelines for nutritional intervention for anorexia nervosa are shown in Table 10–5.

MNT should be targeted at helping the patient understand nutritional needs, as well as help them to begin to make wise food choices by increasing variety in diet and by practicing appropriate food behaviors.[66] One effective counseling technique is cognitive behavioral therapy, which involves challenging erroneous beliefs and thought patterns with more accurate perceptions and interpretations regarding dieting, nutrition, and the relationship between starvation and physical symptoms.[109]

In many cases, monitoring skinfolds can be helpful in determining composition of weight gain, as well as used as an educational tool to show the composition of any weight gain (lean body mass versus fat mass). Percent body fat can be estimated from the sum of four skinfolds measurements (triceps, biceps, subscapular, and suprailiac crest) using the calculations of Durnin and colleagues.[110–111] This method has been validated against underwater weighing in adolescent girls with AN.[111] Bioelectrical impedance analysis has been shown to be unreliable in patients with AN secondary to changes in intracellular and extracellular fluid and chronic dehydration.[113,114]

Dietary supplements may be recommended as needed to meet nutritional needs. Physical activity recommendations need to be based on medical and psychological status and nutritional intake. Physical activity may need to be limited or initially eliminated with the compulsive exerciser who has AN so that weight restoration can be achieved. The counseling effort needs to focus

Table 10–5 Nutrition Intervention in Anorexia Nervosa

A. General Guidelines
1. Provide a nutritionally balanced diet with some individual preferences included (e.g., vegetarian).
2. Provide multivitamin-mineral supplements at recommended dietary allowance (RDA) levels.
3. Provide dietary fiber from grain sources to enhance elimination.
4. Whenever possible, permit small, frequent feedings to reduce sensation of bloating.
5. Use liquid supplements only when the patient cannot achieve goal intake via foods.
6. Provide cold or room-temperature food to reduce satiety sensations.
7. Reduce caffeine intake if appropriate.
8. Parenteral nutrition only in severe cases.
9. Interactive nutritional counseling on an ongoing basis.

B. Energy Recommendations
1. Initial nutrition counseling (outpatient)
   a. determine average kcal intake.
   b. develop nutrition plan with patient that has
      1. three meals and one to two snacks
      2. provides increasing energy levels (50–75% of DRI for energy or approximately 1000–1500 kcal/d). This depends on the current intake. It may take several visits to reach this level of kcal intake because of fears of food and weight gain.
   c. continue to assess for refeeding syndrome.
2. Follow-up counseling
   a. increase diet prescription in small, progressive increments to provide for:
      1. 0.5–1 lb gain /wk—outpatient
      2. 2–4 lb gain /wk—in patient
   b. maintain kcal level as long as appropriate weight gain continues.
   c. increase kcal level if weight gain stops or weight loss occurs.
   d. because of increased energy demands for repair and growth, patients may require higher than expected energy intake ($^1/_2$ to 2 times DRI for energy).
   e. if patient continues to lose or fails to gain on adequate kcal level evaluate for vomiting, discarding food, increased exercise, increased activity.

C. Micronutrients
1. Protein
   a. RDA in g/kg ideal body weight
   b. 15–20% of calories
   c. high biological value
2. Carbohydrates
   a. 50–60% of calories
   b. high fiber for treatment of constipation
3. Fat
   a. 20–25% of calories
   b. Encourage small increasing in fat intake until goal can be attained

D. Micronutrients
1. 100% of RDA for micronutrients with supplements as needed
2. 1300–1500 mg of calcium from food and supplements may help to prevent rapid bone loss
3. Iron supplement may aggravate constipation

E. Physical Activity
1. Monitor physical activity levels, increases in physical activity will affect kcal recommendations
2. Increase physical activity levels as weight restoration occurs
   a. begin with flexibility exercises (~80% expected weight for height)
   b. next add strength exercises (e.g, free weights, pushups, crunches) (~85% expected weight for height)
   c. last add aerobic activities, begin with 10 minutes and increase time as long a weight restoration continues (~88–90% expected weight for height)

on the message that exercise is an activity undertaken for enjoyment and fitness rather than a way to expend energy and promote weight loss. Supervised strength training using low level of weights is less likely to impede weight gain than other forms of activity and may be psychologically helpful for patients.[71] Nutrition therapy must be ongoing to allow the patient to understand his or her nutritional needs as well as to adjust and adapt the nutrition plan to meet the patient's medical and nutritional requirements.

Refeeding Syndrome

During the refeeding phase (especially early in the refeeding process), the patient needs to be monitored closely for signs of refeeding syndrome.[115] Refeeding syndrome is characterized by sudden and sometimes severe hypophosphatemia, sudden drops in potassium and magnesium, glucose intolerance, hypokalemia, gastrointestinal dysfunction, and cardiac arrhythmias.[88,116,117] Water retention during refeeding should be anticipated and discussed with the patient. Guidance with food choices to promote normal bowel function should be provided as well.[65,108] A weight gain goal of 1 to 2 pounds per week for outpatients and 2 to 3 pounds for inpatients is recommended. In the beginning of therapy, the dietitian will need to see the patient on a frequent basis. If the patient responds to medical, nutritional, and psychiatric therapy, nutrition visits may be less frequent. Refeeding syndrome can be seen in both the outpatient and inpatient setting, and the patient should be monitored closely during the early refeeding process. Because more aggressive and rapid refeeding is initiated on the inpatient units, refeeding syndrome is more common.[66,108]

Inpatient

Although many patients may respond to outpatient therapy, others do not. Low weight is only one index of malnutrition; weight should never be used as the only criterion for hospital admission. Most patients with AN are knowledgeable enough to falsify weights through such strategies as excessive water/fluid intake. If body weight alone is used for hospital admission criteria, these behaviors (e.g., excessive water intake) may result in acute hyponutremia or dangerous degrees of unrecognized weight loss.[69] All criteria for admission should be considered. The criteria for inpatient admission are shown on Table 10–6.[68,70,117]

The goals of inpatient therapy are the same as outpatient management, only the intensity increases. If admitted for medical instability, the medical and nutrition stabilization is the first and most important goal of inpatient treatment. This is often necessary before psychological therapy can be optimally effective. Often, the first phase of inpatient treatment is on a medical unit.[70,117,118,119]

The dietitian team member should guide the nutrition plan. The nutrition plan should help the patient, as quickly as possible, to consume a diet that is adequate in energy intake and nutritionally balanced. The energy intake as well as body composition should be monitored to ensure that appropriate weight gain is achieved. As with outpatient therapy, MNT should be targeted at helping the patients understand nutritional needs as well as help them to begin to make wise food choices by increasing variety in the diet and by practicing appropriate food behaviors.[66,119] In very rare instances, enteral or parenteral feeding may be necessary. However, risks associated with aggressive nutrition support in these patients are substantial, including hypophosphatemia, edema, cardiac failure, seizures, aspiration of enteral formula, and death.[66,117] Reliance on foods (rather than enteral or parenteral nutrition support) as the primary method of weight restoration contributes significantly to successful long-term recovery. The overall goal is to help the patient normalize eating patterns and learn that behavior must involve planning and practicing with real food.

BULIMIA NERVOSA

Bulimia Nervosa (BN) occurs in approximately 2–5% of the population. Most patients with BN tend to be of normal weight or moderately overweight and therefore are often undetectable by appearance alone. The average onset of BN occurs between mid-adolescence and the late 20s with a great diversity of socioeconomic status.[120] The

Table 10–6 Indications for Hospitalization in an Adolescent with an Eating Disorder

One or more of the following justify hospitalization:

1. Severe malnutrition (weight under 75% expected weight/height)
2. Dehydration
3. Electrolyte disturbances (hypokalemia, hyponatremia, hypophosphatemia)
4. Cardiac dysrhythmia (including prolonged QT)
5. Physiological instability
   severe bradycardia (heart rate < 50 beats/min)
   hypotension (<80/50 mm Hg)
   hypothermia (body temperature <96° F)
   orthostatic changes in pulse (>20 beats per minute) or blood pressure (>10 mm Hg)
6. Arrested growth and development
7. Failure of outpatient treatment
8. Acute food refusal
9. Uncontrollable binging and purging
10. Acute medical complication of malnutrition (e.g., syncope, seizures, cardiac failure, pancreatitis, etc.)
11. Acute psychiatric emergencies (e.g., suicidal ideation, acute psychoses)
12. Co-morbid diagnosis that interferes with the treatment of the eating disorder (e.g., severe depression, obsessive compulsive disorder, severe family dysfunction).

Source: Data from Position of the American Dietetic Association. Nutrition intervention in the treatment of anorexia nervosa, bulimia nervosa, and eating disorders not otherwise specified (EDNOS). 2001;101(7):810.

individual at risk for the disorder may also have a risk for depression that may be exacerbated by a chaotic or conflicting family, as well as the stress of social expectations.[121,122] A subgroup of BN patients began bingeing before dieting. This group tends to be of a higher body weight.[123]

The patient with BN has an eating pattern, which is typically chaotic with self-imposed rules of what should be eaten, how much, and what constitutes good and bad foods. These considerations occupy the thought process for the majority of the patient's day. Although the amount of food consumed that is labeled a binge episode is subjective, the criteria for bulimia nervosa requires other measures such as the feeling of out of control during the binge (Table 10–2).

The diagnostic criteria for this disorder focuses on the binge/purge behavior; however, much of the time, the person with BN is restricting her or his food intake. The dietary restriction can be the physiological or psychological trigger to subsequent binge eating. Also, the trauma of breaking "the rules" by eating something other than what was intended or more than what was intended may lead to self-destructive binge/purge eating behavior. Any sensation of stomach fullness may trigger the person to purge. Common purging methods consist of self-induced vomiting (with or without the use of syrup of ipecac), laxative use, diuretic use, and excessive exercise. After purging, the patient may feel some initial relief; however, this is often followed by feelings of guilt and shame. Resuming normal eating commonly leads to gastrointestinal complaints such as bloating, constipation, and flatulence. This physical discomfort, as well as the guilt from bingeing, often results in the patient trying to get back on track by restricting once again. The binge/purge behavior is often a means for the person to regulate and manage emotions and to medicate psychological pain.[124]

Medical Symptoms

In the initial assessment, it is important to assess and evaluate for medical conditions that may play a role in the purging behavior. Such conditions as esophageal reflux (GER) and helicobacter pylori may increase the pain and the need for the patient to vomit. Medical interventions for these conditions may help in reducing the vomiting and allow the treatment for BN to be more focused. Nutritional abnormalities for patients with BN depend on the amount of restriction during the nonbinge episodes. It is important to note that purging behaviors do not completely prevent the utilization of calories from the binge; an average retention of 1200 calories occurs from binges of various sizes and contents.[125,126]

Muscle weakness, fatigue, cardiac arrhythmias, dehydration, and electrolyte imbalance can be caused by purging, especially self-induced vomiting and laxative abuse. It is common to see hypokalemia and hypochloremic alkalosis, as well as gastrointestinal problems involving the stomach and esophagus. Some patients may have calluses on one or both hands around the knuckles (Russell signs). This is caused from the teeth hitting the hand when patients use their fingers to induce vomiting. Dental erosion from self-induced vomiting can be quite serious. Although laxatives are used to purge calories, they are quite ineffective. Chronic ipecac use has been shown to cause skeletal myopathy, electrocardiographic changes, and cardiomyopathy with consequent congestive heart failure, arrhythmia, and sudden death.[65,66]

Medical and Nutritional Management of Bulimia Nervosa

As with AN, interdisciplinary team management is essential to care. The majority of patients with BN are treated in an outpatient setting. Indications for inpatient hospitalization include severe disabling symptoms that are unresponsive to outpatient treatment or additional medical problems such as uncontrolled vomiting, severe laxative abuse withdrawal, metabolic abnormalities or vital sign changes, or suicidal ideations.[82]

The main goal for nutrition therapy is to help the patient develop an eating plan to normalize eating. The primary goal of intervention is to normalize eating patterns. Any weight loss that is achieved would occur as a result of a normalized eating plan and the elimination of bingeing. Helping patients combat food myths often requires specialized nutrition knowledge.[127] Bulimic patients of normal or excess body weight often present with a history of attempts to control weight through severe caloric restriction. Foods become categorized as "good" and "bad" or "safe" and "forbidden." Low-fat foods (e.g., fruits, vegetables, rice cakes, nonfat yogurt) become the staples at meals, leading to decreased satiety at meals and an increased vulnerability to bingeing. Food intake patterns are usually quite rigid, and the patient often believes that this seemingly controlled intake is healthy and is the only way to eat to lose or maintain weight. These unrealistic diet restrictions need to be met with clear guidelines that promote satiety, thereby reducing the risk of bingeing. Specific recommendations for nutrition intervention in BN are shown on Table 10–7.

Cognitive-behavioral therapy (CBT) is now a well-established treatment modality for BN.[108,109,128] A key component of the CBT process is nutrition education and dietary guidance. Meal planning, assistance with a regular pattern of eating, and rationale for and discouragement of dieting are all included in CBT. Nutrition education consists of teaching about body weight regulation, energy balance, effects of starvation, misconceptions about dieting and weight control, and the physical consequences of purging behavior. Meal planning consists of three meals a day with one to three snacks per day prescribed in a structured fashion to help break the chaotic eating pattern that continues the cycle of bingeing and purging. Caloric intake should initially be based on the maintenance of weight to help prevent hunger because hunger has been shown to substantially increase the susceptibility to bingeing. One of the hardest challenges of normalizing the eating pattern of the person with BN is to expand the diet to include the patient's self-imposed "forbidden" or "feared" foods. CBT provides a structure to plan for and expose patients to these foods from least feared to most feared, while in a safe, structured, supportive environment. This step is critical in breaking the

Table 10–7 Nutrition Intervention with Bulimia Nervosa

A. General Guidelines
   1. Regularly planned, nutritionally balanced meals and snacks
   2. Adequate but not excessive energy intake
   3. Include warm foods rather than cold or room-temperature foods to increase meal satiety
   4. Avoidance of dieting behavior
   5. Minimize food avoidance
   6. Increase the variety of foods consumed
   7. Dietary fiber for meal satiety and to aid elimination
   8. Develop control strategies for high-risk situations
B. Energy Intake
   1. 75–100% DRI/age/height/weight at physical activity level (PAL) 1(sedentary)
   2. Monitor anthropometric status and adjust caloric intake to ensure weight maintenance
   3. Depending on beginning entry weight, adjust kcal to help patient achieve healthy weight
   4. Initial plans are around 1500 kcal/day
C. Macronutrients
   1. Protein
      a. RDA in g/kg/ideal body weight
      b. 15–20% of total kcal
   2. Carbohydrate
      a. 50–55% of total kcal
      b. Fiber to help with constipation
   3. Fat
      a. 20–30% of total kcal
D. Micronutrients
   1. 100% of RDA through food or supplements

all-or-none behavior that goes along with the deprive-binge cycle.

Discontinuing purging and normalizing eating patterns are key focuses of treatment. A common symptom of stopping purging is fluid retention. The patient needs education and understanding of this temporary, yet disturbing phenomenon. Education should consist of information about the length of time to expect the fluid retention. It is helpful to provide evidence that the weight gain is not causing body fat mass gain. In some cases, utilization of skinfold measurements to determine percent body fat may be helpful in determining body composition changes. The patient must also be taught that continual purging or other methods of dehydration such as restricting sodium or using diuretics or laxatives will prolong the fluid retention. If the patient is laxative dependent, a protocol for laxative withdrawal should be implemented to prevent bowel obstruction. The patient should be instructed on a high-fiber diet with adequate fluids while the physician monitors the slow withdrawal of laxatives.

Self-monitoring tools can be helpful in revealing to the patient his or her food beliefs and eating patterns. Through recognition of certain harmful or self-defeating thoughts and behaviors, choices can be made to find alternatives. Records or journals should include facts, state of mind, and some reflection about his or her emotional world, for example:

1. Type and amount of food eaten
2. Time of day
3. Degree of hunger (low, medium, high) and fullness (low, medium, high)
4. Binge/purge activity

Medication management is more effective in treating BN than in AN and especially with patients who present with comorbid conditions.[82,127] Current evidence sites combined medication management and CBT as most effective in treating BN[129] although research continues looking at effectiveness of other methods and combinations of methods of treatment.

EATING DISORDERS NOT OTHERWISE SPECIFIED

The large group of patients who present with EDNOS consists of subacute cases of AN or BN. The nature and intensity of the medical and nutritional problems and the most effective treatment modality will depend on the severity of impairment and the symptoms. These patients may have met all criteria for anorexia except that they have not missed three consecutive menstrual periods, or they may be of normal weight and purge without bingeing. Although the patient may not present with medical complications, they do often present with medical concerns.

EDNOS also includes binge eating disorder (BED) (Table 10–2) in which the patient has bingeing behavior without the compensatory purging seen in bulimia nervosa. It is estimated that prevalence of this disorder is 1–2% of the population. Binge episodes must occur at least twice a week and have occurred for at least 6 months. Most patients diagnosed with BED are overweight and suffer the same medical problems faced by the nonbingeing obese population such as diabetes, high blood pressure, high blood cholesterol levels, gallbladder disease, heart disease, and certain types of cancer.

The patient with the binge eating disorder often presents with weight management concerns rather than eating disorder concerns. Although researchers are still trying to find the treatment that is the most helpful in controlling binge eating disorder, many treatment manuals exist utilizing the CBT model shown effective for BN.[130–132]

Populations at High Risk

Specific population groups who focus on food or thinness such as athletes, models, culinary professionals, and young people who may be required to limit their food intake because of a disease state are at risk for developing an eating disorder.[81] Additionally, risks for developing an eating disorder may stem from predisposing factors such as a family history of mood, anxiety, or substance abuse disorders. A family history of an eating disorder or obesity, and precipitating factors such as the dynamic interactions among family members and societal pressures to be thin, are additional risk factors.[133,134]

The prevalence of formally diagnosable AN and BN in males is accepted to be from 5% to 10% of all patients with an eating disorder.[135,136] Young men who develop AN are usually members of subgroups that emphasize weight loss. The male anorexic is more likely to have been obese before the onset of the symptoms. Dieting may have been in response to past teasing or criticisms about his weight. Additionally, the association between dieting and sports activity is stronger among males. Both a dietary and activity history should be taken with special emphasis on body image, performance, and sports participation on the part of the male patient. These same young men should be screened for androgenic steroid use. The DSM-IV diagnostic criterion for AN of more than 85th percentile of ideal body weight is less useful in males. A focus on the BMI, nonlean body mass (percent body fat), and the height-weight ratio are far more useful in the assessment of the male with an eating disorder. Adolescent males below the 25th percentile for BMI, upper arm circumference, and subscapular and triceps skinfold thicknesses, should be considered to be in an unhealthy, malnourished state.[136,137]

Although more research is needed into treatment of eating disorders, some strategies to protect adolescents in general from developing an eating disorder or an obsession with weight include:

- Promote the acceptance of a broad range of appearances
- Promote positive self-image and body image
- Educate adolescents and their families about the detrimental consequences of a negative focus on weight

- Educate school personnel, including coaches on risk factors and symptoms for early identification of eating disorders
- Promote a positive focus on sources of self-esteem other than physical appearance, such as academic, artistic, or athletic accomplishments

---

REFERENCES

1. Troiano RP, Flegal KM, Kuczmarski RJ, Campbell SM, Johnson CL. Overweight prevalence and trends for children and adolescents. *Arch Pediatr Adolesc Med.* 1995;149:1085.
2. Must A, Jacques PF, Dallal GE, Bajema CJ, Dietz WH. Long-term morbidity and mortality of overweight adolescents. *N Engl J Med.* 1992;327:1350.
3. Kuczmarski RJ, Flegal KM, Campbell SM, et al. Increasing prevalence of overweight among US adults. *JAMA.* 1994;272:205–210.
4. Gortmaker SL, Must A, Suho AM, et al. Television viewing as a cause of increasing obesity among children in the United States. *Arch Pediatr Adolesc Med.* 1996;150:356–362.
5. Kumanyika S. Ethnicity and obesity development in children. *Ann NY Acad Sci.* 1993;699:81–86.
6. Serdula MK, Ivery D, Coates RJ, et al. Do obese children become obese adults? *Prev Med.* 1993;22:167– 176.
7. Whitaker RC, Wright JA, Pepe MS, Seidel KD, Dietz WH. Predicting obesity in young adulthood from childhood and parental obesity. *N Engl J Med.* 1997;337: 869–873.
8. Ogden CL, Flegal KM, Carroll MD, Johnson CL. Prevalence and trends in overweight among US children and adolescents, 1999–2000. *JAMA.* 2002;288:1728–1732.
9. Centers for Disease Control and Prevention, *Obesity Still on the Rise, New Data Show.* Division of Nutrition and Physical Activity Web site. Retrieved May 15, 2004, from www.cdc.gov.
10. Serdulaa MK, Ivery D, Coates RJ, et al. Do obesity children become obese adults? A review of the literature. *Prev Med.* 1993;22:167–177.
11. Whitaker RC, Wright JA, Pepe MS, Seidel KD, Dietz WH. Predicting obesity in young adulthood from childhood and prenatal obesity. *New England J Med.* 1997;337:869–873.
12. American Academy of Pediatrics: Policy Statement. Prevention of pediatric overweight and obesity. *Pediatrics.* 2003;112(2):424–430.
13. Freedman DS, Dietz WH, Srinivasan SR, Berenson GS. The relationship of overweight to cardiovascular risk factors among children and adolescents: The Bogalusa Health Study. *Pediatrics.* 1999;103(6 pt 1):1175–1182.
14. Gennuso J, Epstein LH, Paluch RA, Cerny F. The relationship between asthma and obesity in urban minority children and adolescents. *Arch Pediatr Adol Med.* 1998; 152:1197–1200.
15. Richards BS. Slipped capital femoral epiphysis. *Pediatr Rev.* 1996;17:69–70.
16. Reaven GM. Banting lecture 1988: Role of insulin resistance in human disease. *Diabetes.* 1988;37:1595–1607.
17. Bray GA, Campagne CM. Obesity and the metabolic syndrome: Implications for dietetics practitioners. *J Am Diet Assoc.* 2004;104:86–89.
18. NHBLI. *Third Report of the National Cholesterol Education Program Expert Panel on Detection, Evaluation and Treatment of High Blood Cholesterol in Adults* (Adult Treatment Panel III). NIH publication no. 01-3670. Bethesda, MD: National Heart, Lung and Blood Institute; May 2001.
19. Alberti KG, Zimmet PZ. Definition, diagnosis and classification of diabetes mellitus and its complications. 1. Diagnosis and classification of diabetes mellitus provisional report of a WHO consultation. *Diabet Med.* 1998;15:539–553.
20. Weiss R, Dziura J, Burget TS, et al. Obesity and the metabolic syndrome in children and adolescents. *N Engl J Med.* 2004;350:2362–2374.
21. American Diabetes Association. Type 2 diabetes. I. children and adolescents. *Diabetes Care.* 2000;286: 1427–1430.
22. Thatcher SS. *Polycystic Ovary Syndrome: The Hidden Epidemic.* Indianapolis, IN: Perspectives Press; 2000.
23. Azziz R, Dewailly D, Nestler JE. *Androgen Disorders in Women.* Philadelphia, PA: Lippincott-Raven; 1997.
24. Polycystic ovary syndrome: Metabolic challenges and new treatment options (1998). *Am J Obstet Gynecol* (supplement);179:S87–S116.
25. Hammer LD, Kraemer HC, Wilson DM, Ritter PL, Dornbusch SM. Standardized percentile curves of body-mass index for children and adolescents. *Am J Dis Child.* 1991;145:259–263.
26. Pietrobelli A, Faith MS, Allison DB, Gallagher D, Chiumello G, Heymsfield SB. Body mass index as a measure of adiposity among children and adolescents: A validation study. *J Pediatrics.* 1998;132:204–210.
27. Whitaker RC, Pepe MS, Wright JA, Seidel KD, Dietz WH. Early adiposity rebound and the risk of adult obesity. *Pediatrics,* 1998;101(5). Available at www.pediatrics.org/cgi/content/full/101-3/e5.
28. Rolland-Cachera MF, Cole TJ, Sempe M, Tichet J, Rossignol C, Charraud A. Body mass index variation: Centiles from birth to 87 years. *Eur J Clin Nutr.* 1991; 45:13–21.

29. Himes JH, Deitz WH. Guidelines for overweight in adolescent preventive services: Recommendations form an expert committee. *Am J Clin Nutr.* 1994;59:307–316.

30. Munoz KA, Drebs-Smith SM, Callard-Barbash R, Cleveland LE. Food intakes of US children and adolescents compared with recommendations (published erratum appears in *Pediatrics* 1998 May;101(5): 952–953). *Pediatrics.* 1997;100(3 p1):323–329.

31. Ludwig DS, Peterson KE, Gortmaker SL. Relation between consumption of sugar-sweetened drinks and childhood obesity: A prospective, observational analysis. *Lancet.* 2001;357(9255):505–508.

32. Zemel MB. Role of dietary calcium and dariy produce in modulating adiposity. *Lipids.* 2003;38:139–146.

33. Skinner JD, Bounds W, Carruth BR, Zeigler P. Longitudinal calcium intake is negatively related to children's body fat indexes. *J Am Diet Assoc.* 2003;103: 1626–1631.

34. US DHHS. *Physical Activity and Health: A Report of the Surgeon General.* Atlanta, GA: US Department of Health and Human Services, Centers for Disease Control and Prevention, Center for Chronic Disease Prevention and Health Promotion; 1996.

35. Rideout VJ, Foehr UG, Robers DF, Brodie M. *Kids and Media@ the New Millennium.* A Kaiser Family Foundation report. November 1999. Retrieved June 1, 2004, from http://kff.org.

36. Robinson TN. Reducing children's television viewing to prevent obesity: A randomized controlled trial. *JAMA.* 1999;282:1561–1567.

37. Barlow SE, Dietz WH. Obesity evaluation and treatment: Expert committee recommendations. *Pediatrics.* 1998;102(3):1–11.

38. Glenny AM, O'Meara S, Melville A, et al. The treatment and prevention of obesity: A systematic review of the literature. *Int. J. Obes.* 1997;21:715–737.

39. Epstein L, Goldfield G. Physical activity in the treatment of childhood overweight and obesity: current evidence and research issues. *Med Sci Sprots Exerc.* 1999; 31(suppl):553–559.

40. Fulton JE, McGuire MT, Caspersen CH, Dietz WH. Interventions for weight loss and weight gain prevention among youth: Current issues. *Sports Med.* 2001;31:153–65.

41. Epstein LH, Myers MD, Raynor HA, et al. Treatment of pediatric obesity. *Pediatrics.* 1998;101:554–570.

42. Epstein LH, Wing RR, Koeske R, et al. Child and parent weight loss in family based behavior modifications programs. *J Consult Clin Phychol.* 1981;49: 674–685.

43. Davis SP, Davis M, Northington L, Moll G, Kolar K. Childhood obesity reduction by school based programs. *ABNF J.* 2002;13:145–149.

44. Sothern MS. Exercise as a modality in the treatment of childhood obesity. *Ped Clin N Am.* 2001;48(4):995–1015.

45. Epstein LH. Family-based behavioural intervention for obese children. *Int J Obes Relat Metab Disord.* 1996; 20:s14–21.

46. Epstein LH, Wing RR, Koeske R, et al. Long-term effects of family-based treatment of childhood obesity. *J Consult Clin Psychol.* 1987;55:91–95.

47. Epstein LH, Valoski AM, Wing RR, et al. Ten-year follow-up of behavioral family-based treatment for obese children. *JAMA.* 1990;264:2519–2523.

48. Epstein LH, Valoski AM, Wing RR, et al. Ten-year outcomes of behavioral family-based treatment for childhood obesity. *Health Psychol.* 1994;13:373–378.

49. Golan M, Fainaru M, Weizman A. Role of behaviour modification in the treatment of childhood obesity with parents as the exclusive agents of change. *Int J Obesity.* 1998;22:1217–1224.

50. Israel AC, Guile CA, Baker JE, et al. An evaluation of enhanced self-regulation training in the treatment of childhood obesity. *J Ped Psychol.* 1994;19:737–749.

51. Brownell KD, Kelman SH, Stunkard AJ. Treatment of obese children with and without their mothers: Changes in weight and blood pressure. *Pediatrics.* 1983;71: 515–523.

52. Epstein LH, Wing RR, Steranchak L, et al. Comparison of family-based behavior modification and nutrition education for childhood obesity. *J Ped Psychol.* 1980; 5:25–36.

53. Epstein L. Treatment of childhood obesity. In: Brownell KD, and Foreyt JP, eds, *Handbook of Eating Disorders.* New York: Basic Books, Inc.; 1986.

54. Society for Nutrition Education, Weight Realities Division. Guidelines for childhood obesity prevention programs: Promoting healthy weight in children. *J Nutr Ed and Behav.* 2003;35:1–5.

55. Kibbe D. *Childhood Obesity—Advancing Effective Prevention and Treatment: An Overview for Health Professionals.* Washington, DC: National Institute for Health Care Management Foundation. 2003;1–44.

56. Kubik MY, Lytel LA, Hannan PJ, Perry CL, Story M. The association of the school food environment with dietary behaviors of young adolescents. *Am J Public Health.* 2003;93(7):1168–1173.

57. Center for Chronic Disease Prevention and Health Promotion. SHPPS 2000: School Health Policies and Programs Study. *J School Health.* 2001;71(7):1–65.

58. Center for Chronic Disease Prevention and Health Promotion. *SHPPS 2004: School Health Policies and Programs Study.* Retrieved June 5, 2004, from www.cdc.gov/HealthyYouth/shpps.

59. French SA. Pricing effects on food choices. *J Nutr.* 2003;133(3):841S–843S.

60. French SA, Story M, et al. Food environment in secondary schools: A la carte, vending machines and food policies and practices. *Am J Public Health.* 2003;93(7): 1161–1168.
61. French SA, Jeffery RW, et al. Pricing and promotion effects on low-fat vending snack purchases: The CHIPS Study. *Am J Public Health.* 2001;91(1)112–117.
62. Story M. School-based approaches for preventing and treating obesity. *Int J Obes Relat Metab Disord.* 1999;23:S43–S51.
63. Ritchie L, Ivey S, Masch M, Woodward-Lopez G, Ikeda J, Crawford P. *Pediatric Overweight: A Review of the Literature.* The Center for Weight and Health, College of Natural Resources, University of California-Berkeley, available at http://nature.berkeley.edu.cwh, June 2001.
64. Adolescent Medicine Committee, Canadian Paediatric Society. Eating disorders in adolescents: Principles of diagnosis and treatment. *Paediatrics and Child Health.* 1998;3(3):189–92.
65. Society for Adolescent Medicine. Eating disorders in adolescents: A position paper of the Society of Adolescent Medicine. *J Adol Health.* 2003;33:496–503.
66. Rock CL. Nutritional and medical assessment and management of eating disorders. *Nutr Clin Care.* 1999;2: 332–343.
67. Kreipe RE, Uphoff M. Treatment and outcome of adolescents with anorexia nervosa. *Adolesc Med.* 1992;16: 519–540.
68. Gralen SJ, Levin MP, Smolak L, et al. Dieting and disorders eating during early and middle adolescents: Do the influences remain the same? *Int J Eating Disorder.* 1990;9:501–512.
69. Kreipe RE, Birndorf DO. Eating disorders in adolescents and young adults. *Med Clin North Am.* 2000; 84(4):1027–1049.
70. Becker AE, Grinspoon SK, Klibanski A, Herzog DB. *N Eng J Med.* 1999;340(14):1092–1098.
71. Kreipe RE, Churchill BH, Strauss J. Longer-term outcome of adolescent with anorexia nervosa. *Am J Dis Child.* 1989;43:1233–1327.
72. Fisher M, Golden NH, Datzman KD, et al. Eating disorders in adolescents: A background paper. *J Adol Health Care.* 1995;16:420–437.
73. American Psychiatric Association. *Diagnostic and Statistical Manual of Mental Disorders,* 4th ed. Washington, DC: APA Press; 2000.
74. Rome ES, Ammerman S, Rosen DS, et al. Children and adolescent with eating disorders: The state of the art. *Pediatrics.* 2003;111:e98–e102.
75. American Academy of Pediatrics Policy Statement. Identifying and treating eating disorders. *Pediatrics.* 2003;111:204–211.
76. Katzman DK, Zipursky RB. Adolescents with anorexia nervosa: The impact of the disorder on bones and brains. In: Jacobson MS, Rees JM, Golden NH, Irwin CE, eds. *Adolescent Nutritional Disorders: Prevention and Treatment.* New York: Annals of the New York Academy of Sciences. 1997;817:127–137.
77. Strober M, Freeman R, Morrell W. The long-term course of severe anorexia nervosa in adolescents: Survival analysis of recovery, relapse and outcome predictors over 10–15 years in a prospective study. *Int J Eat Disord.* 1997;22:339–369.
78. Kreipe RE, Durkarm CP. Outcome of anorexia nervosa related to treatment utilizing an adolescent medicine approach. *J Youth Adolesc.* 1996;25:383–397.
79. Ressler A. A body to die for: Eating disorders and body-image distortion in women. *Int J Fertil Womens Med.* 1998;43(3):133–138.
80. Portilla MG, Smith PD. Diagnosis and treatment of adolescents with eating disorders. *J Ark Med Soc.* 1997;94(5):211–214.
81. Engstrom I, Kroon M, Arvidson CG, et al. Eating disorders in adolescent girls with insulin-dependent diabetes mellitus: A population-based case-control study. *Acta Paediatr.* 1999;88(2):175–180.
82. Hammond KA. Dietary and clinical assessment. *Krause's Food, Nutrition and Diet Therapy,* 11th ed. Philadelphia: WB Saunders; 2004.
83. American Psychiatric Association. Practice guidelines for the treatment of patients with eating disorders. *Am J Psych.* 2000;157(suppl):1–39.
84. Executive Summary of the Clinical Guidelines on the Identification, Evaluation and Treatment of Overweight and Obesity in Adults. *Arch. Intern Med.* 1998;158: 1855–1867.
85. *CDC Growth Charts.* Available at www.cdc.gov/growthcharts; 2000.
86. Nudel DB, Gootman N, Nussbaum MP, Shenker IR. Altered exercise performance in patients with anorexia nervosa. *J Ped.* 1984;105:34–42.
87. Schebendach J, Reichert-Anderson P. Nutrition in eating disorders. In: Mahan K, Escott-Stump S, eds. *Kraus's Nutrition and Diet Therapy.* New York: McGraw-Hill; 2000.
88. Swenne I. Heart risk associated with weight loss in anorexia nervosa and eating disorders: Electrocardiographic changes during the early phase of refeeding. *Acta Paediatr.* 2000;89:447–452.
89. Harris JP, Kreipe RE, Rossback CN. QT prolongation by isoproterenol in anorexia nervosa. *J Adol Health.* 1993;14:390–393.
90. Cooke RA, Chambers JB. Anorexia nervosa and the heart. *Br J Hosp Med.* 1995;54:313–317.
91. Silber T. Anorexia nervosa: Morbidiy and mortality. *Ped. Ann.* 1984; 13:851–859.

92. Web JC, Kiess MS, Chan-Yan CC. Malnutrition and the heart. *Can Med Assoc J.* 1986;135:753–758.

93. Dolan RJ, Mitchell JA. Structural brain changes in patients with anorexia nervosa. *Psychiatr Med.* 1988;18: 349–353.

94. Artmann H, Gruau H, Adelmann M. Reversible and non-reversible enlargement of cerebrospinal fluid spaces in anorexia nervosa. *Neuoradiology.* 1985;27:304–312.

95. Nussbaum M, Shenker I, Marc J, et al. Cerebral atrophy in anorexia nervosa. *J Pediatr.* 1980;96:869–876.

96. Lantzouni E, Frank GR, Golden NH, Shenker RI. Reversibility of growth stunting in early onset anorexia nervosa: A prospective study. *J Adol Health.* 2002;31: 162–165.

97. Fisher M. Medical complications of anorexia and bulimia nervosa. *Adol. Med: State of the Art Reviews.* 1992;3:481–502.

98. Bachrach LK, Guido D, Katzman D, Litt IF, Marcus R. Decreased bone density in adolescent girls with anorexia nervosa. *Pediatrics.*1990;86:440–447.

99. Biller BMK, Saxe V, Herzog DB, et al. Mechanisms of osteoporosis in adult and adolescent women with anorexia nervosa. *J Clin Edocrinol Metab.* 1989;68: 548–554.

100. Bachrach LK, Katzman DK, Litt JF, Buido D, Marcus R. Recovery from osteopenia in adolescent girls with anorexia nervosa. *J Clin Endocrinol Metab.* 1991;72: 602–606.

101. Carmichael KA, Carmichael DI. Bone metabolism and osteopenia in eating disorders. *Medicine.* 1995;74: 254–267.

102. Robinson E, Bachrach KL, Katzman DK. Use of hormone replacement therapy to reduce the risk of osteopenia in adolescent girls with anorexia nervosa. *J Adol Health.* 2000;26:343–348.

103. Rome ES, Ammerman S, Rosen DS, et al. Children and adolescents with eating disorders: The state of the art. *Pediatrics.* 2003;111:e98–108.

104. Devuyst O, Lambert M, Rodhain J, Lefebvre C, Coche E. Hematological changes and infectious complication in anorexia nervosa: A case control study. *Q J M.* 1993;86:791–799.

105. Pomeroy C, Mitchell JE, Eckert ED. Risk of infection and immune function in anorexia nervosa. *Int J Eating Disorder.* 1992;12:47–55.

106. Arden MR, Weiselbert EC, Nussbaum MP, Shenker IR, Jacobson MS, et al. Effect of weight restoration on the dyslipoproteinemia of anorexia nervosa. *J Adol Health.* 1990;11:199–202.

107. Portilla MG, Smith PD. Diagnosis and treatment of adolescents with eating disorders. *Arkansas Med Society.* 1997;94(5):211–214.

108. Sargent J, Liebman R. Outpatient treatment of anorexia nervosa. *Psychosomatics.* 1984;7:235–245.

109. Wilson GT. Cognitive behavior therapy for eating disorder: Progress and problems. *Behav Res Ther.* 1999; 37(suppl 1):S79–S95.

110. Durnin JVGA, Rahaman MM. The assessment of the amount of body fat in the human body from measurements of skinfold thickness. *Br J Nutr.* 1967;21: 681–685.

111. Durnin JVGA, Wormersley J. Body fat assessed from total body density and its estimation from skinfolds thickness: Measurements of 481 men and women aged from 16–72 years. *Br J Nutr.* 1974;32:77–82.

112. Probst M. Body composition in female anorexia nervosa patients. *Br J Nutr.* 1996;76:639–644.

113. Birmingham CL. The reliability of bioelectrical impedance analysis for measuring changes in the body composition of patients with anorexia nervosa. *Int J Eating Disord.* 1996;19:311–313.

114. Scalfi L. Bioimpediance and resting energy expenditure in undernourished and refed anorectic patients. *Eur J Clin Nutr.* 1993; 47:61–68.

115. Solomon SM, Kirby DF. The refeeding syndrome: A review. *J Parenteral Enter Nutr.* 1990;14:90–97.

116. Feldman, R. *Refeeding the malnourished patient. In: Sieisenger and Fordtran's Gastrointestinal and Liver Disease,* 6th ed. New York: WB Saunders Company; 1998.

117. Powers PS, Powers HP. Inpatient treatment of anorexia nervosa. *Psychosomatics.* 1984;25:512–545.

118. Ornstein PM, Golden NH, Jacobson MS, Shenker JR. Hypophosphatemia during nutrition rehabilitation in Anorexia Nervosa: Implications for refeeding and monitoring. *J Adol Health.* 2003;32:83–88.

119. Larocia FEF. An inpatient model for the treatment of eating disorders. *Psychiatr Clin North Am.* 1984;7: 287–298.

120. Hudson JI, Pope HG. *The Psychobiology of Bulimia.* Washington, DC: American Psychiatric Press; 1987.

121. Kirkley BG. Bulimia: Clinical characteristics, development and etiology. *J Am Diet Assoc.* 1986:86:468–475.

122. Heatherington MM, Altemus M, Nelson ML. Eating behavior in bulimia nervosa: Multiple meal analyses. *A J Clin Nutr.* 1994;60:864–873.

123. Haiman C, Devlin MJ. Binge eating before the onset of dieting: A distinct subgroup of bulimia nervosa. *Int J Eating Disorders.* 1999;25:151–157.

124. Mitchell JE, Hatsukami D, Eckert ED, Pyle RL. Characteristics of 275 patients with bulimia. *Am J Psych.* 1985;142:482–485.

125. Kaye WH, Weltzin TE, Hsu LK, McConaha CW, Bolton B. Amount of calories retained after binge eating and vomiting. *A J Psych.* 1993;150:969–971.

126. BoLinn GW, Morawski SG, Fordtran JS. Purging and calorie absorption in bulimic patients and normal women. *Ann Intern Med.* 1983;99:14–17.

127. Boardley D. The treatment of eating disorders: Role of the dietitian. In: Garner DM, ed. *Academy for Eating Disorders Newsletter;* Winter 2000:pp 1–4.

128. Fairburn CG, Jones R, Peveler RC, Hope RA, O'Connor M. Psychotherapy and bulimia nervosa: Longer-term effects of interpersonal psychotherapy, behavior therapy, and cognitive behavioral therapy. *Arch Gen Psych.* 1993;50:419–428.

129. Jimmerson DC, Wolfe BE, Brotman AW, Metzer ED. Medications in the treatment of eating disorders. *Psych Clin N Am.* 1996;19:739–754.

130. Grilo CM, Masheb RM, Wilson GT. A comparison of different methods for assessing and treatment of eating disorders in patients with binge eating disorder. *Journal of Consulting & Clinical Psychology.* 2001;69(2): 317–322.

131. Williamson DA, Martin CK. Binge Eating Disorder: A Review of the Literature After Publication of the DSM-IV. *Eating and Weight Disorders,* 1999;4(3):103–114.

132. Goldfein JA, Devlin JH, Spitzer RL. Cognitive behavioral therapy for the treatment of binge eating disorder: What consititutes success? 2000;157(7):1051–1056.

133. Woodside DB, Field LL, Garfinkel PE, Heinman M. Specificity of eating disorders diagnoses in families of probands with anorexia nervosa and bulimia nervosa. *Compr Psychiatry.* 1998;39(5):261–264.

134. Garner DM, Garfinkle PE. *Handbook of Treatment of Eating Disorders,* 2nd ed. New York: Guilford Press; 1997.

135. Farrow JA. The adolescent male with an eating disorder. *Pedia Ann.* 1992; 21:769–773.

136. Carlat DJ, Camargo CA, Herzog DB. Eating disorders in males: A report on 135 patients. *Am J Psychiatry.* 1997;154(8):1127–1132.

137. Braun D, Sunday SR, Huang A, Halmi KA. More males seek treatment for eating disorders. *Int J Eat Disord.* 1999;25(4):415–424.

CHAPTER 11

Sports Nutrition for Children and Adolescents

Nancy Nevin–Folino

PHYSICAL ACTIVITY

Activity should be encouraged for every child in order to initiate lifetime habits of physical exercise. Physical involvement could determine the long-term health of the population in the future, as well as reduce the burden of disease in adulthood.[1,2] Benefits directly associated with physical activity include reduced incidence of coronary heart disease and other degenerative diseases, maintenance of desired weight for height, and lessened symptoms of anxiety and depression.[3–5] Exercise also provides children opportunities for developing basic communication skills and social interaction, which improves self-esteem and confidence.[3] Table 11–1 outlines a variety of different levels of activity for children and adolescents, with age recommendations, associated dietary comments, fluid needs, and appropriate health assessments.

Attitudes about physical activity and an active lifestyle are often formed in the first 10 years of life. Given the rise in childhood obesity with sedentary behavior as one of the causes, activity should be promoted casually and in organized school programs.[4,6] Children's health fitness is associated with the physical behaviors of parents; therefore, family fitness should be encouraged and promoted.[1]

PHYSIOLOGIC EFFECTS OF EXERCISE

Exercise and training produce many physiologic effects in children. Sports participation should be enjoyable and beneficial to the child and can be so, if the healthy child is matched correctly to the sport.

Cardiorespiratory exercise is recommended for children and adolescents for the following benefits:[2,3,6]

- Improves strength and flexibility
- Conditions the cardiorespiratory system
- Increases endurance
- Develops power, agility, and speed
- Aids in development of muscles
- Exercises neuromuscular skill
- Controls percentage of body fat
- Provides mental well-being
- Promotes bone density

To achieve cardiorespiratory benefits, the exercise should be at least 20 minutes in duration, use large muscles, produce mild perspiration, and cause the heart to beat at 60–80% of maximum rate.[7,8] A cardiorespiratory activity is recommended three to five times a week. See Table 11–2 for heartbeat rates for different ages.

Deleterious consequences of exercise can be prevented. Assessment from a physician and health professionals before exercise or sport involvement is strongly recommended.[8] Determination of the match of maturation age with the sport, injury risk, and general health status should be done prior to training and participation in competitive sports by a pediatrician or a physician trained in sports medicine.[9,10] Education on proper

Table 11–1 Exercise Levels with Age, Nutrition, Fluid, and Health Assessment Guidelines

Definitions	*Examples (not inclusive)*	*Recommended Age*	*Nutrition Comments*	*Fluid Intake*	*Recommended Health Assessment*
1. ROUTINE: The duration of the activity is less than 20 min, and it may or may not reach 60% of maximum heartbeat rate.	Recess play, casual walking, recreational noncontinual sport (i.e., T-ball, volleyball)	Minimum activity level for any age	Normal nutrition for age from the USDA Food Guide.	Normal for age.	Yearly routine exam from a pediatrician or physician for all ages of children.
2. HEALTH FITNESS: 60–80% of maximum heartbeat rate is achieved for greater than 20 min at least three times per week for a minimum of 6 months. The activity should involve muscular strength and flexibility.	Brisk walking, jogging, running, cycling, hiking, swimming, dancing	Preferred level for any age	Normal nutrition for age from the Food Guide Pyramid. If desired weight for height, possibly more calories.	Good hydration, especially in adverse weather. Normal requirements for age and replacement of lost fluid from activity.	Yearly routine exam from a pediatrician or physician for all ages of children. Education from a physician or health professional on healthy practices (diet, fluid, injury prevention, warm-up and cool-down techniques, etc.). Immediate attention from an appropriate health professional for an injury or insult.
3. COMPETITIVE SPORTS: An activity less than or equal to 6 months that consists of team involvement, preseason training, and competing	Swimming, gymnastics, diving, volleyball, wrestling, sprinting, relay,	Junior high age and above	Nutrition assessment, recommendations, and education, preferably from a registered dietitian,	Pre-event, event, and postevent (or prepractice and postpractice) hydration.	Preparticipation assessment by a health team consisting of a physician, dietitian, nurse or

either as a team member or individually at an intramural or interschool level.	football, soccer, basketball, tennis, field hockey, cross-country		for an individual's season intake to achieve weight and body composition for the sport. Recommendations will be dependent on type of activity, duration, and intensity.	Good hydration at other times. Electrolyte replacement may be needed if heavy sweating occurs or in adverse weather conditions.	nurse practitioner, and possibly a physical therapist. Examination as well as education should be given to students at this time. Immediate attention from an appropriate health professional for any injury or insult during the sports season.
3a. Competitive under 6 months: Short endurance—intense activity that lasts for 20 min or less.	Same as 3.	Junior high age and above	2 g pro/kg for growing athletes ≥1 g pro/kg for mature athletes.		
3b. Competitive under 6 months: Long endurance—activity, intense or nonintense, that lasts for longer than 20 min.	Same as 3.	High school age and abcve	May need refueling with carbohydrate during the event if long in duration (more than 4 h).	Electrolyte replacement needs assessed and replacement given if necessary.	
4. COMPETITIVE SPORTS: Longer than 6 months. Same as Competitive, but usually involved at a personal level other than school.	Same as 3, but may include state or national competition	High school age and above	Same as 3.	Same as 3.	Same as 3. It is very important that a physician determine that the maturation age of the participant is appropriate for the sport.
4a. Competitive at least 6 months: Short endurance—same as 4.	Same as 3.				
4b. Competitive at least 6 months: Long endurance—same as 4.	Same as 3.				

continues

Table 11–1 continued

Definitions	*Examples (not inclusive)*	*Recommended Age*	*Nutrition Comments*	*Fluid Intake*	*Recommended Health Assessment*
5. PERFORMING: An activity that requires dedicated practice (several times a week) to perform with a group or individually a routine lasting anywhere from 5 min to 1 hr (or longer) in competition or performance.	Ballet, dance, or gymnastics	Junior high age and above as determined by a physician	Nutrition assessment, recommendations, and education provided, preferably by a registered dietitian due to the usually restricted intake to achieve desired weight for performance.	Normal hydration and replacement of lost fluids from practice or performance.	Preparticipation assessment by a physician, dietitian, and possibly an orthopedist or physical therapist. Injury attention as in competitive sports.
6. MARCHING BAND: Involvement with a band that competes or performs in marching or choreographed performance. Includes preseason training as well as competition or performance.	High school marching or competing bands	Junior high age and above	Nutrition assessment, recommendations, and education, preferably from a registered dietitian a group setting, or individually if necessary.	Same as in 3a and 3b.	Same as in 2 or 3a and 3b. Nutrition attention by a registered dietitian if the participant is less than 85% or greater than 120% of desired weight for height.
7. SEASONAL: Intramural involvement with a team or individual activity, not based heavily on winning but just participation. Practice required. May or may not last longer than 20 min three or more times a week, but activity is not sustained longer than 2 or 3 months.	Soccer, softball, swimming lessons	All ages	Same as in 2.	Same as in 3a and 3b.	Preparticipation assessment by a pediatrician or physician, as in 2. Nutrition attention by a registered dietitian if the participant is less than 85% or greater than 120% of desired weight for height.

Source: Data from references 10–17.

Table 11–2 Suggested Training Heart Rates*

Age (yr)	Heart Rate (beats/min)		
	Maximum	*80%*	*60%*
5–8	220	176	132
10	210	168	126
11	209	167	125
12	208	166	125
13	207	165	124
14	206	165	123
15	205	164	123
16	204	163	122
17	203	162	122
18	202	162	121

*These numbers are taken from a variety of sources and are suggested guidelines initially developed for training athletes. Individuals will vary. If target heart rate seems too hard to maintain, accept a lower one, and conversely, if the target rate does not seem high enough to make one perspire, work harder.

Source: Adapted with permission from *Pediatrics in Review,* Vol. 10, pages 141–148, 1988.

training, diet, and injury prevention should also be given.[8] Coaches and trainers should be conscious of the health consequences of sports and refer team members who develop risks during the season to the appropriate health professional (physician, dietitian, orthopedist, physical therapist, etc.). See Table 11–1 for preparticipation health assessment recommendations.

NUTRITIONAL CONCERNS

Nutritional needs of children involved in routine exercise or sports are for adequate energy supplies that come from the recommended dietary intake for age (see Appendix I). This should include a variety of food products emphasizing a normal, balanced diet. This is an excellent time to educate on the importance of regular eating and snacking with appropriate serving sizes. If extra calories are needed, they should come from healthful food choices within the Food Guide Pyramid[14,18,19] (see Appendix J).

Fluid needs include the amount required for normal hydration for age and weight plus extra for training, participation, and cool-down activity.[18] It is imperative that the school-age athlete is given education on how the young body uses fluid, when the body needs more fluid, and why fluid needs for children are different. Dehydration and its symptoms should be discussed in detail.[14,18,19]

No indication exists that there are increased needs for any other nutrients beyond the Recommended Dietary Allowances (RDAs), although some teens may need more protein during periods of rapid growth (see Chapter 6). The physician or a registered dietitian should evaluate the protein needs of an adolescent athlete on an individual basis.[20] In the initial diet review when deficiencies in an intake are identified—calcium, iron, or any other nutrient—the child or teen athlete should ideally receive individualized nutrition counseling. Independent and arbitrary use of vitamins and minerals is discouraged in youth. Over-the-counter supplements should be evaluated carefully.[14]

Guidelines for base calorie needs are outlined in the DRIs.[12] (See Appendix I.) The need to increase calorie allotments for an activity will depend on the child's age, sex, present weight, desired weight, particular sport, and level of involvement. Many factors for calorie needs vary with each child. Achieving desired weight and maintaining the weight determine the adequacy of calories (see Table 11–3). There is a wide variance in the age of sexual development for children and the connection of body fat composition to development. Evaluation of weight status, body fat content, and weight change goals should be done with caution by experienced pediatric health professionals. Percent of fat content of the child's body can be monitored for changes throughout a sports season, but the importance of the change is emphasized here because of the connection to the rate of maturation.

A skilled professional should do body fat measurements to ensure accurate measurements and evaluation. Instructors and students need guidance in altering weight to ensure that safe practices are followed. Frequent monitoring is recommended if weight change is desired to prevent too rapid a weight gain or loss. Rapid body changes can and will affect performance, so weight changes should be started prior to the sports season.

Fluid requirements should be emphasized to the growing athlete so that performance is not compromised by dehydration.[18,19] Fluids should be consumed before, during, and after sports events. Drinking should be regularly scheduled and not dependent on thirst.[22] (See Table 11–4.)

Water, diluted juice (1 part juice to 7 parts of water), or sports drinks can be used. Coaches, health professionals involved with teams, and parents should stress the importance of proper hydration with physical exertion to begin healthy habits.

EXERCISE RECOMMENDATIONS FOR SPECIFIC GROUPS

Newborns to Age 3

An appropriately stimulating environment for infant activity sets the stage for regular exercise as the child grows. Unstructured, safe play without special exercise equipment can provide all that the infant needs for healthy development.[2] Playpens and walkers restrict babies from exploring and from fully using their muscles or developing their coordination and are not recommended for playtime.

Ages 3 to 8 Years

Exercise interest should be piqued during these years to develop habits of routine participation in enjoyable physical activity.[6] Parental habits will be mimicked, so, ideally, the entire family should be committed to physical activity.[1] Group, as well as unorganized play also fosters normal physical and social development of children. At this age, it is vital that the activities offered focus on participation and not on the end-all goal of winning. Caution should be used so that organized sports at this age are for the children's enjoyment.

Ages 8 to 12 Years

A lifelong pattern of regular exercise using the cardiorespiratory system should be established during the school years. Activity programs should consist of exercise that is fun and can be carried into adulthood.[1] School-age children should be encouraged to participate in casual, unorganized activity; school-sponsored competitive sport; or community sport leagues.[1] The psychosocial and physical benefits of sports lead to continued interest in sports and participation through adolescence.

If a child is considering serious sports involvement and/or competition, his or her maturation level should be determined by a health professional.[10] The vast range of pubertal development is remarkable at this age, and the child that matures early may excel in a sport because of his or her maturity-associated skill and muscular level. This advantage does not always continue as the child gets older.[24] Matching an athlete who has matured early with a one who has not started through puberty could cause the latter to lose interest in sports permanently. Explanation of physiologic changes that occur during puberty should be given to budding athletes to prevent unsafe practices aimed at

Table 11–3 Calorie Requirements*

	Recommended Daily Allowances kcal/lb/d				Competitive‡			Long Endurance§		
Age	Low Calorie	Median Calorie	High Calorie	Health Fitness†	Weight Loss	Weight Stable	Weight Gain	Weight Loss	Weight Stable	Weight Gain
4–6	30	41	52	+3	—	—	—	—	—	—
7–10	27	39	54	+3	—	+8	+16	—	—	—
Males										
11–14	20	27	37	+2	+2	+7	+12	+19	+24	+29
15–18	14	19	27	+2	+1	+5	+8	+13	+16	+20
Females										
11–14	15	22	30	+2	+0	+5	+10	+14	+19	+24
15–18	10	17	25	+1 1/2	+0	+4	+8	+12	+16	+20

*Note: The amounts listed are given in ranges to account for variability of body build and maturational level within an age group. For additional calorie needs for sports to achieve weight maintenance, add figures listed to the daily calorie needs per pound per day. Weight loss or gain is based on 1-lb change per week, with the object of losing body fat or gaining lean muscle mass. These figures are estimates and may need to be adjusted for the individual. Competitive and long-endurance sports are not recommended for 4– to 10– year-olds.

†Based on an average amount of calories expended for four 30-minute periods of exercise per week.
‡Based on an average amount of calories expended for six 2-hour practices per week.
§Based on an average amount of calories expended for seven 3.5-hour practices per week plus three 4-hour competitive events per month.

Source: Data from endnote references 18, 21, and 22.

Table 11–4 Fluid Needs*

Age	*Fluid per Day*†	*Fluid Needs to Replace for Activity*	*Pre-Event*	*Competitive Event*	*Post-event*	*Preferred Fluid for Exercise Hydration*	*Electrolyte Replacement Above Normal Diet*
4–6	26–50 oz	Normal hydration; drinking preferred before and after an activity.				Cold water or diluted beverage	Not necessary
7–10	40–56 oz	As above	12–15 oz 2 hr before; 4–8 oz 15 min before	2–4 oz per 15 min	Weight before minus weight after times 16 oz	Cold water or diluted beverage	Not necessary unless long-endurance activity or profuse sweating. Individual assessment needs to be done, with salt, potassium, and/or chloride to be contained in the diet or a diluted fluid.§
Males 11–15	52–70 oz	As above	15–20 oz 2 hr before; 8–12 oz 15 min before	4 oz per every 15 min	As above	Cold water; sport beverage if needed for long-endurance activity.	As above
Females 11–15	48–64 oz	As above	As above	As above	As above	As above	As above
Males 16–18	60–80 oz	As above	As above	As above	As above	As above	As above
Females 16–18	52–69 oz	As above	As above	As above	As above	As above	As above

*Given in minimum amounts, and individual needs may vary.
†Data in this column from reference 18.
§The American College of Sports Medicine recommends 10 mEq sodium and 5 mEq potassium for adults.

Source: Data from endnote references 18, 21, and 22.

changing body composition for sports participation or appearances.[25]

Ages 13 to 18 Years

At this age, enjoyment and a sense of accomplishment are main motivators in continuing organized sports. Physical activity should continue to be encouraged by health professionals, school staff, and parents. Teenagers are at the highest risk for developing sedentary habits.[1] Exercise should be a year-round activity, not just during a sports season.

Problems may occur in children of this age who are immersed in competitive sports or performing arts, to the exclusion of other interests. The risk of overtraining or obsession can occur. These athletes should be helped to develop other, complementary interests, so that sports or dance are not the only arenas for exercise and social interaction.

Eating habits of teens usually consist of meal-skipping or erratic eating, snacking, reliance on fast foods, and unfounded rituals (see Chapter 6). Normal nutrition education should be emphasized with this group, either in school classes or in conjunction with a sport. Often, students are willing to change their eating behaviors for the outcome of better performance and appearance.[24]

Competitive or Performing Sports

Many of today's youth participate in competitive sports, dance, or gymnastics in grade school. It is important to provide them with routine assessments by appropriate health care professionals.[25] An efficient way to accomplish group assessment of aspiring competitors at one time is to set up a mobile clinic situation in a large room and provide stations for each type of assessment needed. The stations can be staffed with the appropriate professionals. Table 11–1 gives recommendations for the type of health professional who should be included in checkups for different levels of activities.[10] The diet of a participant will give medical information, as well as a prediction of health status and performance potential. A registered dietitian should collect diet and intake data and make diet change recommendations, if needed.[6,19]

Exhibit 11–1 shows a sample of a preparticipation nutrition assessment form. The nutrition assessment questionnaire is most useful if completed by the participant prior to the health assessment. This will allow for individual instruction at the time of the assessment. Adequate nutrition is of major importance for the budding athlete, and education on nutrition needs and safe nutrition practices should begin early.[25] The registered dietitian should also instruct coaches, dance teachers, parents, and students on normal diet needs for age, healthful diet practices for competition, and normal body changes, if necessary. This should help to combat the food fads and quackery often practiced by school-age athletes.

Skinfold measurements, mid-arm circumference measurements, or body mass index should be used to assess body fat.[25] (See Chapters 1 and 2 for additional information.) Registered dietitians are trained specifically to evaluate and measure body fat composition. Body fat results should be used judiciously per individual athlete and should never be used as a criterion for sports participation or classification.[26]

Calcium and iron intake should be checked in all females participating and in other athletes with high needs due to growth because of frequent deficiencies in these population groups. Extra protein needs for the young growing athlete can be easily met in the normal diet that contains milk products and meat/protein servings. The dietitian should individually counsel children who choose to be vegetarian. (See Chapter 8.)

Complex carbohydrates are important to the young athlete, not just for health, but also for performance. This nutrient can efficiently fuel the body before, during, and after sports events or competition. Timing of carbohydrate ingestion is important.[18] Prior to events, meals should consist of complex carbohydrates, low-fat protein, and fluids. See Table 11–5 for timing and food selections. Often, parents or trainers need information about pre-event meals. Meals should be 3 to 4 hours before the event. Easily digested food high in carbohydrate but low in protein and fat can be eaten.

Exhibit 11–1 Preparticipation Nutrition Assessment Questionnaire Form

1. Have you ever been on a diet before? ____________ If yes, why and for how long? ______________
   Has anyone in your immediate family ever been on a diet for (circle appropriate answer/s)
   Blood Pressure Cholesterol Diabetes If so, who? ______________________
2. Do you take a vitamin/mineral supplement? If yes, what and how often? ________________
3. Have you ever tried to (circle the appropriate answer) gain or lose weight before? If yes, how much?
   _____ lbs

---

1. Do you drink milk? Yes No If yes, how often (circle appropriate answer)
   4 glasses/day 1–3 glasses/day 4–6 glasses/week 1–3 glasses/week
2. Do you eat (circle foods eaten) cheese, yogurt, or cottage cheese? How often?
   1 or more times/day 4–6 times/week 1–3 times/week
3. Do you eat meat or protein foods? Yes No How often?
   2 or more times/day 1 time/day 4–6 times/week 1–3 times/week
   List the types of meat or protein foods you eat: ______________________
4. Do you eat vegetables? Yes No How often?
   2 or more times/day 1 time/day 4–6 times/week 1–3 times/week
   List the types of vegetables you eat: ______________________
5. Do you eat fruits or drink 100% fruit juice? Yes No How often?
   2 or more times/day 1 time/day 4–6 times/week 1–3 times/week
   List the types of fruits you eat or juice you drink: ______________________
6. Do you eat (circle foods eaten) bread, cereal, pasta, potatoes, or crackers? How often? (total for foods circled)
   6 or more times/day 1–4 times/day 4–6 times/week 1–3 times/week
7. Do you drink water? Yes No How many glasses per day? ______Size glass? ______
8. Check the foods or beverages you eat or drink and fill in how often in the space provided.
   __ Chips ____ __ Diet pop _____ __ Candy _____
   __ Pop ____ __ Cakes, pies _____ __ Cookies _____

---

1. Are you satisfied with your current weight? Yes No If no, what would you like to weigh? ______ lbs
2. Are you satisfied with your present body composition? Yes No If no, how would you like to change it? ______________________
3. Have you ever not eaten or drunk anything for up to a day before weigh in to make weight?
   Yes No If yes, how often? ______________________
4. Do you ever get so hungry that you eat two to five times more than you usually do and then regret it?
   Yes No If yes, have you ever not eaten the next day or taken laxatives because you felt guilty or did not want to gain weight? ______________________

Dietitian's Information
Student's Name ______________________ Age ____ Sex ____ Intended sport __________
Height: ____ %tile ____ Weight: ____ %tile ____ Comments: ______________
If indicated: Hct/Hgb ____ Cholesterol ____ Blood Pressure ____/____ Other ___________
% Desired weight for height _____% % Fat _____% Means of measurement ______________
Weight change needed ________________ % Body fat change needed ______________
Calorie level ________/day ± ________ Milk Products ± ________ Meat/protein servings
Recommended fluid amounts _____ oz. ± _____ Fruit/vegetable ± _____ Grain group
Exercise time/day needed for weight change ______________________
Other diet needs: ______________________
Comments: ______________________
Recommended body measurement: ________________ How often? ______________

Adequate fluid should be provided, as suggested in Table 11–4. If scheduling of events precludes time for a meal or nervousness makes eating unpleasant, a liquid meal replacement can be considered. Table 11–5 gives examples of sports nutrition supplements. Liquid meal replacements and sports bars also may be used. These supplements can be purchased at drug or grocery stores. Carbohydrates should be offered within 30 minutes after finishing an event to replenish glucose stores. Suggested choices are bagels, grain muffins low in fat, fruit, yogurt, or fruit juice.[19,26] Table 11–6 gives several training and competition scenarios, and suggested eating regimes.

Electrolyte losses in sweat from moderate activity can be easily recovered in a post-event meal. However, if a participant sweats profusely, is involved with a very long endurance event, or participates in adverse weather, electrolyte replacement is recommended.

Some female athletes may need individual counseling because of their tendency to restrict caloric intake because of fear of weight gain. Poor nutrition could affect their performance and their iron and calcium levels, as previously mentioned. A very low body fat status may interfere with normal menstrual cycles. A physician should assess amenorrhea to determine the cause.

It is beyond the scope of this chapter to provide nutrition guidance for those who have chosen to dedicate their time to long endurance or in-depth training for competition at a national or worldwide level. These children need instruction on physical conditioning, nutrition, and training practices similar to what is given to college-age or adult athletes by someone familiar with growth, development, and nutrition.

Obese Children

Calorie intake of obese children may not be significantly different from that of normal-weight children, but their activity level is often lower. Obese children and their family members should be encouraged to participate in appropriate forms of physical activity, as approved by a physician.[27] Family support helps the heavy child to continue with exercise and reinforces fitness as a healthful goal. All health professionals seeing school-age children should address an obesity problem by including exercise in the treatment plan. Physical activity for obese children can serve as a cure for boredom, increase metabolism, and improve feelings of self-esteem and accomplishment, just as it can for other children.[28] The exercise should be cardiorespiratory and calorie burning in nature. This can be accomplished by walking, swimming, or biking three to five times a week for 30 minutes or longer.

Table 11–5 Eating During Competition

3 or More Hours Before	*2–3 Hours Before*	*1–2 Hours Before*	*2–3 Hours After*
Fruit or vegetable juice	Fruit or vegetable juice	Fruit or vegetable juice	Bagel
Fresh fruit	Fresh fruit	Fresh fruit (low fiber such as plums, melons, cherries, peaches)	Pretzels
Bread, bagels	Bread, bagels	Sports drink	Fruit yogurt
English muffins	English muffins		Large banana
Peanut butter, lean meat, low-fat cheese	No margarine or cream cheese		Cranberry-apple juice
Low-fat yogurt			Apple juice
Baked potato			Orange juice
Cereal with low-fat (1%) milk			
Pasta with tomato sauce			

Source: Adapted from Jennings DS, Steen, SN. *Play Hard, Eat Right: A Parent's Guide to Sports Nutrition for Children,* © 1995, John Wiley & Sons, Inc. Adapted with permission of John Wiley & Sons, Inc.

Table 11–6 Eating Well While in Training and Competition

Situation	*Suggestion*
Middle school or high school student eats lunch at 10:30 A.M. and must compete at 4:00 P.M.	Eat a large lunch. Lots of variety; get a quick after-school snack that won't irritate, such as nutrition bars, bagels, banana, as well as plenty of fluid
The same situation but one in which the athlete cannot tolerate any food in stomach just prior to competition.	Definitely eat more lunch and include a little more fat in the meal; good situation for a sports bar, if possible, or a drink in between classes.
Student of any age who has a ball game at 8 or 9 A.M. on a Saturday morning.	Eat a good dinner the night before with lots of carbohydrates. Get to bed a little early and get up a few minutes earlier to eat. Depending on the event, perhaps dry cereal, toast with jelly, and a juice drink may help. Milk and orange juice may not be easily digested.
A track, gymnastics, or swimming athlete who competes at 9 A.M., 1 P.M., and again at 3 P.M. on Saturday.	Eat a good dinner the night before competing. Be prepared. Take a small cooler with foods and fluids. Use foods easily digested such as bagels, bananas and oranges, cheese and crackers, granola bars, and pretzels. Stay away from all chips, greasy fries, and hot dogs. Food choices depend on individual preferences.
An athlete too nervous on game day to eat.	May eat better if in a group; provide favorite finger-foods; periodic snacking is great; pre-event visualization also helps.
A 5- to 10-year-old who has to play in hot, humid weather.	Drink flavored fluids 2 hr before event and water (~1 Cup) within 1 hr of event. Drink fluids during warm-ups and coach's talk. Studies reveal that grape flavoring in fluids resulted in more fluid consumption in kids. Have Popsicles and more fluids afterward.
An athlete who is exhausted after practice every night and falls asleep before eating dinner or while studying.	If poor nutrition is suspected, consult a registered dietitian (RD). Have favorite foods more available—fresh fruit and cut-up veggies with low-fat dip; pack food for after school and before practice; provide favorite juices, meats, carbohydrates, and dairy products. Step up efforts to support nutrition throughout the season.
An athlete who is very concerned about weight gain and refuses to eat lunch or eats only an apple.	Needs at least some education; consult RD. Help athlete by noting calories and fat content; demonstrate healthy choices.
Athletes attending away games.	If no prior arrangements are made, pack a small cooler with a well-balanced meal, plenty of variety, and plenty of fluids.

Source: Reprinted with permission from Habash D, Buell, J. *Nutrition...A Communique to Health and Education Professionals,* Vol. 2, No. 3, © 1998. Columbus, OH: The Ohio State University Extension.

Children with Special Health Care Needs

For the child with a developmental disorder or delay resulting in physical limitations, physical activity at an appropriate level should be encouraged to help the child develop self-esteem and to obtain the benefits of exercise. Regular physical exercise will help to combat the obesity that often comes in later years for children with special health care needs. An appropriate physical activity that can be carried out at accessible facilities with professional guidance should be prescribed for children with special needs.

RECOGNITION AND TREATMENT OF NUTRITION DISORDERS RELATED TO SPORTS

The identification of eating disorders is a responsibility of all professionals involved with sports programs. Preparticipation assessments may single out some students who have eating disorder symptoms or who are at risk for them because of bizarre eating or exercise rituals. Students with anorexia nervosa or bulimia nervosa can concomitantly have a compulsive exercise addiction.[5] (See Chapter 10.) Anyone who is identified, either in preparticipation assessments or during the sports season, to have problems associated with food or exercise control should be referred to an appropriate professional.[5,14] Some of the unhealthful practices associated with efforts to influence weight and body composition changes can be eliminated if a protocol for safe body changes is established by a coach or a registered dietitian at the beginning of the weight training season, with an appropriate time frame to achieve the changes.

ERGOGENIC AIDS AND DRUGS

The drugs abused by young athletes range from steroids and amphetamines to street drugs. The safety and efficacy of sports supplements have not been tested in the pediatric population.[29] Unfortunately, most of the supplements are readily available either in health food stores or on the Internet, which encourages widespread use. These drugs—particularly steroids—have detrimental health effects on the adolescent athlete, and their use is condemned by many of the sports institutions and medical groups (National Football League, National Collegiate Athletic Association, American Academy of Pediatrics, International Olympic Committee, American College of Sports Medicine, etc.).[30] There is a rise in use of ergogenic aids and belief of physical improvement with use over the last decade reported in adolescents as young as the 8th grade.[31,32] Youth do not associate supplement use with "cheating."

Physicians screening athletes, as well as the coach, should be asking in-depth questions about supplement and drug use, dosing, and why the agent is being used. Giving preventive education at early ages is most helpful to establish safe practices.[33] If drug abuse is suspected or identified, referral to appropriate professionals is required.

High intakes of caffeine or caffeine in conjunction with other "performance aids" prior to sports events to hype the athlete is to be discouraged in the school-age population because of its side effects and the illegality of the practice in international competition. Caffeine is widely available, and coaches or sponsors may not be aware of this abuse. The sports participant should be educated about caffeine's effects and the dangers or side effects of high doses.

Ergogenic aids or supplements are popular with adult and endurance athletes, and the use of over-the-counter ergogenic aids to increase performance or muscle ability during prolonged activity is widespread and this is a concern in the pediatric population. Acceptance by respected adult athletes encourages youth to experiment. Many of the products have not had reproducible scientific studies of the initial and/or extrapolated data to make any conclusions as to added benefit. The manufacturers of ergogenic aids advertise miracle changes in performance or endurance, and these must be evaluated for truth, as with any other media promotion.[34] An example is dehydroepiandrosterone (DHEA) that is touted as the "youth hormone" and promoted to improve vigor, health, and well-being. There is a claim that DHEA can be converted to testosterone in the body, which would give some young athletes the notion that the supplement could increase their endurance and strength. Side effects of DHEA are possible acne flare-ups, unwanted hair growth, irritability, and rapid heartbeat with larger doses. The studies on DHEA have shown no beneficial effect on body composition or energy expenditure, and DHEA use has been banned by the U.S. Olympic Committee.[34] Unscrupulous use of this product by adolescents could be useless, expensive, and potentially harmful. Megadoses of specific nutrients or ergogenic aids can be deleterious to health and should not be promoted by coaches or professional athletes to school-age sports participants.

Advertisement and word of mouth tend to be the biggest promoters of ergogenic aids and nutritional supplements. These products fall under the Dietary Supplement and Education Act (DSHEA) and do not require the rigorous testing

Table 11–7 Popular Ergogenic Aids

Ergogenic Aid	*Claim of Advertiser*	*Scientific Evidence*
Protein powders	Facilitate muscle growth, weight gain.	Usual dietary intake provides extra amount needed.
Amino Acids: lysine, arginine orthinine,histidine, methionine, phenylalanine	Stimulate growth hormone and insulin to increase; facilitate muscle growth.	No proof that muscle growth is stimulated; gastrointestinal upset.
Chromium	Affects insulin to increase muscle mass.	Research inconsistent; need controlled studies.
HMB (hydroxymethylbuturate)	Increases muscle mass, increases strength, decreases muscle breakdown.	No data to support this claim.
Creatine	Increases use of fat, spares muscle glycogen, increases endurance.	Some evidence for ability to perform high-intensity muscle contractions (sprinting.)
Vanadium	Has insulin-like effects to increase transport of amino acid into the cell.	No data to support claim.
Boron	Exact function unknown; thought to increase calcium, magnesium, and release of testosterone.	No proof of increased growth.
DHEA (Dehydroepiandrosterone)	Increases strength, lean body mass, and protein synthesis.	No data to support claim; research is ongoing; little known about pediatrics.
Caffeine	Improves high-intensity effort.	Data still inconsistent; can dehydrate.
Anabolic Steroids (synthetic male sex hormone, testosterone)	Increase bulk; at high doses, increase muscle mass and strength.	Multiple serious side effects; banned at all levels of sport; does not increase endurance.

Source: Data from endnote references 29, 30, 31, 32, 35, 36, and 37.

required for sale, as do additives or drugs.[34] Many ergogenic aids are available, and questions should be asked as to their use. Table 11–7 lists ergogenic aids, claims of the advertiser and purported benefits, risks, and available scientific evidence. The coach and/or health professional working with the team should educate the athletes on the risks and evaluation process of ergogenic aids.

EXERCISE PROGRAM RECOMMENDATIONS

All sectors of society should be involved in physical activity the year around.[6] Efforts should be made to provide education opportunities to the public through school systems or community resources about exercise safety, nutrition requirements, and the importance of achieving cardiorespiratory benefits.

REFERENCES

1. U.S. Department of Health and Human Services. *Healthy People 2010. Physical Activity and Fitness Health Indicators.* Retrieved June 22, 2004, from www.healthy people.gov/Document/html/uih/uih_4.htm.
2. President's Council on Physical Fitness and Sports. *Kids in Action: Fitness for Children Birth to Age Five.* Kellogg Company, National Association for Sport and Physical Education, Retrieved July 9, 2004, from http://fitness.gov/funfit/kidsinaction_02.html.
3. The President's Challenge. *It Starts with You.* Retrieved July 9, 2004, from www.presidentschallenge.org/the_challenge/index.aspx.
4. U.S. Department of Agriculture Food and Nutrition Service. *Eat Smart. Play Hard!* Retrieved June 15, 2004, from www.fns.usda.gov.
5. Berg FM. *Afraid to Eat, Children and Teens Afraid to Eat,* 3rd ed. Hettinger, ND: Healthy Weight Publishing Network; 2001.
6. Patrick K, Spear B, Holt K, Sofka D, eds. *Bright Futures in Practice: Physical Activity.* 2001. Retrieved June 10, 2004, from www.brightfutures.org.
7. U.S. Department of Health and Human Services. *Physical Activity in Children and Adolescents.* Objective 22-6. *Healthy People 2010. Physical Activity and Fitness Health Indicators.* Retrieved June 10, 2004, from www.healthy people.gov/Document/html/uih/uih_4.htm.
8. Sady SP. Cardiorespiratory exercise training in children. *Clin Sports Med.* 1986;5:493–514.
9. Emery HM. Considerations in child and adolescent athletes. *Rheum Dis Clin North Am.* 1996:22(3):499–513.
10. Goldberg B, Saraniti A, Witman P, Gavin M, Nicholas JA. Pre-participation sports assessment: An objective evaluation. *Pediatrics.*1980;66:736–745.
11. Luckstead SR. Cardiac risk factors and participation guidelines for youth sports. *Ped Clin N Amer.* 2002;49:4.
12. National Academy of Sciences. *Dietary Reference Intakes/Recommended Dietary Allowances.* Retrieved May 23, 2004, from www.nap.edu.
13. U.S. Department of Agriculture and U.S. Department of Health and Human Services. *Food Guide Pyramid and Guides to Serving Sizes.* Retrieved July 12, 2004, from www.nal.usda.gov/fnic/Fpyr/pyramid.html.
14. Bright Futures. *Nutrition and Sports.* National Center for Education in Maternal and Child Health. 2001. Retrieved June 10, 2004, from www.brightfutures.org.
15. American Academy of Pediatrics Committee on Sports Medicine and Fitness. Medical concerns in the female athlete. *Pediatrics.* 2000;106(3):610–613.
16. Rogoi A. Effects of endurance training on maturation. *Consultant.* 1985;25:68–83.
17. Bar-Or O, Barr S, Bergeron M, Carey R, Clarkson P, Houtkooper L, Rivera-Brown A, Rowland T, Steen S. *Youth in Sport: Nutritional Needs.* Gatorade Sports Science Institute. RT30;8:4. 1997. Retrieved June 22, 2004, from www.gssiweb.com.
18. Sports Nutrition. *Pediatric Nutrition Handbook,* 5th ed. Elk Grove Village, IL. American Academy of Pediatrics; 5th ed. 2004:155–166.
19. Spear BA. Nutrition management of the child athlete. In: Nevin-Folino NL, ed. *Pediatric Manual of Clinical Dietetics.* Chicago: The American Dietetic Association; 2003:113–123.
20. University of Illinois Extension. Questions asked by young athletes. *Sports Nutrition: The Winning Connection.* Retrieved June 22, 2004, from www.urbanext.uiuc.edu/hsnut/hsath3b.html.
21. Nelson WE, Behrman RE, Vaughan VC. *Nelson Textbook of Pediatrics,* 15th ed. Philadelphia, PA: WB Saunders Company; 1995.
22. Steen SN. *How to Ensure that Your Child Gets Adequate Fluids While Playing Sports.* Youth Sports Information for Moms. MomsTeam Media. Retrieved July 9, 2004, from www.momsteam.com.
23. Steen SN. *Fluid Guidelines for Young Athletes. Youth Sports Information for Moms.* MomsTeam Media. Retrieved July 9, 2004, from www.momsteam.com.
24. Rarick GL. The significance of normal patterns of behavior and motor development as important determinants of participation in sports programs. In: *Sports Medicine for Children and Youth, Report of the Tenth Ross Roundtable on Critical Approaches to Common Pediatric Problems.* Columbus, OH: Ross Products; 1979.

25. Berning J. Fueling their engines for the long haul: Teaching good nutrition to young athletes. *J Am Diet Assoc.* 1998;98:418.

26. Steen SN. Nutrition for the school-age child athlete. In: Berning JR, Steen SN, eds. *Nutrition for Sport and Exercise,* 2nd ed. Gaithersburg, MD: Aspen Publishers; 1998:199.

27. Poirier P, Despres JP. Exercise in weight management of obesity. *Cardiol Clin.* 2001;19(3):459–470.

28. Korsten-Reck U, Bauer S, Keul J. Sports and nutrition—An outpatient program for adipose children (long-term experience). *Int J Sports Med.* 1994;15:242–248.

29. Congeni J, Miller S. Supplements and drugs used to enhance athletic performance. *Pediatric Clin N Am.* 2002; 49:435–461.

30. American Academy of Pediatrics. *Steroids: Play Safe, Play Fair.* Retrieved July 9, 2004, from www.aap.org/family/steroids.htm.

31. Stephens MB. Ergogenic supplements and health risk behavior. *J Fam Prac.* 2001;50(8):696–699.

32. Multimedia Public Education. *Initiative Aimed at Reversing Rise in Use of Anabolic Steroids by Teens.* National Institute on Drug Abuse. 2000. Retrieved July 9, 2004, from www.drugabuse.gov.

33. Goldberg L, Elliot DL, Clarke GN, et al. The adolescents training and learning to avoid steroids (AT LAS) prevention program. Background and results of a model intervention. *Arch Pediatr Adolesc Med.* 1996;150(7):713–721.

34. Burke ER. Nutritional ergogenic aids. In: Berning JR, Steen S, eds. *Nutrition for Sports and Exercise,* 2nd ed. Gaithersburg, MD: Aspen Publishers; 1998.

35. Bright Futures in Practice. *Physical Activity. Ergogenic Aids.* National Center for Education in Maternal and Child Health. 2001. Retrieved June 10, 2004, from www.brightfutures.org.

36. Gatorade Sports Science Center. *Dietary Supplements Q & A.* 2002. Retrieved July 8, 2004, from www.gssiweb.com.

37. Clarkson PM. *Nutritional Supplements for Weight Gain.* Gatorade Sports Science Institute. SSE68. 1998;11:1. Retrieved June 22, 2004, from http://www.gssiweb.com.

Chapter 12

Community Nutrition

Vanessa Cavallaro

According to the Institute of Medicine, the mission of public health is to assure conditions in which people can be healthy.[1] The public health approach is different from the clinical or patient-centered model familiar in clinical settings; the public health approach takes a landscape view where the community is the client. More formally, community nutrition is defined as the branch of nutrition that addresses the entire range of food and nutrition issues related to individuals, families, and special needs groups living in a defined geographic area. Community nutrition programs include those programs that provide increased access to food resources, food and nutrition education, and health-related care in a culturally competent manner.[2] The following core functions are attributed to public health in which nutrition is a component:

- Assessing the nutrition needs of a population, monitoring the nutritional status of populations and related systems to care, and processing information back into the assessment functions
- Developing policies, programs, and activities that address highest priority nutritional needs
- Assuring the implementation of effective and sustainable nutrition services[2]

Improving nutritional status helps to improve overall health, which is why nutrition has long been included in public and community health.[3] The rising rates of overweight and obesity and related chronic diseases such as type 2 diabetes and cardiovascular disease are national concerns. Although the program and policy focus may be different, a public health trend throughout the 20th century has been to establish nutrition policy.[4] Today, poor nutrition and physical activity will soon overtake tobacco as the leading cause of premature death in Americans. Overweight and obesity put people at increased risk for four of the nation's top six killers—heart diseases, type 2 diabetes, stroke, and some cancers.[5] An estimated 300,000 American adults die each year from these and other illnesses directly attributable to their weight and lack of fitness.[5] With this, health care costs continue to rise. These facts underscore the need for policies that support healthful living.

COMMUNITY NUTRITION SERVICES IN A CHANGING ENVIRONMENT

The public health professional considers a variety of issues and resources when planning and implementing nutrition services for children. There are national public health initiatives, such as Healthy People 2010[6], that contain nutrition-related objectives, as well as national nutrition surveillance data sources, such as the Pediatric Nutrition Surveillance System (PedNSS)[7], that can guide decision making. Nationally, public health agencies emphasize collaboration, which includes community-based planning, coalition and partnership building, and resource leveraging. Successful community nutritionists have experience in program planning and grant writing, as

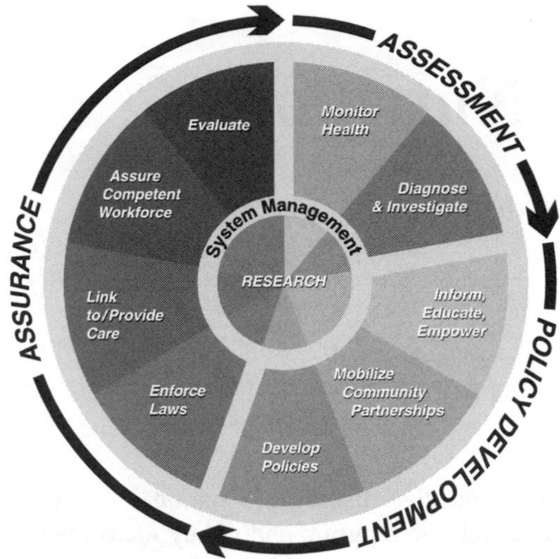

Figure 12–1 Core Functions and Essential Services of Public Health

well as understanding the changing health care environment and its implications. They are knowledgeable about developments in technology.

THE ROLE OF PUBLIC HEALTH DIETITIANS AND COMMUNITY NUTRITIONISTS

Community and public health nutritionists play an increasingly important role in safeguarding the health of children and their families. When setting priorities for services, the nutritional health of children should be considered. To achieve this, public health and community-based dietitians and nutritionists play integral roles in assessing community needs to plan and implement interventions, programs, and services, as well as evaluating their success and how they align with national and state public health initiatives. They are sensitive to the issues affecting the populations they serve, which include socioeconomic, ethnic, cultural, linguistic, and political factors.

Even moderate undernutrition (inadequate or suboptimal nutrient intake) can have lasting effects and compromise cognitive development and school performance.[8] Six- to 11-year-old children from food-insufficient families have been shown to have significantly lower arithmetic scores and are more likely to have repeated a grade. (Families were classified as food deficient if they self-report as sometimes or often not having enough food to eat). In addition, food-insufficient children and teenagers were more likely to have been suspended from school, to have seen a psychologist, and to have difficulty interacting with their peers.[8] Referring eligible families to all appropriate nutrition programs available in their communities is essential to help assure their nutritional and subsequent overall health. In 2001 alone, each day more than 25 million children got their lunch through the National School Lunch Program.[9]

The goal of public health nutrition is to improve the nutritional status of the population served. The public health nutritionist is responsible for identifying the nutrition problems and needs in the community and for developing solutions to the problems.[10,11] This requires a thorough understanding of the effect of economic, social, and political issues on health, the community as a whole, and on community resources.

The roles of community and public health nutritionists are varied. They may work in community-based health or Women, Infant, and Children (WIC) centers, schools, or state and local departments of health, to name a few. For example, in a state department of public health, the role of public health nutritionists emphasizes community-wide wellness promotion and disease prevention. Their responsibilities may include, but are not limited to, coalition building, outreach, and the coordination, implementation, and evaluation of research studies. The title of public health nutritionist is reserved for registered dietitians with graduate-level public health preparation in biostatistics, epidemiology, social-behavioral sciences, environmental sciences, health program planning, management, and evaluation. The term is usually used for an individual with a master's degree in public health.[2]

There also are nutritionists and dietitians based more locally. Their responsibilities include the delivery of programs and services to individuals and groups, which sometimes includes nutrition education. These nutrition professionals may or may not have registration status, but a baccalaureate degree is required.

As health care costs continue to rise, administrators are looking for staff that can multitask. Nutritionists are in demand who have additional training in lactation services, smoking cessation, diabetes education, alcohol and drug issues, social marketing, or community organizing.

Today, in public health and community-based nutrition there is an increasing need for coalition building, establishing public-private partnerships, and supporting sustainable programs and services. Protecting the health and nutritional needs of the community should be a collaborative effort shared by a multidisciplinary team of health care workers.

Advocacy

Advocacy, one of the traditional roles of community nutritionists, is becoming increasingly important in today's political and economic climate. It is often through advocacy that programs are funded, awareness is raised, and policies are changed. The advocacy target may be an agency supervisor or policy maker; another public or private agency, organization, or foundation; or the city, state, or federal legislature. The target, as well as the employing agency, will determine how much of the nutritionist's time will be spend on advocacy issues.

Advocacy involves:[11]

- being well-informed about the needs for the program by having sound statistics on the severity of the problem, the numbers of people affected, and the disadvantages of not having the program
- understanding the views of opponents and being prepared to address them
- knowing alternate funding sources, ways of making the program self-supporting, or other financing mechanisms if financing is a major issue
- obtaining support for the program from appropriate sources, such as other program directors, other agencies, professional organizations or civic groups, influential citizens, or constituents
- building or participating in a coalition with people with similar interests, particularly those with a history of successful advocacy
- communicating effectively with the potential resource on a substantial basis, providing written documentation for the position, and being available to answer questions or to problem solve
- understanding the legislative process if the advocacy target is a legislature, so that verbal and written comment can be appropriate, timely, and adequately prepared
- knowing when hearings are to be held on related regulations or guidelines so that testimony can be presented to include appropriate nutrition services

Whether by pursuing research dollars or supporting new legislation to promote healthier food choices in schools, being an advocate for nutrition and public health services is an essential role for nutrition professionals.

COMMUNITY NUTRITION SERVICES AND PROGRAMS FOR CHILDREN

Many organizations and programs provide nutrition services for children, including federal, state, and local health agencies such as city and county health departments, community health centers, health maintenance organizations (HMOs), hospitals, and clinics. Dietitians in private practice, schools, volunteer organizations, businesses, and industries also provide nutrition services and information.[12] Traditionally, programming has centered on combating undernutrition and hunger; however, the issue of childhood overweight should be considered.

Although seemingly contradictory, the rates of adult obesity and childhood overweight are higher among those with lower levels of education and socioeconomic status.[13,14] Most times, these families are experiencing food insecurity. Making referrals to all appropriate nutrition programs available will not only help assure a family's

Table 12–1 Federal Nutrition Programs

Program	*Purpose(s)*	*For More Information*	*Eligibility*
General Food Assistance Program			
Food Stamp Program	Improve the diets of low-income households by increasing their food purchasing ability.	To be directed to your state food stamp program, visit www.fns.usda.gov/fsp.	Household eligibility and level of assistance are based on income, household size, assets, work requirements, and other factors.
Child Nutrition Programs			
National School Lunch Program	Assist states in providing nutritious, free or reduced-priced lunches and the opportunity to practice skills learned in classroom nutrition education. This program also offers after-school snacks in sites that meet eligibility requirements.	www.fns.usda.gov/cnd/Lunch/default.htm For a listing of state agencies, visit www.fns.usda.gov/cnd and select "Contacts."	• All students attending schools where the lunch program is available can participate. • Children from families with incomes of 130 percent or less of poverty level are eligible for free meals. • Children from families with incomes between 130 and 180 percent of poverty level are eligible for reduced-price meals.
School Breakfast Program	Assist states in providing affordable nutritious breakfasts to promote learning readiness and healthy eating behaviors.	www.fns.usda.gov/cnd/Breakfast/Default.htm For a listing of state agencies, visit www.fns.usda.gov/cnd and select "Contacts."	Eligibility requirements are consistent with those of the National School Lunch Program.
Summer Food Service Program for Children	Provide meals and snacks to children in low-income areas when school is not in session (e.g., during summer and vacation).	www.fns.usda.gov/cnd/Summer/about/index.html For a listing of state agencies, visit www.fns.usda.gov/cnd and select "Contacts."	Any child under 18 years old or anyone over 18 years old who is handicapped and participates in a program for the mentally or physically handicapped may participate.

Programs for Pregnant Women, Infants, and Children			
Special Supplemental Nutrition Program for Women, Infants, and Children (WIC)	To improve the nutritional status of pregnant and lactating females and of children up to 5 years old who are determined to be at nutritional risk by providing, at no cost, supplemental nutritious foods, nutrition education, and referrals.	www.fns.usda.gov/wic For a listing of state agencies, visit www.fns.usda.gov/cnd and select "Contacts."	Pregnant, breastfeeding and postpartum women, infants and children up to five years old are eligible if they are screened to be nutritionally at risk, and they meet an income standard.
WIC Farmers' Market Nutrition Program	Allow WIC participants to purchase fresh produce at authorized farmers' markets; expand consumers' awareness and use of farmers' markets.	www.fns.usda.gov/wic	Consistent with those of the WIC program.
Federal Nutrition Education Programs			
The Extension Food and Nutrition Education Program (EFNEP)	Assist low-income families and youth to acquire the knowledge and skills needed to eat a healthful diet.		Low-income families and youth.
The Head Start Program	Provide comprehensive health education, nutrition, and social services to low-income preschool children and their families.	www2.acf.dhhs.gov/programs/hsb	3- to 5-year-old children from low-income families.
Nutrition Education and Training (NET) Program	Provide nutrition education training to teachers and school food service personnel so that they teach nutrition to children; provide nutrition education materials for use in classrooms and child care settings.		Children eligible to participate in the National School Lunch Program or other child nutrition programs.

Source: Data from endnote reference 16.

nutritional and subsequent overall health, but will also ease the burden of food scarcity. In a 2003 study, food-insecure girls aged 5 to 12 who participated in all three food-assistance programs—Food Stamp Program, School Breakfast, and the National School Lunch Program—had a 68% reduced odds of being overweight compared to food-insecure girls who participated in no programs.[15] See table 12–1 for U.S. government nutrition programs.

FEDERAL FOOD AND NUTRITION EDUCATION RESOURCES

This section is a resource for available community nutrition programs. It summarizes available programs, the purpose of the program, and eligibility requirements. For more information on program availability, contact your state or local department of public health or public health nursing service.

Food and Nutrition Service

The Food and Nutrition Service (FNS) administers the nutrition assistance programs of the U.S. Department of Agriculture (USDA). FNS increases food security and reduces hunger in partnership with cooperating organizations by providing children and low-income people access to food and a healthful diet. FNS also works to empower program participants with comprehensive nutrition education and knowledge of the link between diet and health.[16]

FNS partners with the states to deliver its programs. States are responsible for most administrative details regarding distribution of benefits and eligibility of participants, while FNS provides funding to the states to implement and distribute the programs.

Nutrition Education

FNS also operates the Nutrition Education and Training (NET) Program to support nutrition education in food assistance programs. The U.S. secretary of agriculture allocates NET funds to states each year in the form of grants.

In 1995, the School Meals Initiative for Healthy Children was created with the goal to "improve the health and education of children through better nutrition."[16] The initiative is administered through a national program called Team Nutrition. Through Team Nutrition, FNS also provides:

1. schools with nutrition education materials for children and families
2. technical assistance materials for food service directors, managers, and staff
3. materials to build school and community support for healthy eating and physical activity
4. information and materials for other food assistance programs, such as food stamps and WIC

The program encourages the creation of public-private partnerships, and partners often provide training and technical assistance to support these programs in local schools. For more information on Team Nutrition and how to contact professionals in your area, visit www.fns.usda.gov/tn.

FNS administers the following nutrition assistance and nutrition education programs that benefit children (and adults). To learn more about FNS programs, eligibility requirements or contact information, visit www.fns.usda.gov/fns.

OTHER FOOD RESOURCES IN THE COMMUNITY

Food Pantries and Soup Kitchens

Within many communities, organizations also help to bring food to those who are hungry—for example by providing hot meals or groceries. Local food banks or agencies, grocery stores, and restaurants often donate food. Community members also donate through food drives.

Food Cooperatives

Self Help and Resource Exchange (SHARE), a national food cooperative, is helping many families "stretch" their food dollars. A SHARE is a box of nutritious food that is purchased for approximately $15 at the beginning of the month. The food package is distributed at the end of the month. Sponsoring organizations and volunteers make the program work. Recipients agree to volunteer 2 hours of their time in their communities every month they participate. Local food banks, health departments, or community organizations know how to contact SHARE sites in your area.

COMPONENTS AND SERVICES IN FEDERAL PROGRAMS

Medicaid

This federal health insurance program provides health care for low-income pregnant women and children. States can opt to provide nutrition assessment and counseling as a benefit. The U.S. Department of Health and Human Services (USDHHS) administers the program at the federal level, whereas state health and/or welfare agencies administer it locally. Income eligibility and benefits vary by state. Access to health care providers has been an issue for many years, but recently there has been a trend to provide Medicaid services through managed care plans in an effort to increase access and decrease cost. Medical nutrition therapy (MNT) for Medicare beneficiaries with diabetes and renal disease allows a patient to work with a dietitian to help manage disease progression. The benefit does not cover dietary supplements or foods. Health care providers can help underserved families understand their benefits and navigate the increasingly complex system of health care delivery. Knowing what services are covered can help dietetics professionals advocate for the inclusion of nutrition services in federally funded programs.

For more information or for state-specific information, visit www.cms.hhs.gov/medicaid.

Early and Periodic Screening, Diagnosis, and Treatment (EPSDT)

This is a federally mandated program created to identify and treat health conditions early in low-income children to prevent long-term health problems. The program has set guidelines that require providers of EPSDT services to conduct wellness exams according to a periodicity schedule from birth to age 21. The wellness exam is comprehensive and referrals are made accordingly. There is a list of screening requirements. Nutrition can be integrated through health education, which is a required component of screening services and includes anticipatory guidance. At the outset, the physical and/or dental screening provides the initial context for providing health education. Education and counseling to both parents (or guardians) and children is required. It is designed to assist in understanding what to expect in terms of the child's development and to provide information about the benefits of healthy lifestyles and practices, as well as accident and disease prevention. Case management is an essential component of the program. A designated agency administers the program at the state level (typically, social services or health and welfare agencies). Local county agencies then deliver the administrative and case management services and conduct quality assurance.

Children with Special Health Care Needs (CSHCN)

The USDHHS and a designated state agency administer this program. Funding for such programs, as well as the breadth of services available, varies from state to state. The program provides case management, diagnosis, and treatment for eligible children with special health care needs. It is the position of the American Dietetic Association that persons with developmental disabilities should receive comprehensive nutrition services as part of all heath care, vocational and educational programs.[17]

Early Intervention Program

Early Intervention (EI), a program of the U.S. Department of Education, is administered locally by a designated state agency (state department of health or department of education). It provides health services to prevent or minimize developmental delay in handicapped newborns up to 5 years old. Nutrition consultation may be available to families, depending on a state's EI services.

University-Affiliated Programs (UAP)

Administered locally by universities, these USDHHS programs provide assessment and development of a treatment plan for mentally handicapped or chronically ill children as needed, in an effort to support the training of health professionals. The programs stress multidisciplinary team approaches that typically include a registered dietitian with special training. Major teaching research hospitals around the country may have an affiliated program.

Head Start

Head Start is a national program with over 18,000 sites across the country that provides comprehensive developmental services for this country's low-income, preschool children aged 3 to 5 years and social services for their families.[18] Specific services for children focus on education, socioemotional development, physical and mental health, and nutrition.

Major components of Head Start include:

- Education: Head Start's educational program is designed to meet the needs of each child, the community served, and its ethnic and cultural characteristics. Every child receives a variety of learning experiences to foster intellectual, social, and emotional growth.
- Health: Head Start emphasizes the importance of the early identification of health problems. Every child is involved in a comprehensive health program, which includes immunizations, medical care including mental health, dental care, and nutrition services.
- Parental Involvement: Parents are involved in parent education, program planning, and operating activities. Many parents serve as members of policy councils and committees and have a voice in administrative and managerial decisions. Participation in classes and workshops on child development and staff visits to the home allow parents to learn about the needs of their children and about educational activities that can take place at home.
- Social Services: Services are customized after determining a family's needs and may include community outreach, referrals, recruitment and enrollment of children to other federal assistance programs, and emergency assistance and/or crisis intervention.

For state-specific information, visit www.acf.hhs.gov/programs/hsb/hsweb/index.jsp.

Early Head Start

In 1994, the Head Start Reauthorization Act established a new program for low-income pregnant women and families with infants and toddlers. The program relies on science-based research demonstrating that the period from birth to age 3 is critical to healthy growth and development, as well as a link to later success in school and in life.

The purpose of this program is to enhance children's physical, social, emotional, and cognitive development; to enable parents to be better caregivers and teachers to their children; and to help parents meet their own goals, including that of economic independence.

The program provides early, continuous, intensive, and comprehensive family support services to low-income families with children under the age of 3 years. To ensure continuity of services, projects must coordinate with local Head Start programs. Nutrition is a part of these services. Community nutritionists are involved in the implementation of nutrition guidelines in Early Head Start. For more information and to find state specific information, visit www.ehsnrc.org.

Public Health Nursing Services

State and local health departments employ public health nurses to provide many services, including home visiting, case management of special conditions, pre- and postnatal classes for parents, and community outreach for issues related to lead exposure, immunizations, tuberculosis, and so forth. These nursing services are a valuable resource to local community nutritionists.

School Health, Nursing Services, and Occupational or Physical Therapy

Local school systems assist school staff and food services to meet students' special needs. These services may include nutrition counseling and they can target teens or parenting teens. Partnerships between schools and local health departments can bring variety of nutrition services to children.

Schools also assist children with special health care needs such as feeding problems, food modification needs, adaptive feeding equipment, and special feeding techniques. Nutrition consultation may be available at the district or state levels. See table 12–2 for nutrition education web sites.

Financing Nutrition Services

Potential sources for financing nutrition services include:[19]

- federal, state, and local governmental agencies; block or project grants or contracts
- private sector funding sources, such as foundation or corporate grants or contracts, civic organizations, not-for-profit health-related organizations, or associations
- income from sale of products such as educational materials

Sources of information on funding resources include:[20]

- Federal health, education, and agriculture agencies, especially the U.S. Public Health Service, the Centers for Disease Control and Prevention (CDC), and the USDA. Nutrition personnel of the federal agencies can provide information on specific federal support applicable to nutrition services
- The *Federal Register,* which contains requests for applications (RFAs) on programs funded by the federal government
- The Maternal and Child Health Clearinghouse, which can provide information on projects that have been funded through Maternal and Child Health grants
- State health, mental health, education, and social service agencies, whose employees can identify potential sources of financial support, including reimbursement for services
- Corporations or foundations, which often have a department to deal with corporate giving or community relations
- The Foundation Center, with libraries in

Table 12–2 Relevant Web Sites for Nutrition Education Resources

American Cancer Society	www.cancer.org
American Heart Association	www.americanheart.org
American Dietetic Association	www.eatright.org
American Diabetes Association	www.diabetes.org
Centers for Disease Control and Prevention	www.cdc.gov
Center for Science in the Public Interest	www.cspinet.org
Food and Drug Administration	www.fda.gov
International Food Information Council	www.ific.org
National Dairy Council	www.nationaldairycouncil.org
Tufts Nutrition Navigator	http://navigator.tufts.edu
U.S. Department of Agriculture	www.usda.gov
Access to all U.S. government information on food and nutrition	www.nutrition.gov

New York City; Cleveland; Washington, DC; and San Francisco; and a nationwide network of reference collections with information on foundation grants and workshops for individuals seeking grants
- Private and public insurers, which can provide information on coverage of specific nutrition services

CONCLUSION

Community nutrition practice will continue to expand and change as the community does. Programs and services targeting children and adolescents can have a lasting affect on the health of the nation. Teaching children and adolescents healthy behaviors in their youth will correlate to healthy behaviors in their adult lives. How dietitians respond to new and emerging nutritional needs will be a challenge and an opportunity that makes the work of community nutrition rewarding. Staying informed, staying connected, and bringing diverse skills to the job are essential to truly serve the community.

REFERENCES

1. Institute of Medicine. *The Future of Public Health.* Washington, DC: National Academy Press; 1989.
2. Mixon H, Dodds J, Haughton B. *Guidelines for Community Nutrition Supervised Experiences,* 2nd ed. Public Health/Community Nutrition Practice Group, American Dietetic Association; 2003. Retrieved June 4, 2004, from www.phcnpg.org.
3. U.S. Department of Health and Human Services. *Public Health In America.* Available at www.health.gov/phfunctions/public.htm.
4. Egan M. Public health nutrition: A historical perspective. *J Am Diet Assoc.* 1994;94:298–304.
5. U.S. Department of Health and Human Services. The Surgeon General's call to action to prevent and decrease overweight and obesity. Rockville, MD: U.S. Department of Health and Human Services, Public Health Service, Office of the Surgeon General; 2001.
6. U.S. Department of Health and Human Services. *Healthy People 2010: National Health Promotion and Disease Prevention Objectives.* Retrieved April 16, 2004, from www.cdc.gov/nchs/about/otheract/hpdata2010/abouthp.htm.
7. Centers for Disease Control and Prevention (CDC) Pediatric Nutrition Surveillance System—United States. Retrieved April 16, 2004, from www.cdc.gov/nccdphp/dnpa/PedNSS.htm.
8. Center on Hunger, Poverty, and Nutrition Policy. Statement on the link between nutrition and cognitive development in children. Medford, MA: Friedman School of Nutrition, Science and Policy at Tufts University; 1998.
9. U.S. Department of Agriculture, Food and Nutrition Service. National School Lunch Program. Fact Sheet. Retrieved June 21, 2004, from www.fns.usda.gov/cnd/Lunch/AboutLunch/NSLPFactSheet.htm.
10. Owen AL, Splett P, Owen GM, *Nutrition in the Community: The Art and Sciences of Delivering Services,* 4th ed. Boston, MA: WCB/McGraw-Hill; 1999.
11. Dodds JW, Kaufman M, eds. *Personnel in Public Health Nutrition for the 1990s.* Washington, DC: U.S. Department of Health and Human Services; 1991.
12. Committee on Nutrition, American Academy of Pediatrics. *Pediatric Nutrition Handbook,* 5th ed. Elk Grove Village, IL: American Academy of Pediatrics; 2003.
13. Sobal J, Stunkard AJ. Socioeconomic status and obesity: A review of the literature. *Psychol Bull.* 1989;105: 260–275.
14. Paeratakul S, Lovejoy JC, Ryan DH, Bray GA. The relation of gender, race and socioeconomic status to obesity and obesity comorbidities in a sample of US adults. *Int J Obes Relat Metab Disord.* 2002;26(9):1205–1210.
15. Jones SJ, Jahns L, Laraia BA, Haughton B. Lower risk of overweight in school-aged food insecure girls who participate in food assistance. *Arch Pediatr Adolesc Med.* 2003;157:780–784.
16. U.S. Department of Agriculture, Food and Nutrition Service. Retrieved April 16, 2004, from www.fns.usda.gov/fns.
17. ADA Report. Position of the Am. Diet. Assoc: Providing nutrition services for infants, children, and adults with developmental disabilities and special health care needs. *J Am Diet Assoc.* 2004;104:97–107.
18. U.S. Department of Health and Human Services, Administration for Children, Youth and Families, Head Start Fact Sheet. Retrieved April 16, 2004, from www.acf.hhs.gov/programs/hsb/research/2003.htm.
19. Boyle M, Morria D. *Community Nutrition in Action: An Entrepreneurial Approach.* Boston, MA: West/Wadsworth; 1999.
20. Office of Disease Prevention and Health Promotion. *Locating Funds for Health Promotion Projects.* Washington, DC: U.S. Department of Health and Human Services, Public Health Service; 1993.

CHAPTER 13

Nutrition Support for Inborn Errors

Phyllis B. Acosta

INTRODUCTION

Nutrition support of infants and children with inborn errors of metabolism requires in-depth knowledge of metabolic processes, the science and application of nutrition, growth and development, and food science. When providing nutrition support for patients with inborn errors, the specific nutrient needs of each patient, based on individual genetic and biochemical constitution, must be considered. Nutrient requirements established for normal populations[1] may not apply to individuals with inborn errors of metabolism.[2] Some chemical compounds, normally not considered essential because they can be synthesized de novo, may not be synthesized in patients with a metabolic defect. Consequently, dependent on the inborn error, the subsequent organ damage that accrues and the rate of loss of specific chemicals from the body may make several compounds may become conditionally essential. Among these are the amino acids arginine,[3] carnitine,[4] cystine,[5] and tyrosine[6] and the "vitamins" coenzyme Q10, lipoic acid,[7] and tetrahydrobiopterin.[8] Failure to adapt nutrient intakes to the needs of each patient can result in mental retardation, metabolic crises, neurologic crises, growth failure, and with some inborn errors, death. Quality care is best achieved by an experienced team of specialists in a genetic/metabolic center.

This chapter addresses principles and practical considerations in nutrition support of inborn errors of metabolism; nutrition support of selected inborn errors of amino acid, nitrogen, carbohydrate, fatty acid, lipid, and mineral metabolism; selected areas needing further research; and roles and functions of the dietitian in nutrition support of inborn errors of metabolism. For a detailed guide to nutrition support, see *Nutrition Support Protocols*.[9]

PRINCIPLES AND PRACTICAL CONSIDERATIONS IN NUTRITION SUPPORT

Principles of Nutrition Support

A number of approaches to nutrition support of inborn errors of metabolism are discussed here. The appropriate approach is dependent on the biochemistry and pathophysiology of disease expression. Several therapeutic strategies may be used simultaneously[2]:

1. Enhancing anabolism and depressing catabolism: This involves the use of high-energy feeds, appropriate amounts of amino acid mixtures, and administration of insulin, if needed. Fasting should be prevented. This therapeutic maneuver is important to all inborn errors involving catabolic pathways.
2. Correcting the primary imbalance in metabolic relationships: This correction reduces, through dietary restriction, accumulated toxic substrate(s). Examples are phenylketonuria, maple syrup urine

disease, and galactosemia, where phenylalanine; leucine, isoleucine, and valine; and galactose are limited, respectively.

3. Providing alternate metabolic pathways to decrease accumulated toxic precursors in blocked reaction sequences: For example, innocuous isovalerylglycine is formed from accumulating isovaleric acid if supplemental glycine is provided to drive glycine-N-transacylase. Isovalerylglycine is excreted in the urine.
4. Supplying products of blocked primary pathways: Some examples are arginine in most disorders of the urea cycle, cystine in homocystinuria, tyrosine in PKU, tetrahydrobiopterin in biopterin synthesis defects, and ether lipids[10] and docosahexaenoic acid[11] in patients with some peroxisomal disorders.
5. Supplementing conditionally essential nutrients: Examples are carnitine, cystine, and tyrosine in secondary liver disease[12] or with excess excretion of carnitine in organic acidemias.[13]
6. Stabilizing altered enzyme proteins: The rate of biologic synthesis and degradation of holoenzymes is dependent on their structural conformation. In some holoenzymes, saturation by a coenzyme increases their biologic half-life and, thus, overall enzyme activity at the new equilibrium. This therapeutic mechanism is illustrated in homocystinuria and maple syrup urine disease. Pharmacologic intake of pyridoxine in homocystinuria and of thiamine in maple syrup urine disease increases intracellular pyridoxal phosphate and thiamine pyrophosphate, respectively, and increases the specific activity of any functional cystathionine β-synthase and branched-chain α-ketoacid dehydrogenase complex, respectively.[14,15]
7. Replacing deficient cofactors: Many vitamin-dependent disorders are due to blocks in coenzyme production and are "cured" by pharmacologic intake of a specific vitamin precursor. This mechanism presumably involves overcoming a partially impaired enzyme reaction by mass action. Impaired reactions required to produce methylcobalamin and adenosylcobalamin result in homocystinuria and methylmalonic aciduria. Daily intakes of appropriate forms of milligram quantities of vitamin B12 may cure the disease.[16]
8. Inducing enzyme production: If the structural gene or enzyme is intact but suppressor, enhancer, or promoter elements are not functional, abnormal amounts of enzyme may be produced. The structural gene may be "turned on" or "turned off" to enable normal enzymatic production to occur. In the acute porphyria of type I tyrosinemia, excessive δ-aminolevulinic acid (ALA) production may be reduced by suppressing transcription of the δ-ALA synthase gene with excess glucose.[17]
9. Supplementing nutrients that are inadequately absorbed or not released from their apoenzyme: Examples are zinc in acrodermatitis enteropathica[18] and biotin in biotinidase deficiency.[19]

Practical Considerations in Nutrition Support

Nutrients

Diet restrictions required to correct imbalances in metabolic relationships usually require the use of elemental medical foods. These medical foods are normally supplemented with small amounts of intact protein that supply the restricted amino acid(s). Intact protein seldom supplies more than 50%, and often much less, of the protein requirement of patients with disorders of amino acid or nitrogen metabolism. Other nitrogen-free foods that provide energy are limited in their range of nutrients. Consequently, care must be taken to provide nutrients previously considered to be food contaminants because their essentiality has been demonstrated through long-term use of total parenteral nutrition.[20] Thus in addition to nutrients for which recommended dietary allowances (RDAs)[1] are established, including fat, linoleic acid, and α-linolenic acid, other nutrients must be supplied in adequate amounts. These include trace minerals and vitamins. Most mineral intakes must be greater than RDAs to result in normal nutrition status indices.[9]

Osmolality

Elemental medical foods consist of small molecules that may result in an osmotic load greater than the physiologic tolerance of the patient. Abdominal cramping, diarrhea, distention, nausea, or vomiting may result from use of hyperosmolar feeds. More serious consequences can occur in infants, such as hypertonic dehydration, hypovolemia, hypernatremia, and death. A mathematical formula for estimating approximate osmolality of medical food mixtures is given in *Nutrition Support Protocols*.[9] The neonate should not be fed an elemental formula that contains greater than 450 mOsm/kg water.[9]

Maillard Reaction

Medical foods for inborn errors of amino acid or nitrogen metabolism are formulated from free amino acids, carbohydrate, and often fat. The Maillard reaction is a complex group of chemical reactions in foods in which reacting amino acids, peptides, and protein condense with sugars, forming bonds for which no digestive enzymes are available. The Maillard reaction is accelerated by heat and is characterized in its initial stage by a light brown color, followed by buff yellow and dark brown in the intermediate and final stages. Caramel-like color and roasted aromas develop. Those who prepare medical foods must be able to recognize the Maillard reaction because it causes loss of some sugars and amino acids. For this reason, medical foods should not be heated beyond 100° F (37.8° C).[9]

Introduction of Puréed Foods

Puréed foods (beikost) should be introduced into the diet at about 4 months of age if the infant shows developmental readiness by a decrease in tongue thrust. Beikost is important in the diet to provide unidentified nutrients and fiber, to enhance the infant's acceptance of a variety of tastes and textures, and, when table foods are eaten, to develop jaw muscles important for speech. See "Weaning and Feeding Progression" in Chapter 5.

Changes in Nutrition Support Prescription

As soon as nutrition support is well established in an infant or child, the prescription should be fine-tuned frequently. The frequency depends on the age of the child; infants require at least weekly changes in prescription while children who are growing more slowly may not require a diet change more than monthly or every 2 to 3 months. Small, frequent changes in prescription prevent "bouncing" of plasma amino acid, glucose, organic acid, or ammonia concentrations and allow the intake to grow with the child, thus precluding the child's "growing out of the prescription."[9]

Monitoring

Successful management of inborn errors of metabolism requires frequent monitoring. Frequent monitoring gives the physician and dietitian data that verify the adequacy of the nutrition support prescription. These data also motivate patient/parent compliance with the prescription. Premature and full-term infants to at least 6 months of age require twice weekly monitoring. Thereafter, weekly monitoring may be adequate if the patient is compliant with the diet prescription.

Some centers may wish to draw blood when the patient is fasting to monitor plasma amino acid or ammonia concentrations. Prolonged fasting (over 8 hours) may cause spurious elevations of plasma amino acid concentrations that could lead to unwarranted diet changes,[21] and blood drawn 15 minutes to 1 hour after a meal may also yield spuriously high values.[22]

INBORN ERRORS OF AMINO ACID METABOLISM

The problem of ensuring adequate nutrition for infants and children with inborn errors of metabolism may be decreased by the use of a protocol or plan for treatment.[9] Each patient requires individualized medical and nutrition care. Information in Table 13–1 describes various inborn errors, nutrients to modify, vitamin responsiveness, and medical foods available. Data in Table 13–2 outline recommended nutrient intakes for beginning therapy,[9] while Table 13–3 provides information on nutrition support during acute illness, medications and nutrient interactions, and nutrition assessment parameters.

When specific amino acids require restriction, total deletion for 1 to 3 days only is the best approach to initiating therapy. Longer term deletion or overrestriction may precipitate deficiency of the amino acid(s).[9] The most limiting nutrient determines growth rate, and overrestriction of an amino acid, nitrogen, or energy will result in further intolerance of the toxic nutrient. Results of amino acid and nitrogen deficiencies are described in Table 13–4.

Data outside the parentheses in Table 13–2 describe amounts of amino acids with which to begin nutrition support. For some disorders in which the initial plasma concentration(s) of toxic amino acid is 14 to 20 times the upper limit of the normal reference range, after 2 to 3 days of zero intake of the amino acid, it should be introduced with the lowest recommended amount for age in parentheses.[9] Data within the parentheses indicate the possible range of amino acid requirements, depending on the gene mutation and extent of the enzyme deficit.[83] Only frequent monitoring of plasma concentrations of amino acids and other analytes, nutrient intake, and growth can verify the adequacy of intake.[9]

Protein requirements of infants and children with inborn errors of amino acid metabolism are normal if liver or renal function is not compromised. However, the form in which the protein is administered must be altered in order to restrict specific amino acids. Consequently, medical foods formulated from free amino acids must be used with small amounts of intact protein to provide amino acid and nitrogen requirements.[9] Because nitrogen retention from free amino acid mixes differs from that of amino acids derived from intact protein,[84–86] recommended protein intakes of infants and children with inborn errors of amino acid metabolism are 125–150% greater than RDAs.[1] Medical food and intact protein should be given four to six times daily to enhance nitrogen retention.[84–86] According to Arnold and associates,[87] plasma transthyretin concentrations are positively correlated with linear growth with concentrations of at least 200 mg/L resulting in the greatest height for age. Acosta and colleagues[88] found similar correlations in 2- to 13-year-old children with PKU. Yannicelli and colleagues[45] reported poor linear growth in children with methylmalonic or propionic acidemia who failed to ingest adequate protein and energy. In fact, protein intake as recommended by Acosta and Yannicelli[9] leads to excellent growth with greater phenylalanine tolerance than when RDA for protein is fed.[89] Fat intakes and the essential fatty acids, linoleic and α-linolenic, should meet RDA (1), except in mitochondrial fatty acid oxidation defects. Acosta and others[90] found no essential fatty acid deficiency in patients with PKU undergoing nutrition therapy.

Energy intakes of infants and children with inborn errors of metabolism must be adequate to support normal rates of growth. Provision of apparently adequate amino acids and nitrogen without sufficient energy will lead to growth failure. Pratt and associates[91] suggested that energy requirements are greater than normal when L-amino acids supply the protein equivalent. Maintenance of adequate energy intake is essential for normal growth and development and to prevent catabolism. If RDA[1] for energy cannot be achieved through oral feeds, nasogastric, gastrostomy, or parenteral feeds must be employed. Mathematical formulas for calculating protein and energy requirements for the child with failure to thrive are given in Chapter 18. Amino acid solutions designed for specific

(Text continues on page 267)

Table 13–1 Nutrition Support of Inborn Errors of Metabolism

Key: ALA, alanine, BCAAs, branched-chain amino acids; CYS, cystine; EAAs, essential amino acids (includes conditionally essential cystine and tyrosine); GLY, glycine; GTP, guanosine triphosphate; ILE, isoleucine; IM, intramuscular; LEU leucine; LYS, lysine; MCT, medium-chain triglycerides; MET, methionine; MSUD, maple syrup urine disease; PHE, phenylalanine; PUFAs, polyunsaturated fatty acids; THR, threonine; TRP, tryptophan; TYR, tyrosine; VAL, valine.

Inborn Error and Defect	*Nutrient(s) to Modify*	*Vitamin Responsive*	*Medical Foods Available*
	INBORN ERRORS OF AMINIO ACID METABOLISM **Aromatic Amino Acids**		
Phenylketonuria and hyperphenylalaninemia (phenylalanine hydroxylase)[23]	Restrict PHE, increase TYR.[2,9] Provide protein, mineral, and vitamin intakes greater than RDA.	No	Periflex Phenex-1, -2, -2 Vanilla Phenyl-Free -1, -2, -2HP XP Analog, Maxamaid, Maxamum
Hyperphenylalaninemia (dihydropteridine reductase) GTP cyclohydrolase I; (6-pyruvoyltetrahydropterin synthase)[8]	Same as for phenylketonuria.[8]	Yes. Tetrahydrobiopterin 2 mg/kg/d[8]	Same as for phenylketonuria
Tyrosinemia type I (fumarylacetoacetate hydrolyase)[24]	Restrict PHE and TYR. Provide greater than RDA for protein, energy, mineral, and vitamin intakes.[9,25,26]	No	Tyrex-1, -2 XPHEN, TYR Analog, Maxamaid
Tyrosinemia type II (tyrosine aminotransferase)	Restrict PHE and TYR. Provide protein, mineral and vitamin intakes greater than RDA.[9,27]	No	Same as for tyrosinemia type I.
Tyrosinemia type III (p-OH phenylpyruvic acid dioxygenase)[24]	Same as for tyrosinemia type II.[28]	No	Same as for tyrosinemia type I.

continues

Table 13–1 continued

Inborn Error and Defect	*Nutrient(s) to Modify*	*Vitamin Responsive*	*Medical Foods Available*
	Branched-Chain Amino Acids		
Maple syrup urine disease (branched-chain ketoacid dehydrogenase complex)[29]	Restrict ILE, LEU and VAL.[2,9] Provide protein, energy, mineral, and vitamin intakes above RDA.	Yes. Thiamine-responsive if any residual enzyme activity. Response to thiamine inadequate to alleviate need for restriction of BCAAs.[2]	Acerflex Ketonex-1, -2 MSUD2 MSUD Diet Powder MSUD Analog, Maxamaid, Maxamum
Isovaleric acidemia (isovaleryl-CoA dehydrogenase); β-methylcrotonylglycinuria (3-methylcrotonyl-CoA carboxylase).[30]	Restrict LEU; supplement with L-carnitine and GLY.[9,31] Provide protein, energy, mineral, and vitamin intakes above RDA.	No	I-Valex-1, -2 XLEU Analog, Maxamaid
	Sulfur Amino Acids		
Homocystinuria, pyridoxine-nonresponsive (cystathionine-β-synthase)[32]	Restrict MET[2,9]; increase CYS.[5] Supplement folate, betaine.[33–37] Provide protein, energy, mineral, and vitamin intakes above RDA.	No	HCY powder Hominex-1, -2 XMET Analog, Maxamaid, Maxamum
Homocystinuria, pyridoxine-responsive (cystathionine-β-synthase)[32]	See Chapters 4 and 5 for nutrient needs.	Yes[38]	None may be indicated.
	Other Inborn Errors of Amino Acid Metabolism		
Glutaric acidemia type I (glutaryl-CoA dehydrogenase)[39]	Restrict LYS and TRP.[9,40] Supplement L-carnitine. Provide protein, energy, mineral, and vitamin intakes above RDA.	Yes. Some patients have a partial response to oral riboflavin, 100–300 mg daily.[41] Administer with food.	Glutarex-1, -2 XLys, XTrp Analog, Maxamaid, Maxamum

Methylmalonic acidemia (methylmalonyl-CoA mutase 0 or –)[13]	Restrict ILE, MET, THR, VAL, and long-chain unsaturated fatty acids.[9,42,43] Supplement L-carnitine.[44] Provide greater than RDA for protein, energy, mineral, and vitamin intakes.[45]	No	Propimex-1, -2 XMTVI Analog, Maxamaid, Maxamum
Methylmalonic acidemia (cobalamin reductase; adenosyltransferase)[16]	Minimum restriction of ILE, MET, THR, and VAL. Supplement L-carnitine. See Chapters 4 and 5 for other nutrient needs.	Yes. 1–2 mg hydroxycobalamin daily.[16]	None may be indicated.
Propionic acidemia (propionyl-CoA carboxylase)[13]	Restrict ILE, MET, THR, VAL, and long-chain fatty acids .[9,42,43] Provide greater than RDA for protein, energy, mineral, and vitamin intakes.[45] Supplement L-carnitine.	Questionable. Some clinicians supplement with D-biotin daily.[19]	Propimex-1, -2 XMTVI Analog, Maxamaid, Maxamum
	INBORN ERRORS OF NITROGEN METABOLISM		
Carbamylphosphate synthetase deficiency; Ornithine transcarbamylase deficiency[46]	Restrict protein.[2,9] Supplement with EAAs (47–50), L-carnitine,[51,52] L-arginine, and L-citrulline. Provide greater than RDA for energy, mineral, and vitamin intakes.	No	Cyclinex-1, -2 Pro-Phree Protein-Free Diet Powder WND2
Citrullinemia (argininosuccinate synthetase)[46] Argininosuccinic aciduria (arginonosuccinate lyase)[46]	Restrict protein.[2,9] Supplement with EAAs (47–50), L-arginine, and L-carnitine.[51,52] Provide greater than RDA for energy, mineral, and vitamin intakes. Citrate therapy in ASL deficiency.[53]	No	Cyclinex-1, -2 Pro-Phree Protein-Free Diet Powder WND2
Argininemia (arginase)[46]	Restrict protein.[2,9] Supplement with EAAs (47–50) and L-carnitine.[51] Provide greater than RDA for energy, mineral, and vitamin intakes.	No	Cyclinex-1, -2 Pro-Phree Protein-Free Diet Powder WND2

continues

Table 13–1 continued

Inborn Error and Defect	*Nutrient(s) to Modify*	*Vitamin Responsive*	*Medical Foods Available*
	INBORN ERRORS OF CARBOHYDRATE METABOLISM		
	Galactosemias		
Epimerase deficiency[54]	Delete galactose. Add specific known amount of galactose.[55] Provide RDA for protein, energy, minerals, and vitamins.	No	Isomil powder ProSobee powder
Galactokinase deficiency[54]	Delete galactose. Provide RDA for protein, energy, mineral, and vitamin intakes.	No	Isomil powder ProSobee powder
Galactose-1-phosphate uridyl transferase deficiency[54]	Delete galactose. Provide RDA for protein, energy, mineral, and vitamin intakes.[9,56]	No	Isomil Powder ProSobee Powder
	Glycogen Storage Disease		
Type Ia (glucose-6-phosphatase); Type Ib (defective glucose-6-phosphate transport)[57]	Modify type of carbohydrate and frequency of feeds. Provide RDA for protein, energy, mineral, and vitamin intakes. Avoid lactose, fructose, and sucrose.[9,58,59]	No	ProViMin RCF Uncooked cornstarch
Type III (amylo-1, 6-glucosidase)[57]	Provide high protein,[60] supplement with L-ALA,[61] modify type of carbohydrate and frequency of feeds.[60] Provide RDA for energy, mineral, and vitamin intakes.	No	ProViMin RCF Uncooked cornstarch
Type IV (α-1, 4-glucan: α-1, 4-glucan 6-glucosyltransferase)[57]	Provide high protein unless cirrhosis present; modify type of carbohydrate and frequency of feeds. Provide RDA for energy, mineral, and vitamin intakes.[57,60]	No	ProViMin RCF

Type V (muscle phosphorylase)[57]	Provide high protein, vitamin B6 supplementation. Provide RDA for energy, mineral, and vitamin intakes.[57,60]	No	Mono-and Disaccharide-Free Diet Powder ProViMin RCF
	Hereditary Fructose Intolerance		
Hereditary fructose intolerance (aldolase B)[62]	Restrict fructose[62,63]; restrict protein if liver damage.[64] Provide RDA for energy, mineral, and vitamin intakes.	No	Enfamil Lipil ProViMin, RCF; or whole cow's milk for children Similac Advance
	INBORN ERRORS OF FATTY ACID OXIDATION (MITOCHONDRIAL)		
Carnitine transporter deficiency[65]	Avoid fasting[65]	L-carnitine therapy[65]	None
Carnitine translocase deficiency; Carnitine palmitoyl I transferase I deficiency[65]	Restrict long-chain fats, administer MCT, linoleic and α-linolenic acids, L-carnitine. Uncooked cornstarch for hypoglycemia. Avoid fasting.	No	ProViMin
Very long-chain acyl-CoA dehydrogenase deficiency; Long-chain acyl-CoA dehydrogenase deficiency; Long-chain hydroxyacyl-CoA dehydrogenase deficiency[65]	Restrict long-chain fats, administer MCT, linoleic and α-linolenic acids, L-carnitine. Uncooked cornstarch for hypoglycemia. Avoid fasting.[9]	No	ProViMin
Medium-chain acyl CoA dehydrogenase deficiency[65]	Restrict long-chain and avoid medium-chain fats; administer linoleic and α-linolenic acids, L-carnitine. Uncooked cornstarch for hypoglycemia. Avoid fasting.[9,66]	Yes?	ProViMin

continues

Table 13–1 continued

Inborn Error and Defect	*Nutrient(s) to Modify*	*Vitamin Responsive*	*Medical Foods Available*
Short-chain acyl CoA dehydrogenase deficiency; Short-chain 3-hydroxyacyl CoA dehydrogenase deficiency[65]	Restrict fat; administer linoleic and α-linolenic acids, L-carnitine. Uncooked cornstarch for hypoglycemia. Avoid fasting.[9]	No	ProViMin
Multiple acyl CoA dehydrogenase deficiency (glutaric aciduria type II)[67]	Restrict fat and protein; supplement linoleic and α-linolenic acids, L-carnitine, riboflavin, and glycine.[9,67]	Riboflavin, partial response[67]	ProViMin
	INBORN ERRORS OF LIPOPROTEIN METABOLISM		
Abetalipoproteinemia and hypobetalipoproteinemia (absence and decrease in apoβ)[68]	Restrict triglycerides with long-chain fatty acids. Supplement with vitamins A, D, E, K. Provide RDA for protein, essential fatty acids, energy, mineral and vitamin intakes.	No	MCT ProViMin
	Hyperlipoproteinemias		
Type I (extrahepatic lipoprotein lipase; apo CII absent or decreased)[69]	Restrict fat,[69] supplement with linoleic and α-linolenic acids. See Chapters 4 and 5 for other nutrient needs.	No	MCT ProViMin
Type IIa (LDL receptors absent or defective)[70]	Restrict cholesterol, saturated fat[70]; increase PUFAs. Provide RDA for protein, energy,[71] mineral, and vitamin intakes.	No	Enfamil Lipil ProViMin RCF Similac Advance
Type IIb[70]	Restrict cholesterol, saturated fat, mono- and disaccharides, and alcohol. Increase fiber and PUFAs.[70] Provide RDA for protein, essential fatty acids, energy, mineral, and vitamin intakes.	No	Mono- and Disaccharide-Free Diet Powder ProViMin RCF

Type III (hepatic lipoprotein lipase; homozygous for abnormal apo-E2; remnant receptor defect)[72]	Restrict cholesterol, saturated fat; mono- and disaccharides, and alcohol. Increase PUFAs and fiber. Restrict energy if patient is overweight.[72] Provide RDA for protein, essential fatty acids, mineral, and vitamin intakes.	No	Enfamil Lipil ProViMin RCF Similac Advance
INBORN ERRORS OF MINERAL METABOLISM			
Acrodermatitis enteropathica (defect in intestinal zinc absorption)[18]	Give zinc supplements.[18] Provide RDA for protein and energy intakes. See Chapters 4 and 5 for other nutrient needs.	No	None indicated
Wilson's disease Hepatolenticular degeneration (excessive accumulation of copper)[73]	Restrict dietary copper, supplement zinc. Provide RDA for protein and energy intakes. See Chapters 4 and 5 for other nutrient needs.	No	None indicated

Table 13–2 Recommended Nutrient Intakes (with Ranges) for Beginning Therapy

Key: ARG, arginine; CIT, citrulline; CYS, cystine; GLY, glycine; ILE, isoleucine; LEU, leucine; LYS, lysine; MET, methionine; MUFA, monounsaturated fatty acid; PHE, phenylalanine; PUFA, polyunsaturated fatty acid; THR, threonine; TRP, tryptophan; TYR, tyrosine; VAL, valine.

Nutrients to Modify	*Age (years)* 0.0 < 0.5	0.5 < 1.0	1 < 4	4 < 7	7 < 11	11 < 19
INBORN ERRORS OF AMINO ACID METABOLISM						
Aromatic Amino Acids						
Phenylketonuria and hyperphenylalaninemia[2,9]						
PHE (mg)	55 (70–20)/kg	30 (50–15)/kg	325 (200–450)/d	425 (225–625)/d	450 (250–650)/d	500 (300–750)/d
TYR (mg)	195 (210–180)/kg	185 (200–170)/kg	2800 (1400–4200)/d	3150 (1750–4550)/d	3500 (2100–4900)/d	3850 (2100–5600)/d
Protein (g)	3.5–3.0/kg	3.0–2.5/kg	≥ 30/d	≥ 35/d	≥ 40/d	50–65/d
Energy (kcal)	120/kg	110/kg	900–1800/d	1300–2300/d	1650–3300/d	1500–3300/d
Tyrosinemia type I[2,9,26]						
PHE (mg)	100 (125–65)/kg	80 (105–45)/kg	600 (500–700)/d	650 (550–750)/d	700 (600–800)/d	800 (700–900)/d
TYR (mg)	75 (95–45)/kg	55 (75–30)/kg	400 (300–500)/d	450 (350–550)/d	500 (400–600)/d	550 (450–650)/d
Protein† (g)	3.5–3.0/kg	3.0–2.5/kg	≥ 30/d	≥ 35/d	≥ 40/d	50–65/d
Energy (kcal)	100–120% of RDA					
Tyrosinemia type II, III[2,9,27,28]						
PHE (mg)	100 (125–65)/kg	80 (105–45)/kg	450 (400–500)/d	500 (450–550)/d	550 (500–600)/d	600 (550–700)/d
TYR (mg)	75 (100–40)/kg	55 (80–20)/kg	400 (350–450)/d	450 (400–500)/d	500 (450–550)/d	475 (400–550)/d
Protein (g)	3.5–3.0/kg	3.0–2.5/kg	≥ 30/d	≥ 35/d	≥ 40/d	50–65/d
Energy (kcal)	120/kg	110/kg	900–1800/d	1300–2300/d	1650–3300/d	1500–3300/d
Branched–Chain Amino Acids						
Maple syrup urine disease[2,9]						
ILE (mg)	60 (90–30)/kg	50 (70–30)/kg	50 (70–20)/kg	25 (30–20)/kg	25 (30–20)/kg	25 (30–10)/kg
LEU (mg	80 (100–40)/kg	55 (75–40)/kg	55 (70–40)/kg	50 (65–35)/kg	45 (60–30)/kg	40 (50–15)/kg
VAL (mg)	70 (95–40)/kg	55 (80–30)/kg	50 (70–30)/kg	40 (50–30)/kg	28 (30–25)/kg	22 (30–15)/kg
Protein (g)	3.5–3.0/kg	3.0–2.5/kg	≥ 30/d	≥ 35/d	≥ 40/d	50–65/d
Energy (kcal)	100–125% of RDA					

Isovaleric acidemia and β-methylcrotonyl glycinuria[2,9]						
LEU (mg)	95 (110–65)/kg	75 (90–50)/kg	975 (800–1150)/d	1275 (1050–1500)/d	1445 (1190–1700)/d	1955 (1610–2300)/d
L–carnitine (mg)	300–100/kg	300–100/kg	300–100/kg	300–100/kg	300–100/kg	300–100/kg
GLY (mg)	125 (150–100)/kg	125 (150–100)/kg	125 (150–100)/kg	125 (150–100)/d	125 (150–100)/kg	125 (150–100)/kg
Protein (g)	3.5–3.0/kg	3.0–2.5/kg	≥ 30/d	≥ 35/d	≥ 40/d	50–65/d
Energy (kcal)	100–125% of RDA					
Sulfur Amino Acids						
Homocystinuria, cystathionine-β-synthase deficiency (pyridoxine nonresponsive)[2,9,37]						
MET (mg)	35 (50–20)/kg	28 (40–15)/kg	20 (30–10)/kg	15 (20–10)/kg	15 (20–10)/kg	15 (20–10)/kg
CYS (mg)	300–250/kg	250–200/kg	150 (200–100)/kg	150 (200–100)/kg	150 (200–100)/kg	75 (60–50)/kg
Betaine (g)	1–3/d		3–6/d			
Folate (mg)	0.5–1.0/d		1–3/d			
Protein (g)	3.5–3.0/kg	3.0–2.5/kg	≥ 30/d	≥ 35/d	≥ 40/d	50–65/d
Energy (kcal)	120/kg	115/kg	900–1800/d	1300–2300/d	1650–3300/d	1500–3300/d
Other Amino Acids						
Glutaric acidemia type I[9]						
LYS (mg)	85 (100–70)/kg	65 (90–40)/kg	55 (80–30)kg	50 (75–25)/kg	45 (65–25)/kg	40 (60–20)/kg
TRP (mg)	25 (40–10)/kg	15 (30–10)/kg	12 (16–8)/kg	12 (16–8)/kg	8 (10–5)/kg	6 (8–4)/kg
L-carnitine (mg)	300–100/kg					
Riboflavin (mg)	300–100/d, administer orally with food					
Protein (g)	3.5–3.0/kg	3.0–2.5/kg	≥ 30/d	≥ 35/d	≥ 40/d	50–65/d
Energy (kcal)	120/kg	115/kg	900–1800/d	1300–2300/d	1650–3300/d	1500–3300/d
Propionic acidemia and methylmalonic acidemia[9,45,74,75]						
ILE (mg)	95 (120–60)/kg	70 (90–40)/kg	610 (485–735)/d	795 (630–960)/d	900 (715–1090)/d	1215 (956–1470)/d
MET (mg)	35 (50–15)/kg	25 (40–10)/kg	330 (275–390)/d	435 (360–510)/d	495 (410–580)/d	665 (550–780)/d
THR (mg)	90 (135–50)/kg	55 (75–20)/kg	505 (415–600)/d	660 (540–780)/d	745 (610–885)/d	1010 (830–1195)/d
VAL (mg)	85 (105–60)/kg	55 (75–30)/kg	690 (550–830)/d	900 (720–1080)/d	1020 (815–1225)/d	1380 (1105–1655)/d
D-Biotin (mg)	5–10/d for propionic acidemia					
Hydroxy-cobalamin (mg)	1–2/d for cobalamin-responsive methylmalonic acidemia					
L-carnitine (mg)	300–100/kg	300–100/kg	300–100/kg	300–100/kg	300–100/kg	300–100/kg
Protein (g)	3.5–3.0/kg	3.0–2.5/kg	≥ 30/d	≥ 35/d	≥ 40/d	50–65/d
Energy (kcal)	100–125% of RDA					

continues

Table 13–2 continued

Nutrients to Modify	Age (years) 0.0 < 0.5	0.5 < 1.0	1 < 4	4 < 7	7 < 11	11 < 19
INBORN ERRORS OF NITROGEN METABOLISM						
Citrullinemia; Argininosuccinic aciduria[2,9,47]						
ARG (mg)	700–350/kg	700–350/kg	500–250/kg	500–250/kg	500–250/kg	400–200/kg
Protein‡ (g)	2.2–1.15/kg	1.15–1.0/kg	8.0–12.0/d	12.0–15/d	14.0–17.0/d	20.0–32.0/d
L-carnitine (mg)	100–50/kg	100–50/kg	100–50/kg	100–50/kg	100–50/kg	100–50/kg
Energy (kcal)	125–150% of RDA					
Carbamylphosphate synthetase deficiency; Ornithine transcarbamylase deficiency[2,9,47]						
CIT (mg)	700–350/kg	700–350/kg	500–250/kg	500–250/kg	500–250/kg	400–200/kg
Protein‡ (g)	2.2–1.15/kg	1.15–1.0/kg	8.0–12.0/d	12.0–15/d	14.0–17.0/d	20.0–32.0/d
L-carnitine (mg)	100–50/kg	100–50/kg	100–50/kg	100–50/kg	100–50/kg	100–50/kg
Energy (kcal)	125–150% of RDA					
Argininemia[2,9,47]						
Protein‡ (g)	2.2–1.15/kg	1.15–1.0/kg	8–12/d	12–15/d	14–17/d	20–32/d
L-carnitine (mg)	100–50/kg	100–50/kg	100–50/kg	100–50/kg	100–50/kg	100–50/kg
Energy (kcal)	125–150% of RDA					
INBORN ERRORS OF CARBOHYDRATE METABOLISM						
Galactosemias						
Epimerase deficiency[9,55]						
Galactose (mg)	1000–1500/d		500–1000/d			
Protein (g)	≥ 2.2/kg	≥ 2.0/kg	≥ 23/d	≥ 30/d	≥ 35/d	45–65/d
Energy (kcal)	120/kg	115/kg	900–1800/d	1300–2300/d	1650–3300/d	1500–3300/d
Galactokinase deficiency						
Galactose (mg)	< 50/d	< 50/d	< 100/d	< 100/d	< 100/d	< 100/d
Protein (g)	≥ 2.2/kg	≥ 2.0/kg	≥ 23/d	≥ 30/d	≥ 35/d	45–65/d
Energy (kcal)	120/kg	115/kg	900–1800/d	1300–2300/d	1650–3300/d	1500–3300/d

Galactose-1-phosphate uridyl transferase deficiency[9,56,76]						
Galactose (mg)	< 50/d	< 50/d	< 100/d	< 100/d	< 100/d	< 100/d
Protein (g)	> 2.2/kg	> 2.0/kg	≥ 23/d	> 30/d	≥ 35/d	45–65/d
Energy (kcal)	120/kg	115/kg	900–1800/d	1300–2300/d	1650–3300/d	1500–3300/d
Glycogen Storage Disease[57–60]						
Glucose-6-phosphatase deficiency (von Gierke's disease, type Ia); type Ib						
Carbohydrate	60–70% of energy. Provide at least 50% of carbohydrate as uncooked cornstarch every 4 hours during the day and via continuous tube feeding at night. During the first 3 months of life feed every 2 hours and use Polycose instead of uncooked cornstarch; gradually change to raw cornstarch over 3 months.					
Protein† (g)	≥ 2.2/kg	≥ 2.0/kg	≥ 23/d	≥ 30/d	≥ 35/d	45–65/d
Energy (kcal)	120/kg	115/kg	900–1800/d	1300–2300/d	1650–3300/d	1500–3300/d
Amylo-1, 6-glucosidase deficiency (Cori's disease, type III)[61]						
Protein (g)	4.4/kg	4.0/kg	4.0/kg	3.5/kg	3.0/kg	2.5/kg
L-alanine (mg)	500–400/kg	400–300/kg	300–200/kg	200–100/kg	200–100/kg	200–100/kg
Carbohydrate	40–50% of energy. Provide about one-half as uncooked cornstarch every 6 hours during the day and night. During the first 3 months of life feed every 2 hours and use Polycose instead of uncooked cornstarch; gradually change to raw cornstarch over 3 months.					
Energy (kcal)	120/kg	115/kg	900–1800/d	1300–2300/d	1650–3300/d	1500–3300/d
α-1, 4-glucan: α-1, 4-glucan 6-glucosyltransferase deficiency (Anderson's disease, type IV)[61]						
Protein	High protein as for type III unless cirrhosis present					
Carbohydrate	Uncooked cornstarch every 4–5 hours to maintain normoglycemia. See under type III					
Energy (kcal)	120/kg	115/kg	900–1800/d	1300–2300/d	1650–3300/d	1500–3300/d
Muscle phosphorylase deficiency (McArdle's disease type V)						
Protein	High protein as for type III					
L-alanine	Same as for type III					
Energy (kcal)	120/kg	115/kg	900–1800/d	1300–2300/d	1650–3300/d	1500–3300/d
Hereditary Fructose Intolerance[9,63,64]						
Fructose (mg)	< 10/kg	< 10/kg	< 10/kg	< 20/kg	< 30/kg	< 40/kg
Protein	Restrict only with liver damage					
Energy (kcal)	120/kg	115/kg	900–1800/d	1300–2300/d	1650–3300/d	1500–3300/d

continues

Table 13–2 continued

Nutrients to Modify	Age (years)					
	0.0 < 0.5	*0.5 < 1.0*	*1 < 4*	*4 < 7*	*7 < 11*	*11 < 19*
INBORN ERRORS OF FATTY ACID OXIDATION (MITOCHONDRIAL)						
Carnitine transporter deficiency						
L-carnitine	Administer to maintain normal plasma concentrations					
Carnitine translocase deficiency, carnitine palmitoyl I transferase deficiency, very-long-chain acyl-CoA dehydrogenase deficiency, long-chain acyl-CoA dehydrogenase deficiency, long-chain hydroxyacyl-CoA dehydrogenase deficiency						
L-carnitine	50–100 mg/kg/day					
Long-chain fats	30–40% of energy					
MCT	30–50% of fat					
Linoleic acid	≥ 3% of energy					
α-linolenic acid	≥ 1% of energy					
Uncooked cornstarch	to prevent hypoglycemia					
Protein (g)	RDA					
Energy (kcal)	RDA					
Minerals, vitamins	RDA					
Medium-chain acyl CoA dehydrogenase deficiency, short-chain acyl CoA dehydrogenase deficiency, short chain 3-hydroxyacyl-CoA dehydrogenase deficiency						
L-carnitine	50–100 mg/kg/day					
Fat	20–30% of energy					
Linoleic acid	≥ 3% of energy					
α-linolenic acid	≥ 1% of energy					
Uncooked cornstarch	to prevent hypoglycemia					
Protein (g)	RDA					
Energy (kcal)	RDA					
Minerals, vitamins	RDA					
Multiple acyl-CoA dehydrogenase deficiency (glutaric aciduria type II)						
Fat	25–30% of energy					
L-carnitine	50–100 mg/kg/day					
Riboflavin	50–100 mg/d with meals					
Glycine	50–100 mg/kg/day					

Protein (g)	RDA					
Energy (kcal)	RDA					
Minerals, vitamins	RDA					
INBORN ERRORS OF LIPID METABOLISM						
Abetalipoproteinemia and hypobetalipoproteinemia						
Long-chain fat	13–15% of energy					
Linoleic acid	$\geq$ 3% of energy					
α-linolenic acid	$\geq$ 1% of energy					
Vitamin A	Use water-miscible form to supplement to exceed RDA					
Vitamin E (mg)	1000–2000/d		5000–10,000/d			
Vitamin K	Supplement with water-miscible form if bruising, bleeding, or hypoprothrombinemia present					
Protein (g)	$\geq$ 2.2/kg	$\geq$ 2.0/kg	$\geq$ 23/d	$\geq$ 30/d	$\geq$ 35/d	44–65/d
Energy (kcal)	120/kg	115/kg	900–1800/d	1300–2300/d	1650–3300/d	1500–3300/d
Hyperlipidemias						
Type I						
Long-chain fat	< 15% of energy					
Linoleic acid	$\geq$ 3% of energy					
α-linolenic acid	$\geq$ 1% of energy					
Protein (g)	$\geq$ 2.2/kg	$\geq$ 2.0/kg	$\geq$ 23/d	$\geq$ 30/d	$\geq$ 35/d	44–65/d
Energy (kcal)	120/kg	115/kg	900–1800/d	1300–2300/d	1650–3300/d	1500–3300/d
Type IIa						
Total fat	< 30% of energy					
Cholesterol (mg)	100/1000 kcal. Never > 150/d					
Saturated fat	10% of energy					
PUFAs	15% of energy					
MUFAs	10% of energy					
Protein (g)	$\geq$ 2.2/kg	> 2.0/kg	$\geq$ 23/d	$\geq$ 30/d	$\geq$ 35/d	44–65/d
Energy (kcal)	120/kg	115/kg	900–1800/d	1300–2300/d	1650–3300/d	1500–3300/d
Type IIb						
Cholesterol (mg)	100/1000 kcal. Never > 150/d					
Total fat	30% of energy					
Saturated fat	10% of energy					
PUFAs	15% of energy					

continues

Table 13–2 continued

Nutrients to Modify	*Age (years)* 0.0 < 0.5	0.5 < 1.0	1 < 4	4 < 7	7 < 11	11 < 19
MUFAs	10% of energy					
Fiber	Increase					
Mono- and disaccharides	Restrict					
Protein (g)	≥ 2.2/kg	≥ 2.0/kg	≥ 23/d	≥ 30/d	≥ 35/d	44–65/d
Energy (kcal)	120/kg	115/kg	900–1800/d	1300–2300/d	1650–3300/d	1500–3300/d
Type III						
Cholesterol (mg)	< 100/1000 kcal. Never > 300/d					
Saturated fat	< 10% of energy					
PUFAs	< 15% of energy					
Fiber	Increase					
Protein (g)	≥ 2.2/kg	≥ 2.0/kg/kg	≥ 23/d	≥ 30/d	≥ 35/d	44–65/d
Energy (kcal)	Restrict					
INBORN ERRORS OF MINERAL METABOLISM						
Acrodermatitis enteropathica[18]						
Zinc (mg)	35–100/d elemental zinc; give in 2 or 3 doses with food					
Protein (g)	≥ 2.2/kg	≥ 2.0/kg	≥ 23/d	≥ 30/d	≥ 35/d	45–65/d
Energy (kcal)	120/kg	115/kg	900–1800/d	1300–2300/d	1650–3300/d	1500–3300/d
Wilson's disease[73,77]						
Copper (mg)	0.3/d	0.4/d	0.5/d	0.8/d	1.0/d	1.0/d
Zinc (mg)	20/d	20/d	20/d	30/d	30/d	30/d
Protein (g)	≥ 2.2/kg	≥ 2.0/kg	≥ 23/d	≥ 30/d	≥ 35/d	44–65/d
Energy (kcal)	120/kg	115/kg	900–1800/d	1300–2300/d	1650–3300/d	1500–3300/d
Pyridoxine (mg)	25/d					

†Protein may need to be decreased 5–10% if liver damage with hyperammonemia is present.

‡Total protein intake may be somewhat greater with the use of drugs that enhance waste nitrogen loss.

Table 13–3 Nutrition Support during Acute Illness; Medications and Nutrient Interactions and Nutrition Assessment Parameters

Key: ARG, arginine; ALLO, alloisoleucine; BCAAs, branched-chain amino acics; CBC, complete blood count; CIT, citrulline; CYS, cystine; GLY, glycine; GTP, guanosine triphosphate; HOMOCYS, homocystine; ILE, isoleucine; IV, intravenous; LEU, leucine; LDL, low-density lipoprotein; LYS, lysine; MET, methionine; MUFA, monounsaturated fatty acid; PHE, phenylalanine; PUFA, polyunsaturated fatty acid; RBP, retinol-binding protein; THR, threonine; TRP, tryptophan; TYR, tyrosine; UDP, uridine diphosphate; VAL, valine; VLDL, very low-density lipoprotein.

Inborn Error and Defect	*Nutrition Support During Acute Illness*	*Medications and Nutrient Interaction*	*Nutrition Assessment Parameters*
	INBORN ERRORS OF AMINO ACID METABOLISM **Aromatic Amino Acids**		
Phenylketonuria and Hyperphenylalaninemia (phenylalanine hydroxylase)	Delete dietary PHE 1 to 3 days only. For infant, offer Pedialyte with added Polycose to maintain electrolyte balance if needed. Give sugar-sweetened, caffeine-free soft drinks with added Polycose or Moducal to maintain energy intake at 100% RDA. If necessary, give IV glucose, lipid, and amino acids free of PHE to maintain anabolism. Return to oral medical food and complete diet as rapidly as tolerated.[9]	No medication required with early and continuing therapy throughout life.	Plasma PHE, transthyretin, ferritin, and TYR; dietary intake of PHE, TYR, protein, energy, minerals, and vitamins. Growth.[78,79] See Chapter 2 for other routine assessment parameters and standards.
Hyperphenylalaninemia (dihydropteridine reductase; GTP cyclohydrolase I; 6-pyruvoyltetrahydropterin synthase)	Same as above.		Plasma PHE, TYR, transthyretin, and ferritin; dietary intake of PHE, TYR, protein, energy, minerals, vitamins. Growth.[78,79] See Chapter 2 for other routine assessment parameters and standards.

continues

Table 13–3 continued

Inborn Error and Defect	*Nutrition Support During Acute Illness*	*Medications and Nutrient Interaction*	*Nutrition Assessment Parameters*
Tyrosinemia type I (fumarylacetoacetate hydrolyase)	Delete dietary PHE, TYR, 1 to 3 days only. For infant, offer Pedialyte with added Polycose to maintain electrolyte balance if needed. Give sugar-sweetened, caffeine-free soft drinks with added Polycose or Moducal to maintain energy intake at 120–130% RDA. If necessary, give IV glucose, lipid, and amino acids free of PHE and TYR to maintain anabolism. Return to oral medical food and complete diet as rapidly as tolerated.[9]		Plasma PHE, TYR, transthyretin, ferritin, bicarbonate, phosphate, potassium, alkaline phosphatase, electrolytes; liver enzymes; urinary succinylacetone; dietary intake of PHE, TYR, protein, energy, minerals, and vitamins. Liver imaging studies. Growth. See Chapter 2 for other routine assessment parameters and standards.
Tyrosinemia type II, III (tyrosine aminotransferase, p-OH phenylpyruvic acid dioxygenase)	Same as for tyrosinemia type I.		Plasma PHE, TYR, transthyretin, ferritin, urinary N-acetyl-tyrosine, p-tyramine, p-hydroxyphenylorganic acids; dietary intake of PHE, TYR, protein, energy, minerals, vitamins. Growth. See Chapter 2 for other routine assessment parameters and standards.

	Branched-Chain Amino Acids		
Maple syrup urine disease (branched-chain ketoacid dehydrogenase complex)	Delete dietary BCAAs 1 to 3 days only. For infant, offer Pedialyte with added Polycose to maintain electrolyte balance if needed. Give sugar-sweetened, caffeine-free soft drinks with added Polycose or Moducal to maintain energy intake at 100–125% of RDA. If necessary, give IV glucose, lipid, and amino acids free of BCAAs. Return to oral medical food and complete diet as rapidly as tolerated.[9,80,81]	Anticonvulsants if seizures occur. Phenobarbital and phenytoin lead to accelerated metabolism of vitamin D and vitamin D deficiency that respond to 1,25-dihydroxyvitamin D. Valproate depresses appetite, causes an increase in plasma glycine concentration, and loss of carnitine.[82]	Plasma BCAAs, ALA, ALLO, transthyretin, and ferritin; urine ketoacids of BCAAs. Bone radiographs of lumbar vertebrae, cation/anion gap; dietary intake of BCAAs, protein, energy, minerals, vitamins. Growth. See Chapter 2 for other routine assessment parameters and standards.
Isovaleric acidemia (isovaleryl-CoA dehydrogenase); β-methylcrotonylglycinuria (3-methylcrotonyl-CoA carboxylase)	Delete dietary LEU 1 to 3 days **only**. Increase GLY and L-carnitine. For infant, offer Pedialyte with Polycose to maintain electrolyte balance if needed. Give sugar-sweetened, caffeine-free soft drinks with added Polycose or Moducal to maintain energy intake at 100–125% of RDA. If necessary, give IV glucose, lipid, and amino acids free of LEU. Return to oral medical food and complete diet as rapidly as tolerated.[9]	Benzoates, salicylates are contraindicated.	Plasma BCAAs, carnitine, GLY, isovalerylglycine, transthyretin, ferritin; CBC/differential. Bone radiographs of lumbar vertebrae. Urinary isovalerylglycine, β-hydroxyisovaleric acid, cation/anion gap. Dietary intakes of LEU, protein, energy, minerals, and vitamins. Growth. See Chapter 2 for other routine assessment parameters and standards.

continues

Table 13–3 continued

Inborn Error and Defect	*Nutrition Support During Acute Illness*	*Medications and Nutrient Interaction*	*Nutrition Assessment Parameters*
Sulfur Amino Acids			
Homocystinuria, pyridoxine-nonresponsive (cystathionine-β-synthase)	Delete dietary MET 1 to 3 days **only**. For infant, offer Pedialyte with added Polycose to maintain electrolyte balance if needed. Give sugar-sweetened, caffeine-free soft drinks with added Polycose or Moducal to maintain energy intake at 100% of RDA. If necessary, give IV glucose, lipid, and amino acids free of MET. Return to oral medical food and complete diet as rapidly as tolerated.[2,9]	Anticonvulsants if seizures occur. Phenobarbital and phenytoin lead to accelerated metabolism of vitamin D and cause vitamin D deficiency that responds to 1,25-dihydroxyvitamin D. Valproate depresses appetite, causes an increase in plasma glycine concentration, and loss of carnitine.[82]	Plasma MET, CYS, HOMOCYS; erythrocyte folate; bone radiographs of lumbar vertebrae; dietary intake of MET, CYS, protein, energy, minerals, vitamins.[9] See Chapter 2 for other routine assessment parameters and standards.
Other Inborn Errors of Amino Acid Metabolism			
Glutaric acidemia type I (glutaryl-CoA dehydrogenase)	Delete LYS and TRP 1 to 3 days **only**. For infant, offer Pedialyte with added Polycose to maintain electrolyte balance if needed. Increase L-carnitine. Give caffeine-free soft drinks with added Polycose or Moducal to maintain energy intake at 100% of RDA. If necessary, give IV glucose, lipid, and amino acids free of LYS and TRP. Return to oral medical food and complete diet as rapidly as tolerated.[9]	Baclofen-Geneva Generics, Inc. Valproate depresses appetite, causes an increase in plasma glycine concentration, and loss of carnitine.[82]	Plasma LYS, TRP, transthyretin, ferritin; free carnitine; urinary glutaric acid; dietary intake of LYS, TRP, protein, energy, minerals, and vitamins. Growth. See Chapter 2 for other routine assessment parameters and standards.

Propionic acidemia (propionyl-CoA carboxylase) Methylmalonic acidemia (methylmalonyl-CoA mutase – or °)	Delete ILE, MET, THR, VAL 1 to 3 days **only**. Increase L-carnitine. For infant, offer Pedialyte with added Polycose to maintain electrolyte balance if needed. Give sugar-sweetened, caffeine-free soft drinks with added Polycose or Moducal to maintain energy intake at 100–125% of RDA. If necessary, give IV glucose, lipid, and amino acids free of ILE, MET, THR and VAL to maintain anabolism. Return to oral medical food and complete diet as rapidly as tolerated.[9]	Phenylbutyrate during acute illness if accompanied by elevated blood ammonia. Supplement folate, pantothenate, pyridoxine, and vitamin B12 at three to five times RDA when phenylbutyrate is used. Valproate depresses appetite, causes an increase in plasma glycine concentration, and loss of carnitine.[82]	Plasma ILE, MET, THR, VAL, GLY, free carnitine, blood ammonia, cation/anion gap; urinary metabolites of propionate or methylmalonate, CBC/differential; plasma transthyretin, or RBP. Bone radiographs. Dietary intake of ILE, MET, THR, VAL, protein, energy, minerals, and vitamins. Growth. See Chapter 2 for other routine assessment parameters and standards.
INBORN ERRORS OF NITROGEN METABOLISM			
Urea cycle disorders	Blood NH3 > 200 μmol/L: Delete protein 1 to 3 days **only**. Increase L-ARG or L-CIT if not arginase deficient. Give Pedialyte and sugar-sweetened, caffeine-free soft drinks with added Polycose or Moducal to maintain energy intake at 125–150% of RDA. If necessary, give IV L-ARG or L-CIT, glucose, and lipid to maintain energy intake. Return to oral medical food and complete diet as rapidly as tolerated.[9]	Phenylbutyrate: folate, niacin, pantothenate, pyridoxine, vitamin B12 (administer at three to five times RDA). Anticonvulsants for seizures; phenobarbital and phenytoin lead to accelerated metabolism of vitamin D and vitamin D deficiency that responds to 1,25-dihydroxyvitamin D. Valproate depresses appetite, causes an increase in plasma glycine concentration, and loss of carnitine.[82]	Plasma amino acids, ammonia, transthyretin, and triglycerides; dietary intake of protein, energy, minerals, and vitamins. Growth. See Chapter 2 for other routine assessment parameters and standards.

continues

Table 13–3 continued

Inborn Error and Defect	*Nutrition Support During Acute Illness*	*Medications and Nutrient Interaction*	*Nutrition Assessment Parameters*
INBORN ERRORS OF CARBOHYDRATE METABOLISM			
Galactosemias			
Epimerase deficiency	Same as for normal infant. Avoid drugs containing galactose or lactose.		Dietary intake of galactose, protein, energy, minerals, and vitamins. Growth. See Chapter 2 for other routine assessment parameters and standards.
Galactokinase deficiency	Same as for normal infant. Avoid drugs containing galactose or lactose.		Urinary galactose; routine eye examinations for cataracts. See Chapter 2 for other routine assessment parameters and standards.
Galactose-1-phosphate uridyl transferase deficiency	Same as for normal infant. Avoid drugs containing galactose or lactose.		Erythrocyte galactose-1 phosphate; plasma or urine galactitol; routine eye examinations for cataracts; liver enzymes; dietary intake of galactose, protein, energy, minerals, and vitamins. Growth. Bone radiographs. See Chapter 2 for other routine assessment parameters and standards.

Glycogen Storage Disease			
Type 1a, III, IV	Give oral carbohydrate and/or IV glucose to maintain normoglycemia.		Blood glucose; liver enzymes; dietary intake of carbohydrate, protein, energy, minerals, and vitamins. Growth. See Chapter 2 for other routine assessment parameters and standards.
INBORN ERRORS OF FATTY ACID OXIDATION (MITOCHONDRIAL)			
Carnitine transporter deficiency, carnitine translocase deficiency, carnitine palmitoyl transferase I deficiency, long-chain acyl-CoA dehydrogenase deficiency, medium-chain acyl-CoA dehydrogenase deficiency, very-long-chain acyl-CoA dehydrogenase deficiency	IV glucose 10%, L-carnitine 50–75 mg/kg/day. Uncooked cornstarch as needed to prevent hypoglycemia. 10–15% increase in energy intake.	Valproate depresses appetite, causes an increase in plasma glycine concentration, and loss of carnitine.[82]	Essential fatty acid and carnitine status. Growth.
Multiple acyl-CoA dehydrogenase deficiency	Protein deletion 1 to 3 days **only**. Riboflavin 50–100 mg/day with food.	Valproate depresses appetite, causes an increase in plasma glycine concentration, and loss of carnitine.[82]	Essential fatty acid, carnitine, and protein status. Growth.

continues

Table 13–3 continued

Inborn Error and Defect	*Nutrition Support During Acute Illness*	*Medications and Nutrient Interaction*	*Nutrition Assessment Parameters*
INBORN ERRORS OF LIPOPROTEIN METABOLISM			
Abetalipoproteinemia and hypobetalipoproteinemia (absence and decrease in apoβ)	Same as for normal individual except restrict fat.		Plasma retinol, RBP, α-tocopherol, 1,25-dihydrocholecalciferol, and essential fatty acids; clotting time. Dietary intake of energy, protein, linoleic and α-linolenic acids, total fat, minerals, and vitamins. Growth. See Chapter 2 for other routine assessment parameters and standards.
Hyperlipoproteinemias			
Type I	Same as for normal individual except restrict fat.		Plasma chylomicrons, essential fatty acids; dietary intake of energy, protein, linoleic and α-linolenic acids, total fat, minerals, and vitamins. Growth. See Chapter 2 for other routine assessment parameters and standards.
Type IIa, IIb	Same as for normal individual except restrict cholesterol, saturated fat. Increase PUFAs.	Cholestyramine, colestipol, lovastatin. Cholestyramine and colestipol cause fecal loss of fat, fat-soluble vitamins, folate, vitamin B12 and iron.	Plasma LDL cholesterol, ferritin, folate, RBP; erythrocyte B12; dietary intake of energy, protein, total fat, PUFAs, MUFAs, fiber, mono- and disaccharides, minerals, and vitamins. Growth. See Chapter 2 for other routine assessment parameters and standards.

Type III	Same as for normal individual except restrict cholesterol, saturated fat. Increase PUFAs.	Nicotinic acid, clofibrate, gemfibrozil, mevinolin.	Plasma LDL, VLDL, and cholesterol; blood glucose, uric acid; dietary intake of energy, protein, total fat, PUFAs, mono- and disaccharides, minerals, vitamins, and fiber. Growth. See Chapter 2 for other routine assessment parameters and standards.
INBORN ERRORS OF MINERAL METABOLISM			
Acrodermatitis enteropathica (defect in intestinal zinc absorption)	Same as for normal individual.		Plasma, neutrophil, or urinary zinc; dietary intake of energy, protein, minerals, and vitamins. Growth. See Chapter 2 for other routine assessment parameters and standards.
Wilson's disease Hepatolenticular degeneration (excessive accumulation of copper)	Dependent on etiology of acute illness.	D-penicillamine binds other divalent minerals such as zinc and causes excess excretion. D-penicillamine increases the pyridoxine requirement to 25 mg/day.	Plasma copper, ferritin, and transthyretin. Dietary intake of energy, protein, copper, zinc, other minerals, and vitamins. See Chapter 2 for other routine assessment parameters and standards.

Table 13–4 Results of Amino Acid and Nitrogen Deficiencies

Amino Acid	*Manifestations of Deficiency*
Arginine	Elevated blood ammonia Elevated urinary orotic acid Generalized skin lesions Poor wound healing Retarded growth
Carnitine	Fatty myopathy Cardiomyopathy Depressed liver function Neurologic dysfunction Defective fatty acid oxidation Hypoglycemia Hypertriacylglycerolemia
Citrulline	Elevated blood ammonia
Cysteine	Impaired nitrogen balance Impaired sulfur balance Decreased tissue glutathione Hypotaurinemia
Isoleucine	Weight loss or no weight gain Redness of buccal mucosa Fissures at corners of mouth Tremors of extremities Decreased plasma cholesterol Decreased plasma isoleucine Elevations in plasma lysine, phenylalanine, serine, tyrosine, and valine Skin desquamation, if prolonged
Leucine	Loss of appetite Weight loss or poor weight gain Decreased plasma leucine Increased plasma isoleucine, methionine, serine, threonine, and valine
Lysine	Weight loss or poor weight gain Impaired nitrogen balance
Methionine	Decreased plasma methionine Increased plasma phenylalanine, proline, serine, threonine, and tyrosine Decreased plasma cholesterol Poor weight gain Loss of appetite
Phenylalanine	Weight loss or poor weight gain Impaired nitrogen balance Aminoaciduria

continues

Table 13–4 continued

Amino Acid	*Manifestations of Deficiency*
	Decreased serum globulins Decreased plasma phenylalanine Mental retardation Anemia
Taurine	Impaired visual function Impaired biliary secretion
Threonine	Arrested weight gain Glossitis and reddening of the buccal mucosa Decreased plasma globulin Decreased plasma threonine
Tryptophan	Weight loss or no weight gain Impaired nitrogen retention Decreased plasma cholesterol
Tyrosine	Impaired nitrogen retention Catecholamine deficiency Thyroxine deficiency
Valine	Poor appetite, drowsiness Excess irritability and crying Weight loss or decrease in weight gain Decreased plasma albumin
Nitrogen	No or decreased weight gain Impaired nitrogen retention

metabolic defects may be obtained from PharmaThera (1785 Nonconnah Blvd, Suite 118, Memphis, TN 88132) if parenteral alimentation is required.

Major, trace, and ultratrace mineral and vitamin intakes should exceed RDA for age.[1,88,92–94] If the medical food mixture fails to supply at least 100% of requirements for infants and children, appropriate supplements should be given. In PKU, plasma phenylalanine concentrations greater than 480 μmol/L may lead to loss of bone matrix[95] in spite of adequate calcium intake.

Data in Table 13–5 describes formulations and major nutrient composition of medical foods for inborn errors of metabolism.

INBORN ERRORS OF NITROGEN METABOLISM

The urea cycle normally contributes large amounts of arginine to the body arginine pool. When the urea cycle is nonfunctional, arginine becomes an essential amino acid.[2] Consequently, arginine supplements must be administered in all disorders of the urea cycle except arginase deficiency (Tables 13–1 and 13–2). In carbamyl phosphate synthetase (CPS) or ornithine transcarbamylase (OTC) deficiency, L-citrulline may be given in place of L-arginine. When administered in adequate amounts, these amino acids also enhance waste nitrogen excretion.[96]

(Text continues on page 278)

Table 13–5 Formulation, Nutrient Composition, and Sources of Medical Foods for Selected Inborn Errors of Metabolism

Disorder/ Medical Foods	*Modified Nutrient(s) (mg/100 g)*	*Protein Equivalent (g/100 g), Source*	*Fat (g/100 g), Source*	*Carbohydrate (g/100 g), Source*	*Energy (kcal/100 g)*	*Minerals Not Added*
Inborn Errors of Aromatic Amino Acids						
PKU and Hyperphenylalaninemia						
Periflex*	PHE-0, TYR-1850, TRP-270, L-carnitine-20, taurine-520	20 L-amino acids	17 Canola, hybrid safflower, fractionated coconut oils	40.5 Corn syrup solids	395[b] 411[c]	None
Phenex-1†	PHE-0, TYR-1500, TRP-170, L-carnitine-20, taurine-40	15 L-amino acids	21.7 High-oleic saf-flower, coconut, soy oils	53 Corn syrup solids	480	None
Phenex-2†	PHE-0, TYR-3000, TRP-340, L-carnitine-40, taurine-50	30 L-amino acids	14.0 High-oleic saf-flower, coconut, soy oils	35 Corn syrup solids	410	None
Phenex-2 Vanilla†	PHE-0, TYR-3000, TRP-340, L-carnitine-40, taurine-50	30 L-amino acids	13.5 High-oleic saf-flower, coconut, soy oils	36 Corn syrup solids	410	None
XP Analog*	PHE-0, TYR-1370, TRP-300, L-carnitine-10, taurine-20	13 L-amino acids	20.9 Peanut oil, refined lard, hydro-genated coconut oils	59 Corn syrup solids	475	None

XP Maxamaid*	PHE-0, TYR-2650, TRP-570; L-carnitine-20, taurine-140	25 L-amino acids	< 1.0 None added	62 Sucrose, hydrolyzed corn starch	350	None
XP Maxamum*	PHE-0, TYR-4030, TRP-890, L-carnitine-20, taurine added	39 L-amino acids	< 1.0 None added	45 Sucrose, hydrolyzed corn starch	340	None
Phenyl-Free-1‡	PHE-0, TYR-1600, TRP-290; L-carnitine added, taurine-140	16.2 L-amino acids	26 Palm olein, soy, coconut oils	51 Corn syrup solids, modified corn starch, sugar	500	Chromium Molybdenum
Phenyl-Free-2‡	PHE-0, TYR-2200, TRP-290; L-carnitine, taurine added	22 L-amino acids	8.6 Soy oil	60 Sugar, corn syrup solids, modified corn starch	410	None
Phenyl-Free 2HP‡	PHE-0, TYR-4000, TRP-720; L-carnitine, taurine added	40 L-amino acids	6.3 Soy oil	44 Sugar, corn syrup solids, modified corn starch	390	None

continues

Table 13–5 continued

Disorder/ Medical Foods	Modified Nutrient(s) (mg/100 g)	Protein Equivalent (g/100 g), Source	Fat (g/100 g), Source	Carbohydrate (g/100 g), Source	Energy (kcal/100 g)	Minerals Not Added
Tyrosinemia Types I, II, III						
Tyrex-1†	PHE-0, TYR-0; L-carnitine-20, taurine-40	15 L-amino acids	21.7 High-oleic safflower, coconut, soy oils	53 Corn syrup solids	480	None
Tyrex-2†	PHE-0, TYR-0; L-carnitine-40, taurine-50	30 L-amino acids	14.0 High-oleic safflower, coconut, soy oils	35 Corn syrup solids	410	None
XPHE*, XTyr Analog	PHE-0, TYR-0; L-carnitine-10, taurine-20	13 L-amino acids	20.9 Peanut oil, refined lard, hydrogenated coconut oil	59 Corn syrup solids	475	None
XPHE*, XTyr Maxamaid	PHE-0, TYR-0; L-carnitine-20, taurine-140	25 L-amino acids	< 1.0 None added	62 Sucrose, hydrolyzed corn starch	350	None
Tyros 2‡	PHE-0, TYR-0; L-carnitine, taurine added	22 L-amino acids	8.5 Soy oil	60 Corn syrup solids, modified corn starch, sugar	410	None

Inborn Errors of Branched-Chain Amino Acids

<u>Maple Syrup Urine Disease</u>						
Acerflex*	ILE-0, LEU-0, VAL-0; L-carnitine-20, taurine-140	20 L-amino acids	17 Canola, hybrid safflower, fractionated coconut oils	40.5 Corn syrup solids	395	None
Ketonex-1†	ILE-0, LEU-0, VAL-0; L-carnitine-100, taurine-40	15 L-amino acids	21.7 High-oleic safflower, coconut, soy oils	53 Corn syrup solids	480	None
Ketonex-2†	ILE-0, LEU-0, VAL-0; L-carnitine-200, taurine-50	30 L-amino acids	14.0 High-oleic safflower, coconut, soy oils	35 Corn syrup solids	410	None
MSUD Analog*	ILE-0, LEU-0, VAL-0; L-carnitine-10, taurine-20	13 L-amino acids	20.9 Peanut oil, refined lard, hydrogenated coconut oil	59 Corn syrup solids	475	None
MSUD Diet Powder‡	ILE-0, LEU-0, VAL-0; L-carnitine added, taurine-140	8.8 L-amino acids	20 Corn oil	63 Corn syrup solids, modified corn starch	470	Chromium Molybdenum
MSUD 2 Powder‡	ILE-0, LEU-0, VAL-0; L-carnitine, taurine added	24 L-amino acids	8.5 Soy oil	57 Corn syrup solids, modified corn starch	410	None

continues

Table 13–5 continued

Disorder/ Medical Foods	*Modified Nutrient(s) (mg/100 g)*	*Protein Equivalent (g/100 g), Source*	*Fat (g/100 g), Source*	*Carbohydrate (g/100 g), Source*	*Energy (kcal/100 g)*	*Minerals Not Added*
MSUD Maxamaid*	ILE-0, LEU-0, VAL-0; L-carnitine-10, taurine-140	25 L-amino acids	< 1.0 None added	62 Sucrose, hydrolyzed corn starch	350	None
MSUD Maxamum*	ILE-0, LEU-0, VAL-0; L-carnitine-20, taurine-140	39 L-amino acids	< 1.0 None added	45 Sucrose, hydrolyzed corn starch	340	None
Isovaleric Acidemia						
I-Valex-1†	ILE-430, LEU-0, TRP-170, VAL-480; L-carnitine-900, GLY-1000, taurine-40	15 L-amino acids	21.7 High-oleic safflower, coconut, soy oils	53 Corn syrup solids	480	None
I-Valex-2†	ILE-860, LEU-0, TRP-340, VAL-960; L-carnitine-1800, GLY-3020, taurine-50	30 L-amino acids	14.0 High-oleic safflower, coconut, soy oils	35 Corn syrup solids	410	None
XLEU Analog*	ILE-400, LEU-0, TRP-260, VAL-450; L-carnitine-10, GLY-2500, taurine-20	13 L-amino acids	20.9 Peanut oil, refined lard, hydrogenated coconut oil	59 Corn syrup solids	475	None

XLEU Maxamaid*	ILE-780, LEU-0, TRP-500, VAL-870; L-carnitine-20, GLY-3990, taurine-140	25 L-amino acids	< 1.0 None added	62 Sucrose, hydrolyzed corn starch	350	None
Inborn Errors of Sulfur Amino Acids						
Homocystinuria—Pyridoxine Nonresponsive						
HCY Powder‡	MET-0, CYS-810; L-carnitine, taurine added	22 L-amino acids	8.5 Soy oil	61 Corn syrup solids, modified corn starch	410	None
Hominex-1†	MET-0, CYS-450; L-carnitine-20, taurine-40	15 L-amino acids	21.7 High-oleic safflower, coconut, soy oils	53 Corn syrup solids	480	None
Hominex-2†	MET-0, CYS-900; L-carnitine-40, taurine-50	30 L-amino acids	14.0 High-oleic safflower, coconut, soy oils	35 Corn syrup solids	410	None
XMET Analog*	MET-0, CYS-390; L-carnitine-10, taurine-20	13 L-amino acids	20.9 Peanut oil, refined lard, hydrogenated coconut oil	59 Corn syrup solids	475	None
XMET Maxamaid*	MET-0, CYS-750; L-carnitine-20, taurine-140	25 L-amino acids	< 1.0 None added	62 Sucrose, hydrolyzed corn starch	350	None

continues

Table 13–5 continued

Disorder/ Medical Foods	*Modified Nutrient(s) (mg/100 g)*	*Protein Equivalent (g/100 g), Source*	*Fat (g/100 g), Source*	*Carbohydrate (g/100 g), Source*	*Energy (kcal/100 g)*	*Minerals Not Added*
XMET Maxamum*	MET-0, CYS-1180; L-carnitine-20, taurine-140	39 L-amino acids	< 1.0 None added	45 Sucrose, hydrolyzed corn starch	340	None
			Inborn Errors of Other Amino Acids			
Glutaric Acidemia Type I						
Glutarex-1†	LYS-0, TRP-0; L-carnitine-900, taurine-40	15 L-amino acids	21.7 High-oleic safflower, coconut, soy oil	53 Corn syrup solids	480	None
Glutarex-2†	LYS-0, TRP-0; L-carnitine-1800, taurine-50	30 L-amino acids	13.0 High-oleic safflower, coconut, soy oil	35 Corn syrup solids	410	None
XLYS, TRY Analog*	LYS-0, TRP-0; L-carnitine, taurine-20	13 L-amino acids	20.9 Peanut oil, refined lard, hydrogenated coconut oil	59 Corn syrup solids	475	None
XLYS, TRY Maxamaid*	LYS-0, TRP-0; L-carnitine added, taurine-140	25 L-amino acids	< 1.0 None added	62 Sucrose, hydrolyzed corn starch	350	None

XLYS, TRY Maxamum*	LYS-0, TRP-0; L-carnitine added, taurine-140	39 L-amino acids	< 1.0 None added	45 Sucrose, hydrolyzed corn starch	340	None
<u>Propionic and Methylmalonic Acidemias</u>						
Propimex-1†	ILE-120, MET-0, THR-100, VAL-0; L-carnitine-900, taurine-40	15 L-amino acids	21.7 High-oleic safflower, coconut, soy oil	53 Corn syrup solids	480	None
Propimex-2†	ILE-240, MET-0, THR-200, VAL-0; L-carnitine-1800, taurine-50	30 L-amino acids	13.0 High-oleic safflower, coconut, soy oil	35 Corn syrup solids	410	None
XMTVI Analog*	ILE-trace, MET-0, THR-0, VAL-0; L-carnitine added, taurine-20	13 L-amino acids	20.9 Peanut oil, refined lard, hydrogenated coconut oil	59 Corn syrup solids	475	None
XMTVI Maxamaid*	ILE-trace, MET-0, THR-0, VAL-0; L-carnitine added, taurine-140	25 L-amino acids	< 1.0 None added	62 Sucrose, hydrolyzed corn starch	350	None
XMTVI Maxamum*	ILE-trace, MET-0, THR-0, VAL-0; L-carnitine added, taurine-140	39 L-amino acids	< 1.0 None added	45 Sucrose, hydrolyzed corn starch	340	None

continues

Table 13–5 continued

Disorder/ Medical Foods	*Modified Nutrient(s) (mg/100 g)*	*Protein Equivalent (g/100 g), Source*	*Fat (g/100 g), Source*	*Carbohydrate (g/100 g), Source*	*Energy (kcal/100 g)*	*Minerals Not Added*
		Fatty Acid Oxidation Defects				
ProViMin†	Fat	73.0 Casein, L-amino acids	1.4 Coconut oil	2.0 None added	312	Chromium
		Inborn Errors of Nitrogen Metabolism				
Cyclinex-1†	Nonessential amino acids-0; L-carnitine-190, taurine-40	7.5 L-amino acids	24.5 High-oleic safflower, coconut, soy oils	57 Corn syrup solids	510	None
Cyclinex-2†	Nonessential amino acids-0; L-carnitine-370, taurine-60	15 L-amino acids	17.0 High-oleic safflower, coconut, soy oils	45 Corn syrup solids	440	None
Pro-Phree†	Protein-0; L-carnitine-25, taurine-50	0	31.0 Palm, hydrogenated coconut, soy oils	60 Hydrolyzed cornstarch	520	None
PFD 2‡	Protein-0; L-carnitine, taurine added	0	4.8 Soy oil	88 Corn syrup solids, sugar modified cornstarch	400	None

Protein-Free Diet Powder‡	Protein-0; L-carnitine, taurine added	0	23.0 Corn oil	72 Corn syrup solids, modified tapioca starch	500	Chromium Molybdenum
WND 2	Nonessential amino acids-0; L-carnitine, taurine added	8.2 L-amino acids	6.9 Soy oil	71 Corn syrup solids, modified tapioca starch	410	None

*Scientific Hospital Supplies, North American Division, Gaithersburg, MD.
†Ross Products Division, Abbott Laboratories, Columbus, OH.
‡Mead Johnson Nutritionals Division, Evansville, IN.

Note: Values listed, although accurate at time of publication, are subject to change. The most current information may be obtained by referring to product labels.

Protein (nitrogen) restriction has been the primary approach to prevention of elevated blood ammonia (Tables 13–1 and 13–2). Protein quality is determined by its essential amino acid content. Protein synthesis and nitrogen utilization are more efficient when all essential amino acids are present in appropriate amounts. Severe restriction of intact protein leads to inadequate intake of several essential and conditionally essential amino acids, as well as minerals and vitamins. Because of this, medical foods consisting of essential and conditionally essential amino acids, minerals, and vitamins have been devised (Table 13–5). Carnitine, cystine, taurine, and tyrosine may not be synthesized in adequate amounts when liver parenchymal cells are damaged. Thus, any medical food used for therapy of urea cycle disorders should contain carnitine, cystine, taurine, and tyrosine. Overrestriction of an essential amino acid or nitrogen leads to decreased protein synthesis or body protein catabolism and increased blood ammonia concentration. Thus, to provide adequate amounts of essential amino acids in the protein-restricted diet, about two thirds of the protein prescription should be supplied by medical food.[97] Maintenance of anabolism is essential to prevent hyperammonemia.

Protein quality of medical foods must be evaluated based on their mineral and vitamin content because intact protein sources (dairy products, meat, fish and other seafood, poultry) normally supply large amounts of minerals and vitamins. Intracellular minerals are important for protein synthesis. Medical foods devised for patients with urea cycle disorders must supply all minerals and vitamins not contributed by the small quantities of low-protein breads/cereals, fruits, fats, and vegetables the patient may ingest.

Because protein intake is severely restricted, energy (kcal) intake should be increased to prevent use of muscle protein for energy purposes thereby preventing catabolism of body protein (Table 13–2). Energy is the first requirement of the body and inadequate energy intake for protein synthesis and other needs will lead to elevated blood ammonia concentration.[2]

Waste nitrogen excretion is enhanced through treatment with sodium benzoate, sodium phenylacetate, or sodium phenylbutyrate. Sodium benzoate is conjugated with glycine primarily in hepatic and renal cell mitochondria to form hippurate, which is cleared by the kidney.[96] Sodium phenylacetate conjugates with glutamine in kidney and liver cells to form phenylacetylglutamine, which is excreted by the kidney.[96,97] Phenylacetic acid conjugates with taurine in the kidney.[98] Glycine is readily made from serine. Tetrahydrofolate is required for this reaction to occur. Glycine can also be synthesized from glutamate. Pyridoxal phosphate (PLP) and an aldolase are required for this set of reactions. Because several coenzymes are required to maintain serine, nicotinamide-adenine dinucleotide (NAD), PLP, and glycine pools and the use of CoA in synthesis of hippurate, folate, pantothenate, pyridoxine, and niacin should be administered at three to five times their RDAs[1] for age when sodium benzoate is given therapeutically.[99]

INBORN ERRORS OF CARBOHYDRATE METABOLISM

Galactosemias and Hereditary Fructose Intolerance

Deletion of galactose in most forms of galactosemia and fructose in hereditary fructose intolerance must be accompanied by adequate intakes of protein, energy, minerals, and vitamins (Tables 13–1 and 13–2). Both galactose and fructose bind with phosphate in patients with galactosemia and hereditary fructose intolerance. This intracellular sequestering of phosphorus in combination with excess urinary phosphate loss (Fanconi syndrome) suggests the need for phosphorus intake greater than RDA.[1] Inadequate calcium intake coupled with hypogonadism results in depressed bone mineral density in patients with galactosemia.[100,101]

Therapy of galactosemia due to galactose-1-phosphate uridyl transferase deficiency, although lifesaving, has resulted in less than optimum outcomes. Poor outcomes may be the result of small but significant intakes of naturally occurring galactose in fruits, vegetables, grains, legumes, and other foods[56] or from ongoing deficiencies of riboflavin, phosphorus, and inositol. On the other hand, in vivo synthesis of galactose[102] may be partially responsible for long-term complications in patients with gene mutations resulting in no enzyme activity, while UDP-hexose deficiency[103] and defective galactosylation of proteins, which is depressed by elevated concentrations of erythrocyte galactose-1-phosphate, may contribute.[104] Infant formula powders made from soy protein isolate without added lactose contain significantly less galactose than do liquid soy protein isolate formulas or formulas made from hydrolyzed casein due to the added carrageenan. Milk products and organ meats must be eliminated. Careful label reading for the presence of lactose, casein, or whey and examination of all drug ingredients should be practiced before suggesting the use of any food or drug.[9] Lactobionic acid, found in Neocalglucon®, should not be used in patients with galactosemia due to the presence of galactose.[105] Patients with no enzyme activity may also require deletion of some fruits, vegetables, and legumes from the diet,[2,56] although this is by no means certain.

Glycogen Storage Diseases

Outcomes of patients with glycogen storage disease have been significantly improved by two recent therapeutic approaches.These are continuous nasogastric feeding and administration of raw cornstarch (Table 13–1).[58,60] Both therapeutic modalities aim at maintaining normal blood glucose at all times.[57,59] High-protein diets and L-alanine supplements[58,60,61] have been found beneficial in muscle phosphorylase deficiency (Table 13–2). Uncooked cornstarch should not be added to the diet of infants until about 6 months of age due to inadequate enzyme to digest it. At 6 months of age, slow addition of raw cornstarch is suggested.

INBORN ERRORS OF FATTY ACID OXIDATION (MITOCHONDRIAL)

Fatty acids are a primary fuel for the body when fasting is prolonged and a direct source of fuel for heart and skeletal muscle. Ketones—such as acetoacetate and β-hydroxybutyric acid, obtained during hepatic fat metabolism—are an important energy source for the brain and other tissues.[65] Consequently, all fat must not be removed from the diet and care must be taken to supply required energy and linoleic and α-linolenic acids (Table 13–2). Fat restriction,[66] avoidance of fasting, L-carnitine therapy, and uncooked cornstarch in all disorders of fatty acid oxidation[9,65] and glycine therapy in medium-chain acyl-CoA dehydrogenase deficiency[106] have improved outcomes (Table 13–2).

INBORN ERRORS OF LIPOPROTEIN METABOLISM

Abetalipoproteinemia, hypobetalipoproteinemia, and type I hyperlipoproteinemia all require stringent restriction of dietary fats with long-chain fatty acids.[68,69,107] In all four disorders, adequate linoleic and α-linolenic acids must be provided to prevent deficiency (Table 13–2). Medium-chain triglycerides (MCT) may be used as an energy source. In the abeta- and hypobetalipoproteinemias, all the fat-soluble vitamins require supplementation.[68,69,107] In particular, pharmacologic doses of vitamin E are necessary to prevent myopathy and neurologic degeneration[68] in abetalipoproteinemia.

Restriction of dietary fat, cholesterol, and saturated fat[70,72] is used to treat types IIa, IIb, and III hyperlipoproteinemia. Care must be taken to provide adequate linoleic and α-linolenic acids. Natural fiber in the form of whole grains, legumes, fruits, and vegetables should be increased in the diets of children with types IIb and III hyperlipoproteinemias. Mono- and disaccharides are restricted in the diets of patients with type IIb and type III hyperlipoproteinemias. When cholestyramine or colestipol is used, total dietary fat, fat-soluble vitamins, vitamin B12, and iron may need to be increased in the diet.[99] Great care must be taken to ensure an adequate diet because growth failure and nutritional dwarfing may otherwise result.[71]

INBORN ERRORS OF MINERAL METABOLISM

Acrodermatitis enteropathica—characterized by mental depression, circumoral and acral dermatitis, alopecia, diarrhea, failure to thrive, and death—is a rare inherited disorder affecting zinc absorption.[18] Large supplements of zinc given two to three times daily cure all the symptoms of this disorder (Table 13–2).

Wilson's disease is a rare disorder that results in accumulation of copper in the brain, liver, and kidneys, resulting in neurologic deterioration and liver and renal failure.[73] Therapy includes restriction of foods high in copper and the use of D-penicillamine (Table 13–3). Zinc and pyridoxine supplements should be administered when D-penicillamine is used.[77,108]

AREAS NEEDING FURTHER RESEARCH

In 1988, the National Institutes of Health recognized the need for research on nutrition therapy of inborn errors of metabolism by issuing a request for applications (RFA).[109] The goals listed in the RFA were (1) to improve the effectiveness of currently utilized nutrition therapies of inborn errors by making them safer, more palatable, and less likely to lead to secondary deleterious consequences, and (2) to develop new rational diet therapies based on knowledge of pathogenesis. Research approaches outlined in the following list were identified for support and investigations utilizing these approaches were encouraged. Other approaches for meeting the goals of the RFA were not excluded.

- Investigations of how vitamins may affect active cofactor concentrations and activate specific deficient enzymes.
- Studies of the pathogenesis of the clinical manifestations of inborn errors, designed to develop rationale for better diet therapy.
- Longitudinal studies of the adequacy of nutrition therapies in maintaining normal growth and development while maximizing therapeutic response.
- Studies of the development of secondary nutrient deficiencies in patients on therapeutic diets, due to interference with the availability of other nutrients, such as trace elements.
- Investigation of possible injurious effects of specific components of therapeutic diets.
- Attempts to improve nutrition therapies of inborn errors to eliminate metabolic problems not completely controlled, such as hyperlipidemia and hyperuricemia in glycogen storage disease or carnitine wasting in renal Fanconi syndrome or the organic acidemias.
- Development of methods for improving the palatability or acceptability of nutrition therapy, such as by the substitution of specific amino acid-deficient peptides for amino acid mixtures.
- Development of animal models for the study of nutrition therapies of inborn errors, either by a search for heterozygotes or through use of recombinant DNA methods.

FUNCTIONS OF THE DIETITIAN IN NUTRITION SUPPORT OF PATIENTS WITH AN INBORN ERROR OF METABOLISM

The roles of the dietitian in nutrition support of patients with an inborn error of metabolism are outlined in Table 13-6.[110]

The dietitian, because of her or his central role in therapy, is often the case manager,[111] coordinating clinical care and acting as liaison with the public health nutritionist[112] or home health agency. The crucial role of the dietitian in long-term management of the patient with an inborn error of metabolism mandates excellent interpersonal skills as well as a knowledge base far in excess of entry-level requirements. Without this knowledge and the capability to transmit this knowledge to patients, parents, and professionals, outcomes may be poor or death may occur.

Table 13–6 Functions of the Dietitian in Nutrition Support of Patients with Inborn Errors of Metabolism.

During Diagnosis
Evaluate nutrient intake.
Prepare a nutrition support plan.
Implement a nutrition support plan.
Evaluate the nutrition support plan.
Evaluate nutrition status.
Record findings in the medical records.
Adjust the amino acid prescription (e.g., glycine).
Adjust the selected medications (e.g., sodium benzoate).

During Critical Illness
Recommend the composition of feedings.
Develop tube feedings when needed.
Monitor the nutrition support.
Record in the medical record.
Recommend the amount to feed per hour.
Recommend continuous or intermittent feedings.
Recommend the route of alimentation.
Recommend the necessary laboratory tests.
Recommend peripheral or central line feeding.
Recommend the size of the feeding tube.

During Long-Term Care
Formulate a diet prescription/nutrition care plan.
Record in the medical record.
Monitor for diet compliance.
Revise the nutrition care plan as needed.
Evaluate the effectiveness of the nutrition care plan.
Coordinate with other agencies.
Prepare sample menus.
Modify the diet prescription during illness.
Prescribe medical food.
Prescribe very-low-protein foods.
Recommend methods of feeding.
Evaluate research findings and apply them to the clinical care.
Fill the diet prescription.
Monitor for gastrointestinal complications.
Refer patient to other specialists.
Monitor potential nutrient-drug interactions.
Prepare patient-specific food lists.
Prepare shopping lists.
Review grocery receipts.

REFERENCES

1. Trumbo P, Schlicker S, Yates AA, Poos M. Dietary reference intakes for energy, carbohydrate, fiber, fat, fatty acids, cholesterol, protein and amino acids. *J Am Diet Assoc.* 2002;102:1621–1630.
2. Elsas LJ, Acosta PB. Nutritional support of inherited metabolic diseases. In: Shils ME, Olson JA, Shike M, eds. *Modern Nutrition in Health and Disease,* 9th ed. Baltimore, MD: Williams and Wilkins; 1999: 1003–1056.
3. Goldblum OM, Brusilow SW, Maldonado YA, Farmer ER. Neonatal citrullinemia associated with cutaneous manifestations and arginine deficiency. *J Am Acad Dermatol.* 1986;14:321–326.
4. Borum PR, Bennett SG. Carnitine as an essential nutrient. *J Am Coll Nutr.* 1986;5:117–182.
5. Sansaricq C, Garg S, Norton PM, Phansalkar SV, Snyderman SE. Cystine deficiency during dietotherapy of homocystinemia. *Acta Paediatr Scand.* 1975;64: 215–218.
6. Laidlaw SA, Kopple JD. Newer concepts of the indispensable amino acids. *Am J Clin Nutr.* 1987;46: 593–605.
7. Przyrembel H. Therapy of mitochondrial disorders. *J Inherit Metab Dis.* 1987;10:129–146.
8. Blau N, Thöny B, Cotton RGH, Hyland K. Disorders of tetrahydrobiopterin and related biogenic amines. In: Scriver CR, Beaudet AL, Sly WS, Valle D, eds. *The Metabolic and Molecular Bases of Inherited Disease,* 8th ed. New York: McGraw-Hill, Inc.; 2001:1667–1724.
9. Acosta PB, Yannicelli S. *Nutrition Support Protocols,* 4th ed. Columbus, OH: Ross Products Division; 2001.
10. Holmes RD, Wilson GN, Hajra A. Oral ether lipid therapy in patients with peroxisomal disorders. *J Inherit Metab Dis.* 1987;10(suppl 2):239–241.
11. Martinez M. Docosahexaenoic acid therapy in docosahexaenoic acid-deficient patients with disorders of peroxisomal biogenesis. *Lipids.* 1996;31:S145–S152.
12. Rudman DA, Feller A. Evidence for deficiencies of conditionally essential nutrients during total parenteral nutrition. *J Am Coll Nutr.* 1986;5:101–106.
13. Fenton WA, Gravel RA, Rosenblatt DS. Disorders of propionate and methylmalonate metabolism. In: Scriver CR, Beaudet AL, Sly WS, Valle D, eds. *The Metabolic and Molecular Bases of Inherited Disease,* 8th ed. New York: McGraw-Hill, Inc.; 2001:2165–2193.
14. Elsas LJ, Danner DJ. The role of thiamin in maple syrup urine disease. *Ann N Y Acad Sci.* 1982;378:404–421.
15. Lipson MH, Kraus J, Rosenberg LE. Affinity of cystathionine beta-synthase for pyridoxal 5′-phosphate in cultured cells. A mechanism for pyridoxine-responsive homocystinuria. *J Clin Invest.* 1980;66(2):188–193.
16. Rosenblatt DS, Fenton WA. Inherited disorders of folate and cobalamin transport and metabolism. In: Scriver CR, Beaudet AL, Sly WS, Valle D, eds. *The Metabolic and Molecular Bases of Inherited Disease,* 8th ed. New York: McGraw-Hill, Inc.; 2001:3897–3934.
17. Bonkowsky HL, Magnussen CR, Collins AR, Donerty JM, Ress RA, Tschudy DP. Comparative effects of glycerol and dextrose on porphyrin precursor excretion in acute intermittent porphyria. *Metabolism.* 1976;25: 405–414.
18. Aggett PJ. Acrodermatitis enteropathica. *J Inherit Metab Dis.* 1983;6 (Suppl 1):39–43.
19. Wolf B. Disorders of biotin metabolism. In: Scriver CR, Beaudet AL, Sly WS, Valle D, eds. *The Metabolic and Molecular Bases of Inherited Disease,* 8th ed. New York: McGraw-Hill, Inc.; 2001:3151–3177.
20. Chipponi JX, Bleier JC, Santi MT, Rudman D. Deficiencies of essential and conditionally essential nutrients. *Am J Clin Nutr.* 1982;35:1112–1116.
21. Guttler F, Olesen ES, Wamberg E. Diurnal variations of serum phenylalanine in phenylketonuric children on low phenylalanine diet. *Am J Clin Nutr.* 1969;22: 1568–1570.
22. Stepnick-Gropper S, Acosta PB. The effect of simultaneous ingestion of L-amino acids and whole protein on plasma amino acid concentrations and urea nitrogen concentrations in humans. *J Parenter Enteral Nutr.* 1991;5:48–53.
23. Scriver CR, Kaufman S. The hyperphenylalaninemias. In: Scriver CR, Beaudet AL, Sly WS, Valle D, eds. *The Metabolic and Molecular Bases of Inherited Disease,* 8th ed. New York: McGraw-Hill, Inc.; 2001:1667–1724.
24. Mitchell GA, Grompe M, Lambert M, Tanguay RM. Hypertyrosinemia. In: Scriver CR, Beaudet AL, Sly WS, Valle D, eds. *The Metabolic and Molecular Bases of Inherited Disease,* 8th ed. New York: McGraw-Hill, Inc.; 2001:1777–1805.
25. Lindstedt S, Holme E, Lock EA. Treatment of hereditary tyrosinemia type I by inhibition of 4-hydroxyphenylpyruvate dioxygenase. *Lancet.* 1992;340: 813–817.
26. Holme E, Lindstedt S. Nontransplant treatment of tyrosinemia. *Clin Liver Dis.* 2000;4(4):805–814.
27. Macsai MS, Schwartz TL, Hinkle D, Hummel MB, Mulhern MG, Rootman D. Tyrosinemia type II: Nine cases of ocular signs and symptoms. *Am J Ophthalmol.* 2001;132(4):522–527.
28. Cerone R, Holme E, Schiaffino MC, Caruso U, Maritano L, Romano C. Tyrosinemia type III: Diagnosis and ten-year follow-up. *Acta Paediatr.* 1997; 86(9):1013–1015.
29. Chuang DT, Shih VE. Maple syrup urine disease (branched-chain ketoaciduria). In: Scriver CR, Beaudet AL, Sly WS, Valle D, eds. *The Metabolic and Mo-*

lecular Basis of Inherited Disease, 8th ed. New York: McGraw-Hill, Inc.; 2001:1971–2005.

30. Sweetman L, Williams JC. Branched-chain organic acidurias. In: Scriver CR, Beaudet AL, Sly WS, Valle D, eds. *The Metabolic and Molecular Basis of Inherited Disease,* 8th ed. New York: McGraw-Hill, Inc.; 2001: 2125–2163.
31. Itoh T, Ito T, Ohba S, Sugiyama N, Mizuguchi K, Yamaguchi S, Kodouchi K. Effect of carnitine administration on glycine metabolism in patients with isovaleric acidemia: Significance of acetylcarnitine determination to estimate the proper carnitine dose. *Tohoku J Exp Med.* 1996;179:101–109.
32. Mudd SH, Levy HL, Kraus JP. Disorders of transsulfuration. In: Scriver CR, Beaudet AL, Sly WS, Valle D, eds. *The Metabolic and Molecular Bases of Inherited Disease,* 8th ed. New York: McGraw-Hill, Inc.; 2001:2007–2056.
33. Carey MC, Fennelly JJ, Fitzgerald O. Homocystinuria II: Subnormal serum folate levels, increased folate clearance and effects of folic acid therapy. *Am J Med.* 1968;45:26–31.
34. Matthews A, Johnson TN, Rostami-Hodjegan A, Chakrapani A, Wraith JE, Moat SJ, Bonham JR, Tucker GT. An indirect response model of homocysteine suppression by betaine: Optimising the dosage regimen of betaine in homocystinuria. *Br J Clin Pharmacol.* 2002;54(2):140–146.
35. Singh RH, Kruger WD, Wong L, Pasquali M, Elsas LJ. Cystathionine β-synthase deficiency: Effects of betaine supplementation following methionine restriction in B_6-nonresponsive homocystinuria. *Genet Med.* 2004; 6(2):90–95.
36. Yap S, Naughten ER, Wilcken B, Wilcken DE, Boers GH. Vascular complications of severe hyperhomocysteinemia in patients with homocystinuria due to cystathionine beta-synthase deficiency: Effects of homocysteine-lowering therapy. *Semin Thromb Hemost.* 2000;26(3):335–340.
37. Topaloglu AK, Sansaricq C, Snyderman SE. Influence of metabolic control on growth in homocystinuria due to cystathionine β-synthase deficiency. *Pediatr Res.* 2001;49(6):796–798.
38. Schaumburg H, Kaplan J, Windebank A, Vick N, Rasmus S, Pleasure D, Brown MJ. Sensory neuropathy from pyridoxine abuse. *N Engl J Med.* 1983;309(8): 445–448.
39. Goodman SI, Frerman FE. Organic acidemias due to defects in lysine oxidation: 2-ketoadipic acidemia and glutaric acidemia. In: Scriver CR, Beaudet AL, Sly WS, Valle D, eds. *The Metabolic and Molecular Basis of Inherited Disease,* 8th ed. New York: McGraw-Hill, Inc.; 2001:2195–2204.
40. Hoffmann GF, Zschocke J. Glutaric aciduria type I: From clinical, biochemical and molecular diversity to successful therapy. *J Inherit Metab Dis.* 1999;22(4): 381–391.
41. Lipkin PH, Roe CR, Goodman SI, Batshaw ML. A case of glutaric acidemia type I: Effect of riboflavin and carnitine. *J Pediatr.* 1988;112(1):62–65.
42. Travis S, Mathias MM, Dupont J. Effect of biotin deficiency on the catabolism of linoleate in the rat. *J Nutr.* 1972;102:767–772.
43. North KN, Korson MK, Gopal YR, Rohr FJ, Brazelton TB, Waisbren SE, Warman ML. Neonatal-onset propionic acidemia: Neurologic and developmental profiles, and implications for management. *J Pediatr.* 1995; 126:916–922.
44. Baumgartner ER, Viardot C. Long-term follow up of 77 patients with isolated methylmalonic acidaemia. *J Inherit Metab Dis.* 1995;18:138–142.
45. Yannicelli S, Acosta PB, Velazquez A, Bock HG, Marriage B, Kurczynski TW, Miller M, Korson M, Steiner RD, Rutledge L. Improved growth and nutrition status in children with methylmalonic or propionic acidemia fed an elemental medical food. *Mol Genet Metab.* 2003;80(1-2):181–188.
46. Brusilow SW, Horwich AL. Urea cycle enzymes. In: Scriver CR, Beaudet AL, Sly WS, Valle D, eds. *The Metabolic and Molecular Bases of Inherited Disease,* 8th ed. New York: McGraw-Hill, Inc.; 2001:1909–1964.
47. Acosta PB, Yannicelli S, Arnold G, Marriage B, Bernstein L, Fox J, Miller M. Medical food improves growth and protein status of children with a urea cycle enzyme defect undergoing nutrition management. *J Inherit Metab Dis.* 2003;26(Suppl 2):205A.
48. Berry GT, Steiner RD. Long-term management of patients with urea cycle disorders. *J Pediatr.* 2001;138 (1 Suppl):S56–S60.
49. Leonard JV. The nutritional management of urea cycle disorders. *J Pediatr.* 2001;138(1 Suppl):S40–S44.
50. Summar M. Current strategies for the management of neonatal urea cycle disorders. *J Pediatr.* 2001;138 (1 Suppl):S30–S39.
51. Ohtani Y, Ohyanagi K, Yamamoto S, Matsuda I. Secondary carnitine deficiency in hyperammonemic attacks of ornithine transcarbamylase deficiency. *J Pediatr.* 1988;112(3):409–414.
52. Ohtsuka Y, Griffith OWL. Effect of aminocarnitine on carnitine-dependent metabolism and acute ammonia toxicity. *Biochem Pharmacol.* 1991;41(12):1957–1961.
53. Renner C, Sewell AC, Bervoets K, Forster H, Bohles H. Sodium citrate supplementation in inborn argininosuccinate lyase deficiency: A study in a 5-year-old patient under total parenteral nutrition. *Eur J Pediatr.* 1995;154(11):909–914.
54. Holton JB, Walter JH, Tyfield LA. Galactosemia. In: Scriver CR, Beaudet AL, Sly WS, Valle D, eds. *The*

Metabolic and Molecular Bases of Inherited Disease, 8th ed. New York: McGraw-Hill, Inc.; 2001:1553–1558.

55. Sardharwalla IB, Wraith JE, Bridge C, Fowler B, Roberts SA. A patient with severe type of epimerase deficiency galactosaemia. *J Inherit Metab Dis.* 1988; 11(suppl 2):249–251.
56. Acosta PB, Gross KC. Hidden sources of galactose in the environment. *Eur J Pediatr.* 1995;154(7 Suppl 2):S87–S92.
57. Chen YT. Glycogen storage diseases. In: Scriver CR, Beaudet AL, Sly WS, Valle D, eds. *The Metabolic and Molecular Basis of Inherited Disease,* 8th ed. New York: McGraw-Hill, Inc.; 2001:1521–1551.
58. Wolfsdorf JI, Crigler JF. Cornstarch regimens for nocturnal treatment of young adults with type I glycogen storage disease. *Am J Clin Nutr.* 1997;65:1507–1511.
59. Schwenk WF, Haymond MW. Optimal rate of enteral glucose administration in children with glycogen storage disease type I. *N Engl J Med.* 1986;314:682–685.
60. Parker PH, Ballew M, Greene HL. Nutrition management of glycogen storage disease. *Annu Rev Nutr.* 1993;13:83–109.
61. Slonim AE, Schiff MJ. Alanine is an effective fuel in McArdle's disease. *Clin Res.* 1989;37:461A.
62. Steinmann B, Gitzelmann R, van den Berghe G. Disorders of fructose metabolism. In: Scriver CR, Beaudet AL, Sly WS, Valle D, eds. *The Metabolic and Molecular Bases of Inherited Disease,* 8th ed. New York: McGraw-Hill, Inc.; 2001:1489–1520.
63. Mock DM, Perman JA, Thaler M, Morris RC. Chronic fructose intoxication after infancy in children with hereditary fructose intolerance. *N Engl J Med.* 1983; 309:764–770.
64. Odievre M, Gentil C, Gautier M, Alagille D. Hereditary fructose intolerance in childhood. Diagnosis, management and course in 55 patients. *Am J Dis Child.* 1978; 132:605–608.
65. Roe CR, Ding J. Mitochondrial fatty acid oxidation disorders. In: Scriver CR, Beaudet AL, Sly WS, Valle D, eds. *The Metabolic and Molecular Bases of Inherited Disease,* 8th ed. New York: McGraw-Hill, Inc.; 2001: 2297–2326.
66. Abdenur JE, Chamoles NA, Specola N, Schenone AB, Jorge L, Guinle A, Bernard CI, Levandowskiy V, Lavorgna S. MCAD deficiency: Acylcarnitines (AC) by tandem mass spectrometry (MS-MS) are useful to monitor dietary treatment. *Adv Exp Med Biol.* 1999;466: 353–363.
67. Frerman FE, Goodman SI. Defects of electron transfer flavoprotein and electron transfer flavoprotein-ubiquinone oxidoreductase: Glutaric acidemia type II. In: Scriver CR, Beaudet AL, Sly WS, Valle D, eds. *The Metabolic and Molecular Bases of Inherited Disease,* 8th ed. New York: McGraw-Hill, Inc.; 2001:2357–2365.
68. Kane JP, Havel RJ. Disorders of the biogenesis and secretion of lipoproteins containing the β-lipoproteins. In: Scriver CR, Beaudet AL, Sly WS, Valle D, eds. *The Metabolic and Molecular Bases of Inherited Disease,* 8th ed. New York: McGraw-Hill, Inc.; 2001:2717–2752.
69. Brunzell JD, Deeb S. Familial lipoprotein lipase deficiency, APO C-II deficiency, and hepatic lipase deficiency. In: Scriver CR, Beaudet AL, Sly WS, Valle D, eds. *The Metabolic and Molecular Bases of Inherited Disease,* 8th ed. New York: McGraw-Hill, Inc.; 2001:1913–1932.
70. Goldstein JL, Hobbs HH, Brown MS. Familial hypercholesterolemia. In: Scriver CR, Beaudet AL, Sly WS, Valle D, eds. *The Metabolic and Molecular Bases of Inherited Disease,* 8th ed. New York: McGraw-Hill, Inc.; 2001:2863–2913.
71. Lifshitz F, Moses N. Growth failure: A complication of dietary treatment of hypercholesterolemia. *Am J Dis Child.* 1989;143(5):537–542.
72. Mahley RW, Rall SC. Type III hyperlipoproteinemia (dysbeta-lipoproteinemia): The role of apolipoprotein in normal and abnormal lipid metabolism. In: Scriver CR, Beaudet AL, Sly WS, Valle D, eds. *The Metabolic and Molecular Bases of Inherited Disease,* 8th ed. New York: McGraw-Hill, Inc.; 2001:2835–2862.
73. Culotta VC, Gitlin JD. Disorders of copper transport. In: Scriver CR, Beaudet AL, Sly WS, Valle D, eds. *The Metabolic and Molecular Bases of Inherited Disease,* 8th ed. New York: McGraw-Hill, Inc.; 2001:3105–3126.
74. Feillet F, Bodamer OA, Dixon MA, Sequeira S, Leonard JV. Resting energy expenditure in disorders of propionate metabolism. *J Pediatr.* 2000;136(5):659–663.
75. deKoning TJ, van Hagen CC, Carbasius-Weber E, van denHurk TAM, Oudshoorn A, Dorland L, Berger R. Energy expenditure in patients with propionic and methylmalonic acidemia. *J Inherit Metab Dis.* 2002; 25(Suppl 1):46.
76. Bower BD, Smallpiece V. Lactose-free diet in galactosaemia. *Lancet.* 1955;2:873.
77. Walshe JM. Hudson memorial lecture: Wilson's disease: Genetics and biochemistry—their relevance to therapy. *J Inherit Metab Dis.* 1983;6(suppl 1):51–58.
78. Acosta PB, Yannicelli S, Singh RH, Mofidi S, Steiner R, DeVincentis E, Jurecki E, Bernstein L, Gleason S, Chetty M, Rouse B. Nutrient intakes and physical growth of children with phenylketonuria undergoing nutrition therapy. *J Am Diet Assoc.* 2003;103:1167–1173.
79. Acosta PB, Yannicelli S, Marriage B, Steiner R, Gaffield B, Arnold G, Lewis V, Cho S, Berstein L, Parton P, Leslie N, Korson M. Protein status of infants with phenylketonuria undergoing nutrition management. *J Am Coll Nutr.* 1999;18(2):102–107.
80. Berry GT, Heidenreich R, Kaplan P, Levine F, Mazur A, Palmieri MJ, Yudkoff M, Segal S. Branched-chain

amino acid-free parenteral nutrition in the treatment of acute metabolic decompensation in patients with maple syrup urine disease. *N Engl J Med.* 1991;324(3): 175–179.

81. Thompson GN, Francis DEM, Halliday D. Acute illness in maple syrup urine disease: Dynamics of protein metabolism and implications for management. *J Pediatr.* 1991;119:35–41.

82. Pellock JM. Efficacy and adverse effects of antiepileptic drugs. *Pediatr Clin North Am.* 1989;36:435–448.

83. Guttler F, Guldberg P. Mutations in the phenylalanine hydroxylase gene: Genetic determinants for the phenotypic variability of hyperphenylalaninemia. *Acta Paediatr Suppl.* 1994;407:49–56.

84. Dangin M, Boirie Y, Garcia-Rodenas C, Gachon P, Fauquant J, Callier P, Ballevre O, Beaufrere B. The digestion rate of protein is an independent regulating factor of postprandial protein retention. *Am J Physiol Endocrinol Metab.* 2001;280(2):E340–E348.

85. Herrmann ME, Broesicke HG, Keller M, Moench E, Helge H. Dependence of the utilization of a phenylalanine-free amino acid mixture on different amounts of single dose ingested: A case report. *Eur J Pediatr.* 1994; 153(7):501–503.

86. Schoeffer A, Herrmann ME, Broesicke HG, Moench E. Effect of dosage and timing of amino acid mixtures on nitrogen retention in patients with phenylketonuria. *J Nutr Med.* 1994;4:415–418.

87. Arnold GL, Vladutiu CJ, Kirby RS, Blakely EM, Deluca JM. Protein insufficiency and linear growth restriction in phenylketonuria. *J Pediatr.* 2002;141(2): 243–246.

88. Acosta PB. Growth, plasma amino acids and plasma biochemistries of children with phenylketonuria due to phenylalanine hydroxylase deficiency. Columbus, OH, Ross Products Division, Abbott Laboratories, 2001.

89. Acosta PE, Yannicelli S. Protein intake affects phenylalanine requirements and growth of infants with phenylketonuria. *Acta Paediatr Suppl.* 1994;407:66–67.

90. Acosta PB, Yannicelli S, Singh R, Elsas LJ, Kennedy MJ, Bernstein L, Rohr F, Trahms C, Koch R, Breck J. Intake and blood levels of fatty acids in treated patients with phenylketonuria. *J Pediatr Gastroenterol Nutr.* 2001;33(3)253–259.

91. Pratt EL, Snyderman SE, Cheung MW, Norton P, Holt LE, Hansen AE, Panos TC. The theonine requirement of the normal infant. *J Nutr.* 1955;56:231–251.

92. Acosta PB, Yannicelli S, Singh R, Elsas LJ, Mofidi S, Steiner R. Iron status of children with phenylketonuria undergoing nutrition therapy assessed by transferrin receptors. *Genet. Med.* 2004;6(2):96–101.

93. Yannicelli S, Medeiros DM. Elevated plasma phenylalanine concentrations may adversely affect bone status of phenylketonuric mice. *J Inherit Metab Dis.* 2002;25(5)347–361.

94. Acosta PB, Yannicelli S. Plasma micronutrient concentrations in infants undergoing therapy for phenylketonuria. *Biol Trace Elem Res.* 1999;67:75–84.

95. Pasquali M, Singh R, Kennedy MJ, et al. Pyridinium cross-links: A parameter of bone matrix turnover in phenylketonuria. *Book of Abstracts*, 5th Meeting of the International Society for Neonatal Screening, June 26–29, 2002. Genoa, Italy.

96. Moldave K, Meister A. Synthesis of phenylacetylglutamine by human tissue. *J Biol Chem.* 1957;229: 463–476.

97. Ambrose AM, Powder FW, Sherwin CP. Further studies on the detoxification of phenylacetic acid. *J Biol Chem.* 1933;101:669–675.

98. James MO, Smith RL, Williams RT, Reidenberg M. The conjugation of phenylacetic acid in man, subhuman primates and some non-primate species. *Proc R Soc Lond B Biol Sci.* 1972;182:25–35.

99. Zeman FJ. Drugs and nutritional care. *Clinical Nutrition and Dietetics,* 2nd ed. New York: MacMillan Publishing Co.; 1991:86–116.

100. Kaufman FR, Loro ML, Azen C. Effect of hypogonadism and deficient calcium intake on bone density in patients with galactosemia. *J Pediatr.* 1993;123: 365–370.

101. Rubio-Gozalbo ME, Hamming S, van Kroonenbrugh MJ, Bakker JA, Vermeer C, Forget PP. Bone mineral density in patients with classic galactosaemia. *Arch Dis Child.* 2002;87(1):57–60.

102. Berry GT, Nissim I, Lin Z, Mazur AT, Gibson JG, Segal S. Endogenous synthesis of galactose in normal men and patients with hereditary galactosaemia. *Lancet.* 1995;346:1073–1074.

103. Lai K, Langley SD, Khwaja FW, Schmitt EW, Elsas LJ. GALT deficiency causes UDP-hexose deficit in human galactosemic cells. *Glycobiology.* 2003;13(4)285–294.

104. Charlwood J, Clayton P, Keir G. Defective galactosylation of serum transferrin in galactosemia. Glycobiology. 1998;8:351–357.

105. Harju M. Lactobionic acid as a substrate of β-galactosidases. *Milchwissenschaft.* 1990;45:411–415.

106. Rinaldo P, Schmidt-Sommerfeld E, Posca AP, Heales SJ, Woolf DA, Leonard JV. Effect of treatment with glycine and L-carnitine in medium-chain acyl-coenzyme A dehydrogenase deficiency. *J Pediatr.* 1993;122(4):580–584.

107. Tall AR, Breslow JL, Rubin EM. Genetic disorders affecting plasma high-density lipoproteins. In: Scriver CR, Beaudet AL, Sly WS, Valle D, editors. *The Metabolic and Molecular Bases of Inherited Disease.* ed. 8. New York: McGraw-Hill, Inc., 2001: p 2915–2931.

108. Physicians' Desk Reference. Des Moines, IA: Edward R Barnhart, 1996.
109. Levin EY, de la Cruz F. (eds): *Nutritional therapy of inborn errors of metabolism.* Bethesda, MD: National Institutes of Child Health and Human Development. 1988.
110. Acosta PB, Ryan AS. Functions of dietitians providing nutrition support to patients with inherited metabolic disorders. *J Am Diet Assoc.* 1997;97(7):783–786.
111. Belsten LM, Rarback S, Wellman NS. The metabolic nutritionist as a team member and case manager. *Top Clin Nutr.* 1987;2:76–81.
112. Stephens-Hitchcock E, Walker EJ. The public health approach to the treatment and follow-up of children with metabolic disorders. *Top Clin Nutr.* 1987;2:82–86.

Chapter 14

Developmental Disabilities

Harriet H. Cloud

The nutritional needs of the child with developmental disabilities are variable and primarily involve energy, growth, regulation of the biochemical processes and repair of cells and body tissue. Nutritional risk factors often include growth deficiency, obesity, gastrointestinal disorders, metabolic problems, feeding problems, and drug-nutrient interaction problems. It has been reported by the Centers for Disease Control and Prevention that 17% of children under 18 have some type of developmental disability.[1]

DEFINITION OF DEVELOPMENTAL DISABILITIES

A developmental disability was defined in Public Law 99-101-496 ed (1990 revised in 2000 to PL 106-402), the Developmental Disabilities Assistance and Bill of Rights Act,[2] as a severe chronic disability of a person that is attributable to a mental or physical impairment or combination of mental and physical impairments:

- manifests before the person attains age 22
- likely to continue indefinitely
- results in substantial functional limitations in three or more areas of major life activity (self-care, receptive and expressive language, learning, mobility, self-direction, capacity for independent living, and economic self-sufficiency)
- reflects the person's need for a combination of special interdisciplinary or generic care, treatments, or other services that are lifelong or of extended duration and are individually planned and coordinated

Children with special health care needs are those who have or are at increased risk for a chronic physical, developmental, behavioral, or emotional condition and who require health and related services of a type or amount beyond that required by children generally.[3]

The etiology of developmental disabilities has been traced to chromosomal aberrations such as Down syndrome (trisomy 21) and Prader-Willi syndrome, neurologic insults in the prenatal period, prematurity, infectious diseases, trauma, congenital defects such as cleft lip and palate, neural tube defects such as spina bifida, inborn errors of metabolism, and other syndromes of lesser incidence.[4]

Nutrition considerations that involve the child with developmental disabilities include assessment of growth and the problems surrounding energy balance. This can lead to failure to thrive, obesity, or slow growth rate in height. The second major consideration includes feeding from the standpoint of oral motor problems, developmental delays of feeding skills, inability to self-feed, behavioral problems, and tube feedings. Other areas for nutritional consideration include drug-nutrient interaction, constipation, dental caries, urinary tract infections, allergies, and food or nutrition misinformation the parent has received related to hyperactivity, attention deficit disorders, and treatment of disorders such as Down syndrome and autism with alternative or complementary medicine. Table 14–1 includes a

Table 14–1 Selected Syndromes and Developmental Disabilities: Frequently Reported Nutrition Problems and Factors Contributing to Nutritional Risk

Syndrome/Disability	*Altered Growth Underweight Obesity*	*Altered Energy Need*	*Constipation/ Diarrhea*	*Feeding Problems*	*Others*
Cerebral Palsy A disorder of muscle control or coordination resulting from injury to the brain during its early (fetal, peri-natal, and early child-hood) development. There may be associated prob-lems with intellectual, visual, or other functions.	Growth problems	Failure to thrive	Constipation	Oral/Motor Problems	Central nervous system involvement Orthopedic problems Medication/nutrient interaction related to seizure disorder
Down Syndrome A genetic disorder. Results from an extra #21 chromosome causing development problems such as congenital heart disease, mental retarda-tion, small stature, and decreased muscle tone.	Risk for obesity	Related to short stature and limited activity	Constipation	Poor suck in infancy	Gum disease Increased risk of heart disease Osteoporosis Alzheimer's
Prader-Willi Syndrome A genetic disorder. A disorder characterized by uncontrollable eating habits, inability to distin-guish hunger from appetite, severe obesity, poorly developed geni-talia, and moderate to severe mental retardation.	Risk for obesity	Failure to thrive in infancy	N/A	Weak suck in infancy Abnormal food-related problems	Risk of diabetes mellitus

Autism Classified as a type of pervasive developmental disorder; diagnostic criteria include communication problems, ritualistic behaviors, and inappropriate social interaction.	N/A	N/A	N/A	Limited food selection Strong food dislikes	Pica Medication/nutrient interaction
Spina Bifida Myelomeningocele. Results from a midline defect of the skin, spinal column, and spinal cord. Characterized by hydrocephalus, mental retardation, and lack of muscular control.	Risk for obesity	Altered energy needs based on short stature and limited mobility	Constipation	Swallowing problems caused by the Arnold Chiari malformation of the brain	Urinary tract infections

Source: Adapted from American Dietetic Association. Position of the American Dietetic Association: Providing nutrition services for infants, children, and adults with developmental disabilities and special health care needs. *J Am Diet Assoc.* 2004;104(1):97–107.

list of developmental disorders and their nutrition considerations.

NUTRITIONAL NEEDS OF THE CHILD WITH DEVELOPMENTAL DISABILITIES

Energy needs for the child with developmental disabilities vary as they do for normal children; very little specific information is available for either. A decreased energy need is most apparent in chromosomal aberrations such as Down syndrome, conditions accompanied by limited gross motor activity such as in spina bifida, and syndromes characterized by low muscle tone such as is found in Prader-Willi syndrome, Rubinstein-Tabyi, and Turner's syndrome.

Energy needs of infants and children with other developmental disabilities such as cerebral palsy and Rett syndrome are highly individualized and vary widely.[4]

The new Dietary Reference Intakes are a set of nutrient-based reference values that replace the Recommended Dietary Allowances (RDAs). They were developed in response to a need for a more precise and customized approach to defining nutrient requirements. They consist of an Estimated Average Requirement, Recommended Dietary Allowance, Adequate Intake, Tolerable Upper Intake Level, and an Estimated Energy Requirement (Table 14–2).[5] The adaptability of these reference sets to the special needs population will require further research.

Lowered Energy Needs

For the child with Down syndrome, Prader-Willi syndrome, or spina bifida, the growth rate has been found to be slower and basal energy needs and muscle tone lower, leading to diminished motor activity when compared to the child who is not developmentally disabled.[6] Not to be

Table 14–2 Criteria and Dietary Reference Intake Values for Energy by Active Individuals in the Pediatric Age Group[a]

Life Stage Group	*Criterion*	*Active PAL[b] EER (kcal/d)* Male	Female
0 through 6 months	Energy expenditure plus energy deposition	570	520 (3 mo)
7 through 12 months	Energy expenditure plus energy deposition	743	676 (9 mo)
1 through 2 years	Energy expenditure plus energy deposition	1046	992 (24 mo)
3 through 8 years	Energy expenditure plus energy deposition	1742	1642 (6 years)
9 through 13 years	Energy expenditure plus energy deposition	2279	2071 (11 years)
14 through 18 years	Energy expenditure plus energy deposition	3152	2368 (16 years)
Over 18 years	Energy expenditure plus energy deposition	3067[c]	2403 (19 years)

[a]For healthy moderately active Americans and Canadians.
[b] PAL = physical activity level, EER = estimated energy requirement, TEE = total energy expenditure.
[c]Subtract 10 kcal per day for males and 7 kcal per day for females for each year of age over 19 years.

Source: Institute of Medicine of the National Academies. Dietary Reference Intakes for energy, carbohydrate, fiber, fat, fatty acids, cholesterol, protein and amino acids (macronutrients). Washington, DC: The National Academies Press; 2002.

forgotten is a familial predisposition to obesity. As a result of these factors, children tend to become overweight and obese when fed according to normal standards. Determination of energy needs for children with these developmental disabilities, who tend to be short, led to the recommendation that energy needs be calculated per centimeter of height (see Table 14–3).[7] Recent studies have shown that children with disorders such as Down syndrome are frequently provided food intake greater than the Dietary Reference Intake (DRI).[8]

Higher Energy Needs

Children with cerebral palsy often tend to be seriously underweight for height.[9] Studies have been conducted to estimate the energy needs of the child with cerebral palsy and have utilized indirect calorimetry and the doubly labeled water method. Recent studies have found that adults with cerebral palsy have higher resting metabolic rates than their controls.[10] A previous study by Bandini and colleagues[11] found that the resting energy expenditure of adolescents with cerebral palsy were lower than in adolescent controls. Stallings and associates[12] completed a study of children ages 2 to 12 with spastic quadreplegia cerebral palsy compared with a normal control group. The conclusion was that growth failure and an abnormal pattern of REE are related to inadequate energy intake.[12,13]

Two other methods for determining energy needs of this population include using a nomogram for calculating body surface area and standards based on cal/m2/h (see Appendix G1).[14] This method can be used for males and females 6 years of age and above. Table 14–4 includes basal metabolic rates for infants and children from 1 week of age to 16 years and is based on weight.[14]

The information in determining the basal energy need must be modified for growth and activity level. The DRIs are generally not appropriate to use in determining the energy levels of children with developmental disabilities. A more appropriate strategy would be to utilize basal energy needs with an individualized percentage added for growth rates and energy levels, which encompasses slower growth rates and lowered motor activity. The dearth of research in this area makes it difficult to develop standards and requires that the dietitian and physician evaluate the child's nutritional needs individually.

Table 14–3 Estimated Caloric Needs for Special Conditions

Condition	*Kcal/cm*	*Comments*
Normal Child	16	
Prader-Willi	Maintain growth: 10–11 Slow weight loss: 8.5	For all children and adolescents
Cerebral Palsy		
Mild	14	Reliable for ages 5–11 yr.
Severe, limited mobility	11	Reliable for ages 5–11 yr.
Down Syndrome	Girls: 14.3 Boys: 16.1	Reliable for ages 5–11 yr.
Motor dysfunction		Reliable for ages 5–12 yr.
Nonambulatory	7–11	Reliable for ages 5–12 yr.
Ambulatory	14	
Spina Bifida	Maintain weight: 9–11 Promote weight loss: 7	Over 8 years of age and minimally active

Source: Rokusek C, Heindicles E. *Nutrition and Feeding of the Developmentally Disabled.* Brookings, SD: South Dakota University Affiliated Program, Interdisciplinary Center for Disabilities; 1985. Used with permission.

Table 14–4 Basal Energy Metabolism of Infants and Children

Age 1 week to 10 months Metabolic rate (kcal/hr)		*Age 11–36 Months Metabolic rate (kcal/hr)*			*Age 3–16 Years Metabolic rate (kcal/hr)*		
Weight (kg)	*M/F*	*Weight (kg)*	*M*	*F*	*Weight (kg)*	*M*	*F*
3.5	8.4	9.0	22.0	21.2	15	35.8	33.3
4.0	9.5	9.5	22.8	22.0	20	39.7	37.4
4.5	10.5	10.0	23.6	22.8	25	43.6	41.5
5.0	11.6	10.5	24.4	23.6	30	47.5	45.5
5.5	12.7	11.0	25.2	24.4	35	51.3	49.6
6.0	13.8	11.5	26.0	25.2	40	55.2	53.7
6.5	14.9	12.0	26.8	26.0	45	59.1	57.8
7.0	16.0	12.5	27.6	26.9	50	63.0	61.9
7.5	17.1	13.0	28.4	27.7	55	66.9	66.0
8.0	18.2	13.5	29.2	28.5	60	70.8	70.0
8.5	19.3	14.0	30.0	29.3	65	74.7	74.0
9.0	20.4	14.5	30.8	30.1	70	78.6	78.1
9.5	21.4	15.0	31.6	30.9	75	82.5	82.2
10.0	22.5	15.5	32.4	31.7			
10.5	23.6	16.0	33.3	32.6			
11.0	24.7	16.5	34.0	33.4			

Source: Altman PL, Dittner DS, eds. *Metabolism.* Bethesda, MD: Federation of American Societies of Experimental Biology; 1968. Used with permission.

Protein, Carbohydrates, and Fats

Careful monitoring of protein intake is essential in the child with developmental disabilities. It is generally recommended that 15% to 20% of the total calories come from protein, which may be difficult for the child with an oral motor feeding problem such as a child with cerebral palsy. These children often suffer from serious malnutrition manifested by little or no weight gain and limited growth in height. One recent study of 75 gastrostomy fed children, ages 2 to 6 years, exhibited impressive growth in height and weight at 12 and 18 months after fundoplication surgery and initiation of the gastrostomy feeding.[15]

Carbohydrates are the primary source of energy for all individuals. According to the usual pediatric dietary recommendations, at least 50% of calories should come from carbohydrates with no more than 10% coming from sucrose. Children with developmental disabilities often have a high percentage of their carbohydrate calories coming from foods highly concentrated in sucrose, such as candy, carbonated beverages, cookies, and so forth. Dietary counseling related to better food choices of carbohydrate is frequently required, just as it is for normal children.

Fats should provide 30% to 35% of the total caloric intake, increasing palatability and satiety, as well as providing a supply of the essential fatty acids. For the child who tends to be overweight or obese, fat intake should be carefully evaluated and controlled. For the underweight child, fat can provide an important source of supplemental calories. Infant formulas are now modified to include a higher percentage of the fatty acids arachidonic (ARA) and docosahexanoeic (DHA) based upon research indicating improvement in visual acuity and cognitive development.[16] It should be recommended that these formulas be used for the infant with special needs when the infant is not breastfed.

Vitamins and Minerals

Research findings do not indicate that vitamin and mineral needs for the child with developmental disabilities are higher than normal. Studies have addressed the vitamin needs of the child with Down syndrome, spina bifida, fragile X syndrome, and autism.[17–20]

Numerous studies[17] have searched for nutritional deficiencies as causative factors in Down syndrome. Traditionally, the studies have included numerous vitamins, minerals, fatty acids, digestive enzymes, lipotropic nutrients, and numerous drugs. Recent media coverage has promoted the use of antioxidants (vitamins A, C, E and minerals: zinc, copper, manganese, and selenium) along with the amino acids, glucosamine, tyrosine, and tryptophan. The expected outcomes are improved growth, increased cognition, alertness, and attention span and changed facial features. The key concept in the nutritional intervention is metabolic correction of genetic overexpression. It is reported that presence of the third chromosome 21 causes overproduction of superoxide dismutase and cystathionine beta synthase, which disrupt active methylation pathways. Vitamin supplements of antioxidants are considered key to the treatment. At this point nutritional supplements are considered an expensive, questionable approach. In addition, parents of children with ADHD report that omitting sugar from the diet decreases hyperactivity. Historically this was reported, but is not found in the current literature.[21]

Blue green algae also has been promoted for children with Down syndrome and other developmental disabilities, purportedly to increase attention span and concentration. Of concern is that little monitoring is part of the initiation of these treatments. High-dose supplementation of vitamin B6 and magnesium has been proposed for autism to diminish tantrums and self-stimulation activities, and improve attention and speech.[21] Other proposed treatments include dimethyl glycine (DMG), gluten, and casein-free diets.[22] Limited research is available to substantiate anything other than subjective reports that the child is helped.[23,24]

Studies involving children with spina bifida have involved ascorbic acid saturation and the impact of supplementation of ascorbic acid for producing an acidic urinary pH. Concern was shown in recent studies related to the effect of supplemental ascorbic acid on serum vitamin B12 levels. No evident B12 deficiency developed in one study of 40 children receiving long-term vitamin C supplementation.[21]

Since 1980, the literature reflected the growing interest in vitamin supplementation in the prevention of spina bifida.[25] Nutritional deficiencies identified as possible etiologic factors include folic acid, multivitamins, and zinc.[26] A British study[27] supplemented 234 mothers with a multivitamin/iron preparation 1 month prior to conception. Vitamins included were A, D, thiamine, riboflavin, pyridoxine, niacin, ascorbic acid, and folic acid. Supplemented mothers had a recurrence rate of 0.9% compared to 5.1% of the 219 mothers without supplementation. Homocysteine-methionine metabolism appears to be altered in women with pregnancies affected by neural tube defects; however, the specific mechanisms of causation are not yet known.

As a result of these studies, it was the recommendation of the U.S. Public Health Service that all women between the ages of 14 and 45 get an extra 400 mcg of folate daily.[27] Recent data demonstrate that this public health action is associated with increased folate blood levels among U.S. women of childbearing age and that the national rate of spina bifida has decreased by 20%. The Food and Drug Administration approved fortification of all enriched cereal grain products with folic acid in 1998, although at a level that still requires folic acid supplementation.[28]

An additional concern related to children with spina bifida has been their allergic reaction to latex brought about by multiple surgeries.[29] For those children affected, it has been recommended that they avoid certain foods: bananas, water chestnuts, kiwi, and avocados. Mild reactions can occur from apples, carrots, celery, tomatoes, papaya, and melons.[29]

A special concern regarding adequacy of vitamin and mineral intake is the effect of certain medications commonly prescribed to developmentally disabled children on utilization of certain vitamins and minerals. Among these medications are antibiotics, anticonvulsants, antihypertensives, cathartics, corticosteroids, stimulants, sulfonamides, and tranquilizers (see Table 14–5). Their nutritional effects can include nausea and vomiting, gastric distress, constipation, and interference with the absorption of vitamins and minerals. In some cases,

Table 14–5 Drug Nutrient Interaction

Generic Name	*Brand Name*	*Drug Nutrient Interaction*
Cardiovascular Disease		
Digoxin	Lanoxin	Anorexia Nausea
Furosemide	Lasix	Hyponatremia Hypokalemia Hypomagnesemia Calcium loss
Respiratory Disease		
Prednisone	Deltisone Orasone Liquid Prednisone	Weight gain due to drug induced appetite increase or edema Stunting of growth in children Hyperglycemia
Trimethaprim	Bactrim	Can cause folate depletion Sulfa in the product can cause anemia
Amoxicillin	Amoxil	Absorption provided by increased fluids
Gastrointestinal Disease		
Ranitidine	Zantac	May cause nausea/diarrhea Constipation
Metoclopramide	Reglan	Nausea and diarrhea
Seizure Disorders		
Carbamazepine	Tegretol	Unpleasant taste Anorexia Sore mouth
Phenobarbital	Phenobarbital	Can induce folate deficiency vitamin D deficiency vitamin K deficiency High intake of folic acid (>5mg per day) can interfere with seizure control Folate depletion can lead to megaloblastic anemia
Phenytoin	Dilantin	Same as phenobarbital
Primidone	Mysoline	Folate depletion leading to megaloblastic anemia
Valproic Acid	Depakene and Depakote	Carnitine deficiency Coagulating defects may occur with risk of bleeding and anemia
Hyperactivity		
Methylphenidate	Ritalin	Anorexia when given before a meal

Source: Data from endnote 46.

vitamin and mineral supplements are recommended.[30]

NUTRITION ASSESSMENT

Assessment of the child with developmental disabilities includes all components of nutrition assessment for normal children (as addressed in Chapter 2) plus the inclusion of an evaluation of feeding skills and development. Taking anthropometric measurements of children who are unable to stand and who have gross motor handicaps will require some ingenuity. Weights may be difficult to obtain on standing calibrated balance beam scales for the child with spina bifida or cerebral palsy. Chair and bucket scales are available for use in both clinics and schools, and bed scales are indicated for the severely affected. Recumbent boards can be constructed or commercially obtained. Alternate measures for height measurements include arm span, knee-to-ankle height, or sitting height.[31]

Standards for comparison of weight, height, and head circumference are found on the 2000 Center for Disease Control (CDC) growth charts (see Appendix B).[32] Because these standards were developed using a normal population, the child with developmental disabilities may plot as short, especially when length or height for age is considered. This is particularly true for children with chromosomal aberrations such as Down syndrome[33] or those with a neural tube defect such as spina bifida. Growth curves have been developed for children with a number of disabilities (see Table 14–6) but for the most part the CDC charts are recommended. Copies of the Down syndrome and cerebral palsy curves are in Appendix D1. Proper interpretation is needed.

Weight for age, interpreted for the developmentally disabled, is also an important indicator of nutritional status and requires comparison with height for age. Again, it is the child with Down syndrome, spina bifida, cerebral palsy, Cornelia De Lange syndrome, Prader-Willi, or chromosomal aberrations in general whose height/weight relationship should be carefully monitored. Early identification of inappropriate relationships is critical so that nutrition counseling related to energy balance can be given. The CDC charts include the body mass index (BMI) as an indicator of overweight or risk for overweight. Using the BMI for age can be very helpful for the child with developmental disabilities; however, it may not always identify overweight in children who are overfat because of decreased muscle mass. Skinfold measures also should be used.[34]

Growth velocity is also an important anthropometric measurement (see also Chapters 1 and 2). Growth velocity information assists the dietitian in evaluating changes in rate of growth over a specified period of time. Incremental growth curves are available for plotting growth velocity.[35] Skinfold thickness is a useful measurement for estimating body fat and is recommended along with arm circumference.[34]

Biochemical measures for the child with developmental disabilities should include at minimum hemoglobin and hematocrit levels, complete blood count, urinalysis, and semiquantitative amino acid screening. The inclusion of this test in an assessment would depend upon biochemical testing the child received in the primary health care facility. Other tests may be indicated for children on an anticonvulsant medication who may have low serum levels of folic acid, carnitine, ascorbic acid, calcium, vitamin D, alkaline phosphatase, phosphorus, and pyridoxine. A glucose tolerance test is recommended for the individual with Prader-Willi syndrome.[36] Thyroid levels are part of the protocol for children with Down syndrome.

The methods used to obtain dietary information about the child with developmental disabilities are identical to those used with the normal child. The parent must be interviewed for the infant and young child. Often for the older child who has a degree of mental retardation, it is difficult to obtain the food intake. It is highly recommended that written dietary records be analyzed with computer software.

In addition to dietary information, an assessment of feeding skills and identification of feeding problems that influence the child's food intake is indicated. This part of the evaluation may include such members of the health care

Table 14–6 List of Some Special Growth Charts

Condition	*Reference(s)*	*Printed Copies Available*
Achondroplasia	Horton WA, Rotter JI, Rimoin DL, Scott CI, Hall JG. Standard growth curves for achondroplasia. *J Pediatr.* 1978 Sep;93(3):435–8.	Cedars-Sinai Medical Center Birth Defects Center 444 S. San Vincente Blvd. Los Angeles, CA 90048 (213) 855-2211; Camera-ready copies
Brachman (Cornelia) DeLange syndrome	Kline AD, Stanley C, Belevich J, Brodsky K, Barr M, Jackson LG. Developmental data on individuals with the Brachmann-de Lange syndrome. *Am J Med Genet.* 1993 Nov 15;47(7):1053–8.	
Cerebral Palsy (quadriplegia)	Krick J, Murphy-Miller P, Zeger S, Wright E. Pattern of growth in children with cerebral palsy. *J Am Diet Assoc.* 1996:96:680–685.	Kennedy Krieger Institute 707 N. Broadway, Baltimore, MD 21205; www.kennedykrieger.org
Down syndrome	Cronk CE, Growth of children with Down's syndrome: birth to age 3 years *Pediatrics.* 1978 Arp;61(4):564–8.	
Marfan syndrome	Pyeritz RE. In Emery AH, Rimoirn LD, eds; *Principles and Practice of Medical Genetics.* New York: Churchill Livingstone; 1983. Pyeritz RE, Murphy EA, Lin SJ, Rosell EM. Growth and anthropometrics in the Marfan syndrome. *Prog Clin Biol Res.* 1985;200:355–66.	Camera-ready copies in article
Myelomeningocele	Ekvall, S, ed; *Ped Nutrition in Chronic Disease and Developmental Disorders: Prevention, Assessment and Treatment.* Appendix 2. New York: Oxford Press; 1993.	
Noonan syndrome	Witt DR, Keena BA, Hall JG, Allanson JE. Growth curves for height in Noonan syndrome. *Clin Genet.* 1986;30(3):150–3.	Camera-ready copies in article
Prader-Willi syndrome	Greenswag L and Alexander R. In *Management of Prader-Willi Syndrome,* Second Edition, Appendix B growth chart. New York: Springer-Verlag 1995.	
Sickle cell disease	Phebus CK, Gloninger MF, and Maciak BJ. Growth patterns by age and sex in children with sickle cell disease. *J Pediatr.* 1984;105:28–33. Tanner JM and Davies PS. Clinical longitudinal standards for height and height velocity for North American children, *J Pediatr* 1985;107:317–329.	

team as the physical therapist, occupational therapist, dentist, and the psychologist. Observation of an actual feeding session is critical and may utilize an evaluation tool such as the Developmental Feeding Tool (DFT) from the Boling Center for Developmental Disabilities, University of Tennessee (found in Exhibit 14–1).[37]

The feeding evaluation should include assessment of the oral mechanism, neuromuscular development, head and trunk control, eye-hand coordination, position for feeding, and social-behavioral components, which include the interaction between child and caregiver. Children with developmental disabilities frequently have oral motor feeding problems and positioning problems and tend to be very easily distracted.[37]

Management of Nutrition Concerns

Once the nutritional problems have been identified for the child with developmental disabilities, various types of intervention programs may be implemented. First, however, the motivation level and degree of understanding of the parents and the family must be taken into consideration. Indeed, the guidelines for intervention of the surgeon general's report[38] on case management for children with developmental disabilities specify that all approaches should be family centered, community based, comprehensive, and culturally competent. Intervention should include all aspects of a child's treatment program to avoid issuing an isolated set of instructions relevant only to the treatment goals of one discipline among the many involved in a child's care. This is an important consideration for the dietitian working with this particular population.[39] A parent or other designated family member may be the individual's case manager, or another health care professional may be the case manager. Nutrition intervention would then become a part of the total intervention package rather than something standing alone.

Another important consideration is whether or not the family gives a high priority to a particular intervention procedure. This applies to any discipline, but in this case particularly to nutrition. For example, consider an obese spina bifida child who has frequent urinary tract infections and a major problem with constipation. The family of this child may give a lower priority to weight management until they take care of the other problems. If that is the case, then suggestions should be provided when the family is ready. When it is determined that suggestions should be given to the family related to any kind of nutritional problem, the coping and educational level of the family should be considered. Often parents have difficulty coping with the fact that they have a developmentally disabled child and may not be able to deal with too many suggestions at once. Cultural competence requires sensitivity to the cultural expectations and perspectives related to child care for successful intervention.[40] Increasing numbers of foreign populations are moving into this country and often are non-English speaking, requiring an interpreter to ensure that the family understands and accepts the intervention suggested.

It has been the author's experience that it is better to give one or two specific nutrition activities for a parent to work on at first. More evaluation and suggestions can be given at frequent follow-up visits. Also, it is important to communicate with the parent by telephone for reinterpretation of what was said during the visit. This is particularly true when parents are distraught and find it difficult to follow through on several suggestions given at once. As a result, they may not attempt anything. Increasing numbers of parents have computer access to the Internet, a new avenue for communication.

An important consideration for this particular population is the cost of some of the nutrition intervention suggestions. The nutritionist should determine if there is a community resource or insurance that can help pay. Variability in state coverage requires research on the part of the nutritionist.

The general principle in the management of nutritional concerns is the importance of the interdisciplinary team approach.[39] Again, it has been the author's experience that most children with developmental disabilities have problems that require input from the physician, physical therapist,

Exhibit 14–1 Developmental Feeding Tool

Parent/Guardian ____________________
Address ____________________
City __________ State ______ Zip ______
County __________ Telephone _____ ______
Referrer ____________________
____
____

Date ____________________
Staff member ____________________
Child's name ____________________
Birth date __________ Age _____ Sex ___ Race __________
Head circumference (cm) ___ (%ile NCHS) ___ Hand dominance _____
Height (cm) ___ (%ile NCHS) ___ Weight (kg) ___ (%ile NCHS) _____
Weight for height (%ile NCHS) ____ Hematocrit ____ Urine screen ____

PHYSICAL

Yes No **Size**

___ ___ 1. Weight (Avg. %ile NCHS)
___ ___ 2. Underweight
___ ___ 3. Overweight
___ ___ 4. Stature (Avg. %ile NCHS)
___ ___ 5. Short (Below 5th %ile for ht. NCHS)
___ ___ 6. Tall (Above 95th %ile for ht. NCHS)
___ ___ 7. Abnormal body proportions*
___ ___ 8. Head circumference (Avg. %ile NCHS)
___ ___ 9. Microcephalic
___ ___ 10. Macrocephalic

Laboratory

___ ___ 11. Hematocrit (Normal)
___ ___ 12. Urine screen (Normal)*

Health Status

___ ___ 13. Bowel problems*
___ ___ 14. Diabetes
___ ___ 15. Vomiting
___ ___ 16. Dental caries
___ ___ 17. Anemia
___ ___ 18. Food allergies/intolerance*
___ ___ 19. Medications*
___ ___ 20. Vitamin/mineral supplements*
___ ___ 21. Ingests nonfood items
___ ___ 22. Therapeutic diet*
___ ___ 23. General appearance (Normal)*
___ ___ 24. Head (Normal)*
___ ___ 25. Eyes (Normal)*
___ ___ 26. Ears (Normal)*
___ ___ 27. Nose (Normal)*
___ ___ 28. Teeth/gums (Normal)*
___ ___ 29. Palate (Normal)*
___ ___ 30. Skin (Normal)*
___ ___ 31. Muscles (Normal)*
___ ___ 32. Arms/hands (Normal)*
___ ___ 33. Legs/feet (Normal)*

NEUROMOTOR/ MUSCULAR

Yes No **Tonicity**

___ ___ 34. Body tone (Normal)*

Head and Trunk Control

___ ___ 35. Head control (Normal)*
___ ___ 36. Lifts head in prone
___ ___ 37. Head lags when pulled to sitting
___ ___ 38. Head drops forward
___ ___ 39. Head drops backward
___ ___ 40. Trunk control (Normal)*

Upper Extremity Control

___ ___ 41. Range of motion (Normal)*
___ ___ 42. Approach to object (Normal)*
___ ___ 43. Grasp of object (Normal)*
___ ___ 44. Release of object (Normal)*
___ ___ 45. Brings hand to mouth
___ ___ 46. Dominance established

Reflexes

___ ___ 47. Grossly normal
___ ___ 48. Asymmetrical tonic neck reflex*
___ ___ 49. Symmetrical tonic neck reflex*
___ ___ 50. Moro reflex*
___ ___ 51. Grasp reflex*

Body Alignment

___ ___ 52. Scoliosis
___ ___ 53. Kyphosis
___ ___ 54. Lordosis
___ ___ 55. Hip subluxation or dislocation suspected

Position in Feeding

___ ___ 56. Mother's lap
___ ___ 57. Infant seat
___ ___ 58. High chair
___ ___ 59. Table and chair
___ ___ 60. Wheelchair
___ ___ 61. Other adaptive chair*

ORAL/MOTOR

Facial Expression

___ ___ 62. Symmetrical structure/ function*

Yes No

___ ___ 63. Muscle tone lips/cheeks (Normal)
___ ___ 64. Hypertonic muscle tone of lips
___ ___ 65. Hypotonic muscle tone of lips

Oral Reflexes

___ ___ 66. Gag (Normal)*
___ ___ 67. Bite (Normal)*
___ ___ 68. Rooting (Normal)*
___ ___ 69. Suck/swallow (Normal)*

Respiration

___ ___ 70. Mouth
___ ___ 71. Nose
___ ___ 72. Thoracic
___ ___ 73. Abdominal
___ ___ 74. Regular rhythm*

Oral Sensitivity

___ ___ 75. Inside mouth (Normal)*
___ ___ 76. Outside mouth (Normal)*
___ ___ 77. Hypersensitivity*
___ ___ 78. Hyposensitivity*
___ ___ 79. Intolerance to brushing teeth

FEEDING PATTERNS

Bottle-Feeding

___ ___ 80. Suckling tongue movements
___ ___ 81. Sucking tongue movements
___ ___ 82. Firm lip seal*
___ ___ 83. Coordinated suck-swallow-breathing
___ ___ 84. Difficulty swallowing*

Cup-Drinking

___ ___ 85. Adequate lip closure*
___ ___ 86. Loses less than $^1/_2$ total amount*
___ ___ 87. Wide up-and-down jaw movements
___ ___ 88. Stabilizes jaw by biting edge of cup
___ ___ 89. Stabilizes jaw through muscle control
___ ___ 90. Drinks through a straw

continues

Exhibit 14–1 continued

Yes No	**Feeding Patterns—Spoon-feeding**	Yes No		COMMENTS
___ ___	91. Suckles as food approaches	___ ___	124. Drinks from a cup assisted	
___ ___	92. Cleans food off lower lip	___ ___	125. Finger feeds	
___ ___	93. Cleans food off spoon with upper lip	___ ___	126. Uses a spoon	
___ ___	94. Munching pattern	___ ___	127. Uses a fork	
	Lateralizes Tongue:	___ ___	128. Uses a knife	
___ ___	95. When food placed between molars	___ ___	129. Average rate of eating	
___ ___	96. When food placed center of tongue	___ ___	130. Fast rate of eating	
___ ___	97. To move food from side to side	___ ___	131. Slow rate of eating	
___ ___	98. Vertical jaw movements		**Diet Review**	
___ ___	99. Rotary jaw movements	___ ___	132. Appetite normal	
	Feeding Patterns—Chewing	___ ___	133. Eats 3 meals/day	
___ ___	100. Lip closure during chewing*	___ ___	134. Snacks daily	
	Isolated, Voluntary Tongue Movements		**Dietary Intake, Current**	
___ ___	101. Protrudes/retracts tongue	___ ___	135. Milk/dairy products, 3–4/day	
___ ___	102. Elevates tongue outside mouth	___ ___	136. Vegetables, 2–3/day	
___ ___	103. Elevates tongue inside mouth	___ ___	137. Fruit, 2–3/day	
___ ___	104. Depresses tongue outside mouth	___ ___	138. Meat/meat substitute, 2–3/day	
___ ___	105. Depresses tongue inside mouth	___ ___	139. Bread/cereal, 3–4/day	
___ ___	106. Lateralizes tongue outside mouth	___ ___	140. Sweets/snacks, 1–2/day	
___ ___	107. Lateralizes tongue inside mouth	___ ___	141. Liquids, 2 cups/day	
	Special Oral Problems		**SOCIAL/BEHAVIORAL**	
___ ___	108. Drools*		**Child–Caregiver Relationship**	
___ ___	109. Thrusts tongue when utensil placed in mouth*	___ ___	142. Child responds to caregiver	
___ ___	110. Thrusts tongue during chewing/swallowing*	___ ___	143. Caregiver affectionate to child	
___ ___	111. Other oral-motor problem*		**Social Skills**	
	NUTRITION HISTORY	___ ___	144. Eye contact	
	Past Status	___ ___	145. Smiles	
___ ___	112. Feeding problems birth–1 year*	___ ___	146. Gestures, i.e., waves bye-bye	
___ ___	113. Breast-fed	___ ___	147. Clings to caregiver	
___ ___	114. Bottle-fed	___ ___	148. Interacts with examiner	
___ ___	115. Weaned	___ ___	149. Responds to simple directions	
	Current Status	___ ___	150. Seeks approval	
___ ___	116. Eats blended food	___ ___	151. Toilet trained	
___ ___	117. Eats limited texture	___ ___	152. Knows own sex	
___ ___	118. Eats chopped table foods		**Behavior Problems**	
___ ___	119. Eats table foods	___ ___	153. Self-abusive	
___ ___	120. Feeds unassisted	___ ___	154. Hyperactive	
___ ___	121. Feeds with partial guidance	___ ___	155. Aggressive	
___ ___	122. Feeds with complete guidance	___ ___	156. Withdrawn	
___ ___	123. Drinks from a cup unassisted	___ ___	157. Other*	
			Play	
		___ ___	158. Plays infant games, i.e., pat-a-cake	
		___ ___	159. Solitary play	
		___ ___	160. Parallel play	
		___ ___	161. Cooperative play	
		___ ___	162. Additional comments*	

Source: From Smith MAH, Connolly B, McFadden S, Nicrosi CR, Muckolls J, Russell FF, Wilson WM. *Feeding Management for a Child with a Handicap: A Guide for Professionals*. Memphis, TN: Memphis University of Tennessee Center for the Health Sciences Child Development Center; 1982. Used with permission.

*List or specify on comments section.

occupational therapist, social worker, psychologist, and nurse, in addition to the nutritionist. Pulling that team together is important in order to have successful nutrition intervention. Some examples of the interdisciplinary approach include working with the occupational therapist or speech pathologist in control of oral motor problems and the positioning of the child with a feeding problem or working with a psychologist on behavioral problems. These problems influence how nutrition is addressed. Communication is a key element in the success of the interdisciplinary approach that mandates group discussions, correspondence between groups, and good documentation. The success of an interdisciplinary effort can be phenomenal and bring about positive changes in the nutritional problems, so it is worth the effort to ensure lines of communication are maintained.

MANAGEMENT OF NUTRITIONAL PROBLEMS

Obesity

Weight management of the child with developmental disabilities is indicated for any child who tends to plot higher than the 75th percentile for BMI. Conditions that predispose a child to obesity are low muscle tone, limited physical activity, isolation, lack of knowledge about food, and slow growth in height, all of which are found in children with Down syndrome, Prader-Willi syndrome, spina bifida, Turner's syndrome, Klinefelter syndrome, and mental retardation. The energy needs of such children are outlined in Table 14–3.

Prevention is the best way to avoid obesity. Counseling in appropriate feeding practices, increasing physical activity, and frequent monitoring of height and weight are essential in a prevention program. Important topics to cover in counseling the parent for preventive weight management include:

- assessing growth curves and growth rates
- identifying true hunger cues
- increasing activity
- selecting nutritious low-calorie foods
- identifying food preparation practices
- placing emphasis on food in the family
- estimating serving sizes
- having mealtime structure

Successful programs for the obese individual should be individually planned and include a written meal plan. For the school-age child, successful management will require contact with the child's school to determine which foods are available through the school food service.[4] Often the family is unaware that Section 504 of the 1973 Rehabilitation Act provides for modified school lunches when a prescription is submitted for a child with special needs (see Exhibit 14–2).

Childhood weight management must be carefully planned in order to avoid poor growth or nutritional deficiencies. In the school setting, it should become a part of the individualized education plan (IEP). Dietary records maintained by the parent and others caring for the child such as teachers, day care workers, family, and friends are useful for monitoring intake. The diet plan for the older developmentally disabled child who is also mentally retarded must be presented in a way the child can understand. The interdisciplinary approach of working with a special education teacher to present written or pictorial information in an understandable format is helpful for success in this area.

Lack of exercise is often common in the child or adolescent with developmental disabilities. The availability of exercise programs for such children varies from school system to school system, as does the availability of general community-based programs of exercise. Exploring and coordinating community exercise resources is an important part of the dietitian's role in providing good nutritional care.[38] Special Olympics events exist in almost all states and are associated with school sports in which the child with developmental disabilities can participate and compete.

Behavioral considerations are also an important consideration of weight management programs for the child with developmental disabilities. Important behavioral assessments to make include:

Exhibit 14–2 Diet Prescription for Meals at School

Name of student for whom special meals at school are requested:

____

Disability or medical condition that requires the student to have a special diet.
Include a brief description of the major life activity affected by the student's condition:

____

____

Foods omitted and substitutions. Please check food groups to be omitted. List specific foods to be omitted and suggest substitutions using the back of this form or attach information.

- Meat and Meat Alternates
- Milk and Milk Products
- Bread and Cereal Products
- Fruits and Vegetables

Textures Allowed: Please circle the allowed texture:

Regular Chopped Ground Pureed

Other Information Regarding Diet or Feeding:

I certify that the above named student needs special school meals prepared as described above because of the student's disability or chronic medical condition.

____________________________ ____________________

Physician/Recognized Medical Authority Signature Office Phone Number/Date

Source: Reprinted with permission from CARE. *Manual for School Food Service.* Montgomery, AL: Alabama Department of Education; 1993.

1. speed of eating
2. meal frequency
3. length of time spent eating
4. where meals are eaten

Frequently used behavior strategies to emphasize in the weight management plan include establishing a reward system for compliance with diet, increasing exercise, and targeting eating behaviors to change.

Prader-Willi Syndrome

Intervention for obesity for the child with Prader-Willi syndrome requires special involvement of both the family and health care providers.[41] Total environmental control of food access plus a low-calorie diet combined with consistent behavior management techniques and physical exercise are necessary. Environmental control may include locking the refrigerator, cupboards, and the kitchen. Individuals with Prader-Willi syndrome often hide and hoard food and exhibit emotional outbursts when food is withheld. Physical exercise is challenging due to the hypotonia that is characteristic of the syndrome, a poor sense of balance, and reluctance to exercise. The individual tires easily and often has limited gross motor skills.

It has been estimated that the caloric needs of the child with Prader-Willi syndrome are 37% to 77% of normal for weight maintenance, that weight loss occurs at 8 to 9 calories per centimeter of height, and that maintenance of appropriate weight can be accomplished at 10 to 11 calories per centimeter of height.[40]

Several hypocaloric regimens have been used in various centers with variable success. The use of a modified diabetic exchange list has been successful along with a balanced low-calorie diet, a ketogenic diet, and a protein-sparing modified fast.[36]

Increasing physical activity and exercise is an important strategy, and daily exercise routines should be begun early to prevent problems secondary to hypotonia. Adaptive physical education programs in the school should be used with the school-age child with Prader-Willi. Recent treatment has included growth hormone therapy to increase stature.[42] Short-term studies have shown favorable results of growth hormone therapy. In one Japanese study,[37] clients were assessed for 1 and 5 years and mean height velocity improved significantly.[43] Advances in the early diagnosis of infants with Prader-Willis syndrome is an important factor in beginning an early intervention program that includes working with failure to thrive and then later hyperphagia and weight management concerns.

Failure to Thrive

Failure to thrive, which is defined as inadequate weight gain for height, is frequently found in the child with developmental disabilities. It may result from:

1. impaired oral motor function and resultant feeding problems
2. excessive energy needs, such as occur in cerebral palsy, pulmonary problems, and heart disease
3. gastrointestinal problems such as reflux, diarrhea, and malabsorption
4. infections and frequent illnesses
5. medications that may affect appetite
6. pica consumption leading to lead intoxication or parasites such as giardia
7. parental inadequacy related to feeding

Nutrition intervention must begin with a careful assessment, including a feeding evaluation with the opportunity for observation of parent/caregiver-child interaction and environmental concerns. Management strategies will be individualized, but will generally require increasing calories through providing concentrated formula for the infant, use of supplemental formulas, or providing energy-dense foods through carbohydrate or fat supplements (see Table 14–7).

Some children with developmental disabilities and failure to thrive require medical evaluations to determine the existence of gastroesophageal reflux and aspiration leading to a need for tube feeding or total parenteral nutrition on a temporary basis following a surgical procedure for a gastrointestinal disorder. Usually this will be followed with a return to oral feeding (see Chapter 18).

Constipation

For various reasons, constipation, defined as infrequent bowel movements of hard stools, often afflicts children with developmental disabilities due to lack of activity, generalized hypotonia, or limited bowel muscle function. It can also result from insufficient fluid intake, lack of fiber in the diet, frequent vomiting, and medications. Parents frequently report using laxatives, mineral oil, and enemas on a regular basis to correct the problem. As a rule, laxatives and enemas are not recommended because they can lead to dependency,

Table 14–7 Foods that Can Be Added to Pureed Foods to Increase Calories

Food	*Calories*
Infant cereal	9/tbsp
Nonfat dry milk	25/tbsp
Cheese (melted)	120/oz
Margarine	101/tbsp
Evaporated milk	40/oz
Vegetable oils	110/tbsp
Strained infant meats	100–150/jar
Glucose polymers, powdered or liquid	30/tbsp

and mineral oil decreases the absorption of the fat-soluble vitamins A, D, E, and K.

Treatment includes adjusting the diet to increase fiber and fluid content. Usual recommendations are as follows:

- Maintain adequate fluid intake, exceeding the daily requirement for age, including water and diluted fruit juice.
- Increase fiber content of the diet by replacing white bread and canned fruits with whole-grain breads and cereals, raw vegetables, fresh fruits, dried fruits, commercial fiber-rich beverages, and cereals fortified with 1 to 2 tablespoons of unprocessed bran.
- Increase daily exercise.

Feeding Problems

Feeding problems are defined as the inability or refusal to eat certain foods because of neuromotor dysfunction, obstructive lesions, or psychosocial factors. Most feeding problems are the result of oral motor difficulties (see Table 14–8) caused by neuromotor dysfunction, developmental delays, positioning problems, a poor mother-child relationship, and sensory defensiveness.[37] All of these problems may contribute to such behavioral problems as a refusal to eat, mealtime tantrums, resistance to texture changes, and the like.

Intervention for feeding problems lends itself best to the team approach, utilizing occupational therapy, physical therapy, speech, nursing, psychology, nutrition, and social work.[37] A single written care plan developed by the team, prioritized with the parent's assistance according to the child's needs, should be provided. Nutritional intervention may involve increasing calories, altering the texture of foods offered, and determining tube-feeding formulas. Additional nutrition education and counseling, oral motor therapy, and behavior management counseling are part of the feeding plan.

Dental Disease

Dental health care contributes to overall improved nutritional status but is often an unmet need in children and adolescents who are developmentally disabled. Dental caries and gum disease are prevalent in this population and are caused by plaque formation, tooth susceptibility, sugar consumption, and medication. Prevention includes home care, professional treatment, and nutritional intervention.

Nutritional intervention involves decreasing the sucrose intake of the diet by eliminating candy, sugar-containing gum, sugar-containing carbonated beverages, cookies, cakes, and highly sweetened foods. Supplying adequate fluoride in the drinking water is helpful in the prevention of

Table 14–8 Common Feeding Problems

Problem	*Description*
Tonic bite reflex	Strong jaw closure when teeth and gums are stimulated
Tongue thrust	Forceful and often repetitive protusion of an often bunched or thick tongue in response to oral stimulation
Jaw thrust	Forceful opening of the jaw to the maximal extent during eating, drinking, attempts to speak or general excitement
Tongue retraction	Pulling back the tongue within the oral cavity at the presentation of food, spoon, or cup
Lip retraction	Pulling back the lips in a very tight smile-like pattern at the approach of the spoon or cup toward the face
Sensory defensiveness	A strong adverse reaction to sensory input (touch, sound, light)

Source: Modified from Lane SJ, Cloud HH. Feeding problems and intervention: An interdisciplinary approach. *Topics in Clinical Nutrition.* 1988;3(3):26. Copyright Aspen Publishers, Inc., Gaithersburg, MD.

caries. In communities where the water supply is not fluoridated, toothpaste and topical application of fluoride can be used. Bottled water is utilized by many families and may not contain fluoride; however some manufacturers are now adding fluoride and list it on the food label.

Gingival disease is often found where dental hygiene is poor. Children taking Dilantin for seizures may suffer gingival hyperplasia, a side effect of the drug. Nutrition counseling to decrease sucrose intake, increase intake of raw fruits and vegetables, and improve snacking practices, coupled with good dental hygiene instruction from the dentist and regular dental care, are important components of dental intervention problems. One additional concern for the child with developmental disabilities is late weaning from the bottle and extended use of the "sippy" cup filled with juice, tea, or other sweetened beverages. Permitting a child to constantly drink from this cup can contributed to an increase in dental caries.

OTHER NUTRITIONAL CONSIDERATIONS

The ketogenic diet has been developed and used in the treatment of epileptic seizures nonresponsive to anticonvulsants.[44] Traditionally, the diet is recommended for children under age 5 with myoclonic, absence, and atonic seizures that are medically nonresponsive. This diet is high in fat and very low in protein and carbohydrates designed to increase the body's reliance on fatty acids rather than glucose for energy. The classic fat to carboyhydrate ratio is 4:1. It is thought that the ketosis produced by the high fat to low carbohydrate ratio decreases the number and severity of the seizures. Typically, the diet provides 1 gram of protein per kg body weight, although protein can be increased if linear growth slows unacceptably.[44] To achieve dehydration and reduce urinary loss of ketones, fluids are limited. Historically, the diet is high in saturated fat content; however, in recent years corn oil and MCT oil have been used, but protocols also contain whipping cream, bacon, butter, margarine, and mayonnaise.[44] A powdered formula is now available (Ketocal; Scientific Hospital Supplies). One study of 58 children showed excellent results in seizure control.[45] Daily carbohydrate-free vitamin and mineral supplements are required because the diet is low in calcium, magnesium, iron, vitamin C, and other water-soluble vitamins and minerals. The expense of the diet, compliance problems, and lack of palatability have made its use controversial. Concerns have been raised related to growth.

Like all children on metabolic diets, the child requires close monitoring and frequent follow-up visits. Routine laboratory studies are required at clinic visits following initiation on months 1, 2, 6, 9, and 12, including urinalysis, electrolytes, transaminates, bilirubin, glucose, serum calcium, lipid profile, and prealbumin. The diet may be discontinued for children who are seizure-free for 2 years. Although this diet is high in fat and low in protein and carbohydrates, it is different from the Atkins diet and parents should be so advised.

CONCLUSION

The nutritional needs of the child with developmental disabilities are important considerations in treatment and program planning. The goal is to ensure a nutritional intake adequate for growth and to provide enough energy for participation in therapy. Research is needed to better define the nutritional requirements of this population and the use of the DRIs for this population.

Dietitians in programs serving this population are challenged to defend the cost effectiveness of nutritional care and to develop nutrition education materials and programs specifically adapted for these children and adolescents, in collaboration with special education professionals.

REFERENCES

1. Centers for Disease Control and Prevention. *Developmental Disabilities.* Retrieved August 21, 2003, from www.cdc.gov/ncbddd/dd/default.htm.
2. Developmental Disabilities Assistance and Bill of Rights Act, Public Law 106-402;2000.

3. McPherson M, Arango P, Fox H, Lauaver C, McManus M, Newacheck PW, Perrin JM, Shonkogg JP, Strickland B. A new definition of children with special health care needs. *Pediatrics.* 1998;102:137–140.
4. Cloud H. Update on Nutrition for the Children with Special Needs. *Top Clin Nutr.* 1997;13(1)21–32.
5. Institute of Medicine of the National Academies. *Dietary Reference Intakes for Energy, Carbohydrate, Fiber, Fat, Fatty Acids, Cholesterol, Protein and Amino Acids.* Washington, DC: The National Academies Press; 2002.
6. Luke A, Roizen NJ, Sutton M, Schoeller DA. Energy expenditure in children with Down syndrome: Correcting metabolic rate for movement. *J Pediatr.* 1994;125: 829–838.
7. Heinricks E, Rokusek C. *Nutrition and Feeding for the Developmentally Disabled.* Vermillion: South Dakota Department of Education and Cultural Affairs; 1992.
8. Luke A, Sutton M, Raizen NJ, Schoeller DA. Nutrient intake and obesity in prepubescent children with Down syndrome. *J Am Diet Assoc.* 1996(12):1262–1267.
9. Sullivan PB, Juszczak E, Lambert BR, Rose M, Ford-Adams ME, Johnson A. Impact of feeding problems on nutritional intake and growth: Oxford Feeding Study II. *Dev Med Child Neurol.* 2002;44(7):461–467.
10. Johnson RK, Goran MI, Ferrara MS, Poehlman ET. Athetosis raises resting metabolic rate in adults with cerebral palsy. *J Am Diet Assoc.* 1996;96:145–148.
11. Bandini LG, Schneller DA, Fukagana NK, Wykes L, Dietz WH. Body composition and energy expenditure in adolescents with cerebral palsy or myelodysplasia. *Pediatr Res.* 1991;29:70–77.
12. Stallings VA, Cronk CE, Zemme BS, Charney EB. Body composition in children with spastic quadriplegic cerebral palsy. *J of Ped.* 1995;126(5):833–839.
13. Stallings VA, Zemel BS, Davies JC, Cronk CE, Charney EB. Energy expenditure of children and adolescents with severe disabilities: A cerebral palsy model. *Am J Clin Nutr.* 1996;64 (4):627–634.
14. Walker WA, Hendricks KM. Estimation of energy needs. In: *Manual of Pediatric Nutrition.* Philadelphia, PA: WB Saunders; 1985.
15. Corwin DS, Isaacs JS, Georgeson KE, Bartolucci A, Cloud HH, Craig CB. Weight and length increases in children after gastrosomy placement. *J Am Diet Assoc.* 1996;96(9):874–879.
16. San Giovanni JP, Berkey CS, Dwyer JT, Colditz GA. Dietary essential fatty acids, and visual resolution acuity in health fully term infants: A systematic review. *Early Hum Dev.* 2000;54:165–188.
17. Bennett FC, McClelland S, Kriegsmann E, Andrus L, Sells C. Vitamin and mineral supplementation in Down's syndrome. *Pediatrics.* 1983;72:707–713.
18. Bidder RT, Gray P, Newcombe RG, Evans BK, Hughes M. The effects of multivitamins and minerals on children with Down syndrome. *Dev Med Child Neurol.* 1989;31: 532–537.
20. Pueschel SM. General health care and therapeutic approaches. In: *Biomedical Concerns in Persons with Down Syndrome,* Pueschel SM and Pueschel JK, eds. 1992. Baltimore, MD: Paul H. Brooks Publishing Co; 273–287.
21. Ekvall SW. Myelomeningocele. In: Ekvall SW, ed. *Pediatric Nutrition in Chronic Diseases and Developmental Disorders.* New York: Oxford Press; 1993:111–113.
22. Patterson B, Ekvall SW, Mays SD. Autism. In: Ekvall SW, ed. *Pediatric Nutrition in Chronic Diseases and Developmental Disorders.* Oxford Press: 1993, New York: 131–136.
23. Cornish E. Gluten and casein free diets in autism: a study of the effects on food choice and nutrition. *J Hum Nutr Diet.* 2002;15(4):261–269.
24. Quinn HP. Nutrition concerns for children with pervasive developmental disorder/autism. *Nutrition Focus.* Seattle: University of Washington, Center on Human Development and Disability; 1995;10(5):1–7.
25. Lawrence KM, James N, Campbell H. Blood folate levels and quality of the maternal diet. *Br Med J.* 1980; 285:216.
26. Bergman KE, Makoseh J, Tews KH. Abnormalities of hair zinc concentrations in mothers of newborn infants with spina bifida. *Am J Clin Nutr.* 1980;33:2145–2150.
27. Smithells RN, Nevin NC, Seller MJ, et al. Further experience of vitamin supplementation for prevention of neural tube defect recurrences. *Lancet.* 1983;1:1027.
28. Green NS. Folic acid supplementation and prevention of birth defects. *J Nutr.* 2002;132(8Suppl):2356S–2360S.
29. Pittman T. Latex allergy in children with spina bifida. *Ped Neurosurgery.* 1995;22(2):96–100.
30. Stevenson RD. Nutrition and feeding of children with developmental disabilities. *Ped Annals.* 1995;24(5): 255–260.
31. Chumlea WC, Guo SS, Steinbaugh ML. Prediction of stature from knee height for black and white adults and children with application to mobility–impaired or handicapped persons. *J Am Diet Assoc.* 1994;94(12): 1385–1388.
32. National Center for Health Statistics in collaboration with the National Center for Chronic Disease Prevention and Health Promotion, 2000. Available at www.cdc.gov/growthcharts.
33. Cronk C, et al. Growth charts for children with Down syndrome: 1 month to 18 years of age. *Pediatrics.* 1988; 81:102.
34. Frisancho AR. New norms of upper limb fat and muscle areas for assessment of nutritional status. *Am J Clin Nutr.* 1981;34:2540–2545.
35. Roche AF, Hines JH. Incremental growth charts. *Am J Clin Nutr.* 1980; 33:2041–2052.

36. Cassidy SB. Prader-Willi syndrome. *J Med Genetics.* 1997;34(11):917–923.

37. Smith MAH, Connolly B, McFadden S, et al. Developmental feeding tool. In: *Feeding Management for a Child with a Handicap.* Memphis, TN: The Boling Child Development Center, University of Tennessee Center for Health Sciences; 1982:69.

38. U.S. Department of Health and Human Services, Public Health Service. *Surgeon General's Report: Children with Special Health Care Needs*. DHHS publication no. (HRS) D/MC, 87-2.

39. American Dietetic Association. Providing nutrition services for infants, children and adults with developmental disabilities and special health care needs. *J Am Diet Assoc.* 2004;104(1):97–106.

40. Terry RD. Needed: A new appreciation of culture and food behavior. *J Am Diet. Assoc.* 1994;95(5):501–503.

41. Hoffman CJ, Abeltman D, Pipes P. A nutrition survey of and recommendations for individuals with Prader-Willi who live in group homes. *J Am Diet Assoc.* 1992;92(7): 823–830.

42. Hauffa BP. One-year results of growth hormone treatment of short stature in Prader-Willi syndrome. *Acta Paedia.* Supplement. 1997;423:63–65.

43. Obata K, Sakazume S, Yoshino A, Murakami N, Sakuta R. Effects of 5 years' growth hormone treatment in patients with Prader-Willi syndrome. *J Pediatr Endocrinol Metab.* 2003;16(2):155–162.

44. Kelly MT, Hays TL. Implementing the ketogenic diet. *Top Clin Nutr.* 1997;13(1):53–61.

45. Freeman JM, Vining EP, Pillas DJ, Pyzik PL, Casey JC, Kelly LM. The efficacy of the ketogenic diet—1998: A prospective evaluation of intervention of 150 children. *Pediatrics.* 1998;102:1358–1363.

46. Pronsky ZM, Redfern CM, Crowe J, Epstein J, Young V. *Food Medication Interactions,* 12th ed. Birchrunville, PA: 2002.

Chapter 15

Pulmonary Diseases

Nancy H. Wooldridge

Promoting optimal growth and development is an important outcome criterion for any child, but it is especially important for the child with chronic pulmonary disease. In this chapter, the nutritional management of cystic fibrosis, bronchopulmonary dysplasia, and asthma is discussed. Adequate nutrition in the care of the child with cystic fibrosis or bronchopulmonary dysplasia plays an important prognostic role in the outcome of these diseases. A discussion on asthma is included because it is the most common chronic disease of childhood and nutrition may play an important role in its management.

CYSTIC FIBROSIS

Cystic fibrosis (CF), a genetic disorder of children, adolescents, and young adults characterized by widespread dysfunction of the exocrine glands, is the most common lethal hereditary disease of the Caucasian race.[1] Characteristic of the disease is an abnormality in the CF transmembrane conductance regulator (CFTR) protein, causing an increased sodium reabsorption and a decreased chloride secretion. The result is the production of abnormally thick and viscous mucus, which affects various organs of the body. In the lungs, the thick mucus clogs the airways, causing obstruction, subsequent bacterial infections, and progressive lung disease. In the pancreas, the thick mucus prevents the release of pancreatic enzymes into the small intestine for the digestion of foods. Blockage of ducts eventually causes pancreatic fibrosis and cyst formation. About 85% of CF patients have pancreatic involvement, exhibited by such gastrointestinal symptoms as frequent, foul-smelling stools; increased flatus; and abdominal cramping. In a small percentage of patients, 6.1 % according to the 2002 CF Foundation Patient Registry,[2] the ducts and tubules of the liver are obstructed by mucus, resulting in liver disease which may progress to cirrhosis. Another complication is CF-related diabetes (CFRD), seen particularly in the adolescent and young adult population. A unique characteristic of CF is an increased loss of sodium and chloride in the sweat. Sterility in males and decreased fertility in females is also seen.

The life expectancy of CF patients has greatly improved since the disease was first described as a distinct clinical entity by Andersen in 1938.[3] During the 1930s to 1950s, CF patients usually died at an early age, secondary to malabsorption and malnutrition. Pancreatic enzyme therapy, antibiotic therapy, nutrition therapy, and earlier diagnosis have been major contributory factors to the improvement in the prognosis for patients with CF. The CF Foundation currently reports the median age of survival to be 31.6 years.[2]

Genetics/Incidence

CF is transmitted as an autosomal recessive trait. Both parents are carriers of the defective gene but exhibit no symptoms of the disease themselves. Each offspring of two carriers of the defective gene has a 25% chance of having the disease, a 50% chance of being a carrier of the defective gene, and a 25% chance of neither having the disease nor being a carrier.

The CF gene was discovered in 1989 on the long arm of chromosome 7.[4] The CF gene product is a protein called the CFTR, which is a cyclic adenosine monophosphate (cAMP)-regulated chloride channel and regulator of secondary chloride and sodium channels normally present in epithelial cells.[5–10] The most common mutation is called ΔF508 and accounts for about 67% of CF alleles among the Caucasian population worldwide.[11] However, over 1,000 mutations of the CFTR gene have been identified, which accounts for the variability of disease symptoms and severity that is seen among patients with CF. It is hoped that these genetic discoveries will lead to improved treatment including gene therapy and ultimately a cure for the disease.

The incidence of CF in Caucasians is in the range of 1 in 2,500 to 3,200 live births, with a carrier rate of 1 in 20.[10,12] The incidence is 1 in 15,000 births among African-Americans. The disease is rarely seen in the Asian or Native American populations.[12]

Manifestations/Diagnosis

Manifestations of the disease are numerous and are quite variable from patient to patient, due in part to the large numbers of mutations of the defective gene. A summary of common pulmonary and gastrointestinal manifestations of CF is depicted in Table 15–1. Any child who repeatedly exhibits any of these symptoms should be tested for CF. In addition, CF should be considered when a child tastes salty when kissed or experiences heat prostration. Other manifestations of CF include the bilateral absence of the vas deferens in males and decreased fertility in females.

According to the consensus statement on the diagnosis of CF published by the CF Foundation,[13] the diagnosis of CF should be based on the presence of one or more characteristic features of the disease:

1. evidence of chronic sinopulmonary disease
2. evidence of gastrointestinal and nutritional abnormalities
3. evidence of salt-loss syndromes
4. evidence of obstructive azospermia in males
5. family history of the disease
6. a positive newborn screening test result plus an elevated sweat chloride test

Sweat chloride is measured by a quantitative pilocarpine iontophoresis sweat test. A sweat chloride concentration greater than 60 mmol/L is indicative of the diagnosis of CF. The diagnosis can now also be made with the identification of CF mutations on both alleles of the CFTR gene.[13] The demonstration of abnormal nasal epithelial ion

Table 15–1 Manifestations of Cystic Fibrosis

Pulmonary	*Gastrointestinal*
Chronic cough	Failure to thrive
Repeated bronchial infections	Steatorrhea
Increased work of breathing	Hypoalbuminemia
Digital clubbing	Rectal prolapse
Bronchospasm	Frequent, foul-smelling stools
Cyanosis	Abdominal cramping
Chronic pneumonia	Voracious appetite
Nasal polyps	Anemia
Chronic sinusitis	Intussusception of the small and large bowel
	Vitamin deficiencies

transport is being investigated as a method of diagnosis but is presently limited to research centers.

Health care practitioners in the community have become more familiar with CF and with the many ways the disease may manifest itself. Several centers are investigating the use of newborn screening for CF and the impact of early diagnosis on the course of the disease. According to the 2002 CF Patient Registry, the median age at diagnosis was 6 months and the mean age at diagnosis was 3.2 years.[2] Because of the variability of the disease, the diagnosis may not be recognized in some patients until adolescence or young adulthood.

Management

Rigorous daily management is required to control the symptoms of the disease. Daily chest percussion therapy and postural drainage, along with aerosolized medications, help to clear the airways of mucus, improve existing lung compromise, and retard future deterioration. Aerosolized, oral, or intravenous antibiotics are used to control pulmonary infections. Pancreatic enzyme replacement therapy is a crucial part of the management of the gastrointestinal symptoms. In pancreatic-insufficient patients, enzymes are required with each meal and snack. Dosage is individualized, depending on factors such as the extent of pancreatic involvement, the patient's dietary intake, and the patient's age. Vitamin, mineral, and salt supplementation is also recommended and is discussed in detail in the nutrition management section on page 323 of this chapter. Providing adequate nutrition for normal growth and development is one of the primary goals of disease management in CF. The complex and multifaceted nature of the disease requires an interdisciplinary team approach with patient and family involvement in decision making for proper management.

Effects of CF on Nutritional Status

Chronic Energy Deficit

Many aspects of the disease of CF stress the nutritional status of the patient directly or indirectly by affecting the patient's appetite and subsequent intake. Aspects of pulmonary and gastrointestinal involvement affecting nutritional status are summarized in Table 15–2. CFRD and liver disease impact nutritional status. Bile salts and bile acid losses contribute to fat malabsorption. Gastrointestinal losses occur in spite of pancreatic enzyme replacement therapy. Also, catch-up growth after diagnosis requires additional calories. The energy metabolism of CF patients has been studied and generally an increase in resting energy expenditure has been found, as compared with controls and/or predicted resting energy expenditure.[14–18] All of these factors can contribute to a chronic energy deficit which, if left untreated, can lead to a marasmic type of malnutrition. The primary goal of nutritional therapy is to overcome this energy deficit and to promote normal growth and development for CF patients.

Table 15–2 Aspects of Cystic Fibrosis that Affect Nutritional Status

Pulmonary	*Gastrointestinal*
Increased work of breathing	Malabsorption of fat
Chronic cough	Loss of fat-soluble vitamins
Cough-emesis cycle	Loss of essential fatty acids
Chronic antibiotic therapy	Malabsorption of protein
Fatigue, anxiety	Anorexia
Decreased tolerance for exercise	Gastroesophageal reflux/esophagitis
Repeated pulmonary infections	Bile salts and bile acid loss
	Distal intestinal obstructive syndrome (DIOS)
	Fibrosing colonopathy

Appetite

Many references have been made to the voracious appetites of CF patients. This may be true of undiagnosed and untreated patients, particularly infants. In practice, however, dietetics professionals often deal with patients with CF who have very poor appetites. Table 15–2 delineates some aspects of CF that can contribute to poor appetite and failure to thrive. Psychosocial issues that the patient may be dealing with may cause depression, anxiety, fatigue, and anorexia that will also impact appetite and nutritional status. Behavioral issues related to eating and ineffective parenting strategies may play a role in a child's poor appetite and intake. Studies of the use of medications for appetite stimulation, such as megastrol acetate, as part of therapy for CF have been conducted with positive short-term results.[19] However, more study is needed to determine the long-term effects of megastrol acetate on growth, pulmonary function, and clinical stability in CF.[19]

Growth

Growth studies have found CF patients to be smaller and lighter than their age- and sex-matched peers. For example, Sproul and Huang[20] found the 50th percentile for CF patients from infancy to adolescence for height and weight to be between the 3rd and 10th percentiles on the growth charts for healthy children. These same investigators noted an absence of the adolescent growth spurt in the CF population. Growth deficiencies significantly correlated with the severity of respiratory disease but did not correlate with pancreatic insufficiency. A more recent study based on the 1993 National CF Patient Registry found that children with CF continue to have poorer growth at all ages when compared to healthy peers.[21] In this study, the median height-for-age percentile and weight-for-age percentile for children with CF was at the 20th percentile of the NCHS growth charts. The largest differences were found in the infant population and the preadolescent population. These investigators believe that this finding may be reflective of the high energy and nutrient requirements of infancy and adolescence.[21] This study did not correlate factors such as severity of respiratory disease or pancreatic insufficiency with growth.[21] According to the 2002 CF Foundation Patient Registry, 17.3% of patients with CF had weights under the 5th percentile and 15.8% had heights less than the 5th percentile of the National Center for Health Statistics/Centers for Disease Control (NCHS/CDC) growth curves.[2,22]

In contrast, the Toronto CF clinic reported that its patients conform to the normal distribution for height in both males and females and for weight in males.[23] This clinic has advocated a high-calorie diet, with 40% of total calories as fat, coupled with high doses of pancreatic enzymes, as part of its routine medical care since the early 1970s. The CF Foundation has recognized the importance of nutritional care that promotes normal growth at the patient's genetic potential.[24,25]

Nutrition as a Prognostic Indicator

More and more studies are indicating that nutritional status is an important prognostic indicator in the outcome of CF. For example, Konstan and associates[26] evaluated the 1990s data from the Epidemiologic Study of Cystic Fibrosis (ESCF) and found that better growth parameters at age 3 were associated with better pulmonary function at age 6 years. Furthermore, patients whose growth parameters improved between the ages of 3 and 6 had better pulmonary function at age 6.[26] Peterson and colleagues[27] found that children who weighed more and who steadily gained weight at an appropriate and uninterrupted rate had better pulmonary function as measured by forced expiratory volume at 1 second (FEV_1) than did those children with CF who experienced periodic weight losses. Data from the German CF quality assurance project found a positive association of weights-for-heights with lung function.[28] Patients with CF who had weights-for-heights less than 90% of predicted had significantly lower values on pulmonary function tests than those patients with more normal weights-for-heights.[28] Beker and colleagues[29] found height to be an important prognostic indicator of survival for both male and female patients with CF. All of these studies point to an association between growth parameters and lung function. Because progressive lung disease is usually what causes the morbidity and mortality of CF, aggressive nutrition follow-up and therapy to promote normal growth, which in turn may impact lung function, is warranted.

Nutritional Screening and Assessment

Because nutrition plays such an important role in the treatment of CF, routine nutritional screenings and thorough assessments are very important. In this section, anthropometric, biochemical, clinical, dietary, and drug-nutrient interaction evaluations will be discussed. The CF Foundation has published a consensus report on the pediatric nutrition for patients with CF as well as the *Clinical Practice Guidelines for Cystic Fibrosis,* which include nutrition management information.[24,25,30] Refer to Exhibit 15–1 for the CF Foundation's recommendations for nutritional status assessment.

Anthropometric

Monitoring growth parameters is an important component of the screening, assessment, and follow-up of CF patients. As with any child, CF patients should be weighed and measured routinely by trained individuals and using appropriate techniques and equipment, such as those described by Fomon[31] and the CF Foundation.[24,25] For children less than 36 months of age, weight-for-age, recumbent length-for-age, weight-for-height, and head circumference-for-age should be accurately measured and plotted on the National Center for Health Statistics (NCHS) growth curves at each clinic visit or hospitalization.[22] For children 2 years of age or greater who are measured standing, weight-for-age, height-for-age, and BMI-for-age should be measured, plotted, and calculated. (See Chapter 2 for additional information.) It is also recommended that the registered dietitian annually calculate weight as a percent of ideal weight for height.[24,25,30] This can be done by obtaining the patient's height age or the age at which the patient's height is at the 50th percentile and noting a corresponding weight from the growth chart. Percent ideal body weight is calculated by dividing the patient's current weight by ideal weight for height $\times$ 100.[24,25] Exhibit 15–2 depicts the CF Foundation's definitions of nutritional failure and at risk for nutritional failure for patients with CF and outlines appropriate action.[24,25]

Growth charts are simple and readily accessible screening and assessment tools. Although they are intended for use with a healthy population of children, NCHS growth charts provide a way to monitor the growth of CF patients. Their use also seems appropriate when taking into consideration the fact that the CF patients will be comparing themselves to their peers.

According to the CF Foundation, anthropometric measurements, including mid-arm circumference and triceps skinfold thickness, should be obtained by a registered dietitian at least once a year on all patients greater than 1 year of age according to standard procedures.[24,25,30,32] From these measurements, mid-arm muscle circumference, mid-arm muscle area (mm2) and mid-arm fat area (mm^2) should be calculated and compared with gender and age specific normative data.[33] These measurements provide information about fat and somatic protein stores and are particularly beneficial when monitoring the effects of nutrition intervention over time.

Mid-Parental Height. It is important to determine if patients with CF are achieving their full genetic potential in terms of height growth. One method is to determine mid-parental height, plot this height on the growth chart at age 20, and use this percentile as the target for the individual patient. The CF Foundation suggests calculating target height as follows. Add 13 centimeters to the mother's height if the patient is a boy, or subtract 13 centimeters from the father's height if the patient is a girl. Obtain the average of the 2 heights. To calculate the patient's target height range, adjust $\pm$ 10 cm for a boy and $\pm$ 9 cm for a girl.[24,25]

Biochemical

Laboratory monitoring of nutritional status as recommended by the CF Foundation at diagnosis and annually is outlined in Exhibit 15–3.

Exhibit 15–1 Nutritional Assessment in Routine CF Center Care

	At Diagnosis	Every 3 Months Birth to 24 Months	Every 3 Months	Annually
Head circumference	x[a]	x		
Weight (to 0.1 kg)	x	x	x	
Length (to 0.1 kg)	x	x		
Height (to 0.1 cm)	x		x	
Mid-arm circumference (MAC) (to 0.1 cm)	x			x
Triceps skinfold (TSF) (to 1.0 mm)	x[b]			x
Mid-arm muscle area, mm^2 (calculated from MAC and TSF)	x[b]			x
Mid-arm fat area, mm^2 (calculated from MAC and TSF)	x[b]			x
Biological parents' heights[c]	x			
Pubertal status, female				x[d]
Pubertal status, male				x[e]
24–hour diet recall				x
Nutritional supplement intake[f]				x
Anticipatory dietary and feeding behavior guidance		x	x[g]	x

[a]If younger than 24 months of age at diagnosis
[b]Only in patients older than 1 year of age
[c]Record in cm and gender-specific height percentile; note patient's target height percentile on all growth charts
[d]Starting at age 9 years, annual pubertal self-assessment form (patient or parent and patient) or physician examination for breast and pubic hair Tanner-stage determination; annual question as to menarchal status. Record month and year of menarche on all growth charts
[e]Starting at age 12 years, annual pubertal self-assessment form (patient or parent and patient) or physician examination for genital development and pubic hair Tanner-stage determination
[f]A review of enzymes, vitamins, minerals, oral and enteral formulas, herbal, botanical, and other CAM products
[g]Routine surveillance may be done informally by other team members, but the annual assessment and every 3 month visits in the first 2 years of life and quarterly visits for patients at nutritional risk should be done by the center's registered dietitian

Source: Used with permission of the Cystic Fibrosis Foundation. Consensus Conference: Concept in CF Care, Pediatric Nutrition for Patients with Cystic Fibrosis. Bethesda, MD: Cystic Fibrosis Foundation; 2001;1–39.

Protein Status. Undiagnosed infants, particularly those who are breast-fed, often present with hypoalbuminemia and subsequent edema. The malabsorption that occurs in undiagnosed CF causes inadequate absorption of protein. The low protein content of breast milk as compared with modified cow's milk formulas further compromises the infant's protein status. Upon diagnosis of CF and the initiation of pancreatic enzyme therapy, hypoalbuminemia is usually corrected because the infant is no longer malabsorbing protein. It is wise to check an albumin level in newly diagnosed infants. Any time an inadequate protein intake is suspected, it may be

Exhibit 15–2 Definition of Nutritional Failure in Patients with CF and Those at Risk

Nutritional Status	Length or Height	Percentage IBW[1] All Ages	Weight-for-Length Percentile[2] 0 to 2 Years	BMI Percentile[3] 2 to 20 Years	Action
Acceptable	Normal growth	≥90%	>25th	>25th	Continue to monitor with usual care
At risk[4]	Not at genetic potential	≥90%, with weight loss or weight plateau[5]	10th to 25th	10th to 25th	Consider nutritional and medical evaluation; some but not all patients in this category are at risk for nutritional failure
Nutritional failure	<5%ile	<90%	<10th	<10th	Treat nutritional failure

[1]From Moore, et al. and 1992 committee report, with 2001 committee report of cut-points.
[2]From 2000 NCHS/CDC growth charts (weight-for-length) available for children, ages 0 to 2 years.
[3]From 2000 NCHS/CDC growth chart, available for children and adolescents, ages 2 to 20 years.
[4]Delayed puberty also should be considered a marker of patients at risk for nutritional failure (no breast development past age 13 in girls; no menarche by age 16 or more than 5 years after the start of breast development in girls; no testicular enlargement or genital changes by age 14 in boys).
[5]Weight plateau is defined as no increase in weight for >3 months in a patient younger than 5 years of age, or no increase in weight for >6 months in a patient older than 5 years of age.

Moore BJ, Durie PR, Forstner GG, Pencharz PB. The assessment of nutritional status in children. *Nutr Res* 1985; 57:97–99.

Ramsey BW, Farrell PM, Pencharz P, Consensus Committee. Nutritional assessment and management in cystic fibrosis: A consensus report. *Am J Clin Nutr.* 1992;55:108–16.

Source: Used with permission of the Cystic Fibrosis Foundation. Consensus Conference: Concept in CF Care, Pediatric Nutrition for Patients with Cystic Fibrosis. Bethesda, MD: Cystic Fibrosis Foundation; 2001;1–39.

beneficial to assess the albumin or prealbumin level. However, it is important to remember that other potential causes of an abnormal albumin value include infection and other physiologic stress, fluid overload, congestive heart failure, and severe hepatic insufficiency.[34] CF patients, who chronically have inadequate calorie intakes, usually have a marasmic type of malnutrition. Their visceral protein levels are usually in the normal range, whereas somatic protein stores are low.[34]

Iron Status. Hemoglobin and hematocrit are checked annually. If there is evidence of anemia, further iron studies should be obtained, including serum iron, iron-binding capacity, ferritin, and reticulocyte count.[30] A trial of iron therapy will help determine if the anemia is caused by iron deficiency or anemia of chronic disease. Serum

Exhibit 15–3 Laboratory Monitoring of Nutritional Status

	How Often to Monitor			
	At Diagnosis	**Annually**	**Other**	**Tests**
Beta Carotene			At physician's discretion	Serum levels
Vitamin A	x[1]	x		Vitamin A (retinol)
Vitamin D	x[1]	x		25-OH-D
Vitamin E	x[1]	x		α-tocopherol
Vitamin K	x[1]		If patient has hemoptysis or hematemesis; in patients with liver disease	PIVKA-II (preferably) or prothrombin time
Essential Fatty Acids			Consider checking in infants or those with FTT	Triene; tetraene
Calcium/Bone Status			>age 8 years if risk factors are present (see page 317)	Calcium, phosphorus, ionized PTH, DEXA scan
Iron	x	x	Consider in-depth evaluation for patients with poor appetite	Hemoglobin, hematocrit
Zinc			Consider 6-month supplementation trial and follow growth	No acceptable measurement
Sodium			Consider checking if exposed to heat stress and becomes dehydrated	Serum sodium; spot urine sodium if total body sodium depletion suspected
Protein Stores	x	x	Check in patients with nutritional failure or those at risk	Albumin

[1]Patients diagnosed by neonatal screening do not need these measured.

Source: Used with permission of the Cystic Fibrosis Foundation. Consensus Conference: Concept in CF Care, Pediatric Nutrition for Patients with Cystic Fibrosis. Bethesda, MD: Cystic Fibrosis Foundation; 2001;1–39.

transferrin receptor levels are not affected by inflammation and would be a good measure of iron status, but this test is not available commercially.[24,25]

Fat-Soluble Vitamins. Even patients who are adequately treated with pancreatic enzymes may continue to malabsorb fat and consequently fat-soluble vitamins and that is why the CF Foundation recommends routine monitoring of fat-soluble vitamins (Exhibit 15–4).[24,25] Vitamin A levels should not be drawn during an acute illness because vitamin A is a negative acute phase reactant and will be decreased with acute illness and inflammation.[24,25] Many CF patients, especially those in northern latitudes, among certain cultures, or with limited sun exposure, may not be exposed to enough sunlight to meet vitamin D needs. Measuring 25-hydroxy vitamin D annually in the late fall is also recommended for monitoring bone disease (see the bone health section on page 317).[24,25] Reports of low vitamin E levels and symptomatic deficiency states have been reported.[24,25]

The long-term antibiotic therapy, common in the treatment of CF, alters the gut flora. Because an important source of vitamin K is microbiologic synthesis in the gut, vitamin K status is affected. For this reason, it is important preferably to monitor proteins induced by vitamin K absence or antagonism (PIVKA-II) or, if not available, prothrombin times routinely. Prothrombin time may also be a useful measure of hepatic synthetic function in patients with nutritional failure or biliary cirrhosis.[24,25]

Essential Fatty Acids

Patients with CF are also at risk of essential fatty acid deficiency. The triene to tetraene ratio falls in patients with essential fatty acid deficiency. This ratio should be checked in infants or other patients who are failing to grow (see Exhibit 15–3).

CF-Related Diabetes Screening. With the increased life expectancy of CF patients, the frequency of glucose intolerance in this population has increased.[35] According to CF Foundation statistics, 14.2% of CF patients greater than 13 years of age are treated with insulin for diabetes.[2] It is estimated that as many as 50% of patients with CF may have abnormal glucose tolerance.[35] CFRD is a distinct clinical entity because it has features of both type 1 and type 2 diabetes.[35–37]

The CF Foundation convened a consensus conference on CFRD and issued recommendations for monitoring glucose intolerance.[36,37] On an outpatient basis, it is recommended that a casual glucose level be obtained annually.[35–37] Based on the results, decisions should be made as follows[35–37]:

1. If casual blood glucose is $<$126 mg/dl, no further action is required.
2. If casual blood glucose is ≥126 mg/dl (7.0 mM), measure fasting blood glucose (FBG).
3. If FBG ≥126 mg/dl (7.0 mM) and is confirmed by a second FBG or in conjunction with a casual glucose level of ≥200 mg/dl (11.1 mM), this is diagnostic for CFRD.
4. An oral glucose tolerance test (OGTT) should be performed in all patients with

Exhibit 15–4 Recommendations for Vitamin Supplementation

In addition to a standard, age-appropriate dose of nonfat-soluble multivitamins, the following should be given:

	Individual Vitamin Daily Supplementation			
	Vitamin A (IU)	Vitamin E (IU)	Vitamin D (IU)	Vitamin K (mg)
0–12 months	1500	40–50	400	
1–3 years	5000	80–150	400–800	
4–8 years	5000–10000	100–200	400–800	At least 0.3 mg*
>8 years	10000	200–400	400–800	

*Currently, commercially available products do not have ideal doses for supplementation. In a recent review, no adverse effects have been reported at any dosage level of vitamin K. Clinicians should try to follow these recommendations as closely as possible until better dosage forms are available. Prothrombin time or, ideally, PIVKA-II levels should be checked in patients with liver disease, and vitamin K dose titrated as indicated.

Source: Used with permission of the Cystic Fibrosis Foundation. Consensus Conference: Concept in CF Care, Pediatric Nutrition for Patients with Cystic Fibrosis. Bethesda, MD: Cystic Fibrosis Foundation; 2001;1–39.

symptoms of diabetes, including weight loss, delayed puberty, polyuria, and polydipsia, in spite of a normal FBG. A value ≥200 mg/dl (11.1 mM) is diagnostic of CFRD.

For inpatients, all CF patients with pancreatic insufficiency should have a casual glucose level measured on the first and third days of hospitalization.[35–37] Decisions should be made as follows[35–37]:

1. If FBG ≥126 mg/dl (7.0 mM) in either measurement, a FBG and a 2-hour postprandial glucose should be performed the next morning.
2. If FBG <126 mg/dl (7.0 mM) and 2-hour post-prandial glucose <200 mg/dl (11.1 mM), no further action is required.
3. If repeated FBG ≥126 mg/dl (7.0 mM), it should be repeated the next morning. If fasting hyperglycemia persists for more than 48 hours, insulin treatment of diabetes should be begun.
4. If FBG <126 mg/dl (7.0 mM) but 2-hour post-prandial glucose is >200 mg/dl (11.0 mM), patients are not usually started on insulin.

CFRD can be classified as CFRD with fasting hyperglycemia (FBG >126 mg/dl) or CFRD without fasting hyperglycemia.[35,36]

Pancreatic Function. Pancreatic insufficiency is often inferred based on symptoms of malabsorption. Tests that can be performed to document pancreatic insufficiency include:

1. duodenal intubation with stimulations
2. 72-hour fecal fat balance
3. immunoreactive trypsinogen after 8 years of age
4. fecal elastase-1 determination.

Patients who at diagnosis are determined to be pancreatic sufficient can become pancreatic insufficient over time, especially those who have an identified mutation that is associated with pancreatic insufficiency, and should be evaluated annually.[24,25]

Clinical

An assessment of the patient's overall health status should be obtained. Questions about activity and energy levels should be asked. Any missed school or work days should be noted. It is recommended that a description of the patient's body habitus and sexual maturity rating (SMR) be noted.[24,25,30] A general review of systems should be performed by the physician and/or nurse. Comorbid medical conditions such as active pulmonary or sinus disease, gastroesophageal reflux disease (GERD), CFRD, hepatobiliary disease, history of gut resection, and the like should be noted.[24,25,30] These conditions will also have a direct impact on the patient's nutritional status by affecting appetite, intake, and disease state. Questions about the patient's use of alternative/complementary medicine therapies should be asked.

Stool Pattern. Information about the patient's stool pattern should be monitored carefully at each clinic visit because this is a good indication of the adequacy of the enzyme therapy. Questions to be asked during a nutrition screening and assessment should include the following:

1. number of stools per day
2. consistency of stools
3. presence of oily discharge
4. rectal prolapse
5. foul-smelling, floating stools and/or flatus
6. abdominal cramping
7. protruding abdomen

Enzyme Therapy. Important aspects of enzyme replacement therapy that need to be checked every clinic visit and hospitalization are:

1. type
2. brand
3. amount taken
4. when taken
5. method of administration
6. timing with meals
7. calculation of units of lipase/kilogram body weight/meal

Refer to the dosage section on page 324 in this chapter and Table 15–3 for additional information. It is important to ask about constipation as well as malabsorptive symptoms. Constipation can be a symptom of distal intestinal obstructive syndrome (DIOS), which is also a complication of pancreatic insufficiency. The patient with persistent malabsorption symptoms should be evaluated for nonpancreatic causes of malabsorption such as lactose intolerance, bacterial overgrowth of the small intestine, Giardia or other parasites, celiac disease, or inflammatory bowel disease.[24,25]

Other Medications. It is important to note other medications the patient may be taking at each clinic visit, including antibiotics, bronchodilators, H_2 blockers, antacids, prokinetic agents, steroids, diuretics, cardiac medications, vitamins, and minerals.

Pulmonary Status. The pulmonary status of the patient will directly influence the patient's nutritional status. The dietetics professional should note the presence of an acute pulmonary exacerbation and chronic disease. CF patients older than about 6 years of age will be able to perform pulmonary function tests to assess the extent of their pulmonary involvement.

Bone Health Indices

Patients with CF are at risk for developing osteopenia and osteoporosis. Risk factors for bone disease in patients with CF include[38]:

1. low weight-for-height (<90th percentile ideal body weight or BMI <25th percentile or weight-for-length <25th percentile)
2. low physical activity
3. use of corticosteroids (more than 90 days in past year)
4. delayed skeletal or sexual maturation
5. illness severity (FEV_1 <50%)
6. low dietary calcium and/or vitamin D intake
7. suboptimal vitamin K status
8. 25-hydroxy vitamin D level <30 ng/ml
9. inflammation

Patients older than 8 years of age who have a positive screen for one of the risk factors for bone disease should have a dual X-ray absorptiometry (DXA) as a measure of bone mineral density. Normative data is not available for children younger than 8 years of age. All patients should have DXA scans by age 18 years if the scans have not been previously obtained for other reasons.

Dietary

As part of the nutritional assessment, dietary analysis provides important information about what, where, and how much the CF patient is eating. Several methods of gathering the data can be utilized, including a 24-hour dietary recall, a 3- to 5-day food record, and a food frequency questionnaire. The dietetics professional should analyze the diet's adequacy in terms of energy, protein, and other key nutrients such as calcium and iron by looking for a variety of foods in adequate amounts. During this interview, information about the patient's appetite, eating patterns, consumption of sweetened beverages, and behavioral issues related to feeding should be noted.[24,25,30] The Behavioral Pediatrics Feeding Assessment Scale, which is a self-report measure of meal time problems, may be administered to identify and evaluate behavioral issues related to eating.[24,25,39]

Drug Nutrient Interactions

Prolonged antibiotic therapy can alter the gut flora and subsequently influence vitamin K status. Some of the intravenous antibiotics can cause nausea in some patients. CF patients with an asthma component of their disease may be on bursts of steroids. As the CF patient's pulmonary disease progresses cor pulmonale may develop. Diuretics may be prescribed at this point. Electrolyte and fluid status need to be carefully monitored.

Nutritional Management

The overall goal of nutrition management is to promote normal growth and development for the patient with CF, which may be an important prognostic indicator. The main components of nutrition management in CF are the provision of

Table 15–3 Examples of Pancreatic Enzymes

Product	*Form*	*Lipase USP Units*	*Protease USP Units*	*Amylase USP Units*
Creon 5 (Solvay Pharmaceuticals)	Delayed Release Mini-microspheres	5,000	18,750	16,600
Creon 10	Delayed Release Mini-microspheres	10,000	37,500	33,200
Creon 20	Delayed Release Mini-microspheres	20,000	75,000	66,400
Pancrease (Ortho-McNeil)	Enteric-coated Microspheres	4,500	25,000	20,000
Pancrease MT4	Enteric-coated Microtablets	4,000	12,000	12,000
Pancrease MT10	Enteric-coated Microtablets	10,000	30,000	30,000
Pancrease MT16	Enteric-coated Microtablets	16,000	48,000	48,000
Pancrease MT20	Enteric-coated Microtablets	20,000	44,000	56,000
Pancrecarb MS-4 (Digestive Care, Inc.)	Enteric-coated Microspheres with bicarbonate buffer	4,000	25,000	25,000
Pancrecarb MS-8 (Digestive Care, Inc.)	Enteric-coated Microspheres with bicarbonate buffer	8,000	45,000	40,000
Ultrase (Axcan-Scandipharm)	Enteric-coated Microspheres	4,500	25,000	20,000
Ultrase MT12	Enteric-coated Minitablets	12,000	39,000	39,000
Ultrase MT18	Enteric-coated Minitablets	18,000	58,500	58,500
Ultrase MT20	Enteric-coated Minitablets	20,000	65,000	65,000
Viokase Powder	Powder ($^1/_4$ tsp or 0.7 g)	16,800	70,000	70,000
Viokase 8 Tablet	Tablet	8,000	30,000	30,000
Viokase 16 Tablet	Tablet	16,000	60,000	60,000

adequate energy, protein, and nutrients; pancreatic enzyme therapy; and vitamin and mineral supplementation.

Adequate Diet for Normal Growth and Development

In the past, the gastrointestinal symptoms of the disease, such as increased number of bulky, foul-smelling stools; increased flatus; and abdominal cramping, were treated with a low-fat diet. Today, with the advent of better enzyme replacement therapy, fat restriction is no longer routinely imposed on all patients. Health professionals now appreciate the tremendous energy demands of the disease, although the specific energy, protein, and nutrient requirements of CF patients have not been determined quantitatively. It is difficult to meet the high energy needs within the confines of a fat restriction. It is generally recommended that the diets of patients with CF derive up to 40% of total calories from fat based on the individual patient's tolerance.[40] It is appropriate to encourage the use of polyunsaturated fats that are good sources of the essential fatty acids, linoleic and alpha-linoleic acids, rather than saturated fats. Vegetable oils such as flax, canola, and soy and cold-water marine fish are high in calories and a good source of these fats.[24,25]

According to the CF Consensus Conference on pediatric nutrition, patients with CF may be able to grow normally on the Dietary Reference Intakes (DRIs) for age for energy.[41] The report also includes a method for determining estimated energy needs based on the World Health Organization (WHO) equation for basal metabolic rate,[42] an activity factor, and pancreatic insufficiency factor for patients who do not thrive on the DRIs for energy.[24,25] Several reports have advocated 120–150% of the previous RDAs for energy based on age and gender for CF patients.[43–46]

Age-specific considerations in the nutritional management of CF are summarized in Exhibit 15–5. Infants with CF may be successfully breastfed, as long as pancreatic enzymes are administered prior to each feeding. Standard iron-fortified infant formulas are alternatives to breast milk but also require the administration of pancreatic enzymes prior to each feeding. A study of newly diagnosed infants with cystic fibrosis compared nutrition and growth parameters of those infants fed standard infant formula with those fed a protein hydrolysate formula.[47] There was no significant difference in growth parameters between the two groups of infants. Therefore, these researchers concluded that their research failed to support the use of the more expensive protein hydrolysate formula for the routine care of newly diagnosed infants with CF.[47]

In practice, it is easy for a CF patient to achieve a high protein intake because the average American diet is so high in protein. It is much more difficult to achieve the calorie intake that is recommended. A 3-year longitudinal study of dietary intakes of CF patients reported that these patients did not meet the recommended 120% RDA for energy or a high-fat, 40% of energy diet.[48] In practice, this is a common observation.

To close the gap between energy needs and the amount of calories the patient is able to consume, energy-dense foods can be added to the patient's diet. Margarine, cheese, sour cream, and cream cheese can easily be added to the patient's favorite foods, as tolerated by the patient. Exhibit 15–6 depicts one approach to increasing calories and protein.

A meta analysis of the literature on treatment approaches to the nutrition management of CF patients including oral supplementation, enteral nutrition, parenteral nutrition, and behavioral intervention and their effectiveness on weight gain was reported. Weight gain was produced in CF patients with all interventions. The behavioral interventions were found to be as effective as more invasive medical procedures.[49] The best choice of intervention for a CF patient needs to be made on an individual basis.

Pregnancy. With the increased life expectancy of patients with CF, more women with the disease are becoming pregnant. In addition to the usual nutrient recommendations of CF, the increased energy needs of pregnancy must be taken into consideration. Emphasis needs to be put on proper weight gain. In addition to the usual vitamin therapy, one prenatal vitamin per day is

Exhibit 15–5 Nutritional Management of CF Patients

1. Infant
   - Breast milk or standard iron-fortified infant formula should be recommended. Special formulas such as Alimentum* and Pregestimil+ (protein hydrolysate formulas containing medium-chain triglycerides) can be recommended for infants in special situations, such as gut resection or increased fat malabsorption.
   - Pancreatic enzymes should be given prior to feedings with any of the milks or formulas just listed (see page 323).
   - Vitamin supplements and a source of fluoride should be given.
   - Introduction of solid foods and advancement of diet should proceed as with an infant who does not have CF. Some high-calorie, starchy vegetables and dessert baby foods can also be added to the diet to increase energy intake.
   - Salt should be added to breast milk or infant formula, particularly in hot weather (see specific recommendations on page 323). When solid foods are added to the infant's diet, salt should be added to these foods.
   - Referrals to community programs such as the WIC program should be made.
2. Toddler
   - Toddlers' diets should be based on a normal healthy diet for age with a variety of foods.
   - Parents should be forewarned of the normal decrease in growth and appetite during this age.
   - Regular meal and snack times should be encouraged.
   - Constant snacking or "grazing" should be discouraged.
   - Drinking of sweetened beverages should be discouraged.
   - Pancreatic enzymes and vitamins are continued.
   - Continue communication with community programs such as the WIC program.
3. Preschool and school age
   - A normal healthy diet with a variety of foods should continue to form the basis of the diet.
   - Limit sweetened beverages.
   - Parents lose control of what child eats away from home at preschool, child care, and school.
   - Arrangements need to be made for child to take enzymes during the school day.
   - Vitamin therapy is continued.
   - Diet prescriptions for a high-calorie, high-protein, high-salt diet can be sent to the school.
4. Adolescent
   - Patients are exercising more independence in food choices.
   - Parents can provide appropriate food environment at home.
   - Patients can be taught to include quick-to-prepare high-calorie foods in daily diet.
   - Snack and fast foods can add a significant amount of calories to the diet and should not be discouraged.
   - Limit sweetened beverages.
   - Importance of high-calorie intake and enzyme and vitamin therapy should be emphasized by health professionals directly to the patient and not via the parents.
   - Nutrition needs increase prior to and during adolescent growth spurt.

*Ross Laboratories, Columbus, Ohio

+Mead Johnson Nutritionals, Mead Johnson and Company, Evansville, Indiana

Exhibit 15–6 Instructional Handout on Increasing Calories

Calorie-Protein BOOSTERS

—Some ways to hide extra calories and protein—

Powdered milk (33 cal/tbsp, 3 gm pro/tbsp)
Add 2–4 tbsp to 1 cup milk. Mix into puddings, potatoes, soups, ground meats, vegetables, and cooked cereal.

Eggs (80 cal/egg, 7 gm pro/tbsp)
Add to casseroles, meat loaf, mashed potato, cooked cereal, and macaroni & cheese. Add extra to pancake batter and french toast. (Do not use raw eggs in uncooked items.)

Butter or margarine (45 cal/tsp)
Add to puddings, casseroles, sandwiches, vegetables, and cooked cereal.

Cheeses (100 cal/oz, 7 gm pro/oz)
Give as snacks or in sandwiches. Add melted to casseroles, potatoes, vegetables, and soup.

Wheat germ (25 cal/tbsp)
Add a tablespoon or two to cereal. Mix into meat dishes, cookie batter, casseroles, etc.

Mayonnaise or salad dressings (45 cal/tsp)
Use liberally on sandwiches, on salads, as a dip for raw vegetables, or sauce on cooked vegetables.

Evaporated milk (25 cal/tbsp, 1 gm pro/tbsp)
Use in place of whole milk, in desserts, baked goods, meat dishes, and cooked cereals.

Sour cream (26 cal/tbsp)
Add to potatoes, casseroles, dips; use in sauces, baked goods, etc.

Sweetened condensed milk (60 cal/tbsp, 1 gm pro/tbsp)
Add to pies, puddings, milkshakes. Mix 1–2 tbsp with peanut butter and spread on toast.

Peanut butter (95 cal/tbsp, 4 gm pro/tbsp)
Serve on toast, crackers, bananas, apples, and celery.

Carnation Instant Breakfast (130 cal/pckt, 7 gm pro/pckt)
Add to milk and milkshakes.

Gravies (40 cal/tbsp)
Use liberally on mashed potatoes and meats.

High Protein Foods

* MEATS—Beef, Chicken, Fish, Turkey, Lamb
* MILK & CHEESE—Yogurt, Cottage Cheese, Cream Cheese
* EGGS
* PEANUT BUTTER (with Bread or Crackers)
* DRIED BEANS & PEAS (with Bread, Cornbread, Rice)

Source: Courtesy of Pediatric Pulmonary Center, ©1990, University of Alabama at Birmingham, Birmingham, Alabama.

usually added to the regimen. Mothers with CF have successfully breast-fed their infants.[50] Breastfeeding further increases the energy demands on the patient with CF and needs to be considered on an individual basis.

CF-Related Diabetes. As with any patient with CF, the treatment goal of CFRD is to provide a diet that promotes optimal growth and development in children and adolescents, achievement and maintenance of normal weight in adults, and optimal nutritional status.[35–37] Other treatment goals include controlling hyperglycemia to reduce diabetes complications, avoiding severe hypoglycemia, and assisting the patient in adapting to another chronic illness from a psychological standpoint.[36] The patient with CFRD should be allowed as much flexibility as possible in the nutrition management of these two diseases.[36] The primary goal remains meeting the patient's energy needs.[35] Because carbohydrates have the most effect on glycemic index, emphasis should be placed on total amount of carbohydrate eaten rather than the carbohydrate source.[36] Simple sugars can be included in the diet plan but regular sodas and other sweetened beverages should be discouraged. The patient needs to learn how to recognize the carbohydrate content of foods, such as with the "carbohydrate counting" method.[35–37] Patients should also be encouraged to spread their carbohydrate intake throughout the day.[35] Eating protein and fat-containing foods along with simple sugars slows the absorption of the simple sugars from the intestinal tract. Fat should continue to contribute about 40% of total calories, and protein intake should provide about 20% of total calories.[35]

Patient/Family Education. Patient and family education on nutrition management and its importance in the patient's overall health care is an integral component of the individual patient's care plan. A qualified, registered dietitian should be available to the patient and family to assist them in meeting the nutritional needs of the patient in the least invasive way possible. Information about the nutrient content of foods and suggestions for increasing the patient's caloric intake should be available.

Luder and Gilbride[51] studied the effects of nutrition counseling that was provided quarterly for a 4-year period, based on self-management skills in a group of patients with CF. These patients had significant increases in their energy intakes as well as in their body mass index values, without decline in pulmonary function over this time period.[51] More and more emphasis is being placed on anticipatory guidance as an integral part of nutrition management.[24,25,30]

Feeding issues are prominent in this patient population and the health professional needs to provide anticipatory guidance to the parents/caretakers of these patients to try and avoid battles over eating.[52,53] The importance of behavioral programs in the nutritional care of CF patients is receiving more and more recognition.[54]

Supplemental Nutrition. Milkshakes and other high-calorie drinks can be used as supplemental feedings. Commercial oral feedings can also be used to boost calories but they require additional expense and, in some instances, they may be difficult for the family to obtain.

Oftentimes, in spite of vigorous efforts by the patient, the patient's family, and dietetics professionals, it is very difficult to meet the patient's energy needs by the oral route alone. The CF Consensus Conference on pediatric nutrition for patients with CF suggests that the use of supplemental tube feedings be considered when optimization of feeding behaviors and addition of oral supplements have not achieved the desired weight gain or when the patient's growth parameters fall within the nutritional failure category (see Exhibit 15–2).[24,25] The patient and family need to be given the facts about available adjunct therapies in a positive way and be involved in the decision making.[24,25] CF centers have reported using various forms of tube feedings, including nasogastric, gastrostomy, and jejunostomy feedings. Tube feedings are sometimes administered on a continuous basis while the patient is asleep. Some centers use a partially predigested formula with or without enzymes; others use a nonelemental formula with enzymes. A study by Erskine and associates[55] showed no difference in absorption between a predigested formula and a nonelemental formula with enzyme replacement. Predigested formulas, however, are more costly than nonelemental formulas.

Enzyme administration poses a problem with nocturnal tube feedings. Mixing enzymes directly into the feeding causes the product to begin to break down and may clog the feeding tube. The CF Foundation recommends that patients take their usual premeal dose of pancreatic enzymes prior to the initiation of the feeding.[24,25] Some patients may need additional doses during the night or at the end of the feeding.[24,25]

Vitamin and Mineral Supplementation

Vitamins. Recommendations of the CF Consensus Conference for pediatric nutrition for patients with CF for vitamin supplementation can be found in Exhibit 15–4.[24,25] There are multivitamin preparations available on the market that contain water-miscible forms of the fat-soluble vitamins A, D, E, and K: ADEK (Scandipharm; Birmingham, AL), SourceCF Softgel Multivitamins (SourceCF; Huntsville, AL), and Vitamax (CF Pharmacy Services, Inc.; Bethesda, MD). ADEK is available in drops and a chewable tablet. SourceCF Softgel Multivitamin is a capsule. Vitamax is available in a cherry-flavored drop and in grape-, orange-, or cherry-flavored chewable tablets. The use of these products may simplify the vitamin regimen and improve patient compliance.[30] Not all of the commercially available products contain the recommended level of vitamin K, so vitamin K status needs to be carefully monitored.[24,25]

The CF Foundation has specific recommendations in regard to treating a 25-OH vitamin D level that is less than 30 ng/ml.[38] The recommendation is to treat with vitamin D for 8 weeks according to the following dosing schedule: 12,000 IU biweekly for patients less than 5 years of age and 50,000 IU biweekly for patients over 5 years of age. If after 8 weeks, the 25-OH vitamin D level is still less than 30 ng/ml, an additional 8 weeks of treatment is recommended at the same levels. If after this additional treatment, the levels are still less than 30 ng/ml, then phototherapy or increased sunlight exposure should be considered or a referral to endocrinology for consideration of use of more polar vitamin D supplements, which may be better absorbed.[38]

Minerals. Minerals such as zinc, iron, and selenium have been studied in the CF population.[56] Additional study is needed before specific supplementation recommendations can be made. A trial of zinc supplementation may be initiated for patients with CF who have poor growth.[24,25] All patients with CF should be encouraged to consume at least the DRIs for calcium for their age group. For example, the DRI for calcium for children greater than 9 years of age is 1300 mg.[57] CF patients who are on steroids, who have decreased dietary intake of calcium, and/or who are found to have decreased bone density may benefit from calcium supplementation. These minerals as well as other macro- and micronutrients, are important in the overall nutritional status of the patient with CF. Therefore, eating a variety of foods should be encouraged.

Additional salt should be added to the diet during times of increased sweating, such as

1. during hot weather
2. with fevers
3. during strenuous physical activity
4. with profuse diarrhea

The additional salt compensates for the increased losses of sodium and chloride through perspiration. In most instances, liberal use of the salt shaker and the inclusion of high-salt foods in the diet will supply the needed sodium and chloride. Salt supplements may be used in instances of very heavy sweating. Both breast-fed and formula-fed infants need supplementation with sodium chloride, particularly during hot weather.[24,25] Infants without CF require 2 to 4 mEq/kg/day of sodium and infants with CF are likely to require the upper end of this normal range even when not exposed to heat stress.[24,25]

Pancreatic Enzyme Replacement Therapy

Types of Available Enzymes. Many different brands and types of pancreatic enzymes are available (Table 15–3) and they contain varying amounts of lipase that breaks down fat; protease that breaks down protein; and amylase which breaks down carbohydrate.

The nonproprietary names of these products are pancrelipase and pancreatin. Most of the products feature an enteric coating that protects the enzymes from inactivation in the acid environment of the stomach. The enzymes become activated in the alkaline pH of the duodenum. Pancreatic enzymes are also available in powder and capsule forms.

Dosage/Administration. There is a CF consensus statement on the use of pancreatic enzyme supplements.[58,59] Extremely high doses of pancreatic enzymes have been associated with fibrosing colonopathy or strictures in the colon in CF patients.[60,61] A recommended starting dose for infants is 2,000 to 4,000 units of lipase per 120 ml of formula or breastfeeding.[58,59] Another proposed weight-based enzyme dosing schedule is 1,000 units of lipase/kg body weight/meal for children younger than 4 years of age and 500 units of lipase/kilogram body weight/meal for those over age 4.[58,59] The usual enzyme dose for snacks is one half of the mealtime dose. The recommendations are not to exceed a dose of 2500 units of lipase/kilogram body weight/meal and are based on a usual intake of three meals plus 2 to 3 snacks per day.[58–60] It is the amount of lipase presented to the gut at any one time that appears to be important in the context of fibrosing colonopathy. Calculating units of lipase/kilogram body weight/meal has become an integral component of routine care. For example, a 10-year-old child weighing 35.7 kg who takes a mealtime dose of three capsules of a pancreatic enzyme preparation containing 20,000 units of lipase per capsule will receive 1681 units of lipase/kg body weight/meal (60,000 units of lipase divided by 35.7 kg = 1681 units of lipase/kg body weight/meal). Careful monitoring of the patient's growth, stool pattern, and the absence or presence of gastrointestinal symptoms is necessary to determine the adequacy of therapy. Monitoring and adjusting the dosage as needed should be continued throughout the patient's treatment. If the patient with CF is still exhibiting symptoms of malabsorption after reaching a maximum enzyme dose, it may be because the stomach contents are too acidic when reaching the small intestine and are inactivating the enzymes. In these cases, the addition of bicarbonate or other drugs that inhibit gastric acidity may be helpful.[58,59] Nonpancreatic reasons for malabsorption should also be considered.

Enzymes should be taken within the hour prior to meals and snacks to be most effective. The enterically coated enzymes should not be chewed or crushed. Most of the enzymes are available in capsule form. For infants and small children who are unable to swallow a capsule, the capsule can be broken open and the contents mixed with a soft, acidic food such as applesauce. Enzymes mixed with food should be used within 30 minutes of mixing. When the enterically coated enzymes are mixed with a higher pH food such as pudding or milk, the enzymes will become activated and begin breaking down the food. Powdered enzymes are already in an activated form. Mixing enzymes directly into a tube feeding or infant formula causes the feeding enzymatic digestion to begin. This may cause the feeding to take on an unpleasant color, taste, or odor.

Patient Compliance. Administering enzymes to an extremely young infant can be a frustrating endeavor for the parent or caretaker, primarily because of the young infant's natural extrusion reflex. After a few months of age, taking enzymes becomes part of a patient's daily routine. Parents of toddlers should be warned against allowing the child to "graze" throughout the day because this makes enzyme dosing difficult. In the preadolescent and adolescent age groups, patient compliance with enzyme administration can become a big issue. Some schools require the child to come to the school office for medications and this may be a source of embarrassment and alienation from peers for the child with CF. The lack of compliance needs to be discussed with the child and a solution must be found that is agreeable to the child, parents, and school authorities.

Pancreatic enzyme therapy is very expensive and contributes significantly to the overall cost of this disease. Enzymes are often covered by third-party payers and state programs for children with special health care needs.

Referral to Food/Nutrition and Other Resources

Referral to food and nutrition resources such as the USDA's Special Supplemental Nutrition Program for Women, Infants, and Children (WIC) program and the Food Stamp Program should be made based on the individual's needs. In some states, referrals can be made to the state program for children with special health care needs for aid in obtaining supplemental feedings, enzymes, and vitamins. Children who participate in the Child Nutrition Program at their school will need diet prescriptions for high-calorie, high-protein diets sent to their schools.

CF has a tremendous impact on patients and their families emotionally, physically, and financially. Most CF centers provide an interdisciplinary team approach to the care of these children and their families to better help them meet their many needs.

Alternative/Complementary Medicine

As with other chronic diseases, the use of alternative/complementary medicine in CF care has sparked the interest of patients with CF, their families, and health professionals. For example, the use of docosahexaenoic acid (DHA) has received recent attention because of animal research in this area and because of DHA's anti-inflammatory properties. However, DHA supplementation for patients with CF is not recommended at this time because of the lack of clinical trials in this area.

To date, little published science-based research exists in the area of alternative and complementary medicine in CF care. More and more CF centers are surveying their patients to ascertain the extent of alternative medicine practices. Currently, CF patients are obtaining a lot of their information from the Internet, with many CF Internet sites having links to alternative medicine sites. CF centers will need to study alternative medicine practices further so that CF caregivers can advise patients and their families as to the safety and efficacy of various therapies.

The entire population of CF patients followed at Case Western Reserve University and Rainbow Babies and Children's Hospital in Cleveland, Ohio, participated in a survey of the use of nonmedical treatment.[62] The results indicated that nonmedical treatment was used by 66% of the population; 57% of the population used at least one religious treatment; 27% used at least one nonreligious treatment.[62] Group prayer (48%) was the most common nonmedical therapy, and 92% of those participating in group prayer perceived benefit. Chiropractors were consulted by 14% with 69% of these patients perceiving benefit. Nutrition modalities other than those prescribed by the CF caretakers were employed by 11% of the population; 78% of these patients used these treatments frequently (over 5 times); 87% perceived benefit. Meditation was used by 5% with 94% reporting perceived benefit.

It is important for CF caregivers to include questions about alternative/complementary medicine practices when interviewing CF patients and their family members, especially in regard to ingested substances. This is especially important information to obtain from patients who may be participating in studies with experimental drugs because the possibility exists that substances such as unregulated botanical products may confound the study results.

Identification of Areas Needing Further Research

There are many unanswered questions about CF in general and, more specifically, in regard to nutrition. Additional research is needed to determine specific nutrient requirements of patients with CF in regard to energy, protein, vitamins, minerals, and essential fatty acids. The most appropriate method for delivering these nutrients must be determined. Further study on the psychosocial and emotional benefits and drawbacks of invasive nutritional therapy and the effect of improved nutritional status on body composition and the progression of the pulmonary disease would be beneficial. More study is needed on the role of anabolic agents such as insulin and growth hormone and on appetite stimulants, such as megastrol acetate, to determine the cost/benefits of these adjunct therapies. With lung transplantation becoming more available to CF patients, appropriate nutrition management pre- and posttransplantation will need further study.

CF is a complicated disease, affecting many organs of the body, and the disease process is highly variable. Proper nutritional care is an integral part of its therapy. Therefore, every patient and family deserve individualized treatment and support from an interdisciplinary team of health professionals, including a qualified dietetics professional, trained in the care of patients with CF.

BRONCHOPULMONARY DYSPLASIA

Bronchopulmonary dysplasia (BPD) was first described by Northway and colleagues[63] in 1967 as a form of chronic lung disease seen in infants with severe hyaline membrane disease who required mechanical ventilation and high concentrations of oxygen for prolonged periods of time. Since that time, a commonly accepted definition of BPD has been a chronic lung disease with abnormal chest radiographic findings that requires the use of supplemental oxygen on the 28th day of life.[64] Over the years, clinical practice has advanced resulting in a decrease in lung injury in larger (greater than 1200 gram birth weight) and more mature infants. At the same time, more and more premature infants are surviving at earlier gestational ages and lower birth weights. The National Institute of Child Health and Human Development/National Heart, Lung and Blood Institute refined the definition of BPD to reflect differing criteria for infants born at less than or greater than 32 weeks gestation.[65] The expanded definition includes different diagnostic criteria for mild, moderate, and severe forms of the disease.[65] For example, the definition of severe BPD for an infant with a gestational age of less than 32 weeks is the need for 30% oxygen or more and/or positive pressure at 36 weeks postmenstrual age or discharge, whichever comes first.[65]

Today's definition of BPD includes infants who have had an acute lung injury with minimal clinical and radiographic findings, as well as those with major radiographic abnormalities. BPD represents a continuum of lung disease. This chronic disease is seen in young infants, the vast majority being premature infants, who require respiratory support during the first 2 weeks of life or longer for neonatal respiratory distress. Full-term infants can also develop BPD as a result of conditions such as respiratory distress syndrome, meconium aspiration pneumonia, congenital heart disease, and congenital neuromuscular disorders.[66] The pathogenesis of BPD is multifactorial but includes severe, diffuse, acute lung injury and an early inflammatory response. The lungs are damaged by the barotrauma from the use of intermittent positive pressure ventilation (IPPV) and by oxygen toxicity from the high concentrations of oxygen required by these infants early in life.[64,67,68] Infection may play a role in the pathogenesis of BPD.[64,67] Other factors that may contribute to the development of the disease include increased fluids contributing to pulmonary edema[69] and inadequate early nutrition impeding lung reparative processes.[70,71]

Today, younger and smaller preterm infants are surviving with the aid of mechanical ventilation. Consequently, BPD has become one of the most common sequelae of newborn intensive care unit stays. The incidence of BPD is about 30% of infants with birth weight under 1000 grams and is higher in lower birth weight infants. BPD has become rare in premature infants weighing 1500 grams or more with uncomplicated respiratory distress syndrome. This is due to the use of antenatal steroids, surfactant replacement therapy, gentler ventilation which reduces barotrauma, better nutrition, and careful use of supplemental oxygen.[66,72] As BPD patients are followed over time, chronic lung disease remains a major clinical problem for many of these patients into late childhood and early adolescence.[67,73]

Signs of respiratory distress, such as chest retractions, tachypnea, crackles, and wheezing, characterize BPD. Supplemental oxygen therapy may be required, and there will be changes on the patient's chest radiograph. Pulmonary complications of BPD may include recurrent atelectasis, pulmonary infections, and respiratory failure requiring mechanical ventilation. Other complications of BPD include pulmonary edema, cor pulmonale, poor growth, neurodevelopmental delays including delayed feeding skills, and cardiovascular problems.

The primary goal of BPD management is to provide the patient with the necessary pulmonary support during the acute and chronic phases of the disease to minimize lung damage and to maintain optimal oxygen saturation. This may include mechanical ventilation, supplemental oxygen, anti-inflammatory and β-adrenergic aerosols, and diuretic therapy. Of equal importance is the provision of adequate nutrition, not only for growth and development, but also to compensate for the demands of the disease. Growth of new lung tissue can occur in humans until about 8 years of age. Theoretically, a BPD patient can "outgrow" the disease if adequate pulmonary and nutritional support can be provided.

Increased Nutrient Requirements

Effects of Prematurity

Considering the fact that most babies who develop BPD are premature infants, it is easy to see that these infants have little fat, glycogen, or other nutrients in reserve, particularly iron, calcium, and phosphorus. Faced with the demands of prematurity and the stress of BPD, the infant can quickly develop a state of negative nutrient balance.

Effects of Bronchopulmonary Dysplasia

Several factors increase the energy and nutrient requirements of BPD patients including:

1. increased basal metabolic rate
2. increased work of breathing
3. chronic hypoxia
4. chronic illness/infections
5. respiratory distress/metabolic complications
6. tissue repair/catch-up growth
7. drug/nutrient interactions

Weinstein and Oh[74] report that resting oxygen consumption was approximately 25% higher in eight infants with BPD, when compared with controls. Kurzner and colleagues[75] found that infants with BPD and growth failure had increased resting oxygen consumption, as compared with control infants and infants with BPD and normal growth. Other investigators have also found an increase in resting energy expenditure in infants with BPD as compared to controls, ranging from 125–150%.[76–78]

Treatment of the BPD patient usually includes a wide array of medications, including diuretics and bronchodilators. The impact of these drugs on the patient's nutritional status is further discussed in the drug-nutrient interaction section on page 329 of this chapter.

Decreased Nutrient Consumption

Infants with BPD are extremely fluid sensitive because of the acute lung disease and the possible complication of cor pulmonale, or right-sided heart failure. When fluid restrictions are imposed, this places a limitation on the provision of energy and nutrients. Yeh and associates[77] showed that infants with BPD had significantly lower energy intakes, as compared to controls.

Frequent intubations and mechanical ventilation interfere with the normal feeding sequence and feeding-skill development. Therefore, these infants may be poor oral feeders and develop adversive oral behavior.[64] Also, these patients may experience fatigue or decreased oxygen saturation during feeding because of their underlying pulmonary disease.[79,80]

Growth of Infants with BPD

It is unrealistic to expect true growth to occur when life-threatening events, such as respiratory failure, necrotizing enterocolitis, or other serious problems of prematurity, are taking place. The patient must be fairly stable in order for growth to occur. Growth failure has been recognized as a complication of BPD. Shankaran and associates[81] found a poor pattern of growth in BPD patients to be related to the severity of pulmonary disease.

Similarly, Kurzner and colleagues[75] found resting metabolic rate to be inversely correlated with body weight in infants with BPD. These investigators also compared BPD infants with growth failure with BPD infants with normal growth and found that the infants in the growth failure group had significantly lower birth weights, younger gestational ages, increased duration of oxygen therapy, and increased duration of mechanical ventilation as compared to those infants with normal growth.[75] Yeh and colleagues[77] found a significantly smaller rate of weight gain (grams/day) in infants with BPD as compared to controls, who were premature infants who had mild transient pulmonary problems and did not require mechanical ventilation.

DeRegnier and colleagues[82] studied 16 very-low-birth-weight infants who developed BPD and compared them to birth-weight-matched control infants without BPD during the first 6 postnatal weeks. At the end of the study period, the infants with BPD had lower Z scores for weight and head circumference, as well as lower arm muscle area and arm fat area, as compared with controls. Length Z scores were not significantly different between the two groups. When the BPD infants achieved full enteral feedings, they gained at the same rate as the controls but did not achieve catch-up growth. These investigators speculate that early reductions in muscle and fat accretion and growth velocity may contribute to the long-term growth failure of BPD patients, and they emphasize the importance of delivering optimal nutrition early in the postnatal period.[82]

Johnson and associates[83] studied 40 infants with BPD for 7 months after initial hospital discharge. During this study period, 73% of the infants experienced a decrease in weight-for-age Z score; 20% experienced a decrease in length-forage Z score; and 65% experienced a decrease in weight-for-length Z score. Low socioeconomic status, days of postdischarge illness, and "suspect" development were associated with a significantly increased risk of growth failure. Another study of preterm infants with BPD found that they had significantly lower weights, lengths, total body fat, and fat-free mass than controls at 6 weeks after term. Fat-free mass and total body fat of the BPD patients remained low as compared with healthy infants during the first year of life.[84]

In more long-term follow-up of BPD patients, Giacoia and associates[73] studied 12 school-aged children with BPD and compared them with a preterm control group matched for birth weight, gestational age, and gender, as well as with an age-matched control group. Both the BPD group and the preterm group were shorter than the healthy term control group. The BPD group had lower lean-body mass, compared with the term control group, and had lower bone mineral content when compared to both control groups.[73] Another study of school-aged children with BPD was performed by Vrlenich and colleagues,[85] who compared children who had been born prematurely with and without the development of BPD. The children with BPD were significantly smaller in weight and head circumference but not height. However, when possible confounders that are known to be correlates of poor growth were applied, the differences were no longer significant. These investigators suggest that the poor growth reported in children with BPD may be related to other factors besides BPD.[85]

Adequate oxygenation must be maintained in the patient with BPD for growth to occur. Studies have shown that desaturation may occur during feeding and during sleeping.[79,80,86] Moyer-Mileur and colleagues[86] demonstrated positive growth trends in infants with BPD who maintained an oxygen saturation of greater than 92% while sleeping. These investigators also found that short-term pulse oxygen saturation studies were not always reliable predictors of oxygen saturation during prolonged periods of sleep. Groothuis and Rosenberg[87] found that BPD patients who were maintained on home oxygen therapy maintained their original weight percentiles whereas those infants who discontinued oxygen therapy experienced significant decreases in weight gain.

Nutritional Screening and Assessment

Anthropometric

Obtaining daily weights in a BPD patient is essential during the early hospitalization(s) and critical stages of the disease. Weight data help to identify fluid overload in a patient, as well as growth.

Monitoring weight, length, and head circumference on a regular basis during the follow-up period will provide the necessary data to assess whether the patient is achieving expected growth. Measurements should be made using appropriate techniques and equipment (see Chapter 2) and be plotted on appropriate growth charts, using either the NCHS growth charts and correcting for gestational age or growth charts that allow assessment of infants of varying gestational age, such as those by Babson and Benda.[22,88] Additional measurements that may be useful in monitoring nutritional status include the mid-arm circumference and triceps skinfold.

Biochemical

Biochemical monitoring of the BPD patient is individualized based on the patient's clinical status, the type and amount of diuretic therapy, and the protocol of the individual institution. If the patient is on diuretic therapy, electrolytes need to be monitored, especially sodium, chloride, and potassium. Mineral status should be monitored including calcium, phosphorus, and magnesium. Other helpful measurements include prealbumin or albumin as a measure of visceral protein stores, a complete blood count, alkaline phosphatase for monitoring for rickets of prematurity, and urine specific gravity, especially if the patient is fluid restricted and/or a concentrated formula is being given.

Clinical

The patient's pulmonary status will have an impact on nutritional needs and intake. Noting the patient's pulmonary status is an important component of the nutrition assessment. If a BPD patient is ventilator dependent, this is an indication of respiratory failure and of severe lung disease. Ventilator-dependent BPD patients require close follow-up because it may be difficult initially to determine their nutritional needs. Many chronic ventilator-dependent patients with BPD have very low energy needs and yet their other nutrient needs are the same as other infants with BPD. For these patients, feedings must be adjusted to meet nutrient needs without providing too many calories, which often requires vitamin and mineral supplementation. A patient who has a low arterial partial pressure of oxygen is not properly oxygenating tissue, which may contribute to growth failure. These patients may require supplemental oxygen for tissue oxygenation and for growth. Noting a patient's oximetry reading is important. An increase in pulmonary symptoms such as the presence of tachypnea, rales, rhonchi, and bronchiolitis/pneumonia is indicative of active pulmonary disease. The presence of chronic pulmonary disease and acute pulmonary exacerbations in BPD patients increases energy needs and at the same time may increase their sensitivity to fluids.

Other medical conditions, such as cor pulmonale, gastroesophageal reflux with or without aspiration, esophagitis, repeated emesis, and the patient's medication regimen, should also be noted. Table 15–4 lists drug-nutrient interactions of medications commonly prescribed for BPD patients. It is important to note a patient's input and output to complete the clinical assessment.

Dietary

The BPD patient's dietary intake needs to be evaluated for calories, protein, fluid, electrolytes, key minerals such as calcium, phosphorus, and iron, and caloric distribution of fat, protein, and carbohydrate. The type of feeding—enteral versus parenteral—should be noted, as well as the route of administration and vitamin and mineral supplementation. This can then be compared to the patient's estimated nutrient and fluid requirements.

Of particular importance in the nutrition assessment of BPD patients is careful monitoring of the patient's ability to suck and swallow and the patient's feeding skill development. The sucking reflex does not develop until about 34 weeks gestation. Alternate methods of feeding are required until this reflex develops. Neurologic impairment may prevent the patient from being able to coordinate sucking and swallowing. Noxious stimuli to the patient's mouth, such as frequent intubations and suctioning, may seriously affect

Table 15–4 BPD Drug-Nutrient Interactions

Medication	*Nutrients Affected (lowers all)*	*Other Effects*
Diuretics (e.g., furosemide)	Na, K, Cl, Mg, Ca, Zn	Volume depletion Metabolic alkalosis Anorexia Diarrhea Hyperuricemia Gastrointestinal irritant
Bronchodilators (e.g., theophylline)		Gastrointestinal distress Nausea Vomiting Diarrhea
Steroids (e.g., dexamethasone)	Ca, P	Growth suppression

normal feeding skill development. Maintaining adequate oxygenation during feedings is essential.[79,80] It is important to note whether the patient tires during feedings and whether he or she turns blue around the mouth or fingertips, indicating a drop in oxygen saturation. It is imperative that these problems be identified early and appropriate intervention instituted.

Nutrition Management

Nutrients of Concern

Energy and Protein. As has already been discussed, the patient with BPD has high energy and nutrient needs. Estimations of the increase in resting energy expenditure of infants with BPD as compared to controls range from 125–150%.[76–78] At the same time, numerous constraints are placed on the delivery of the appropriate amount of energy and nutrients, such as fluid restrictions, gastrointestinal immaturity, and renal immaturity. Oh[89] describes three phases of nutritional management of infants with BPD, which are summarized here. The estimated energy requirements of each phase and the components of the energy expenditure are depicted in Table 15–5.

Acute Phase. The BPD patient during this phase is critically ill and at risk for clinical morbidities, such as patent ductus arteriosus and necrotizing enterocolitis. No calories are needed for specific dynamic action or for growth. Efforts should be made to keep thermal losses to a minimum. Possible feeding complications during this phase include fluid overload and hyperglycemia. The BPD patient has decreased fluid tolerance because of pulmonary edema and reduced cardiac output. Caloric provision is often relegated to secondary importance, behind these two problems and electrolyte imbalance.

Intermediate Phase. This phase is characterized by a period of clinical improvements and a gradual introduction of oral feeding. Again, thermal losses should be kept to a minimum. Fluid overload continues to be a possible complication, but generally the BPD patient is able to tolerate an increase in fluid during this phase.

Convalescent Phase. This is a period of recovery. Usually, but not always, the patient is exclusively feeding orally. Minimizing thermal losses continues to be important, as well as monitoring activity, growth, and adequate oxygenation of tissues. Continued monitoring of intake, growth, and development is important. Nutritional recommendations must be individualized according to each patient's needs.

Adequate protein is necessary to achieve growth, but the immature kidney cannot handle high-protein loads. Protein should constitute about 8% to 12% of the total calories, with the

Table 15–5 Calorie Requirements (kcal/kg/d) of Infants with Bronchopulmonary Dysplasia at Various Stages of Nutritional Management

Component	*Acute*	*Intermediate*	*Convalescent*
Basal metabolic rate	45	60	60
Stool losses	0–10	10	60
Thermal stress	0–10	0–10	10
Activity	5	5	10
Specific dynamic action	0	0–5	10
Growth allowance	0	20–30	20–30
Total	50–70	95–120	120–130

Acute = clinical illness, oral feeding difficult; intermediate = clinical improvement, gradual introduction of oral feeding; convalescent = recovery, oral feeding exclusively.

Source: Used with permission of Ross Products Division, Abbott Laboratories, Inc., Columbus, OH 43216. From *Bronchopulmonary Dysplasia and Related Chronic Respiratory Disorders*, © 1986, Ross Products Division, Abbott Laboratories, Inc.

remainder of the calories evenly divided between carbohydrate and fat.[90]

Vitamins A and E. Many studies have examined the role of vitamin A (retinol) in animals and premature infants who develop chronic lung disease.[91] Vitamin A is essential in the respiratory tract for maintenance of the integrity and differentiation of epithelial cells. Deficiency of vitamin A results in loss of cilia and other changes in the airways, which resemble the changes seen in BPD. Robbins and colleagues[92] showed that vitamin A adequacy may decrease the incidence of BPD in infants with very low birth weight. With vitamin A supplementation, monitoring of plasma levels is essential.[92] Studies have been conducted administering 5000 IU vitamin A intramuscularly three times a week to infants at risk for developing BPD with positive results and no adverse effects.[93,94] Some newborn intensive care units administer vitamin A in an attempt to protect against BPD.[95]

Adequate vitamin E status is particularly important in premature infants with BPD who are on oxygen therapy because vitamin E is a major antioxidant. Vitamin E acts as an oxygen-free radical scavenger and membrane stabilizer, protecting lipid-containing cell membranes from oxidation. Infants are most likely to receive adequate vitamin E when fed human milk or commercial formulas. Large doses of vitamin E appear to offer no additional protection against BPD.[96] If, for medical reasons, the infant is not fed parenterally or enterally, the premature infant with BPD is at increased risk for developing vitamin E deficiency. Also at risk for vitamin E deficiency is the infant maintained by parenteral nutrition that includes large amounts of polyunsaturated fatty acids but little vitamin E.

Trace Minerals. Particular attention should be given to the following trace minerals, which are components of an antioxidant enzyme system: copper, zinc, selenium, and manganese.[90] No specific recommendations for these minerals have been established for the infant with BPD. Zinc can be decreased with diuretic therapy (refer to Table 15–4) and often premature infants are in negative zinc balance.[97] Infants with BPD may be at risk for toxic accumulation of certain trace elements, such as copper and manganese, especially if the patient has cholestasis or other liver disease.[90]

Iron. The recommended iron intake is 2 to 4 mg of elemental iron/kg/day,[98] and the supplementation should begin no later than 2 months of age. Iron can be provided through a supplement or through the use of iron-fortified formulas. Adequate iron status is especially important in patients with BPD in order to maximize tissue oxygenation and minimize oxygen consumption.[68]

Calcium and Phosphorus. As previously stated, infants born prematurely are born without the benefit of the calcium and phosphorus accretion of the third trimester of gestation. In addition, the calcium and phosphorus status of premature infants with BPD is further compromised by diuretic therapy, steroid therapy, long-term use of parenteral nutrition, and feeding delays. Consequently, infants with BPD are at risk for developing rickets of prematurity or osteopenia, which is diagnosed by decreased bone density on X-rays and an alkaline phosphatase over 400 units/L. Therefore, the adequacy of calcium and phosphorus intake requires special attention. Preterm human milk can be fortified with a commercial human milk fortifier. Premature formulas provide higher concentrations of these minerals. Adequate vitamin D (400 IU/d) intake is also important.[98]

Electrolytes. Electrolyte imbalance may result, especially when the infant is receiving diuretic therapy. The BPD infant can usually tolerate a sodium intake of 1.5 to 3.5 mEq/kg/d.[68] Potassium (3 mEq/kg/d) and chloride may need to be supplemented depending on the diuretic therapy.[68,69] Careful monitoring is a must when sodium chloride and/or potassium chloride are being added to feedings.

Barriers to Meeting Increased Needs

Many barriers must be overcome in order to meet the increased nutrient needs of the infant with BPD. These barriers include:

1. fluid restriction for infants with cor pulmonale with or without right-sided heart failure and those who are fluid sensitive
2. gastrointestinal limitations such as an immature gut and gastroesophageal reflux
3. immature renal function, making renal solute load of feedings an issue
4. chronic hypoxia, especially during feedings and during sleep
5. feeding difficulties, including lack of sucking reflex and feeding aversions

Meeting Nutritional Needs

Translating these energy, protein, and other nutrient needs into a feeding order can be difficult in light of the restrictions just described. This discussion on meeting nutritional needs of the infant with BPD will be divided into parenteral and enteral routes of feeding.

Parenteral Nutrition. During the acute phase of BPD, parenteral nutrition is often employed. Refer to Chapter 4 for specific guidelines for parenteral nutrition in the early postnatal period for premature infants.

Studies have raised concern about the effect of intravenous fat in pulmonary-compromised patients.[100,101] Other studies have shown that the possible adverse effect of lipid infusion is related to the maturity of the infant and the rate of the infusion.[102,103] The American Academy of Pediatrics recommends starting lipids in the low-birth-weight infant at 0.5 to 1.0 g/kg/d and slowly increasing to a maximum of 2.0 to 3.0 g/kg/d.[98] Serum triglyceride levels should be kept below 150 mg/dl.[98]

For preterm infants, the American Academy of Pediatrics recommends starting glucose infusions at a rate less than 6 mg/kg/minute and steadily increasing to an infusion rate of 11 to 12 mg/kg/minute.[98] High-glucose loads in BPD patients have been shown to increase resting energy expenditure, increase basal oxygen consumption, and increase carbon dioxide production.[76] Infants with borderline respiratory function may not be able to excrete this additional carbon dioxide, and respiratory acidosis can result.

Enteral Nutrition. Enteral feedings must be begun at a slow rate to allow the immature intestine of the premature infant to adapt to the feedings (refer to Chapter 4). During this transitional phase, parenteral nutrition is often continued in order to meet the increased energy needs of the patient. It is very important to maintain the delivery of adequate energy and protein while tolerance to enteral feedings is being established.

This transitional phase can become very complicated. An infant must be hungry before an oral feeding will be readily accepted. Continuous infusions of nutritional solutions may suppress natural hunger sensations. Hunger is particularly important when feeding skills are being developed. An appropriate schedule of parenteral feedings, enteral tube feedings, and oral feedings must be determined by members of the interdisciplinary health care team, including family members and caregivers, to best suit the individual patient's needs.

Fortified breast milk or premature infant formulas, which have higher concentrations of vitamins and minerals, may be used initially. The infant should continue with breast milk fortified with a human milk fortifier or with premature formula until reaching a weight of 2000 to 2500 g. At this point, the infant can most likely be transitioned to a premature follow-up formula or a standard infant formula concentrated to 22 or 24 Kcal/oz. Both premature formulas and premature follow-up formulas have the fatty acids docosahexaenoic acid (DHA) and arachidonic acid (ARA) added. To meet some infants' very high energy needs, it may become necessary to further concentrate the formula to 26 to 30 Kcal/oz. Currently, there is some controversy as to the best approach for further concentration of the formula. Some registered dietitians prefer to further concentrate the formula by adding less water. The proponents of this method argue that by concentrating formula in this manner, protein, vitamins, and mineral contents per volume are not diluted. Another approach is using a 24 Kcal/oz formula as a base and adding carbohydrate in the form of glucose polymers or rice cereal and/or lipids. When modulating formulas in this manner, it is important to maintain a proper balance of nutrients. Caloric distribution should continue to be approximately 8% to 12% protein, 40% to 50% carbohydrate, and 40% to 50% fat.[90] An example of a modulated formula is given in Table 15–6. When modulating formulas, care should be taken not to dilute the protein content to a level that is inadequate for growth.[99] Fat should not provide more than 60% of total calories because ketosis may be induced. Fat delays gastric emptying and a high fat content may be contraindicated in patients who have gastroesophageal reflux.[99] Boehm and associates[104] showed decreased fat absorption in patients with BPD that may contribute to inadequate weight gain. Regardless of the approach taken, excessive osmolality and renal solute load should be avoided. It is important to maintain adequate vitamin and mineral intakes. Once an infant is on standard formula or breast milk, a supplement of a standard infant multivitamin preparation may be recommended until the infant is taking about 1 L of formula. The usual recommendation is 1 cc of a standard infant multivitamin with breast milk or formula intakes over 16 ounces per day and .5 cc for intakes between 16 and 30 ounces per day.[105]

Brunton and colleagues[106] performed a prospective double-blind, randomized trial in which preterm infants with BPD received either a standard formula or an enriched formula. The

Table 15–6 Examples of a Modulated Formula

	Carbohydrate (g)	*Protein (g)*	*Fat (g)*
30 mL NeoSure ADVANCE 24*	2.49	0.69	1.32
1 g Polycose* powder	0.94	—	—
1 mL Microlipid⁺	—	—	0.50
Total	3.43	0.69	1.82
Kilocalories per gram	× 4	× 4	× 9
Kilocalories	13.72	2.76	16.38
% Total kilocalories	42	8	50

Total kilocalories = 32.86/31 mL
1.06 kilocalories/mL

*Ross Laboratories, Columbus, Ohio

⁺Microlipid, Mead Johnson, Evansville, Indiana

enriched formula had the same caloric concentration as the standard formula (27 Kcal/oz), but had higher concentrations of protein, calcium, phosphorus, and zinc. The study was conducted from 37 weeks postmenstrual age to 3 months chronological age. The results included greater linear growth, greater radial bone mineral content, and greater lean mass in the infants who were fed the enriched formula. This study suggests that, in addition to calories, greater concentrations of protein and selected minerals may be necessary for catch-up growth in patients with BPD.[106]

When infants are receiving high-calorie formulas, careful monitoring is warranted. Increasing the caloric density may increase the potential renal solute load if fluid intake is limited. When the infant is growing and nitrogen is being utilized to form new tissue, the infant usually handles the solute load. However, if growth ceases or if there is increased fluid loss, such as with a febrile illness, renal solute load may become a problem for these infants, and azotemia may result. Urine specific gravity should be monitored. [99]

The infant may be unable to consume an adequate amount of formula by mouth. It may be necessary to deliver the balance of the formula via tube feeding to achieve adequate intake. Oral gastric or nasogastric feedings are commonly used for short-term supplementary feedings, whereas gastrostomy feedings are used for long-term tube feeding.

Addressing Feeding Difficulties

The patient's ability to suck and swallow must be assessed. Abnormalities in the developmental patterns of suck-and-swallow rhythms during feeding in preterm infants with BPD have been reported.[107] Feeding behavior should be assessed for age appropriateness based on corrected age.

BPD patients are susceptible to developing feeding difficulties because of their usual prematurity and because of the nature of the life-sustaining respiratory therapy that they receive. Intubations and suctioning are noxious stimuli to the oral area and can interfere with normal feeding development. Supplemental oxygen is usually delivered by nasal cannula and does not interfere with oral feedings.

Occupational therapists and speech pathologists identify feeding problems and design treatment plans. Nonnutritive sucking can be instituted during a tube feeding so that the infant can begin to associate feelings of satiety with sucking. In some instances, feedings thickened with rice cereal may be easier for infants to handle. Overlooking problems in the development of feeding skills can result in serious aversions to eating or decreased and inadequate intake.

When critical steps in feeding skill development have been missed, it may be necessary to design a program that breaks eating down into small steps and to orient the child to each step. Instead of feeding according to chronological age, it is more important to feed the child according to the stage of feeding development. A behavioral program may be necessary to help the patient overcome fears related to eating or when food refusal is used manipulatively.

Singer and associates[108] found that mothers of infants with BPD spent more time prompting the infants to feed, but these infants took in less formula and spent less time sucking than the two control groups of premature infants without BPD and term infants. In the Johnson and colleagues study, parents often expressed concern about getting their infant with BPD to take enough food and reported long feeding times.[83] Problematic feeding interactions between the caregiver and the infant may develop. It is important that the health care professional be aware of this potential problem and provide the family with anticipatory guidance in this area. If the patient's oral intake is not adequate to meet nutritional needs, then tube feedings are necessary. A plan for balancing tube feedings with oral feedings must be designed to establish hunger and appetite for feedings by mouth but providing the balance of nutrition via the tube feeding. Tube feedings can be nasogastric, oral gastric, trans pyloric, or gastrostomy. For long-term tube feedings gastrostomy feedings are usually chosen. Drip, bolus, or a combination tube feeding schedule can be developed based on the patient's individual needs.

Family/Caretaker Education

The home care of the patient with BPD can be quite complex and may include supplemental oxygen and multiple medications and therapies as well as nutrition management. Family and caretaker education by a registered dietitian is an important component of the nutrition care plan, and adequate time must be devoted to education during the discharge-planning process. Written instructions for mixing formulas in common household measures for volumes that will be used in 24 hours or less should be given to families. It is best to have the family member or caretaker demonstrate the proper mixing of formulas, especially formula that is being concentrated or contains additives. Reinforcement of these instructions needs to take place on an ongoing basis in outpatient follow-up.

Referral to Food/Nutrition Resources

Caring for a BPD patient can be very draining for the patient's family from emotional, physical, and financial standpoints. It is important to assess the patient's and family's needs with regard to food and nutrition resources. Appropriate referrals must be made. Often, this can be done in cooperation with the nurse and/or social worker (see also Chapter 12).

Medical and Nutrition Follow-up

After discharge from the hospital, the infant with BPD will require regular medical and nutrition follow-up. Feedings will need to be adjusted as the patient grows and develops. Many patients benefit from being enrolled in early intervention programs, which can provide nutrition, occupational therapy, physical therapy, and speech therapy as needed by the individual patient.

Identification of Areas Needing Further Research

Effects of early onset of respiratory failure and vigorous ventilator support on nutrient and energy requirements for BPD patients should be assessed at various stages of the disease, particularly regarding energy, protein, vitamins A and E, and minerals such as calcium, phosphorus, and zinc. Assimilation and absorption of nutrients in BPD patients and whether or not a deficiency of one of these nutrients plays a role in the etiology of the disease also must be determined. General growth studies, including studies that establish appropriate growth for BPD patients at various stages of the disease, would provide guidance for health care practitioners. Nutritional requirements of BPD patients at various stages of the disease and appropriate methods and timing of nutrition intervention in BPD treatment require further study. The long-term sequelae of BPD and its current treatment modalities require ongoing investigation.

ASTHMA

Asthma is the most common chronic disease of childhood, affecting an estimated 6.3 million children from birth to 17 years of age.[109] The prevalence of childhood asthma has been increasing, as it has for adults, since 1980 and has become a major public health problem.[110] Asthma is the most common cause of school absenteeism in the United States with about 14 million lost school days per year.[110] In 2000, children up to 17 years old had 4.6 million outpatient doctor's visits, over 700,000 emergency department visits, and over 200,000 hospitalizations because of asthma.[110] Disparities exist among racial/ethnic populations with a higher prevalence seen in non-Hispanic blacks, American Indian/Alaskan Natives, and multiracial, non-Hispanic groups.[111] Puerto Ricans also have a high prevalence of asthma.[111] Non-Hispanic blacks have more emergency department visits, more hospitalizations, and an increase in asthma mortality, which are not explained entirely by higher asthma prevalence.[111] There is increased prevalence in childhood among males, children of lower socioeconomic groups, African-Americans, and those with a family history of asthma or allergies.[112,113] Underdiagnosis and inappropriate treatment are major contributors to morbidity and mortality.[113]

Eight objectives of the Healthy People 2010[114] health objectives for the nation are related to asthma. These objectives are:

1. reduce asthma deaths (objective 24-1)
2. reduce hospitalizations for asthma (objective 24-2)
3. reduce hospital emergency department visits for asthma (objective 24-3)
4. reduce activity limitations among persons with asthma (objective 24-4)
5. reduce number of school or work days missed (objective 24-5)
6. increase the proportion of persons with asthma who received formal patient education (objective 24-6)
7. increase the proportion of persons with asthma who receive appropriate care (objective 24-7)
8. establish in at least 15 states a surveillance system for tracking asthma data (objective 24-8).

Asthma is defined by the National Heart Lung and Blood Institute (NHLBI) in its publication *Expert Panel Report 2: Guidelines for the Diagnosis and Management of Asthma*[115] as a chronic inflammatory disorder of the airways. Symptoms of this inflammation include recurrent episodes of wheezing, breathlessness, chest tightness, and cough, particularly at night and early in the morning. These asthma episodes are associated with widespread but variable obstruction of airflow, which is often reversible either spontaneously or with treatment. Inflammation of the airways also causes an associated increase in airway responsiveness to a variety of stimuli.[115] Inflammation causes airway narrowing and increased airway secretions. Chronic inflammation can lead to airway remodeling, which can cause progressive loss of pulmonary function.[113] Airway obstruction is caused by bronchoconstriction, airway edema, chronic mucus plug formation, and airway remodeling.[113,115]

According to the NHLBI guidelines,[115] asthma management consists of four components:

1. Assessment and monitoring
   a. Initial assessment and diagnosis of asthma
   b. Periodic assessment and monitoring
2. Control of factors affecting severity
3. Pharmacologic therapy
4. Education for a partnership in asthma care

The diagnosis of asthma can be made when the clinician determines that episodic symptoms of airflow obstruction are present, that airflow obstruction is at least partially reversible, and when alternative diagnoses have been excluded.[115] Diagnostic tools available to the clinician include obtaining a thorough history; spirometry, which measures pulmonary function but is not feasible to measure in young children up to 5 to 6 years of age; chest radiograph; and pulse oximetry, a measure of oxygen saturation, to evaluate hypoxemia during an acute episode. Other diagnostic tests available include allergy testing, nasal and sinus evaluation, and gastroesophageal reflux assessment.[113] Differential diagnoses include aspiration, cystic fibrosis, cardiac or anatomical defects, and upper and lower respiratory tract infections.[113] The NHLBI guidelines include a classification system of asthma severity: mild intermittent, mild persistent, moderate persistent, and severe persistent. These classifications reflect the clinical manifestations of asthma and are based on frequency of daytime and nighttime symptoms, on spirometry if available, and severity of asthma flare-ups.[115]

According to the NHLBI guidelines, the goals of asthma therapy are to:[115]

1. Prevent chronic symptoms
2. Maintain normal or near normal pulmonary functions
3. Maintain normal activity levels
4. Prevent recurrent exacerbations
5. Provide optimal pharmacotherapy with minimal or no side effects
6. Meet patient's and family's expectations and satisfaction with asthma care

A major goal of asthma treatment is to reduce inflammation. The first step toward this is for the patient to recognize and avoid the triggers of asthma. Triggers may include indoor allergens such as dust mites, cockroaches, mold, and animal dander, and outdoor allergens such as trees, grasses, weeds, and pollens.[113] Environmental tobacco smoke and air pollutants are major precipitants of asthma symptoms in children.[115] Viral respiratory infections are the primary cause of severe asthma flare-ups. Other factors contributing to asthma severity include rhinitis, sinusitis, gastroesophageal reflux, and sulfite sensitivity.[115] In some children, weather or humidity changes, or exercise—especially in cold and dry air—may produce inflammation of the airways.[113] Food allergies may also cause asthma symptoms, although this is rare.[116]

In addition to reducing factors that increase the patient's asthma symptoms, pharmacologic therapy is an important component of asthma management.[115,117] The choice of specific medicines is based on asthma severity and the classification of asthma. The goal is to optimize pharmacotherapy while minimizing side effects. Long-term control medicines are taken daily to achieve and maintain control of persistent asthma by reducing inflammation. Long-term control medicines include inhaled corticosteroids, long-acting $beta_2$ agonists, cromolyn sodium and nedocromil sodium (mast cell stabilizers), methylxanthine, leukotriene modifiers, oral corticosteroids, and inhaled corticosteroids and long-acting $beta_2$ agonists in combination. Quick-relief medications, inhaled short-acting $beta_2$ agonists, anticholinergics, and short-course systemic corticosteroids are used to treat acute symptoms and exacerbations. Additionally, short-acting $beta_2$ agonists are used to pretreat exercise-induced asthma.[113,115,117]

Patient and family education in asthma care is another integral part of treatment. As the NHLBI guidelines[115] recommend, a partnership with the patient and family must be built by the health care professional. The patient and family need to be involved in problem solving for appropriate solutions for asthma trigger control and medication options. They should be able to recognize asthma symptoms and to treat appropriately and early. The patient and family members should demonstrate the proper use of inhalers and exhibit understanding of the proper use of other medications. Written instructions should be provided.[115,117] Long-term follow-up is essential to adjust medication as needed and for education reinforcement. Tobacco smoke is a common irritant and asthma trigger; therefore, smoking cessation information and counseling should be made available to family members.[113,115]

Food Allergies and Asthma

According to Sampson,[116] the confirmed incidence of adverse reactions to food is probably 1% to 2% in young children and 4% to 6% in infants (see Chapter 9). The role of food allergies in asthma is controversial.[118] In a study by Adler and associates,[119] 14.5% of children with asthma were reported by their parents to have food-provoked asthma symptoms. Several studies have been reported in the scientific literature investigating the true incidence of asthma symptoms caused by food allergies using double-blind, placebo-controlled food challenges.[120–122] The results of these investigations thus far include findings that IgE-mediated reactions to food can cause respiratory symptoms, including wheezing, but that this is uncommon, even in children with histories of other adverse reactions to food. Even when respiratory symptoms are exhibited after food ingestion, the changes in pulmonary function are not significant.[118] Further investigation in this area is needed before strong conclusions can be drawn, but based on currently available data, food allergies do not appear to contribute significantly to the burden of asthma in the population.

Milk and Mucus

It is a common misconception among lay people that drinking milk causes an increased production of mucus and may be a trigger for asthma. However, there is no scientific evidence to support this claim. This belief may persist because milk, particularly whole milk, coats the tongue and mouth and some people may have the sensation that they have an increase in mucus production or that their mucus is thicker after milk consumption. In an Australian study, believers and nonbelievers of the milk-mucus connection were studied.[123] Clearing their throats was the most common symptom described by both the believers and nonbelievers after drinking milk. Words commonly used to describe the sensation associated with drinking milk were "thick," "blocked," and "clogged."[123] These same researchers administered chocolate cow's milk or chocolate soy milk in a randomized trial.[124] They found that the same type of sensory perceptions of milk were described by believers and nonbelievers of the milk-mucus connection theory for both types of milk. These researchers concluded that these same perceptions extended to milk substitute beverages as well as milk. Further studies found no effect of the ingestion of a cow milk solution powder dissolved in a strawberry-flavored beverage versus placebo on the pulmonary function in a group of adult mild asthmatics in a double-blind placebo-controlled study.[124,125] Individuals may have bona fide milk allergy but these numbers are relatively low. Indiscriminate elimination of a whole food group such as dairy products from the diet of a child with asthma may be totally unnecessary and may deprive the child of an important source of nutrients such as calcium.

Role of Breastfeeding in the Prevention of Asthma

The relationship of breastfeeding in asthma prevention has been studied using data from NHANES III with conflicting interpretations. One group of investigators found that breast-fed children as compared to never breast-fed children "may" have a delay in the onset of asthma or recurrent wheeze or they "may" actually be actively protected against asthma.[126] However, Rust and colleagues[127] found that breastfeeding "did not appear" to have an impact on asthma prevention or a reduction in its severity. According to the NHANES III data, the relationship between breastfeeding and asthma prevention is not strong. Wright and associates[128] found that longer durations of exclusive breastfeeding increased the risk of reported asthma among children with asthmatic mothers.

Relationship Between Asthma and Obesity

Both asthma and obesity have been increasing at alarming rates in the United States. This epidemiological observation prompted studies conducted during the 1980s, which generated the hypothesis of an association between asthma and obesity.[129] This association has been studied in adults and children.

Findings in Adult Studies

Studies in adults have found that obesity does affect pulmonary function. The prospective Nurses' Health Study II found that BMI was a strong, independent, positive risk factor for the onset of asthma.[130] Other investigators in Finland have shown improvements in lung function, symptoms, morbidity, and health status with weight reduction in obese patients with asthma.[131] Possible explanations for the association between asthma and obesity include the possibilities that gastroesophageal reflux as a result of obesity exacerbates asthma, that physical inactivity may promote both diseases, and that the high fat diets of obese patients may promote airway inflammation and asthma.[129]

Findings in Pediatric Studies

The relationship between asthma and obesity has been studied in the pediatric population. Many of these studies have been conducted with inner city, minority populations because these populations have the highest prevalence of asthma and are at the greatest risks of experiencing the morbidity and mortality of this chronic disease.

Luder and associates[132] compared a group of inner city children with asthma to a group of their peers. The prevalence of overweight was significantly higher in children with moderate to severe asthma than in their peers. In the asthma group, a higher BMI was associated with significantly more severe asthma symptoms, such as lower pulmonary function measurements, more school absenteeism, and a greater number of prescribed asthma medications.[132] These investigators recommend studying the effect of weight reduction in asthma patients with a high BMI on asthma symptoms. Gennuso and colleagues[133] studied urban minority children and adolescents who had asthma and nonasthma controls. These investigators found an increase in obesity among children with asthma for both sexes and across ages as compared to controls. The severity of asthma was not related to obesity. These investigators concluded that asthma is a risk factor for obesity in children. As part of the National Cooperative Inner City Asthma Study, Belamarich and colleagues[134] found that 19% of the asthma patients ages 4 to 9 years had BMIs over the 95th percentile as compared to 11% of all children in the National Health and Nutrition Examination Survey (NHANES) III. The investigators also found that obese children with asthma required more asthma medication, reported more days of wheezing, and visited the emergency departments more than nonobese children with asthma.

The Tucson Children's Respiratory Study found that female subjects who were overweight or obese between 6 and 11 years of age were seven times more likely to develop new asthma symptoms at age 11 and 13 years.[135] These investigators hypothesized that being overweight may influence female sex hormones, which in turn increase asthma risk. Gilliland and associates[136] studied almost 4,000 school-age children in the longitudinal Children's Health Study which was conducted in southern California between 1993 and 1998. These investigators found that overweight was associated with increased risk of new onset asthma in boys and in nonallergic children. Tantisira and colleagues[137] studied children with mild to moderate asthma who were enrolled in the Childhood Asthma Management Program (CAMP). They found that although an increasing BMI was associated with an increase in forced expiratory volume in 1 second (FEV_1) and forced vital capacity (FVC), the ratio of FEV_1 to FVC was reduced. There was a positive association between BMI and cough/wheeze with exercise. This study does not support the hypothesis that an increase in BMI increases asthma severity, but the increase in exercise-induced bronchospasm with increasing BMI suggests a relationship between increased airway responsiveness and BMI.

The conclusions that can be drawn regarding the association of overweight and asthma from these studies in pediatrics include:

1. There is a higher prevalence of overweight in children with asthma.
2. Overweight children with asthma have increased asthma symptoms.
3. Overweight may influence asthma risk.

Effects of Nutrients on Asthma

Because asthma affects the lives of so many adults and children, much research has been done in the area of asthma treatment and the prevention of asthma exacerbations, including the impact of nutrition on asthma patients. Many studies have been performed investigating the role of various nutrients in protecting against asthma, as well as their effects on improving asthma symptoms. Nutrients that have been studied include vitamin C, fish oils, selenium, and electrolytes, including sodium and magnesium.[118]

Vitamin C

Antioxidants protect cell membranes from damage caused by free radicals and chemical oxidants. Of the antioxidant vitamins, vitamin C has received the most attention, with most of the studies involving adult subjects. According to the NHANES I, lower dietary vitamin C intakes were associated with lower FEV_1. However, the difference in this pulmonary function test between the highest and lowest levels of dietary vitamin C was not great and the clinical significance of this finding was questioned.[138] Other studies of adult subjects showed that asthma patients had low blood levels of vitamin C and that low vitamin C intake was associated with weaker lung function.[118] In one pediatric study, children ages 8 to 11 years who never ate fresh fruit had 4.3% lower pulmonary function and had a 25.3% higher incidence of wheezing than did children who ate fruit more than once a day.[139] However, vitamin C intake was not specifically analyzed in this study. Other studies have suggested possible short-term protective effects of vitamin C on airway responsiveness.[118] No conclusive evidence links vitamin C levels to asthma or identifies the role that vitamin C may play in the treatment of asthma.[118] This area warrants further investigation before routine supplementation can be recommended for asthma patients. However, encouraging children with asthma to include a daily source of vitamin C in their diets is sound advice.

Fish Oils

The ingestion of fish oils, which contain omega-3 fatty acids, causes arachidonic acid (AA) to be replaced by eicosapentaenoic acid (EPA) and docosahexaenoic acid (DHA) in cell membranes. This replacement leads to a decrease in the production of the inflammatory metabolites of AA, including leukotrienes. It is thought that this change in metabolites could have potential effects on airway inflammation, which is why fish oil ingestion and its relationship to asthma has been studied.[118,140]

As with the antioxidants, most of the studies have been with adult asthma patients.[118] A positive relationship between dietary fish intake and higher pulmonary function was found when the data from the NHANES I was examined.[141] Two studies of Australian school children found an association between oily fish intake (tuna, salmon, herring) and a reduction in prevalence of increased airway responsiveness and a reduction in the incidence of asthma.[142,143] This same group of investigators compared the clinical effects of fish oil supplementation and a diet that increases omega-3 polyunsaturated fatty acids with a diet enriched in omega-6 fatty acids in a double-blind, randomized trial of 39 children with asthma. No significant changes in clinical severity of asthma were found.[144] Another group of investigators found decreased asthma symptoms when fish oil capsules were given to 29 children with asthma who participated in a randomized controlled trial in a controlled environment in terms of inhalant allergens and diet.[145] The majority of the studies do not show significant clinical improvement in asthma patients with the use of fish oils, despite some changes seen in inflammatory cell functions.[146] Another question that remains is whether dietary fatty acids play a role in the development of asthma.[146] The data is inconclusive at this point and does not support the use of fish oil in the treatment of asthma.[118] Further investigation is warranted but recommending the inclusion of fatty fish in the diets of children with asthma is simply consistent with current healthy diet recommendations.

Selenium

The relationship of selenium to asthma has been studied because of selenium's role as an antioxidant. No current data demonstrate a beneficial effect of selenium supplementation on pulmonary function tests in asthma patients. Although some studies have indicated a possible correlation between low serum levels of selenium and asthma symptoms, there is not sufficient evidence to advocate the use of selenium supplementation in the treatment of asthma.[118]

The role that specific nutrients may play in asthma has sparked much interest in the scientific community. More research in this area is needed before specific recommendations can be made. The interest in this area will probably continue to grow, especially as the practice of alternative/complementary medicine receives more attention. The data gathered to date reinforces the importance to asthma patients of a diet containing a variety of food sources.

Electrolytes

The relationship of increased sodium intake and asthma has been investigated by several groups of researchers.[118] These studies have been performed because it has been hypothesized that diets high in salt may increase bronchial reactivity. Although the data have shown small adverse effects of increased sodium intake on bronchial reactivity, no significant effects on the clinical symptoms of asthma have been found.[118] Also, the data from many of the studies are confounded by other variables, such as other dietary constituents. Currently, there is little scientific data to support the use of low-salt diets in the treatment of asthma.[118]

Magnesium and its role in asthma have been studied in adult asthma patients. Clinical trials have been conducted on the effect of magnesium infusion during acute asthma exacerbations.[118] Small, transient improvements in pulmonary functions were observed with the magnesium infusions, but these changes were not as great as those seen with $beta_2$ agonist inhalation therapy.[118] One study in England by Britton and associates[147] studied the relationship of magnesium intake, assessed from food frequency questionnaires, with pulmonary function FEV_1, airway reactivity to methacholine, and self-reported wheezing. A magnesium intake of 100 mg per day or higher was associated with a 27.7 ml higher FEV_1, a reduction in relative odds of airway hyperresponsiveness of 0.82, and a reduction in wheeze symptoms.[147] These studies indicate that although intravenous magnesium supplementation may have a minimal role in the treatment of acute asthma, further study is needed of the role of magnesium supplementation in the treatment of chronic asthma.[118]

Effects of Asthma Treatment on Nutritional Status

Most of the effects of asthma treatment on the nutritional status of patients are related to the use of oral steroids and high-dose inhaled steroids. According to the NHLBI guidelines, medium- to high-dose inhaled corticosteroids may be needed daily for long-term control in patients whose disease is classified as moderate persistent.[115] For patients whose disease is in the severe persistent classification, long-term control may require high-dose inhaled corticosteroids as well as a long-acting bronchodilator plus oral corticosteroids.[115] The primary goal is to treat the asthma with the smallest doses of medicines that will control the symptoms in order to minimize side effects.

Linear Growth

According to the NHLBI guidelines, poorly controlled asthma may delay growth in children.[115] In general, children with asthma tend to have longer periods of reduced growth rates prior to puberty.[115] However, this delay in puberty does not appear to affect final adult height.[148] This delay in puberty is also not associated with the use of inhaled corticosteroids.[149] The potential for adverse effects on linear growth from inhaled corticosteroids appears to be dose-dependent.[115,149–151] High doses of inhaled corticosteroids have greater potential for growth suppression than lower doses.[115] When inhaled corticosteroids are used as recommended, the majority of studies report no change in expected growth velocity.[150,151] In contrast, a few studies have demonstrated a small growth delay in children on inhaled corticosteroids, but the delay in growth velocity is not sustained, is not progressive, and may be reversible.[115,117] A meta-analysis of the effect of inhaled steroids found decreased growth velocity with inhaled steroids, but the effect on final adult height was unknown.[152] A study by Agertoft and Pedersen[153] in Denmark showed that expected adult height was attained for asthma patients on inhaled steroids. This is an area of asthma management that warrants further study, especially in young, preschool-aged children.[154] Using high doses of inhaled corticosteroids with children having severe persistent asthma has less potential for decreasing linear growth than does using oral systemic corticosteroids.[115] The use of oral corticosteroids on a prolonged basis does stunt linear growth.[148]

Bone Density

Chronic corticosteroid use does induce osteoporosis.[155] Corticosteroids decrease calcium absorption from the gastrointestinal tract and decrease renal calcium reabsorption, which leads to a decrease in plasma calcium. At the same time, there is an increase in parathyroid hormone secretion and an increase in bone resorption, all of which lead to osteoporosis. That is why it is important that the smallest possible dose be used to control asthma symptoms. Many studies—again mainly in adults—have been performed on the effect of inhaled corticosteroids on bone density, with varying results reported. Short-term effects on markers of bone turnover, such as osteocalcin, have been reported, but the long-term risk of osteoporosis is not clear.[156,157]

Collagen turnover was found to be reduced in children receiving long-term (over 12 months) inhaled steroid treatment.[158] Martinati and colleagues[159] found no adverse effect on bone mass in prepubertal children with mild-moderate asthma when treated with beclomethasone dipropionate, as compared to children treated with cromolyn sodium, a nonsteroidal anti-inflammatory drug. Most long-term studies indicate that there is negligible, if any, effect on bone mineral density of inhaled corticosteroids.[154] However, more research is needed before there is agreement as to the effect of the dose and duration of inhaled corticosteroids on bone density in patients, especially children with asthma.

Investigators conclude that attention should be given to the maintenance of adequate calcium and vitamin D intake in patients on chronic steroid therapy.[155] Calcium supplementation may be necessary in some patients, especially if dietary intake of calcium is low.[157] Calcium supplementation alone may be insufficient to completely block the progression of corticosteroid-dependent osteoporosis.[160] Other factors that may benefit the patient are weight-bearing exercise and the avoidance of other inhibitors of osteoblast production, such as alcohol excess.[154] In a study of adult asthmatic patients, Gagnon and associates[161] did find a significant positive correlation between bone density and calcium intake in asthmatic patients. This is another compelling reason why indiscriminate elimination of dairy products from the diet of a child with asthma may be harmful.

Excessive Weight Gain

Common, well-known side effects of oral corticosteroid therapy include appetite stimulation, central distribution of fat, sodium and fluid retention, and steroid-induced glucose intolerance. For the asthma patient whose disease is in the persistent severe classification and who may require chronic oral steroid therapy to control asthma symptoms, anticipatory dietary guidance as to how to combat some of these side effects, such as limiting salt intake or limiting concentrated sweets, will be beneficial.

Nutritional Management

The growth of children with asthma should be monitored on a regular basis (see Chapter 2). Any deviation in growth parameters should be investigated. BMI should be calculated and the BMI for age growth charts used to monitor at risk for overweight and overweight in asthma patients.[22] Nutrition counseling and lifestyle changes need to be emphasized by the health care practitioner at the first sign that an asthma patient may be at risk for overweight.

Based on the available data, a diet that provides a variety of foods, including fruits, vegetables, and dairy products, should be encouraged. Educational tools such as the USDA/HHS *Food Guide* Pyramid[162] or the USDA/HHS *Dietary Guidelines for Americans*[163] can be utilized. Patients and family members should be warned against eliminating whole food groups from the diet indiscriminately. Preadolescent and adolescent patients should receive information about healthy weight control practices, including regular exercise. Chronically ill adolescents, including asthma patients, were found to have increased body dissatisfaction and to be at increased risk of engaging in unhealthy weight-loss practices.[164]

Some patients with asthma who have a true food allergy will require an allergen elimination diet (see Chapter 9, Food Hypersensitivities).

Combating Steroid Side Effects

For those asthma patients who must take oral corticosteroids on a regular basis, additional factors should be more closely monitored. An adequate calcium intake is essential. These patients should be receiving at least the Dietary Reference Intakes (DRIs)[57] for calcium and in some instances may require calcium supplementation. Adequate vitamin D intake is also important.[155] The patient may need to modify kilocalorie intake to maintain weight control. The registered dietitian can assist the patient in identifying ways to accomplish a healthy diet, especially if the patient develops steroid-induced hyperglycemia. Moderate exercise should be encouraged because this will help maintain bone density and will assist with weight control.

Alternative/Complementary Medicine

Many asthma patients and their families have turned to alternative/complementary medicine therapies. Relaxation techniques, such as biofeedback training and yoga, are commonly practiced. Herbs, such as ma huang, echinacea, Asian mushrooms, and ginseng have been used by asthma patients.[165] It is important to ask about the use of these products when obtaining a diet history. These substances require scientific study before their effects on asthma are known. Asthma patients have also tried acupuncture and chiropractic spinal manipulation in attempts to control this chronic disease.[165]

Identification of Areas for Further Research

The areas needing further research have been indicated throughout this section. Additional scientific study of the role of specific nutrients in asthma must be done before precise recommendations for supplementation can be made. The effects of chronic steroid therapy and chronic inhaled steroid therapy on growth in children, especially in infants and young children, and on bone density require continued study. The relationship between being overweight and asthma requires further investigation. It is exciting to realize that nutrition may play a major role in the treatment of this significant public health problem.

REFERENCES

1. Welsh MJ, Tsui L, Boat TF, Beaudet AL. Cystic fibrosis. In: Scriver CR, eds. *The Metabolic Basis of Inherited Disease*. McGraw-Hill, NY, NY. 1989;3799–3876.
2. Cystic Fibrosis Foundation. *Cystic Fibrosis Foundation Patient Registry 2002 Annual Data Report*. Bethesda, MD: Cystic Fibrosis Foundation; September 2003.
3. Andersen DH. Cystic fibrosis of the pancreas and its relation to celiac disease: A clinical and pathologic study. *Am J Dis Child*. 1938;56:344–399.
4. Riordan JR, Rommens JM, Kerem B, et al. Identification of the cystic fibrosis gene: Cloning and characterization of complementary DNA. *Science*. 1989;245: 1066–1073.
5. Anderson MP, Gregory RJ, Thompson S, et al. Demonstration that CFTR is a chloride channel by alteration of its anion selectivity. *Science*. 1991;253:202–205.
6. Bear CE, Li CH, Kartner N, et al. Purification and functional reconstitution of the cystic fibrosis transmembrane conductance regulator (CFTR). *Cell*. 1992; 68:809–818.
7. Cheng SH, Rich DP, Marshall J, et al. Phosphorylation of the R domain by cAMP-dependent protein kinase regulates the CFTR chloride channel. *Cell*. 1991; 66:1027–1036.
8. Schwiebert EM, Egan ME, Hwang TH, et al. CFTR regulates outwardly rectifying chloride channels through an autocrine mechanism involving ATP. *Cell*. 1995;81: 1063–1073.
9. Stutts MJ, Canessa CM, Olsen JC, et al. CFTR as a cAMP-dependent regulator of sodium channels. *Science*. 1995;269:847–850.
10. Welsh MJ, Smith AE. Molecular mechanisms of CFTR chloride channel dysfunction in cystic fibrosis. *Cell*. 1993;73:1251–1254.
11. Cystic Fibrosis Genetic Analysis Consortium. Population variation of common cystic fibrosis mutations. *Hum Mutat*. 1994;4:167–177.
12. Hamosh A, FitzSimmons SC, Macek M, et al. Comparison of the clinical manifestations of cystic fibrosis in black and white patients. *J Pediatr*. 1998;132:255–259.
13. Rosenstein BJ, Cutting GR, Cystic Fibrosis Foundation Consensus Panel. The diagnosis of cystic fibrosis: A consensus statement. *J Pediatr*. 1998;132:589–595.
14. Tomezsko JL, Stallings VA, Kawchak DA, et al. Energy expenditure and genotype of children with cystic fibrosis. *Pediatr Res*. 1994;35:451–460.
15. O'Rawe A, McIntosh I, Dodge JA, et al. Increased energy expenditure in cystic fibrosis is associated with specific mutations. *Clin Sci*. 1992;82:71–76.
16. Murphy M, Ireton-Jones CS, Hilman BC, et al. Resting energy expenditures measured by indirect calorimetry are higher in preadolescent children with cystic fibrosis than expenditures calculated from prediction equations. *J Am Diet Assoc*. 1995;95:30–33.
17. Shepherd RW, Vasques-Velasquez L, Prentice A, et al. Increased energy expenditure in young children with cystic fibrosis. *Lancet*. 1988;135:1300–1303.
18. Vaisman N, Pencharz PB, Corey M, et al. Energy expenditure of patients with cystic fibrosis. *J Pediatr*. 1987;111:137–141.
19. Eubanks V, Koppersmith N, Wooldridge N, et al. Effects of megestrol acetate on weight gain, body composition, and pulmonary function in patients with cystic fibrosis. *J Pediatr*. 2002;140:439–1444.

20. Sproul A, Huang N. Growth patterns in children with cystic fibrosis. *J Pediatr.* 1964;65:664–676.

21. Lai HC, Kosorok MR, Sondel SA, et al. Growth status in children with cystic fibrosis based on the National Cystic Fibrosis Patient Registry data: Evaluation of various criteria used to identify malnutrition. *J Pediatr.* 1998;132:478–485.

22. Centers for Disease Control and Prevention. National Center for Health Statistics. CDC growth charts: United States. Retrieved April 1, 2004, from www.cdc.gov/nchs/about/major/nhanes/growthcharts/charts.htm.

23. Corey M, McLaughlin FJ, Williams M, Levison H. A comparison of survival, growth, and pulmonary function in patients with cystic fibrosis in Boston and Toronto. *J Clin Epidemiol.* 1988;41:583–591.

24. Cystic Fibrosis Foundation. Pediatric nutrition for patients with cystic fibrosis. Consensus Conferences: Concept in CF Care. Bethesda, MD: Cystic Fibrosis Foundation; 2001;1–39.

25. Borowitz D, Baker RD, Stallings V. Consensus report on nutrition for pediatric patients with cystic fibrosis. *J Pediatr Gastro and Nutr.* 2002;35:246–259.

26. Konstan MW, Butler SM, Wohl MEB, et al. Growth and nutritional indexes in early life predict pulmonary function in cystic fibrosis. *J Pediatr.* 2003;142:624–630.

27. Peterson ML, Jacobs DR, Milla CE. Longitudinal changes in growth parameters are correlated with changes in pulmonary function in children with cystic fibrosis. *Pediatrics.* 2003;112:588–592.

28. Steinkamp G, Wiedemann B, on behalf of the German CFQA Group. Relationship between nutritional status and lung function in cystic fibrosis: Cross sectional and longitudinal analyses from the German CF quality assurance (CFQA) project. *Thorax.* 2002;57:596–601.

29. Beker LT, Russek-Cohen E, Fink RJ. Stature as a prognostic factor in cystic fibrosis survival. *J Amer Diet Assoc.* 2001;101:438–442.

30. Cystic Fibrosis Foundation. *Clinical Practice Guidelines for Cystic Fibrosis*. Bethesda, MD: Cystic Fibrosis Foundation; 1997.

31. Fomon SJ. *Nutrition of Normal Infants*. Philadelphia, PA: Mosby; 1993.

32. Grant A, DeHoog S. *Nutritional Assessment and Support,* 5th ed. Seattle, WA: Anne Grant/Susan DeHoog; 1999.

33. Frisancho AR. New norms of upper limb fat and muscle areas for assessment of nutritional status. *Am J Clin Nutr.* 1981;34:2540–2545.

34. Heimburger DC, Weinsier RL. *Handbook of Clinical Nutrition*, 3rd ed. St. Louis, MO: Mosby; 1997.

35. Hardin DS. The diagnosis and management of cystic fibrosis related diabetes. *The Endocrinologist.* 1998; 8:265–272.

36. Moran A. Highlights of the February 1998 consensus conference on CFRD. *Pediatr Pulmonology.* October 1998; Supplement 17:104–105.

37. Cystic Fibrosis Foundation. Consensus document diagnosis, screening, and management of cystic fibrosis related diabetes mellitus. Consensus Conferences: Concept in CF Care, Bethesda, MD: Cystic Fibrosis Foundation; 1999;1–26.

38. Cystic Fibrosis Foundation. Guide to bone health and disease in cystic fibrosis consensus conference report. Consensus Conferences: Concept in CF Care, Bethesda, MD: Cystic Fibrosis Foundation; 2002;1–35.

39. Crist W, McDonnell P, Beck M, et al. Behavior at mealtimes in the young child with cystic fibrosis. *J Devel Behav Pediatr.* 1994;15:157–161.

40. Bell L, Durie P, Forstner GG. What do children with cystic fibrosis eat? *J Pediatr Gastroenterol Nutr.* 1984; 3(Suppl 1):S137–S146.

41. Institute of Medicine, Food and Nutrition Board. Dietary reference intakes for energy, carbohydrate, fiber, fat, protein and amino acids. Washington, DC: National Academy Press; 2003.

42. World Health Organization. Energy and protein requirements. *WHO Tech Report.* Ser. No. 724, 1985; 924:5–206.

43. National Research Council. *Recommended Dietary Allowances*, 10th ed. Washington, DC: National Academy Press; 1989.

44. Daniels L, Davidson GP, Martin AJ. Comparison of the macronutrient intake of healthy controls and children with cystic fibrosis on low fat or nonrestricted fat diets. *J Pediatr Gastroenterol Nutr.* 1987;6:381–386.

45. Pencharz PB, Durie PR. Nutritional management of cystic fibrosis. *Annu Rev Nutr.* 1993;13:111–136.

46. Roy CC, Darling P, Weber AM. A rational approach to meeting macro- and micronutrient needs in cystic fibrosis. *J Pediatr Gastroenterol Nutr.* 1984;3(Suppl.1): S154–S162.

47. Ellis L, Kalnins D, Corey M, et al. Do infants with cystic fibrosis need a protein hydrolysate formula? A prospective, randomized, comparative study. *J Pediatr.* 1998;132:270–276.

48. Kawchak DA, Zhao H, Scanlin TF, et al. Longitudinal, prospective analysis of dietary intake in children with cystic fibrosis. *J Pediatr.* 1996;129:119–129.

49. Jelalian E, Stark LJ, Reynolds L, Seifer R. Nutrition intervention for weight gain in cystic fibrosis: A meta analysis. *J Pediatr.* 1998;132:486–492.

50. Michel SH, Mueller DH. Impact of lactation on women with cystic fibrosis and their infants: A review of five cases. *J Am Diet Assoc.* 1994; 94:159–165.

51. Luder E, Gilbride JA. Teaching self-management skills to cystic fibrosis patients and its effect on their caloric intake. *J Am Diet Assoc.* 1989;89:359–364.

52. Stark LJ, Jelalian E, Mulvihill MM, et al. Eating in preschool children with cystic fibrosis and healthy peers: Behavioral analysis. *Pediatrics*. 1995;95:210–215.
53. Stark LJ, Mulvihill MM, Jelalian E, et al. Descriptive analysis of eating behavior in school-age children with cystic fibrosis and heathy control children. *Pediatrics*. 1997;99:665–671.
54. Stark LJ, Mulvihill MM, Powers SE, et al. Behavioral intervention to improve calorie intake of children with cystic fibrosis: treatment vs. waitlist control. *J Pediatr Gastroenterol Nutr*. 1996;22:240–253.
55. Erskine JM, Lingard CD, Sontag MK, Accurso FJ. Enteral nutrition for patients with cystic fibrosis: Comparison of a semi-elemental and nonelemental formula. *J Pediatr*. 1998;132:265–269.
56. Farrell PM, Hubbard VS. Nutrition in cystic fibrosis: Vitamins, fatty acids and minerals. In: Lloyd-Still JD, ed. *Textbook of Cystic Fibrosis*. Littleton, MA: John Wright; 1983.
57. Institute of Medicine, Food and Nutrition Board. Dietary reference intakes for calcium, phosphorus, magnesium, vitamin D, and fluoride. Washington, DC: National Academy Press; 1997.
58. Cystic Fibrosis Foundation. Use of pancreatic enzyme supplements for patients with cystic fibrosis in the context of fibrosing colonopathy. Consensus Conferences: Concepts in Care, Bethesda, MD: Cystic Fibrosis Foundation; 1995;1–11.
59. Borowitz DS, Grand RJ, Durie PR, Consensus Committee. Use of pancreatic enzyme supplements for patients with cystic fibrosis in the context of fibrosing colonopathy. *J Pediatr*. 1995;127:681–684.
60. FitzSimmons SC, Burkhart GA, Borowitz D, et al. High-dose pancreatic enzyme supplements and fibrosing colonopathy in children with cystic fibrosis. *N Eng J Med*. 1997;336:1283–1289.
61. Schwarzenberg SJ, Wielinski CL, Shamieh I, et al. Cystic fibrosis-associated colitis and fibrosing colonopathy. *J Pediatr*. 1995;127:565–570.
62. Stern RC, Canda ER, Doershuk CF. Use of nonmedical treatment by cystic fibrosis patients. *J Adol Health*. 1992;3:612–615.
63. Northway WH, Rosan RCC, Porter DY. Pulmonary disease following respiratory therapy of hyaline membrane disease. *N Engl J Med*. 1967;276:357–368.
64. Farrell PA, Fiascone JM. Bronchopulmonary dysplasia in the 1990s: A review for the pediatrician. *Curr Probl Pediatr*. 1997;27:129–163.
65. Jobe AH, Bancalari E. Bronchopulmonary dysplasia. National Institute of Child Health and Human Development National Heart Lung and Blood Institute Office of Rare Diseases Workshop Summary. *Am J Respir Crit Care Med*. 2001;163:1723–1729.
66. American Thoracic Society. Statement on the care of the child with chronic lung disease of infancy and childhood. *Am J Respir Crit Care Med*. 2003;168: 356–396.
67. Abman SH, Groothius JR. Pathophysiology and treatment of bronchopulmonary dysplasia. Current issues. *Pediatr Clinics*. 1994;41:277–315.
68. Cox JH. Bronchopulmonary dysplasia. In: Groh-Wargo S, Thompson M, Cox J, eds. *Nutritional Care for High-Risk Newborns*, 3rd ed. Chicago: Precept Press, Inc.; 2000;369–390.
69. Tammela OKT, Lanning FP, Koivisto ME. The relationship of fluid restriction during the 1st month of life to the occurrence and severity of bronchopulmonary dysplasia in low birth weight infants: A 1-year radiological follow up. *Eur J Pediatr*. 1992;151: 367–371.
70. Wilson DC, McClure G, Halliday HL, et al. Nutrition and bronchopulmonary dysplasia. *Arch Dis Child*. 1991;66:37–38.
71. Frank L, Sosenko IR. Undernutrition as a major contributing factor in the pathogenesis of bronchopulmonary dysplasia. *Am Rev Respir Dis*. 1988;138:725–729.
72. Northway WH. Bronchopulmonary dysplasia: Thirty-three years later. *Pediatric Pulmonology*. 2001; Suppl 23:5–7.
73. Giacoia GP, Venkataraman PS, West-Wilson KI, Faulkner MJ. Follow-up of school-age children with bronchopulmonary dysplasia. *J Pediatr*. 1997;130: 400–408.
74. Weinstein MR, Oh W. Oxygen consumption in infants with bronchopulmonary dysplasia. *J Pediatr*. 1981; 99:958–960.
75. Kurzner WI, Garg M, Bautista DB, et al. Growth failure in infants with bronchopulmonary dysplasia: Nutrition and elevated resting metabolic expenditure. *Pediatrics*. 1988;81:379–384.
76. Yunis KA, Oh W. Effects of intravenous glucose loading on oxygen consumption, carbon dioxide production, and resting energy expenditure in infants with bronchopulmonary dysplasia. *J Pediatr*. 1989;115:127–132.
77. Yeh TF, McClenan DA, Ajayi OA, Pildes RS. Metabolic rate and energy balance in infants with bronchopulmonary dysplasia. *J Pediatr*. 1989;114:448–451.
78. deGamarra E. Energy expenditure in premature newborns with bronchopulmonary dysplasia. *Biol Neonate*. 1992;61:337–44.
79. Singer L, Martin RJ, Hawkins SW, et al. Oxygen desaturation complicates feeding in infants with bronchopulmonary dysplasia after discharge. *Pediatrics*. 1992;90:380–384.
80. Garg M, Kurzner SI, Bautista DB, Keens TG. Clinically unsuspected hypoxia during sleep and feeding in infants with bronchopulmonary dysplasia. *Pediatrics*. 1988; 81:635–642.

81. Shankaran S, Szego E, Eizert D, Siegel P. Severe bronchopulmonary dysplasia: Predictors of survival and outcome. *Chest*. 1984;86:607.

82. deRegnier RA, Guilbert TW, Mills MM, Georgieff MK. Growth failure and altered body composition are established by one month of age in infants with bronchopulmonary dysplasia. *J Nutr*. 1996;126:168–175.

83. Johnson DB, Cheney C, Monsen ER. Nutrition and feeding in infants with bronchopulmonary dysplasia after initial hospital discharge: Risk factors for growth failure. *J Am Diet Assoc*. 1998;98: 649–656.

84. Huysman WA, deRidder M, deBruin NC, et al. Growth and body composition in preterm infants with bronchopulmonary dysplasia. *Arch Dis Child Fetal Neonatal Ed*. 2003;88:F46–F51.

85. Vrlenich LA, Bozynski ME, Shyr Y, et al. The effect of bronchopulmonary dysplasia on growth at school age. *Pediatrics*. 1995;95:855–859.

86. Moyer-Mileur LJ, Nielson DW, Pfeffer KD, et al. Eliminating sleep-associated hypoxemia improves growth in infants with bronchopulmonary dysplasia. *Pediatrics*. 1996;98: 779–783.

87. Groothuis JF, Rosenberg AA. Home oxygen promotes weight gain in infants with bronchopulmonary dysplasia. *AJDC*. 1987;141: 992–995.

88. Babson SG, Benda GI. Growth graphs for the clinical assessment of infants of varying gestational age. *J Pediatr*. 1976;89:814–820.

89. Oh W. Nutritional management of infants with bronchopulmonary dysplasia. In: Farrell PM, Taussig LM, eds. *Bronchopulmonary Dysplasia and Related Chronic Respiratory Disorders*. Columbus, OH: Ross Laboratories; 1986;96–101.

90. Niermeyer S. Nutritional and metabolic problems in infants with bronchopulmonary dysplasia. In: Bancalari E, Stocker JT, eds. *Bronchopulmonary Dysplasia*. Washington, DC: Hemisphere Publishing Corp.; 1988;313–336.

91. Zachman RD. Role of vitamin A in lung development. *J Nutr*. 1995;125:1634S–1638S.

92. Robbins ST, Fletcher AB. Early vs. delayed vitamin A supplementation in very-low-birth-weight infants. *JPEN*. 1993;17:220–225.

93. Kennedy KA, Stoll BJ, Ehrenkranz RA, et al. Vitamin A to prevent bronchopulmonary dysplasia in very-low-birth-weight infants: Has the dose been too low? *Early Human Dev*. 1997;49:19–31.

94. Tyson JE, Wright LL, Oh W, et al. Vitamin A supplementation for extremely-low-birth-weight infants. *New Eng J Med*. 1999;340:1962–1968.

95. Shenai JP. Vitamin A supplementation in very low birth weight neonates: Rationale and evidence. *Pediatrics*. 1999;104:1369–1374.

96. Atkinson SA. Special nutritional needs of infants for prevention of and recovery from bronchopulmonary dysplasia. *J Nutr*. 2001;131:942S–946S.

97. Higashi A, Ikeda T, Iribe K, Matsuda I. Zinc balance in premature infants given the minimal dietary zinc requirement. *J Pediatr*. 1988;112:262–266.

98. American Academy of Pediatrics, Committee on Nutrition. Kleinman RE, ed., *Pediatric Nutrition Handbook*, 5th ed. Elk Grove Village, IL: American Academy of Pediatrics; 2004.

99. Reimers KJ, Carlson SJ, Lombard KA. Nutritional management of infants with bronchopulmonary dysplasia. *Nutr Clin Prac*. 1992;7:127–132.

100. Green HL, Hazlett D, Demarec R. Relationship between intralipid-induced hyperlipemia and pulmonary function. *Am J Clin Nutr*. 1976;29:127–135.

101. Friedman Z, Marks KH, Maisels J, et al. Effect of parenteral fat emulsion on the pulmonary and reticuloendothelial systems in the newborn infant. *Pediatrics*. 1978;61:694.

102. Perira GR, Foxx WW, Stanely CA, et al. Decreased oxygenation and hyperlipemia during intravenous fat infusions in premature infants. *Pediatrics*. 1980;66:26–30.

103. Stahl GE, Spear MC, Egler JM, et al. The effect of lipid infusion rate on oxygenation in premature infants. *Pediatr Res*. 1984;18:406A.

104. Boehm G, Bierbach U, Moro G, Minoli I. Limited fat digestion in infants with bronchopulmonary dysplasia. *J Pediatr Gastroenterol Nutr*. 1996;22:161–166.

105. Johnson, D. *Gaining and Growing: Assuring Nutritional Care of Preterm Infants*. University of Washington. Available at http://depts.washington.edu/growing.

106. Brunton JA, Saigal S, Atkinson SA. Growth and body composition in infants with bronchopulmonary dysplasia up to 3 months corrected age: A randomized trial of a high-energy nutrient-enriched formula fed after hospital discharge. *J Pediatr*. 1998;133:340–345.

107. Gewolb IH, Bosma JF, Taciak VL, Vice FL. Abnormal developmental patterns of suck and swallow rhythms during feeding in preterm infants with bronchopulmonary dysplasia. *Dev Med Child Neur*. 2001;43: 454–459.

108. Singer LT, Davillier M, Preuss L, et al. Feeding interactions in infants with very low birth weight and bronchopulmonary dysplasia. *J Dev Behav Pediatr*. 1996; 17:69–76.

109. Centers for Disease Control, National Center for Health Statistics. Asthma prevalence, health care use and morbidity, 2000–2001. Retrieved April 1, 2004, from www.cdc.gov/nchs/products/pubs/pubd/hestats/asthma/asthma.htm.

110. Mannino DM, Homa DM, Akinbami LJ, et al. Surveillance for asthma—United States, 1980–1999.

In: *Surveillance Summaries*, March 29, 2002. *MMWR*. 2002;51:1–13.

111. Centers for Disease Control and Prevention. Asthma prevalence and control characteristics by race/ethnicity—United States, 2002. *MMWR*. 2004;53:145–148.

112. Rodriguez MA, Winkleby MA, Ahn D, et al. Identification of population subgroups of children and adolescents with high asthma prevalence. *Arch Pediatr Adolesc Med*. 2002;156:269–275.

113. Johnston J. Lower respiratory disorders. In: Millonig VL, Mobley C. eds. *Pediatric Nurse Practitioner Certification Review Guide,* 4th ed. Potomac, MD: Health Leadership Associates, Inc.; 2004.

114. U.S. Department of Health and Human Services. *Healthy People 2010* (Conference edition, in two volumes). Washington, DC: USDHHS; January 2000.

115. National Heart, Lung, and Blood Institute. *Highlights of the Expert Panel Report 2: Guidelines for the Diagnosis and Management of Asthma*. NIH Publication No. 97-4051A. Bethesda, MD: NHLBI; 1997.

116. Sampson HA. IgE-mediated food intolerance. *J Allergy Clin Immunol*. 1988;81:495–504.

117. National Asthma Education and Prevention Program, National Heart, Lung, and Blood Institute. *Expert Panel Report: Guidelines for the Diagnosis and Management of Asthma—Update of Selected Topics 2002*. Publication no. 02-5075. Bethesda, MD: National Institutes of Health; 2002.

118. Monteleone CA, Sherman AR. Nutrition and asthma. *Arch Intern Med*. 1997;157:23–34.

119. Adler BR, Assadullahi T, Warner JA, Warner JO. Evaluation of a multiple food specific IgE antibody test compared to parental perception, allergy skin tests and RAST. *Clin Exp Allergy*. 1991;21:683–688.

120. Bock SA. Respiratory reactions induced by food challenges in children with pulmonary disease. *Pediatr Allergy Immunol*. 1992;3:188–194.

121. James JM, Berhisel-Broadbent J, Sampson HA. Respiratory reactions provoked by double-blind food challenges in children. *Am J Respir Crit Care Med*. 1994;149:59–64.

122. Onorato J, Merland N, Terral C, et al. Placebo-controlled double-blind food challenge in asthma. *J Allergy Clin Immunol*. 1986;78:1139–1146.

123. Arney WK, Pinnock CB. The milk mucus belief: Sensations associated with the belief and characteristics of believers. *Appetite*. 1993;20:53–60.

124. Pinnock CB, Arney WK. The milk-mucus belief: Sensory analysis comparing cow's milk and a soy placebo. *Appetite*. 1993;20:61–70.

125. Nguyen MT. Effect of cow milk on pulmonary function in atopic asthmatic patients. *Ann Allergy Asthma Immunol*. 1997;79:62–64.

126. Chulada PC, Arbes SJ, Dunson D, Zeldin DC. Breastfeeding and the prevalence of asthma and wheeze in children: Analyses from the Third National Health and Nutrition Examination Survey. *J Allergy Clin Immunol*. 2003;112:328–336.

127. Rust GS, Thompson CJ, Minor P, Davis-Mitchell W, et al. Does breastfeeding protect children from asthma? Analysis of NHANES III survey data. *J Nat Med Assoc*. 2001;93:139–148.

128. Wright AL, Holberg CJ, Taussig LM, Martinez F. Maternal asthma status alters relation of infant feeding to asthma childhood. *Advances in Exper Med & Biol*. 2000;478:131–137.

129. Chinn S. Obesity and asthma: Evidence for and against a causal relation. *J of Asthma*. 2003;40:1–16.

130. Camargo CA, Weiss ST, Zhang S, Willett WC, Speizer FE. Prospective study of body mass index, weight change, and risk of adult-onset asthma in women. *Arch Intern Med*. 1999;159:2582–2588.

131. Stenius-Aarniala B, Poussa T, Kvarnstrom J, et al. Immediate and long term effects of weight reduction in obese people with asthma: randomized controlled study. *BMJ*. 2000;320:827–832.

132. Luder E, Melnik TA, DiMaio M. Association of being overweight with greater asthma symptoms in inner city black and Hispanic children. *J Pediatr*. 1998;132: 699–703.

133. Gennuso J, Epstein LH, Paluch RA, Cerny F. The relationship between asthma and obesity in urban minority children and adolescents. *Arch Pediatr Adolesc Med*. 1998;152:1197–1200.

134. Belamarich PF, Luder E, Kattan M, et al. Do obese inner-city children with asthma have more symptoms than nonobese children with asthma? *Pediatrics*. 2000;106:1436–1441.

135. Castro-Rodriguez JA, Holbert CJ, Morgan WJ, Wright AL, Martinez FD. Increased incidence of asthmalike symptoms in girls who become overweight or obese during the school years. *Am J Respir Crit Care Med*. 2001;163:1344–1349.

136. Gilliland FD, Berhane K, Islam T, et al. Obesity and the risk of newly diagnosed asthma in school-age children. *Amer J Epi*. 2003;158:406–415.

137. Tantisira KG, Litonjua AA, Weiss ST, Fuhlbrigge AL, for the Childhood Asthma Management Program Research Group. Association of body mass with pulmonary function in the Childhood Asthma Management Program (CAMP). *Thorax*. 2003;58:1036–1041.

138. Schwartz J, Weiss ST. Relationship between dietary vitamin C intake and pulmonary function in the first National Health and Nutrition Examination Survey (NHANES I). *Amer J Clin Nutr*. 1994;59:110–114.

139. Cook DG, Carey IM, Whincup PH, et al. Effect of fresh fruit consumption on lung function and wheeze in children. *Thorax.* 1997;52:628–633.

140. Spector SL, Surette ME. Diet and asthma: Has the role of dietary lipids been overlooked in the management of asthma? *Ann Allergy Asthma Immunol.* 2003;90:371–377.

141. Schwartz J, Weiss ST. The relationship of dietary fish intake to level of pulmonary function in the first National Health and Nutrition Examination Survey (NHANES I). *Eur Respir J.* 1994;7:1821–1824.

142. Peat JK, Salome CM, Woolcock AJ. Factors associated with bronchial hyperresponsiveness in Australian adults and children. *Eur Respir J.* 1992;5:921–929.

143. Hodge I, Salome CM, Peat JK, et al. Consumption of oily fish and childhood asthma risk. *Med J Austr.* 1996;164:137–140.

144. Hodge L, Salome CM, Hughes JM, et al. Effect of dietary intake of omega-3 and omega-6 fatty acids on severity of asthma in children. *Eur Respir J.* 1998;11:361–365.

145. Nagakura T, Matsuda S, Shichijyo K, et al. Dietary supplementation with fish oil rich in omega-3 polyunsaturated fatty acids in children with bronchial asthma. *Eur Respir J.* 2000;16:861–865.

146. Morris A, Noakes M, Clifton PM. The role of n-6 polyunsaturated fat in stable asthmatics. *J of Asthma.* 2001;38:311–319.

147. Britton J, Pavord I, Wisniewski A, et al. Dietary magnesium, lung function, wheezing, and airway hyperreactivity in a random adult population. *Lancet.* 1994;344:357–363.

148. Price JF. Asthma, growth and inhaled corticosteroids. *Resp Med.* 1993;87:23–26.

149. Merkus PJFM, van Essen-Zandvliet EEM, Duiverman EJ, et al. Long-term effect of inhaled corticosteroids on growth rate in adolescents with asthma. *Pediatrics.* 1993;91:1121–1126.

150. Agertoft L, Pedersen S. Effects of long-term treatment with an inhaled corticosteroid on growth and pulmonary function in asthmatic children. *Resp Med.* 1994;88:373–381.

151. Allen DB, Bronshky EA, LaForce CF, et al. Growth in asthmatic children treated with fluticasone propionate. *J Pediatr.* 1998;132:472–477.

152. Sharek PJ, Bergman DA. The effect of inhaled steroids on the linear growth of children with asthma: A meta-analysis. *Pediatr.* 2000;106. Retrieved February 1, 2002, from www.pediatrics.org/cgi/content/full/106/1/e8.

153. Agertoft L, Pedersen S. Effect of long-term treatment with inhaled budesonide on adult height in children with asthma. *N Eng J Med.* 2000;343:1064–1069.

154. Allen DB. Inhaled corticosteroid therapy for asthma in preschool children: Growth issues. *Pediatrics.* 2002;109:373–380.

155. Hosking DJ. Effects of corticosteroids on bone turnover. *Resp Med.* 1993;87:15–21.

156. Barnes NC. Safety of high-dose inhaled corticosteroids. *Resp Med.* 1993;87:27–31.

157. Boner AL, Piacentini GL. Inhaled corticosteroids in children. Is there a "safe" dosage? *Drug Safety.* 1993;9:9–20.

158. Crowley S, Trivedi P, Risteli L, et al. Collagen metabolism and growth in prepubertal children with asthma treated with inhaled steroids. *J Pediatr.* 1998;132:409–413.

159. Martinati LC, Bertoldo F, Gasperi E, et al. Effect on cortical and trabecular bone mass of different anti-inflammatory treatments in preadolescent children with chronic asthma. *Am J Respir Crit Care Med.* 1996;153:232–236.

160. Picado C, Luengo M. Corticosteroid-induced bone loss. *Drug Safety.* 1996;15:347–359.

161. Gagnon L, Boulet LP, Brown J, Desrosiers T. Influence of inhaled corticosteroids and dietary intake on bone density and metabolism in patients with moderate to severe asthma. *J Amer Diet Assoc.* 1997;97:1401–1406.

162. U.S. Department of Agriculture. *Food Guide Pyramid: A guide to daily food choice.* Home and Garden Bulletin No. 252. Washington, DC: USDA, Human Nutrition Information Service; 1992.

163. U.S. Department of Agriculture and U.S. Department of Health and Human Services. *Dietary Guidelines for Americans,* 2000, 5th ed. Home and Garden Bulletin No. 232, Washington, DC: www.nal.usda.gov/fnic/dguide95.html.

164. Neumark-Sztainer D, Story M, Resnick MD, et al. Body dissatisfaction and unhealthy weight-control practices among adolescents with and without chronic illness: A population-based study. *Arch Pediatr Adolesc Med.* 1995;149:1330–1335.

165. Dinsmoor R. Alternative therapies—Are they effective in treating asthma? In: *Asthma,* Butler RE, ed. Newton, MA: Sept./Oct. 1998.

RESOURCES

Books

Advance, newsletter of the Asthma and Allergy Foundation of America, 1125 15th St. NW, Suite 502, Washington, DC 2005;202-466-7643;800-7-ASTHMA; www.aafa.org

Bowser EK, Farris R, Johnson D, Luder E, Marcus M, Sondel SA, Walker S, Wooldridge N, Zerzan J. *Chronic Pulmonary Conditions in Children: Case Studies for Nutrition Management.* Chicago, IL: Pediatric Nutrition Practice Group, American Dietetic Association; 1999.

Hardin DS, Brunzell C, Schissel K, Schindler T, Moran A. *Managing Cystic Fibrosis Related Diabetes (CFRD). An Instruction Guide for Patients and Families.* Bethesda, MD: Cystic Fibrosis Foundation; 1999.

Cookbooks

A Way of Life: Cystic Fibrosis Nutrition Handbook and Cookbook, 2nd ed., 1997. Available from Pediatric Pulmonary Center, Food and Nutrition Services, University of Wisconsin Hospital and Clinics, 600 Highland Avenue, Room F4/120, Madison, WI 53792–1510.

Web Pages

www.cff.org. The Cystic Fibrosis Foundation home page has general information about CF, patient education materials, and archived virtual patient education days.

http://depts.washington.edu/growing. Gaining and Growing: Assuring Nutritional Care of Preterm Infants, initiated by Donna Johnson, PhD, RD, University of Washington. This site was funded by a grant from the Maternal and Child Health Bureau, Health Resources and Services Administration, U.S. Department of Health and Human Services.

www.mchneighborhood.ichp.edu/ppc. Pediatric Pulmonary Centers, Maternal and Child Health Bureau, Health Resources and Services Administration, Department of Health and Human Services.

CHAPTER 16

Gastrointestinal Disorders

Jacqueline Jones Wessel and Patricia Queen Samour

The gastrointestinal tract—that may be thought of as a tube that processes and absorbs nutrients—is the site of the assimilation of macro- and micronutrients, vitamins, and minerals. The function of the gastrointestinal tract may be disrupted by disease and result in alterations in nutritional requirements. Many nutrients are absorbed throughout the intestinal tract, while others are absorbed only from specific sites. Absorption of the latter class of nutrients is particularly vulnerable to disease or surgical resection. In Figure 16–1, the principal sites of absorption of macro- and micronutrients, vitamins, and minerals are presented.

Most symptoms of gastrointestinal disease can arise from disorders located in a specific region of the bowel, the entire bowel, or distant sites (e.g., vomiting can occur due to pyloric stenosis, gastroenteritis, or a brain tumor). In Figure 16–2, conditions that involve portions of the gastrointestinal tract rather than the entire tract are presented. In Table 16–1, common symptoms are grouped according to their most common location of origin. The differential diagnosis of these symptoms and treatment of the etiology of symptoms are presented.

DIAGNOSTIC TESTS

A myriad of tests is available to evaluate gastrointestinal function. The tests most commonly performed are presented in Table 16–2. For each test, the procedure and potential diagnoses are listed.

Acute Diarrhea

Acute diarrhea, namely, diarrhea of less than 7 days duration, is among the most common reasons for seeking the assistance of a pediatrician. Under most circumstances, a normal diet should be continued throughout the illness. When dehydration is imminent, the use of maintenance glucose-electrolyte solutions may prevent progression of the illness. When patients become dehydrated, oral rehydration solutions or intravenous fluids may be required. The composition of commonly used oral maintenance and rehydration solutions is presented in Table 16–3.

Nutrition Management

The American Academy of Pediatrics recommends that infants or children with mild to moderate dehydration be rehydrated within 4 to 6 hours, then offered age-appropriate foods, with resumption of breastfeeding for breast-fed infants.[1] For bottle-fed infants, there is controversy regarding whether a lactose-free formula is necessary.[1–6] The most practical solution would seem to be if a child's diarrhea worsens upon returning to a lactose-containing formula, lactose-free feedings should be used until the illness has resolved.[7] Full-strength formula should be used because dilution of formula has not shown to improve outcome.[8] A soy protein, lactose-free formula with added soy polysaccharide fiber has been used in the treatment of acute diarrhea. The fiber-containing formula decreased the duration of diarrheal symptoms significantly in two studies on infants and toddlers.[9,10]

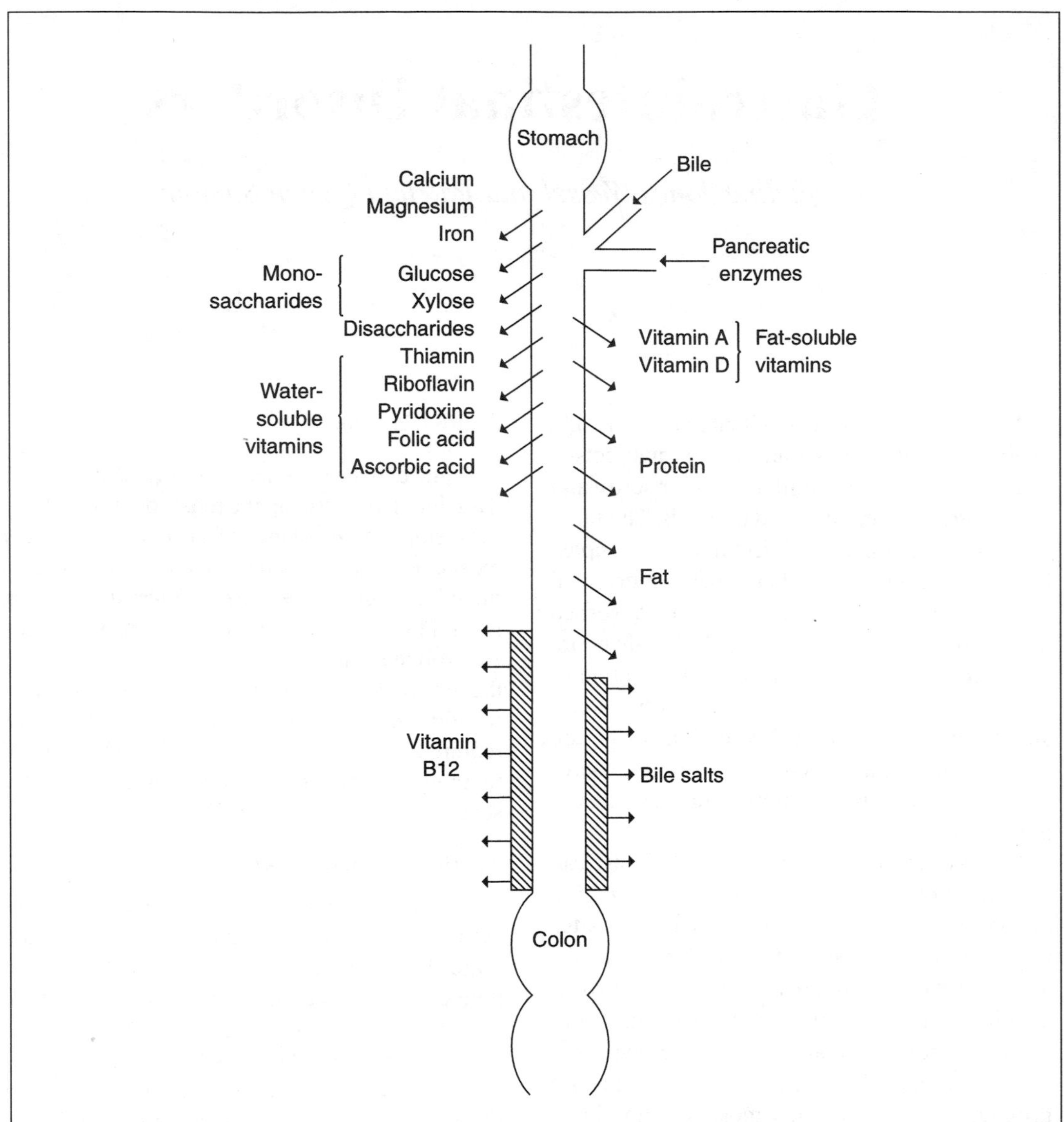

Figure 16–1 Principal Sites of Absorption of Nutrients. *Source:* Reprinted from *Handbook of Physiology*, vol. 3, ed. 6 by CC Booth with permission of the American Physiological Society, © 1968.

Chronic Diarrhea of Infancy

Chronic diarrhea of infancy, also called protracted diarrhea of infancy, is a reversible clinical condition,[11] and considered to be a nutritional disorder.[12,13] As with all diarrheal illnesses in infants, chronic diarrhea is dangerous if not treated promptly and appropriately, because it can result in dehydration and severe malnutrition.[14] Chronic diarrhea is most commonly seen in the first 6 months of life and occurs typically after an acute bout of diarrhea. The pathogenesis is largely unknown, and most likely has

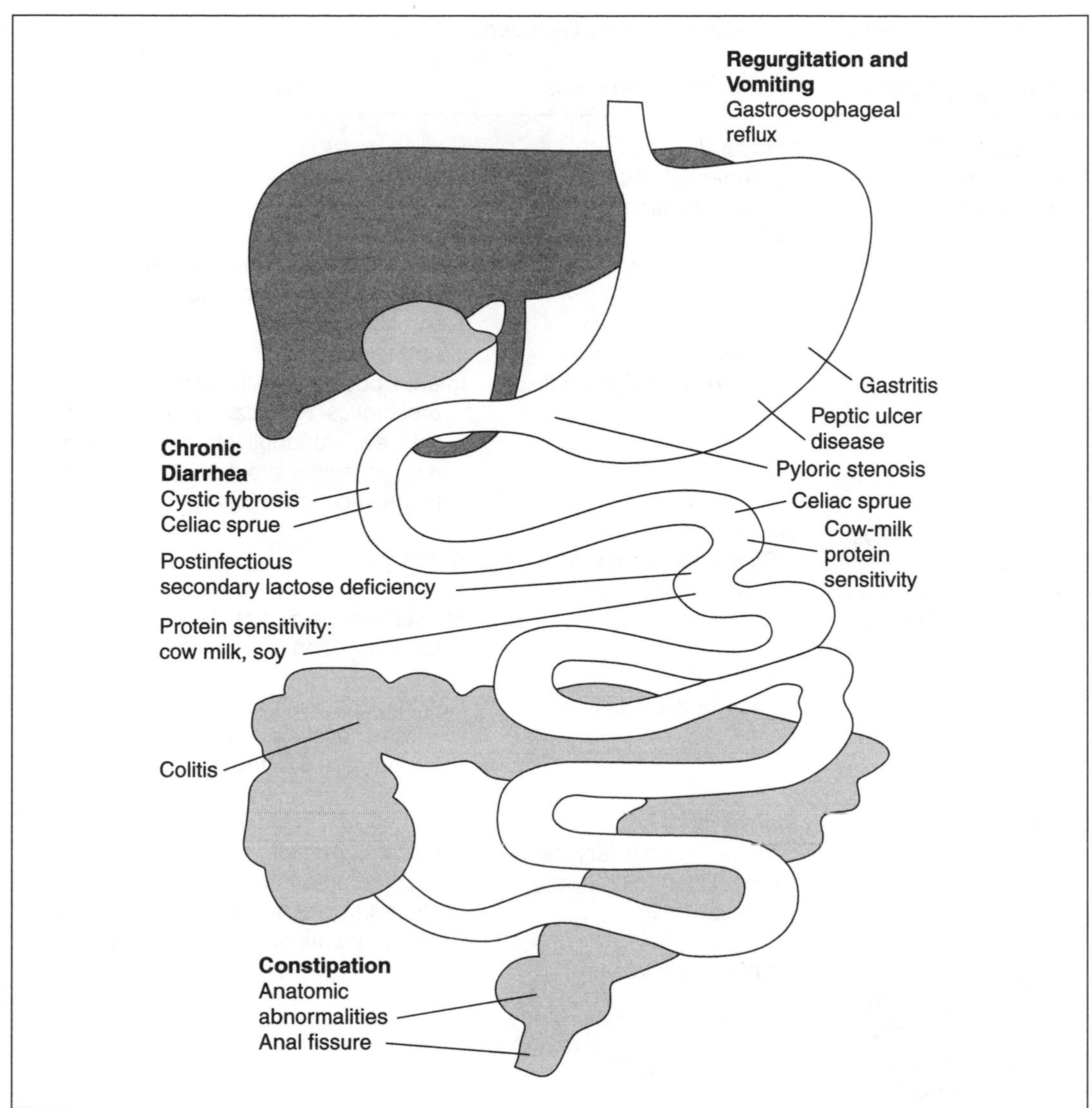

Figure 16–2 The Site of Pathology Within the Gastrointestinal Tract Varies with the Disease Process. *Source:* Used with permission of Ross Products Division, Abbott Laboratories, Inc., Columbus, OH 43216. From *Problems Relating to Feedings in First Two Years*, © 1977, Ross Products Division, Abbott Laboratories, Inc.

many contributing factors. Chronic diarrhea results in a malnourished infant with a characteristic large volume, acidic, and often gassy diarrhea.[11]

Nutrition Management

In an effort by the family to reduce stooling, the diet is usually restricted and malnutrition results.[14] As discussed earlier, the recommendations for diet therapy for diarrhea are to resume normal diet after 4 to 6 hours of rehydration.[1] The typical treatment, however, is bowel rest, then clear liquids, followed by a restrictive diet such as the BRAT diet (bananas, rice, apple juice, and toast).[15] Restrictive diets are usually nutritionally

Table 16–1 Common Pediatric Gastrointestinal Disorders

Presenting Symptom	*Differential Diagnosis*	*Treatment*
Stomach and Esophagus	*Structural:*	
Vomiting/ regurgitation	Congenital anomaly of the gastrointestinal tract	Surgery
	Inflammatory:	
	Peptic disease	Medications, e.g., antacids; avoid caffeine-containing foods, alcohol, smoking
	Functional:	
	Gastroesophageal reflux	Infants: positioning, thickened feeds, prokinetics. Surgical treatment if above fails, e.g., fundoplication. Medications, e.g., antacids; avoid caffeine-containing foods, alcohol, smoking
Dysphagia (choking after eating), odynophagia (pain with swallowing)	*Structural:*	
	Congenital anomalies	Surgery
	Inflammatory:	
	Peptic strictures	Medications, e.g., antacids; dilatation, fundoplication
	Functional:	
	Esophageal spasms	Calcium channel blockers and nitrates; avoid extreme temperatures in foods
Pancreas and Liver	*Structural:*	
Jaundice	Extrahepatic biliary tract obstruction, e.g., biliary atresia	Surgical correction; fat-soluble vitamin supplementation (fat source: MCT); choleretic agents, e.g., phenobarbital, cholestyramine, ursodeoxycholate
Failure to tolerate feeds, persistent bilious vomiting, and distended upper abdomen	Annular pancreas	Surgery
Recurrent abdominal pain, jaundice	Gallstones	Surgery, lithotripsy, dissolution therapy
	Choledochal cyst	Surgery
Anorexia, nausea, vomiting, jaundice	*Inflammatory:*	
	Hepatitis	Diet as tolerated; steroids for autoimmune hepatitis
Abdominal pain	Pancreatitis	NPO; nasogastric suctioning; TPN if prolonged course. Medications: pain control (e.g., meperidine), H_2 antagonists (i.e., cimetadine), pancreatic enzyme replacement. When improved, high-CHO, low-fat diet. Elemental diet may be beneficial.

continues

Table 16–1 continued

Presenting Symptom	*Differential Diagnosis*	*Treatment*
	Functional:	
	Hereditary metabolic disorders	See Chapter 13
Meconium ileus, failure to thrive, chronic diarrhea	Pancreatic insufficiency, e.g., cystic fibrosis, Shwachman/ Diamond syndrome	Enzyme replacement therapy; fat-soluble vitamin supplementation; high-calorie, high-fat diet
Small bowel and colon	*Structural:*	
Failure to thrive, diarrhea	Short bowel syndrome	TPN progressing to MCT-predominate hydrolysate formula; vitamin and mineral supplements
Abdominal distention, steatorrhea	Lymphangiectasia, protein-losing enteropathy	Surgical excision, if possible. Fat-soluble vitamin supplementation. High-calorie, high-protein, low-LCT diet; high-MCT diet or TPN may be necessary.
Anemia, gastrointestinal bleeding	Congenital malformations, e.g., Meckel's diverticulum, duplication cysts	Surgery
	Inflammatory:	
Diarrhea, vomiting	Infectious enteropathies	Oral rehydration solutions, followed by lactose and/or sucrose restrictions*
Failure to thrive, abdominal distention, steatorrhea	Gluten-sensitive enteropathy (celiac disease)	Gluten-free diet
Failure to thrive, vomiting, diarrhea	Dietary protein intolerance	Hydrolysate formula, elimination diet
Postprandial abdominal pain	Inflammatory bowel disease, small bowel (Crohn's) disease	High-calorie diet; B12 supplementation if ileum affected
Rectal bleeding, diarrhea, tenesmus	Ulcerative colitis or Crohn's disease of the colon	High-calorie diet; folate supplementation; low-residue diet,† if strictures or active colitis; other foods as tolerated
Fermentive diarrhea after introduction of sucrose-containing foods	*Functional:* Congenital enzyme deficiency, e.g., sucrase/isomaltase deficiency	Dietary restrictions of sucrose-containing foods

continues

Table 16–1 continued

Presenting Symptom	*Differential Diagnosis*	*Treatment*
Severe, watery diarrhea from first day of life	Lactase deficiency	Dietary restrictions with calcium supplement or enzyme replacement, i.e., Lactaid, Lactrase
Chronic diarrhea, normal growth pattern	Irritable bowel syndrome (chronic nonspecific diarrhea, toddler's diarrhea, or spastic colon)‡	Normal diet for age, increased fiber intake, decreased intake of sorbitol-containing beverages (apple and pear juice)
Constipation	*Structural:* Hirschsprung's disease; post-NEC strictures	Surgery
	Functional: Constipation	Complete bowel clean out using saltwater enemas, mineral oil; high-fiber diet, bowel habit training. In infants, increase CHO content of diet using sucrose, dextrimaltose

LCT, long-chain triglycerides; MCT, medium-chain triglycerides; NEC, necrotizing enterocolitis; TPN, total parenteral nutrition.

* The use of oral rehydration solutions should be closely monitored. Oral rehydration solutions should be used for 6–8 hours, then infant refeeding should begin to prevent further weight loss. To refeed, oral rehydration solutions may be alternated with a full-strength lactose-free formula for the first few feedings, or a concentrated formula may be reconstituted with the rehydration solution. Studies have shown that early refeeding does not exacerbate the diarrhea, and the child recovers more quickly. Frequently, the cow milk–based formula the child may have been consuming prior to the enteropathy may be used instead of a lactose-free formula. If a lactose-free formula is preferred, the previous formula may be reintroduced after a period of 1 or more weeks.

†The use of milk or a low-residue diet should be dictated by the individual tolerance of the patient.

‡This disorder often follows a bout of infectious enteropathy or antibiotic therapy and is exacerbated by increased fluid intake or strict elimination diets. A good rule of thumb is to "feed the child, not the diarrhea."

Source: Reprinted from Boyne LJ, Heitlinger LA, Gastrointestinal disorders. In: Queen PM, Lang CE, eds., *Handbook of Pediatric Nutrition.* © 1993, Aspen Publishers, Inc.

incomplete and deficient in protein, calories, vitamins, and minerals. Severe malnutrition can result if the restrictions are followed for an extended period of time.[14]

In chronic diarrhea, the enterocyte is damaged and the absorptive ability of the intestine is compromised. There is a downward spiral as the infant becomes weak and compromised from malnutrition. Voluntary oral intake decreases and the infant becomes more dehydrated and more malnourished, and the enterocyte cannot heal. In the acute phase, small intestinal mucosal biopsy reveals villous atrophy.[16] Mucosal disaccharidase activity is significantly decreased with lactase most severely affected, then sucrase, and glucoamylase the least affected.[17] The intestinal absorptive capacity is decreased by approximately tenfold[11] and there is a linear relationship with the ability to absorb glucose.[16]

Treatment

The treatment for chronic diarrhea of infancy is completely nutritional.[11] The first step is appropriate fluid resuscitation. Next, cautious refeeding through enteral feedings or enteral and parenteral nutrition is started slowly due to the possibility of metabolic alterations from refeeding syndrome.[18] Carbohydrate should be increased

Table 16–2 Common Diagnostic Tests for Pediatric Gastrointestinal Disorders

Test	*Procedure*	*Diagnosis*
Barium swallow	Swallow barium sulfate; upper gastrointestinal tract and small bowel visualized by fluoroscopy. NPO 4 hours.	Hiatal hernia, stricture, dysmotility disorders, varices
Esophageal pH monitoring	8 French tube with pH sensor on end, inserted for 24 hours. Infants fed 1/2 formula, 1/2 apple juice every 4 hours. Older child fed applesauce, and apple juice added to diet.	Gastroesophageal reflux
Esophago-gastro-duodenoscopy (EGD)	Fiberoptic tube into upper gastrointestinal tract; lining visualized and biopsies taken. NPO.	Esophagitis, gastritis, duodenitis, peptic ulcer disease, caustic substance ingestions
Upper GI with small bowel follow-through	Swallow barium sulfate; look for strictures and mucosal lesions by fluoroscopy. NPO.	Inflammatory and structural lesions
Breath hydrogen	Oral sugar load of 1 g/kg to a maximum of 25 g. End expiratory breath collection. NPO.	Lactose or other sugar intolerance; peak after 90 minutes, rise of >20 ppm is positive
D-xylose	D-xylose administered in morning after fast after midnight. Dose: 0.35 g/kg. Blood drawn 1 hour after administration.	Malabsorption syndrome; normal if > 20 mg/dL
Quantitative fecal fat	Diet with > 30% total calories as fat for 2 days prior to stool collection. Three-day stool collection after charcoal marker noted in stool. (Do not use diaper creams, e.g., A&D ointment. Reverse disposable diaper for easier collection.)	Pancreatic insufficiency, e.g., cystic fibrosis; mucosal atrophy, e.g., celiac disease
Barium enema	Barium sulfate by enema. Lumen and mucosa of colon visualized by fluoroscopy.	Colitis, polyps, Hirschsprung's disease
Colonoscopy	Insertion of flexible fiberoptic tube via anus into large bowel. Visual examination of colonic lining, biopsies obtained (alternative to barium enema). NPO.	Colitis, polyps
Liver and pancreas tests		
Bilirubin	Blood (serum) test to determine excretory function of liver.	Hepatitis, biliary tract disease

continues

Table 16–2 continued

Test	*Procedure*	*Diagnosis*
Biliary tract nuclear scan	Intravenous injection of a bile salt analogue; images obtained over liver and bowel for 24 hours.	Obstructive lesions of biliary tree (e.g., impacted gall stones, biliary atresia); poor uptake is indicative of hepatitis
Plasma ammonia level	Blood (plasma) test to determine *detoxification* capabilities of liver.	Hepatic encephalopathy, hepatic failure, Reye's syndrome
Prothrombin time	Blood (whole blood) test to determine *synthetic* function of liver; vitamin K dependent, clotting factors.	If prothrombin time is prolonged and patient is not on antibiotics, hepatic protein synthesis diminishes
Ultrasonography	Study to determine gross structure of liver, evaluate liver and biliary systems.	Gallstones, pancreatic pseudocysts, biliary tract anomalies, biliary tract obstructions, hepatic tumors
Aminotransferase levels	Blood (serum) test to determine inflammation of liver due to virus, toxin.	Infectious, toxic, or autoimmune hepatitis
Serum amylase and lipase levels	Blood (serum) test to determine pancreatic inflammation or obstruction.	Acute or chronic pancreatitis. Amylase is elevated in mumps, pregnancy and lactation, pelvic inflammatory disease, and small bowel disease
Liver-spleen nuclear scan	Intravenous injection of a marker of blood flow. Poor uptake by liver and uptake by spleen, lung, and bone marrow indicative of portal hypertension.	Obstruction of extrahepatic blood vessels (e.g., portal vein thrombosis), cirrhosis, hepatic failure
Computed tomography scan of abdomen	Multiple radiographs of abdomen with or without intraluminal and/or intravenous contrast. Computer reconstructs multiple images to generate "slices" through the abdomen. NPO.	Demonstration of organ size, consistency, blood flow, and function (kidney); identification of tumors and areas of inflammation (e.g., abscess)

Source: Reprinted from Boyne LJ, Heitlinger LA, Gastrointestinal disorders in *Handbook of Pediatric Nutrition:* Queen PM, Lang CE, eds., © 1993, Aspen Publishers, Inc.

Table 16–3 Composition of Oral Electrolyte-Glucose Solutions (Concentration When Reconstituted)

Solution	*Na⁺ (mEq/l)*	*K⁺ (mEq/l)*	*Cl⁻ (mEq/l)*	*Carbohydrate (g/l)*	*Osmolality (mOsM/l)*
Rehydration					
WHO-ORS*	90	20	80	20[1]	310
Rehydralyte†	75	20	65	25[1]	310
Maintenance					
Infalyte‡	50	25	45	0[1]	200
Ricelyte§	50	25	45	20[2]	290
Pedialyte†	45	20	35	25[1]	270
Resol‖	50	20	50	20[1]	269
Other clear liquids					
Cola¶	2	0.1		50–150[3]	550
Ginger ale¶	3	1		50–150[3]	540
Apple juice¶	3	28		100–150[4]	700
Chicken broth	250	8		0	450
Tea	0	0		0	5

*Continued use of this product without the addition of free water could lead to hypernatremia.
†Ross Laboratories, Columbus, OH.
‡Pennwalt, Rochester, NY.
§Mead Johnson, Evansville, IN.
‖Wyeth-Ayerst Laboratories, Philadelphia, PA.
¶These products also contain fructose.
[1]Containing glucose.
[2]Containing rice-syrup solids.
[3]High-fructose syrup.
[4]Sucrose.

Source: Reproduced with permission from *AAP News,* vol. 5, p. 5, 1989.

gradually; however, adequate normal levels of protein, lipid, and vitamins can be given.[19]

Electrolyte and Mineral Repletion

For the first week, daily serum potassium, phosphorus, glucose, and magnesium levels must be part of the laboratory monitoring if refeeding syndrome is a possibility.[20] Supplementation of potassium and phosphorus is often necessary. When a malnourished patient is rapidly refed by either the enteral or parenteral route, metabolic and clinical problems may occur as the result of the reversal of the adaptive mechanism to starvation.[21] Fluid and electrolyte shifts result; as the body becomes anabolic, minerals shift from extracellular to intracellular, and serum levels decrease. Hypophosphatemia, hypokalemia, and hypomagnesemia may develop as a result, which can lead to respiratory failure and circulatory collapse.[22] Mezoff and associates looked at the incidence of hypophosphatemia in children during nutritional recovery and found that abnormal anthropometric measurements, arm circumference, and arm muscle circumference under the 5th percentile may be predictive of patients at risk for refeeding syndrome.[23]

Parenteral and Enteral Nutrition

Parenteral nutrition is sometimes necessary if a child is extremely malnourished. This is often combined with enteral nutrition. In infants with intestinal problems, absorption of many nutrients may be improved by using continuous enteral feedings. A crossover study in infants with protracted diarrhea showed greater absorption of zinc, calcium, copper, fat, and nitrogen during continuous feedings than with bolus feedings.[24] Small bolus oral feedings may be retained for oral motor stimulation. The calories needed for catch-up growth may be in the range of 140–200 kcal/kg.[25] Supplemental zinc is added for diarrheal losses[26] in the amount of 8000 mcg/L if administered through parenteral nutrition, or two to three times the RDA if given orally.[27] Supplemental vitamin A may have a role in the nutritional therapy for chronic diarrhea.[28,29] Cereal and other infant foods should be continued as tolerated; however, juices should be avoided due to high osmolality. A lactose-free formula may be better tolerated in some infants, because studies in the treatment of acute diarrhea show shorter duration of acute bouts of diarrhea with a lactose-free formula compared to a lactose-containing formula.[30] For infants more severely affected, a semielemental protein hydrolysate formula such as Alimentum (Ross Products) or Pregestimil (Mead Johnson) may be used. Although elemental formulas are commonly used in many hospitals because short peptides are absorbed better than an equimolar amount of amino acids,[31,32] a semielemental formula may be superior to an elemental amino acid–based formula such as Neocate (Scientific Hospital Supply) or Elecare (Ross Products).

As the infant improves, parenteral nutrition or IV hydration, if needed, is weaned, and enteral nutrition gradually increased in the form of continuous feedings. Larger bolus oral feedings are added gradually as tolerated. If this period of progressing from parenteral to enteral nutrition is prolonged, the transition from continuous feeding to oral bolus feedings can often be accomplished in the home setting.

Breastfeeding

As the enterocytes heal, calorie needs gradually decrease as absorption improves. If the infant was breast-fed and the mother is willing to express milk for a continuous feeding regimen, breast milk can be used. Because there is calorie loss from continuously infused breast milk through loss of protein and lipids,[33,34] consideration of this factor should be made in the calorie determinations. Alterations in the continuous infusion-feeding method can be made to maximize nutrient delivery by using the shortest amount of tubing available and slanting the feeding syringe.[35] Another option is to use a formula in combination with breast milk for the continuous infusion for greater lipid delivery,[36] saving the expressed breast milk for oral feedings.

Fiber

No published studies to date have been conducted using a formula with fiber for the treatment of chronic diarrhea as has been used in acute diarrhea in infants.[9,10] Fiber has been used as part of a food-based regimen in several studies in underdeveloped countries. The World Health Organization has developed an algorithm for the treatment of persistent diarrhea using locally available foods and simple clinical guidelines for use in underdeveloped countries.[37] Kolacek and colleagues compared a modular diet using food with a semielemental infant formula in the treatment of chronic diarrhea. The modular diet was found to decrease the duration of diarrhea and decrease the time to nutritional recovery.[38] In another study, infant formula fermented with Lactobacillus bulgaris and Streptococcus thermophilus was compared to standard infant formula in the treatment of persistent diarrhea. Clinical treatment failure occurred in 45% of the formula group as compare to 15% of the "yogurt" formula group.[39] These creative studies based on the culture or available foods illustrate that the U.S. traditional formula-based plan is not the only method of treatment.

Incidence

Recent reports indicate that the incidence of chronic diarrhea has declined in the United States over the past two decades due to better treatment of acute diarrheal episodes.[11] Severe malnutrition, however, is still seen as a result of the management of diarrhea.[14] Education of parents and medical personnel as to the nutritional ramifications of the treatment of diarrhea may continue to improve patient outcomes.

Celiac Disease

Celiac disease is an immune-mediated enteropathic condition triggered in genetically susceptible individuals by the ingestion of gluten. Celiac disease is also called gluten-induced enteropathy because it is an intolerance to gliadin, a constituent of the protein gluten. This disease is a form of malabsorption primarily affecting the proximal portion of the small intestine with destruction of the villi. The incidence of celiac disease is now in 1 out of every 133 people in the United States according to a landmark study conducted by the Center for Celiac Research in 2003.[40] Celiac disease is often difficult to diagnose because some of the symptoms are not obvious—such as anemia and behavior problems. Celiac disease is diagnosed by intestinal biopsy. This biopsy is done if the antibody tests, endomysial (EMA) and tissue transglutaminase (TTG), come back positive. The principal therapy is the removal of gluten-containing foods from the diet. The infant foods to use and avoid are presented in Table 16–4. Traditionally wheat, rye, barley, and possibly oats are removed from the diet. There has been debate concerning whether or not to exclude oats from the diet.[41] Osteoporosis is a common finding in adult patients with celiac disease. Recently a study examined bone-mineral density in children and

Table 16–4 Gluten-Free Diet for Infants with Celiac Disease

	Use	*Avoid*
Formula	Breast milk or iron-fortified infant formula	None
Dry cereal	Beech-Nut, Mead Johnson: Rice Cereal; Gerber: Rice Cereal with Bananas; Heinz: Instant Rice Cereal	All others
Jarred cereal	Beech-Nut, Gerber: Strained Rice with Applesauce and Bananas; Gerber: Junior Rice with Mixed Fruit; Heinz: Instant Rice Cereal with Bananas and Apple Juice, Rice Cereal with Pears and Apple Juice; Mead Johnson: Bananas 'n Rice	All others
Fruits, juices	All plain	None
Vegetables	All except those to avoid, plus Mead Johnson: Peas 'n Rice, Carrots 'n Rice	Gerber: Mixed Vegetables, Strained Creamed Spinach, Junior Creamed Green Beans
Protein	All plain meats, egg yolks	None
	Beech-Nut: Chicken Rice Dinner, Turkey Rice Dinner, Vegetable Chicken Dinner, Cottage Cheese with Pineapple	All other dinners and high-meat dinners
Teething, finger foods	Gluten-free rice wafers, rice cakes; Gerber: Turkey, Chicken, or Meat Sticks	

Note: Gluten or possible gluten-containing foods are those that have the following ingredients listed on a food label: wheat, rye, oats, barley; flour or cereal products; malt, malt flavor; hydrolyzed vegetable or plant protein; modified food starch; or gluten-containing flavorings, vegetable gums, emulsifiers, or stabilizers. Gluten may be present in foods, either as a basic ingredient or added during preparation/processing by the manufacturer. Reading food labels is very important in strict adherence to a gluten-free diet.

Source: Reprinted with permission from Merritt RJ and Hack S, Infant feeding and enteral nutrition, in *Nutrition in Clinical Practice* (1988;3:47–64), Copyright © 1988, American Society for Parenteral and Enteral Nutrition.

adolescents at diagnosis. The celiac-diagnosed patients exhibited significantly lower bone density than control children. However, after 1 year of a gluten-free diet, their studies had normalized.[42] At diagnosis, it is not uncommon for anthropometric, biochemical, and bone-density data to be significantly abnormal. Another study has shown normalization of body mass composition after 1 year of a gluten-free diet.[43] These studies emphasize the need for early diagnosis and prompt treatment to restore optimal nutritional status. The key is diagnosis and adherence to a gluten-free diet.

Inflammatory Bowel Disease (IBD)

The two major diseases of inflammatory bowel disease (IBD) are Crohn's disease (CD) and ulcerative colitis (UC). Crohn's disease may occur in any portion of the gastrointestinal tract. UC is by definition confined to the colon with minimal involvement of the terminal ileum.[44] Other diseases that do not fit in either category are termed indeterminate colitis.[45] The two diseases have many features in common: diarrhea, gastrointestinal blood and protein loss, abdominal pain, weight loss, anemia, and growth failure. Approximately 30% of children with IBD will have growth failure; children with Crohn's disease are three times more likely to have permanent growth stunting than patients with UC. Children with IBD have growth failure due to inadequate intake, malabsorption, excessive nutrient losses, and increased nutrient needs. Inadequate intake may be due to abdominal discomfort, effort to decrease diarrhea, and lack of interest in a restricted diet. Altered taste perceptions can occur in children with zinc deficiency.[27] Medications such as metronidazole may also affect intake by changing taste perceptions. Children with Crohn's disease have dietary intakes significantly less than nonaffected peers.[46]

Nutrient Deficits-IBD

Nutrient deficits have been noted in 30–40% of adolescents and children with IBD.[46] Malabsorption can occur as a result of inflammation of the mucosa. Protein-losing enteropathy may result. Malabsorption may also occur as a result of bacterial overgrowth due to altered motility or strictures. Bile salt malabsorption can alter lipid absorption. Lactose intolerance is seen in approximately one sixth of children with CD and UC.[27] Patients who have had bowel resections may also malabsorb as a result of their shortened bowel length. Patients with resections or disease in the terminal ileum may not be able to absorb sufficient vitamin B12 and will need evaluation by the Schilling test and intramuscular supplementation, 1 mg every 3 months, if results are abnormal.

Other single nutrient deficiencies seen in IBD are folic acid and iron. Multiple deficiencies are more common and include protein, calcium, magnesium, zinc, vitamin D, and vitamin B12. Folic acid deficiency has been reported in 38% of patients with CD and 58% of those with UC. Zinc deficiency may be a result of malabsorption and losses from diarrhea and/or fistula drainage; clinical signs of deficiency are sometimes seen. Magnesium deficiency can also occur due to increased losses and may complicate active disease.[47–53]

Food-Drug Interactions

Drug-nutrient interactions from the pharmacotherapy used in the treatment of IBD may affect nutrition. Sulfasalazine (azulfidine) interferes with folate absorption.[27] Corticosteroid therapy interferes with absorption of calcium, phosphate, and zinc; doses greater than 12 mg/m^2 of body surface area can induce catabolism and affect linear growth.[54]

Malnutrition

Malnutrition appears to be the primary cause of growth failure in IBD.[44] Several nutritional rehabilitation studies have demonstrated the beneficial effect of supplemental nutrition therapy on growth. After supplementation, growth velocity equaled or exceeded normal controls. Some studies have used parenteral nutrition[55–58]; others have been successful with enteral supplementation.[59–65] Although both methods increased the rate of growth, parenteral nutrition is associated with greater complications and cost. The concept of using the gastrointestinal tract for nutritional rehabilitation in IBD is a milestone for enteral nutrition therapy.

Nutrition Management

Nutrition support appears to have both a primary and adjunctive role in the treatment of IBD.[46] Primary nutrition therapy appears to be more effective in the treatment of Crohn's disease than of ulcerative colitis.[46,49] Uncontrolled studies in children have used elemental formulas (with either amino acids or peptides) administered via nasogastric tube with immunosuppressive drugs. Hypoallergenic foods were gradually introduced. Symptoms resolved, growth rates improved, and corticosteroid doses were reduced by two- to fourfold. A 70% remission rate continued for 12 to 18 months after nutrition therapy was initiated.[44,66–68] Controlled studies were conducted in children with Crohn's disease comparing enteral formula against immunosuppressive drugs and sulfasalazine in the treatment of active disease.[69–71] The enteral formulas contained either amino acids, protein hydrolysate, or intact protein (casein) and were administered orally or by nasogastric tube for 1 to 2 months. Hypoallergenic foods were introduced gradually into the diet. The two groups were comparable in terms of markers of disease activity and remission lasted approximately 10 months. Height velocity was superior in the enteral nutrition group despite more sustained energy intake in the medications group.[44] Despite these positive studies in children and several others in adults comparing altered diet to the use of medications,[72–74] the European Cooperative Crohn's Disease study found opposite results using a semielemental formula. Medications were compared to a protein hydrolysate formula. Significantly higher remission and return to work rates at 6 weeks were displayed in the medication group.[75] Ludvigsson and associates found in a randomized controlled trial that a polymeric enteral formula and an elemental formula were similar in inducing remission in children with Crohn's disease. The children given a polymeric diet, however, had better weight gain.[76] In a study with adult CD patients, elemental formula was more effective in inducing remissions than semielemental formula.[77] Elemental diet and nutrition education in perforating and nonperforating Crohn's disease in adults was found to reduce the incidence of second resections.[78] Elemental diets with varying amounts of long-chain triglycerides were examined by the Bamba group.[79] Diets with high fat had a 25% rate of remission, medium fat 40% rate, and low-fat diets had an 80% rate of remission.[79]

Fatty Acids

Marine oils have been discussed as primary therapy for ulcerative colitis. These oils, which are high in omega-3 long-chain fatty acids, appear to modulate the immune response of the large bowel. In adult studies, a reduction in disease activity and reduction in corticosteroids was noted in patients receiving omega-3 oils in patients with UC but not CD.[80–82] Histological samples showed a difference in the fatty acid composition of the colon and a reduction in the number of inflammatory cells and inflammatory mediators.[80,82,83] There was, however, no difference in the relapse rate between treatment and control groups.[83]

Enteral Support

Although enteral feeding has been shown to reduce inflammation and improve well-being, nutrition, and growth, there has been discussion about what exactly affects the change. A study done by Bannerjee and associates showed that the improvement in growth and growth-related proteins were due to the anti-inflammatory effect of the enteral nutrition.[84]

Nutritional Rehabilitation

Nutritional rehabilitation requires increased calories and protein with 140–150% of RDA for age.[27] Multivitamin and folate, zinc, and iron supplementation should be considered and vitamin B12 sufficiency assessed. A high-calorie, high-protein, well-balanced diet should be encouraged. Restrictions should be based on individual tolerance rather than the potential hazard of various foods. There is little evidence that eating or avoiding specific foods affects the frequency of relapses or the severity of the disease.[43] Olestra, the fat-free fat substitute, has been studied in adult patients with IBD in remission; it did not affect the disease activity in this study.[85] Although there does not seem to be a role for a fat substitute in the day-to-day diet of a pediatric patient with IBD, it is helpful to know that it does not appear to be harmful if ingested occasionally. Controlled studies have not supported the use of a low-residue, high-fiber, or low-refined sugar diet to maintain remission of Crohn's disease.[86–88] Dairy products need not be restricted in all patients with IBD; however, lactose malabsorption is more common in patients with small bowel Crohn's disease than in patients with disease involving the colon or UC. Advice concerning the intake of dairy products should be individualized to avoid unnecessary dietary restrictions.[89] During periods of illness or weight loss, oral nutritional supplementation can be useful. The choice of the formula used depends on disease activity and tolerance. If voluntary intake is insufficient, nasogastric nocturnal continuous or intermittent enteral supplementation may be considered. If there is no evidence of gastric Crohn's disease, a skin level or button gastrostomy may be useful and more acceptable than an indwelling or intermittent nasogastric tube. Parenteral nutrition should be reserved for patients who have bowel obstructions or short-bowel syndrome, or are unable to tolerate sufficient quantity of enteral nutrition because of active disease.

Role of Nutritionist

Nutritional issues are sometimes given inadequate attention in the management of IBD.[90] The pediatric nutritionist should play an integral role in the treatment plan for both ulcerative colitis and Crohn's disease. The nutritionist should assess each patient for vitamin and mineral status, especially iron, folate, B12, calcium, magnesium, and zinc. See the latest version of ASPEN's nutrition support practice manual for the most current recommendations.[27] Further research is needed to better define the benefits of nutrition therapy as adjunctive therapy and investigate the role of specific nutrients in the primary treatment of IBD.

Lactose Intolerance

Lactose intolerance (LI) is the most common of all of the syndromes of carbohydrate malabsorption. It is characterized by bloating, flatulence, and diarrhea after ingestion of a lactose-containing food. The most commonly used diagnostic test of LI is the breath hydrogen test, which is done after a test dose of lactose has been given. Carbohydrate that is malabsorbed in the small intestine is fermented by colonic bacteria and hydrogen gas is released. Intermittent samples are taken and analyzed.[92]

Lactose intolerance may be primary or secondary. Secondary disorders are most common in infancy. There are three primary disorders of primary lactose intolerance: developmental, congenital, and late onset.[91]

Developmental Lactose Intolerance

Lactase activity develops late in the third trimester of pregnancy,[93] so premature infants typically have lower levels of lactase activity.[94] There is no evidence to suggest lactase can be induced—that by giving infants lactose that there is a more rapid development of lactase activity.[93] Premature infant formulas contain a combination of lactose and glucose polymers as the carbohydrate composition.[95] A study of premature infants were studied with breath hydrogen tests to assess the degree of lactose intolerance. Although the infants had positive breath tests, they did not have clinical symptoms of LI such as diarrhea. The infants gained weight appropriately and had low mean stool output.[96] In practice, most infants do quite well.[95] Malabsorption may be normal for premature infants, and salvage of carbohydrate by the colon is operational in premature infants. This process may in fact be beneficial; associated with the development of fecal flora, which prevents the colonization of the colon with enteropathogens.[91]

Congenital Lactose Intolerance

Congenital lactase deficiency is extremely rare; lactase activity remains abnormal throughout life in this disorder.[91] As a result, individuals with this condition must severely restrict or omit lactose in their diet.

Late Onset Lactose Intolerance

The other primary disorder, late onset LI, is also known as adult onset lactose intolerance. In the world, only a small number of people have the developmental lactase deficiency in adulthood, so in the global perspective, late onset LI is the norm.[91] Lactose intolerance is common among different racial and ethnic backgrounds. LI is common among adult Eskimos, American Indians, Asians, some Africans, and Semitics.[97] It is uncommon in Northern Europeans and several tribes in Africa and India.[98] In the United States, it is seen in up to 70% of African-Americans[99] beginning between the age of 6 and the teenage years.[100] In the Caucasian population, LI is less common with less than 20% affected.[99] A good rule of thumb is that if evidence (by breath hydrogen or lactose tolerance test) of LI is found in an African-American child under 3 years of age or a Caucasian child under 5 years that the possibility of damage to the intestinal mucosa be considered.[101]

Secondary Lactose Intolerance

Most cases of secondary lactose intolerance are caused by an acute diarrheal disease[102–104] and the deficiency is temporary.[98–99] Lactose can generally be reintroduced into the diet after several weeks. Rotavirus, the leading cause of diarrhea in older infants and toddlers, is likely to be associated with temporary lactose intolerance.[103] Secondary LI is also seen with chronic diarrhea of infancy, food-protein intolerance, parasitic infections, and gluten-sensitive enteropathy.[92]

Low-Lactose Diet

Infant formulas such as Lactofree (Mead Johnson) and soy formulas such as Isomil (Ross Products) and Prosobee (Mead Johnson) can be used for infants. For older children, milk and dairy products may need to be eliminated from the diet temporarily. Because these foods are an excellent source of calcium, protein, and other vitamins and minerals, it is best not to eliminate these foods permanently unless absolutely necessary. If a lactose-free infant formula is substituted, the diet can be sufficient. All milk substitutes or "imitation" milk products are not equal; some do not contain the nutrients normally found in milk. Pellagra, beriberi, iron deficiency anemia, and zinc and essential fatty acid deficiencies were found in an infant consuming an "imitation" milk product that contained less than 2% of the RDA for B complex, zinc, iron, and essential fatty acids.[105] Milk-free diets often need calcium and other mineral and vitamin supplementation. Calcium supplements are available in carbonate, gluconate, lactate, and citrate. Dolomite and bone meal calcium supplements should be avoided because they have been linked with lead poisoning.[106] Stoker and Castle describe a method for testing the physical ability of a calcium supplement to be absorbed by placing a tablet in a glass of vinegar for 30 minutes. If it has not dissolved in 30 minutes, they do not classify it as an easily absorbed source of calcium.[106]

Many children and adolescents can better tolerate a low-lactose diet because they have some lactase activity. Some foods with lactose are better tolerated than others, and factors such as the fat content of the food or beverage, amount consumed, and timing—whether it is ingested by itself, or with a meal—are important. Ingesting small amounts at a time and taking the lactose-containing food with a larger meal reduces the chance of side effects and malabsorption. Higher fat lactose-containing foods sometimes are tolerated better than low or fat-free products. When reintroducing new foods into the diet, a recommendation is to wait 48 hours before each new food or change in amount of food to check whether it is tolerated.[106] Commercially available lactase enzymes can be taken during a meal containing lactose or products such as Lactaid milk can be purchased and consumed. The package insert directions should be followed for the needed (70% or 90%) lactose reduction. Reduced lactose ready-to-consume milks are also available. Naturally aged cheese such as blue, brie, cheddar, and Swiss seem to be tolerated; increased aging improves tolerance.[106]

Constipation

Constipation is common in childhood. High-fiber diets with adequate fluids are recommended as the first line of therapy. When fiber alone fails, lubricants and laxatives may be required. The fiber content of common foods is presented in Table 16–5. Inadequate fluid intake can also be a cause of constipation.[107] Medications such as phenytoin may slow peristalsis or diuretics that alter fluid balance may cause constipation as well.[107]

When stooling is chronically difficult or painful, children may withhold stool aggravating the existing problem. Encopresis may result due to the stretched rectal wall, allowing softer stool to leak out involuntarily.[107] A bowel program after a thorough clean out may include a high-fiber diet, adequate fluid, and increased physical activity.

Iron in Diet

Iron contained in formula may be perceived by mothers to cause constipation. They may make this association because of their experience with iron supplementation in pregnancy,[107] but iron in formula has not been associated with adverse side effects including constipation.[108–111] Iron-fortified formula is recommended by the American Association of Pediatrics for the first year of life to prevent anemia.[111] If parents choose a low-iron formula, an iron supplement is necessary by 4 to 6 months when iron stores become depleted.[112]

Pancreatic Insufficiency and Cholestatic Liver Disease

Fat-soluble vitamin malabsorption is a problem that occurs with pancreatic insufficiency and cholestatic liver disease. Supplementation at levels exceeding the recommended dietary allowances (RDAs) for normal healthy children is recommended for children with these disorders. The

Table 16–5 Good Sources of Dietary Fiber

Food	*Grams of Fiber*
Apple, 1 med. w/ skin	2.2
Apple, 1 med. w/o skin	2.0
Apricot, dried, 3 oz	7.8
Blueberries, 1 cup raw	4.4
Dates, dried, 10	4.2
Kiwi, 3 oz	3.4
Pear, 1 med. raw	4.1
Prunes, dried, 3 oz	7.2
Prunes, stewed, 3 oz	6.6
Raisins, 3 oz	5.3
Raspberries, 1 cup	5.8
Strawberries, raw, 1 cup	2.8
Avocado, California, raw, 1 med.	3.0
Beans, black, boiled, 1 cup	7.2
Beans, great northern, boiled, 1 cup	6.0
Beans, kidney, boiled, 1 cup	6.4
Beans, lima, boiled, 1 cup	6.2
Beans, baby lima, boiled, 1 cup	7.8
Beans, navy, boiled 1 cup	6.6
Beans, green, canned 1/2 cup	6.8
Broccoli, boiled, 1/2 cup	2.2
Chickpeas (garbanzo beans), 1 cup	5.7
Cowpeas (blackeye peas), 1 cup	4.4
Lentils, boiled, 1 cup	7.9

continues

Table 16–5 continued

Ready-to-Eat Cereal	*Fiber Grams*	*Serving*
Fiber One	13	1/2 c
All Bran	10	1/2 c
Shredded Wheat and Bran	8	1 1/4 c
100% Bran	8	1/3 c
Raisin Bran	8	1 c
Multi Bran Chex	7	1 c
Cracklin' Oat Bran	6	1 3/4 c
Mini Wheats	6	1 c
Mini Wheats with raisins	5	3/4 c
Mini Wheats with strawberries	5	3/4 c
Shredded Wheat	5	1 c
Grape Nuts	5	1/2 c
Fruit n Fiber	5	1 c
Wheat Chex	5	1 c
Complete Wheat	5	3/4 c
Bran Flakes	5	3/4 c
Great Grains	4	2/3 c
Banana Nut Crunch	4	1 c
Raisin Bran Crunch	4	1 c
Cranberry Almond Crunch	3	1 c
Healthy Choice Low Fat Granola	3	1/2 c
Grape Nut Flakes	3	3/4 c

Source: Data for sections on fruits and vegetables from references 166 and 167; data for section on ready-to-eat cereals from a supermarket survey of manufacturer's labels as of April 1999.

recommended dosage for supplementation of fat-soluble vitamins is presented in Table 16–6.

Nutrition Management

Unfortunately, parenteral nutrition-associated cholestasis is common in pediatrics.[113,114] Infants or children with cholestasis who are receiving parenteral nutrition should have levels of copper and manganese decreased because these nutrients are excreted through the biliary system. (Parenteral nutrition is discussed in detail in Chapter 25.) For infants receiving enteral formulas, those containing 50–60% medium-chain triglycerides (MCT) and 40–50% long-chain triglycerides (LCT) are typically recommended. For premature infants, premature formulas such as Similac Special Care (Ross Products) or Enfamil Premature (Mead Johnson) have this lipid profile. For term infants, Alimentum (Ross Products) or Pregestimil (Mead Johnson) contain MCT/LCT in this mix. In cholestasis, there is insufficient bile for micelle formation for optimal LCT absorption; MCTs do not require bile for absorption. MCTs do not, however, provide essential fatty acids or aid in the absorption of fat-soluble vitamins;[115] thus, a source of linoleic acid is essential. Essential fatty acid deficiency has been seen with the use of a high MCT formula such as Portagen (Mead Johnson) in an infant with hepatobiliary disease and presumed LCT malabsorption.[116]

Short Bowel Syndrome

Short Bowel Syndrome (SBS) is a condition in which the patient has an anatomic or functional loss of more than 50% of the expected small intestine.[117] These patients have difficulty sustaining appropriate growth and development with

Table 16–6 Vitamin Supplementation in Cystic Fibrosis and Hepatic Disorders

Vitamin Needed	*Dose*
Cystic fibrosis	
Vitamin A	1–2 × RDA
Vitamin D	1–2 × RDA
Hepatic disorders	
Vitamin A (Aquasol A)	5000 IU/d
Vitamin D	2,000–10,000 IU/d
or	
25-Hydroxycholecalciferol	50 μg/d
Vitamin E	50–400 IU/d
Vitamin K	2.5–5 mg/d

Source: Adapted with permission from Merritt RJ and Hack S, Infant feeding and enteral nutrition, in *Nutrition in Clinical Practice* (1988;3:47–64), Copyright © 1988, American Society for Parenteral and Enteral Nutrition.

normal age appropriate enteral nutrition. Although most patients have had a significant bowel resection, SBS cannot be solely described by an arbitrary length of remaining small intestine. Some patients may have had a rather small amount of bowel resected, but the entire bowel was damaged, causing difficulty with enteral nutrition.[118] The injury may be a result of necrotizing enterocolitis (NEC), volvulus, intestinal atresias, gastroschisis, ruptured omphalocele, or vascular infarct.[117] The result of the injury and/or resection is decreased small intestine surface area, which leads to malabsorption and large volume watery diarrhea. The degree of malabsorption varies with the area and extent of missing or injured bowel. Recovery depends on the degree of functional intestinal adaptation.

Nutrient and Fluid Absorption

Absorption of fluids and nutrients occurs throughout the small intestine, but half of the mucosal surface is contained within the proximal one-fourth of the small intestine.[118] The duodenum and jejunum are the primary sites of digestion and absorption of proteins, carbohydrates, lipids, and most vitamins and minerals. Vitamin B12 is an exception; it is only absorbed in the ileum. Bile salts are also absorbed in the ileum; this is necessary for enterohepatic circulation. If the bile acid pool becomes depleted, there is decreased fat and fat-soluble vitamin absorption.[119] Many gut hormones are produced in the ileum, including enteroglucagon and peptide YY that affect gastrointestinal motility. Resection of the ileum can impair nutrient-regulated gut motility.[120] The ileum can adapt to take the place of the jejunum; however, due to some of these specific roles of the ileum, the jejunum cannot adapt to the role of the ileum.[119]

The presence of the ileocecal valve is very important; it slows transit time and acts as a barrier to bacteria moving into the small bowel from the colon. Bacterial overgrowth in the small bowel can be a major problem and lead to increased diarrhea and malabsorption.[117] The colon absorbs water, can salvage malabsorbed carbohydrate, and absorbs sodium. Patients with a jejunostomy or ileostomy will have watery stomal output high in sodium, zinc, and other minerals. There are different schools of thought in the surgical community as to whether or not to perform a primary anastomosis, putting the bowel back together to create continuity, at the time of a bowel resection. Sometimes patients are also too labile, and a temporary ostomy is created. Although having all the bowel in continuity maximizes the gastrointestinal surface area for absorption of nutrients, there are advantages of an ostomy. Fluid management is easier to monitor because it is easy to measure ostomy output and analyze it as needed for electrolytes, carbohydrate, and the like. Measuring urine output is easily done by weighing the urine-only diapers. After an anastomosis, output is difficult to gauge because it is reported as mixed stool and urine. When a patient is stooling heavily and fluid intake is inadequate, stool and urine can look very similar, further complicating assessment. The use of urine-specific gravity, obtained by putting cotton balls in the urine area of the diaper, becomes a useful tool to assess hydration status.

Parenteral Nutrition

The first phase in the treatment of a new patient with SBS is parenteral. Total parenteral nutrition (TPN) should be started as soon as possible. Due to the possible long-term aspect of this form of nutrition, consideration should be given to central vein access. Initially, gastric contents are drained. Gastric drainage may consist of 140 mEq/L of sodium, 15 mEq/L of potassium, and 155 mEq/L of chloride.[121] Replacement fluids should be used to replace gastrointestinal losses for easier fluid and electrolyte management. Initial parenteral calorie needs vary from infant to infant but are around 100–105 kcal/kg with 3 to 3.5 gm/kg protein and 3.0 gm/kg lipid. As soon as stooling begins, additional sodium, magnesium, and zinc are needed to compensate for stool or ostomy losses.

Ileostomy output may contain 80–140 mEq/L of sodium, 15 mEq/L of potassium, 40mEq/L of bicarbonate, 115mEq/L of chloride[121] and 12 mg of zinc/L.[122] Patients without an ostomy but with diarrhea may lose considerable amounts of zinc and selenium.[123] Zinc loss in diarrhea may equal 16 mg/L.[124] Monitoring zinc status is not easy as serum and leukocyte measurements of zinc may be unreliable.[125] Significant quantities of magnesium may be lost in small intestinal ostomies.[126] As magnesium deficiency may occur despite a normal serum magnesium, it may be useful to measure urine magnesium loss.[126,127] Magnesium deficiency can cause calcium deficiency as hypomagnesemia impairs the parathyroid hormone release.[128] Because all infants on parenteral nutrition are not receiving optimal calcium intake and most patients with SBS are in a negative calcium balance,[129] this is important to note. TPN should be monitored carefully to minimize complications associated with all parenteral nutrition therapy. TPN-associated cholestasis is a major cause of death in patients with SBS.[114] (See Chapter 25.)

Gastric acid hypersecretion can occur after a large bowel resection. It is seen most often after a large resection when enteral feedings are initiated.[130] IV ranitidine can be effective in inhibiting acid secretion[131] and can be put in the TPN as an additive. A normal dosage should be used at first, the gastric pH checked, and the dosage titrated for effective therapy with the assistance of the clinical pharmacist. Hypersecretion is usually transitory so the periodic review of medications and dosages should include gastric pH testing. Ranitidine may decrease intrinsic factor secretion that can affect vitamin B12 absorption. The potential for bacterial contamination of the bowel may be increased with the long term use of H_2 blockers.[118]

Enteral Nutrition

Enteral nutrition is the next phase and should be started as soon as the patient is stable and gastrointestinal motility has returned.[132] Enteral nutrition is necessary to promote intestinal adaptation. Adaptation with cellular hyperplasia, villous hypertrophy, intestinal lengthening, and motility improvement may take 1 year or more.[133] There is great controversy as to the ideal formula for infants and toddlers with SBS. Breast milk is tolerated well (if available) and animal studies suggest it stimulates mucosal growth.[134] Premature infants with smaller resections may do well with premature infant formulas. Premature infants have developmental lactase deficiency,[93] and their illness could also affect lactase activity. Premature infant formulas such as Similac Special Care (Ross Products) or Enfamil Premature (Mead Johnson), with a carbohydrate source of approximately 50% lactose and 50% glucose polymers and lipid mix of MCT and LCT,[94] have been used successfully in SBS. Protein hydrolysate formulas such as Alimentum (Ross Products) and Pregestimil (Mead Johnson) are the traditional formula of choice for infants and toddlers with SBS. In general, they are tolerated well, but will not have the additional protein, mineral, and vitamin content suitable to a premature infant. Although most protein is absorbed as di- or tripeptides, such as are found in protein hydrolysates,[120] sometimes there appears to be an allergic component as well as SBS and amino acid–based formulas such as Neocate (Scientific Hospital Supply) or Elecare (Ross Products) are tolerated well.[135] For older infants and toddlers, fiber-containing complex formulas[120] such as Pediasure with Fiber (Ross Products) are tolerated well. Full-strength breast milk or formula can typically be used starting at 1 cc/hr and progress as tolerated. Some centers prefer to use dilute formulas.[136,137]

Enteral Tube Feeding

Continuous gastric feeding is the preferred feeding method for infants and toddlers with SBS due to the studies showing greater absorption of nutrients and clinical experience.[24,137] Orogastric tubes may be used in premature infants because they are obligate nose breathers[138] with indwelling nasogastric tubes used in older infants. If infants will be using tube feedings for longer than 3 months, a surgically placed gastrostomy tube is preferable. If infants have a proximal high ostomy and a mucous fistula connected to a substantial portion of bowel, refeeding the mucous fistula with the proximal bowel content has been done to prevent disuse atrophy.[139] Until the infant is able to eat by mouth, an oral motor stimulation program should be in place. Specially trained occupational therapists or speech pathologists can work with the nursing staff and parents on a plan. As soon as the team feels the infant is developmentally ready and can tolerate small amounts of bolus feedings, small volume oral feeding should begin. Continuous feedings should continue to be the preferred enteral route of nutrition, but oral stimulation is very important for development of feeding skills. Feeding aversion in patients with SBS is very difficult to treat.[140] Preventing aversive feeding behavior is extremely important.

Introduction to Solid Food

When the infant is 4 to 6 months, solids can be added. Cereals are tolerated well as are most starches, especially those higher in fiber. Fruit juices are avoided because they may cause increased diarrhea. Most fruits, vegetables, and meats are tolerated but there is considerable individual variation on specific food intolerances. Only one new food should be tried at a time, waiting at least 2 days before adding a new food. Some centers report a greater number of food allergies in their patients with SBS and use greater caution with the introduction of hyperallergenic foods. Lactose need not be omitted from the diet forever; at least one study has shown tolerance to a diet with 20 gm/day later in the course of therapy.[141]

Transition from TPN to Enteral Feedings

The transition from parenteral nutrition to all enteral nutrition may be slow. Malabsorption is common with enteral feedings and calorie needs increase per kg as the percent of enteral nutrition increases. Lifshitz uses a guideline that for every 3 cc increase in enteral nutrition, the parenteral rate can be decreased by 1 cc, keeping the IV lipid rate the same. At least 20% to 30% of the enteral formula may be malabsorbed.[136] Calorie needs are difficult to estimate, but may be 120 to 150 cal/kg or higher. As stooling increases with the introduction of enteral feedings, sodium and zinc loss from ostomy output should be considered. Additional zinc can be given by parenteral (up to 8000 mcg/L) or enteral route. Several articles have been written documenting poor growth and abnormal labs from sodium loss from ileostomy drainage.[142–144] Similar losses could occur in a patient with a subtotal proximal colon resection and a primary anastomosis. Urine sodium values can be used to titrate the amount of additional sodium needed in combination with stool volume; supplementation can be initiated using the average stool output and the midrange estimate of 110 mEq/L of sodium contained in ileostomy fluid. Assuming normal renal function, enteral or parenteral sodium is added until the urine contains sodium. Usually sodium chloride is used, but if the patient has bicarbonate loss and is acidotic, a combination of sodium chloride and sodium citrate can be used. Prior to correction, all factors that could cause acidosis should be examined.

Bacterial Overgrowth

Small bowel bacterial overgrowth can develop when the ileocecal valve is absent, when there is slow motility, or when there is a partial small bowel obstruction.[136] Symptoms of overgrowth are diarrhea and/or air within the bowel wall.[136] Antibiotic treatment is available and some centers routinely cycle patients on an antibiotic such as metronidazole (Flagyl) for 1 to 2 weeks every month for overgrowth treatment. Metabolic acidosis can occur from the absorption of d-lactic acid produced by bacteria from malabsorbed carbohydrate. This has been seen in young children who are eating a mixed diet that can cause drowsiness and mental confusion.[145,146]

Vitamin and Mineral Supplementation

For patients who have successfully been weaned from parenteral nutrition, vitamin supplementation is often necessary. Vitamin B12 may need to be supplemented with an intramuscular administration of 1 mg every 3 months. Iron, folate, and magnesium may also need to be supplied.[27] An assessment for vitamin and mineral supplements should be made for each child.

Infants and children may need supplemental continuous enteral infusion for an extended period of time. Very small enteral pumps using a back or fanny pack are available for home use. The palatability of some enteral formula becomes an issue during the transition to oral feedings. Some patients take one formula by mouth and use another for gastric feeds. Some patients who are off of parenteral nutrition still need daily IV hydration. Portable IV pumps can contribute to making their lifestyle more normal.

For patients who do not seem to be making progress weaning from parenteral nutrition, there are other options. Growth hormone, glutamine, and a modified diet have been used in a supervised treatment plan in adults to enhance nutrient absorption and decrease dependence on parenteral therapy.[147] However, others were not able to duplicate these results[148–149] and found no improvement in absorption. Patients also developed peripheral edema on this regimen, which resolved after therapy was discontinued.[148–149] New research with adults has shown positive findings for the use of glucagon-like peptide-2 (GLP-2) in decreasing energy malabsorption and stoma output.[150]

Cholestasis occurs in 30% to 60% of children with SBS; liver failure develops in 3% to 19% of children who acquired SBS in the neonatal period.[151–153] Although it has always been assumed that parenteral nutrition was the leading culprit in the etiology, a recent study points out the close association between cholestasis and bacterial or fungal infections.[154] Alternative surgical procedures such as bowel lengthening or tapering enteroplasty may be considered for those patients who are not making progress.[120,155–157]

Intestinal Transplantation

Bowel transplantation is now clinically feasible and may offer hope for patients who have no other options. Combined liver and bowel transplantation is reserved for those patients with life-threatening progressive liver disease.[158] Although there has been much progress made in bowel transplantation over the past 5 years, better immunosuppressive drugs and more donors are needed to improve outcomes.[158]

Care for the posttransplant patient varies from center to center. The majority of bowel transplants to date have been done in 5 centers.[159] Currently, there are no randomized controlled trials with outcome-based endpoints in the literature. Simon Horslen surveyed the major transplant centers to describe optimal management.[159] His conclusions showed variation in many aspects of care. Enteral feedings were started in a range from as soon as possible to 2 weeks. The formulas used were predominately elemental. One center started with clear liquids for 2 days; another used diluted formula at first. Mode of feeding was often jejunal, because poor gastric emptying was a common finding. Progression was made to oral feedings as tolerated (depending on the incidence of feeding aversion). Some centers reported using a fat restriction for 1 month; one center restricted for the first year. Fruit juice and high-sugar foods were also restricted.[159]

Liver Transplantation

The most common disease requiring liver transplantation in childhood is biliary atresia (over 50% of cases); other less prominent causes are inherited metabolic disorders (e.g., α-1-antitrypsin deficiency, glycogen storage disease, Wilson's Disease, tyrosinemia), intrahepatic cholestasis syndromes (e.g., Alagille, Byler), chronic hepatitis with cirrhosis, and fulminant viral or toxic hepatitis. Indications for transplantation include hepatic failure, intractable ascites, recurrent variceal hemorrhage, and hypersplenism.

The patient with end-stage liver disease awaiting transplantation presents a formidable challenge to the medical team. The particular liver disease involved, the magnitude of liver dysfunction, the presence of complications, and the transplantation procedure itself combine to present a complex treatment process including meeting nutritional needs for healing and growth.[160]

Pretransplant Nutrition Assessment

Pretransplant nutritional care involves both assessment of current status and development of a therapeutic diet tailored to the liver disease and degree of debilitation. Assessment parameters the dietitian should follow include:[161–163]

1. Anthropometrics: height/length, weight, triceps skinfolds, mid-arm circumference, abdominal girth
2. Laboratory studies: complete blood count with differential; platelet count; prothrombin and partial thromboplastin times; serum levels of total and direct bilirubin, alanine aminotransferase, aspartate aminotransferase, alkaline phosphatase, total protein, prealbumin, albumin, ammonia, electrolytes, calcium, inorganic phosphorus, blood urea nitrogen, creatinine, serum bile salts, and vitamins A, D, and E; serologic testing for titers of hepatitis A and B, Epstein-Barr virus, cytomegalovirus, herpes virus, human immunodeficiency virus
3. Radiology: ultrasound (to check for patency of vascular structures)

Pretransplant Diet

Generally, the pretransplant diet should be as follows. Calories should be provided at 140% of the RDA for age. Adding glucose polymers or medium-chain triglyceride oil to feedings can help boost energy intake to these levels. Enteral drip feedings (intermittent or 24-hour long) may be necessary to ensure intake (however, enteral drip feedings may be contraindicated if the prothrombin time is prolonged or the platelet count is low). Protein should be provided at 2.0 to 2.5 g/kg of dry weight if parenteral nutrition is being employed or at 2.5 to 3.0 g/kg of dry weight if enteral feeding is used. The parenteral nutrition solution used should contain a balanced amino acid mixture; the enteral solution should be low in sodium. If the patient is encephalopathic, the protein intake should be reduced to 1.0 to 1.5 g/kg of dry weight. Branched-chain amino acid solutions may also be considered in this setting. Water-miscible fat-soluble vitamins should be used. Zinc and iron are provided as needed, and sodium is restricted to 0.5 to 1.0 mEq/kg to help control ascites.[161,162]

Post-transplant Nutrition Management

Immediately after transplantation, TPN is begun using a balanced amino acid solution with dextrose and an appropriate intravenous lipid source. Pediatric multivitamins and trace elements are added to the solution based on age. It is suggested the formula provide nutrients at the following specified levels: protein 2.0 to 2.5 g/kg of dry weight; lipid 2 to 3 g/kg of dry weight; and nonprotein calories 80 to 100 kcal/kg of dry weight.[162] Sodium, potassium, calcium, and phosphorus amounts are based on serum levels.

Routine posttransplant care includes monitoring fluid balance closely, which requires strict intake and output measurements and daily weights. Many laboratory tests may need to be monitored. These include complete blood count and differential and levels of blood and urine glucose, triglycerides, electrolytes, calcium, phosphorus, magnesium, albumin, and liver enzymes. When bowel movements resume, stools should be checked for pH, reducing substances, and occult blood.[163,164]

Enteral feedings may begin when the postoperative ileus has resolved. This is usually exhibited by the patient having bowel sounds or having bowel movements. Enteral feedings should be gradually increased as the patient is gradually weaned from TPN. For the younger child, continuous nasogastric feeding using MCT-oil predominant formula may be preferred. Feedings should be advanced as tolerated to an oral regular formula as the stooling pattern normalizes. For the older child, use either continuous nasogastric feedings or oral-defined diets. Diet can then be advanced to a soft low-residue diet, and then to a regular diet, as tolerated. All children should routinely receive multivitamin supplements, but each child's need for zinc, iron, and vitamin E will depend on his or her serum levels. A mild sodium restriction should be used in all children to prevent fluid retention caused by steroid use.[164,165]

Possible problems in resumption of oral feeding include oral defensiveness due to prolonged use of TPN and developmental delay in sucking and chewing skills in infants. Appropriately trained occupational therapists or speech pathologists should be consulted to devise an interdisciplinary treatment plan for these problems.

The postdischarge follow-up of liver transplant recipients includes assessment of anthropometric values and the patient's dietary intake record at each clinic visit. In the long term, the transplant patient should receive dietary supplements only if indicated. Problems the dietitian should be alert for in this population include fat malabsorption, metabolic bone disease, dental caries, hypertension, and anemia.[165] Referrals can then be made to the appropriate care teams.

Formula Change and Acceptance

When a change in formula is indicated as part of the treatment of a GI problem, there is concern about acceptance. As infant formulas become more elemental, the taste becomes less sweet and more bitter and sour; they also have a less pleasant odor and an unpleasant aftertaste.[168] Amniotic fluid and breast milk are sweet and variable in flavor based on the mother's diet.[169] A difference has been noted by clinicians between an infant who is initially offered a hydrolysate formula (and accepts it well) versus an older infant who is changed to the formula (who does not accept it well). The rejection does not occur until after 4 months of age. An interesting study by Mennella and associates looked at acceptance of a protein-hydrolysate formula after initially being given either a hydrolysate or a milk-based formula. Infants who were given a hydrolysate throughout infancy continued to accept it at 7.5 months (and disliked the better tasting cow milk–based formula) whereas an infant who is switched to it at 7.5 months rejects the hydrolysate.[168] Their research indicates that responses to olfactory components of flavor are influenced by experience.[170] This is also shown in 4- to 5-year-old children who were fed hydrolysates as infants and had more positive responses to them years later.[170,171] Adolescents with phenylketonuria who went off of their formula have been shown to be able to go back to the formula with some difficulty but with fewer problems than those who were not exposed as infants.[172] Infants will readily drink hydrolyzed formulas if introduced before 4 months of age. If required at this age, it should be mixed with a formula that is already accepted while gradually increasing the proportion of hydrolysate.[168] The parent needs to work closely with a dietitian to make this transition acceptable to the child.

REFERENCES

1. American Academy of Pediatrics, Committee on Nutrition. Use of oral fluid therapy and posttreatment feeding following enteritis in children in a developed country. *Pediatrics*. 1985;75:358–361.
2. Wall CR, Webster J, Quirk P, et al. The nutritional management of acute diarrhea in young infants: Effect of carbohydrate ingested. *J Pediatr Gastroenterol Nutr*. 1994;19:170–174.
3. Liftshitz F, Maggioni A. The nutritional management of acute diarrhea in young infants. *J Pediatr Gastroenterol Nutr.* 1994;19:148–150.

4. Brown KH. Dietary management of acute childhood diarrhea: Optimal timing of feeding and appropriate use of milks and mixed diets. *J Pediatr*. 1991;118:S92–98.

5. Santosham M, Foster S, Reid R, et al. Role of soy-based, lactose-free formula during treatment of acute diarrhea. *Pediatrics*. 1985;76:292–298.

6. Santosham M, Goepp J, Burns B, et al. Role of soy-based lactose-free formula in the outpatient management of diarrhea. *Pediatrics*. 1991;87:619–622.

7. Goepp JG. Acute diarrhea. In: Walker WA, Watkins JB. *Nutrition in Pediatrics: Basic Science and Clinical Applications*. Hamilton: ON Decker; 1997;594.

8. Chew F, Penna FJ, Peret Filho LA, et al. Is dilution of cow's milk formula necessary for dietary management of acute diarrhoea in infants aged less than 6 months? *Lancet*. 1993;341:194–197.

9. Brown KH, Perez F, Peerson JM, et al. Effect of dietary fiber (soy polysaccharide) on the severity, duration, and nutritional outcome of acute, watery diarrhea in children. *Pediatrics*. 1993;92:241–247.

10. Vanderhoof JA, Murray ND, Paule CL, et al. Use of soy fiber in acute diarrhea in infants and toddlers. *Clinical Pediatrics*. 1997;36:135–139.

11. Klish WJ. Chronic diarrhea. In: Walker WA, Watkins JB. *Nutrition in Pediatrics: Basic Science and Clinical Applications*. Hamilton: ON Decker; 1997;603.

12. Lo CW, Walker WA. Chronic protracted diarrhea of infancy: A nutritional disorder. *Pediatrics*. 1983;72:786.

13. Editorial. Chronic diarrhea in children: A nutritional disorder. *Lancet*. 1987;1:143.

14. Baker SS, Davis AM. Hypocaloric oral therapy during an episode of diarrhea and vomiting can lead to severe malnutrition. *J Pediatr Gastroenterol Nutr*. 1998;27:1–5.

15. Bezerra JA, Stathos TH, Duncan B, et al. Treatment of infants with acute diarrhea: What's recommended and what's practices. *Pediatrics*. 1994;80:1–4.

16. Klish WJ, Udall JN, Rodriguez JT, et al. Intestinal surface area of infants with acquired monosaccharide intolerance. *J Pediatr*. 1978;92:566–571.

17. Calvin RT, Klish WJ, Nichols BL. Disaccharidase activities, jejunal morphology and carbohydrate tolerance in children with chronic diarrhea. *J Pediatr Gastroenterol Nutr*. 1985;4:949–953.

18. Solomon SM, Kirby KF. The refeeding syndrome: A review. *J Parenter Enteral Nutr*. 1985;85:28–36.

19. Lee PC, Werlin SL. Carbohydrates. In: Baker RD Jr, Baker SS, Davis AM. *Pediatric Parenteral Nutrition*. New York: Chapman and Hall; 1997;103.

20. Blackman JA, Nelson CLA. Reinstituting oral feedings in children fed by gastrostomy tube. *Clin Pediatr*. 1985; 24:434.

21. Heymsfield S. Metabolic changes associated with refeeding. *ASPEN Update* 1982;4:1–2.

22. Weisner RL, Krumdieck CL. Death resulting from overzealous total parenteral nutrition: The refeeding syndrome revisited. *Am J Clin Nutr*. 1981;34:393–399.

23. Mezoff AG, Gremse DA, Farrell MK. Hypophosphatemia in the nutritional recovery syndrome. *Am J Dis Child*. 1989;143:1111.

24. Parker P, Stroop S, Greene H. A controlled comparison of continuous versus intermittent feeding in the treatment of infants with intestinal disease. *J Pediatr*. 1987;99:360.

25. Thobani S, Molla AM, Snyder JD. Nutritional therapy for persistent diarrhea. In: Baker SS, Baker RD Jr., Davis AM. *Pediatric Enteral Nutrition*. New York: Chapman and Hall; 1994;291.

26. Sachdev HPS, Mittal NK, Mittal SK, et al. A controlled trial on utility of oral zinc supplementation in acute dehydrating diarrhea in infants. *J Pediatr Gastroenterol Nutr*. 1988;7:877.

27. Davis AM, Baker SS, Baker RD, Jr, et al. Pediatric gastrointestinal disorders. In: Meritt RM, ed., *The ASPEN Nutrition Support Practice Manual*. Silver Spring, MD: ASPEN; 1998;27–30.

28. Rahmathullah L, Underwood BA, Thulasiraj RD, et al. Reduced mortality among children in Southern India receiving a small weekly dose of vitamin A. *N Eng J Med*. 1990;323:929.

29. Brown KH. Appropriate diets for the rehabilitation of malnourished children in the community setting. *Acta Paediatr Scand*. 1991;374(Suppl):151.

30. Wall CR, Webster J, Quirk P, et al. The nutritional management of acute diarrhea in young infants: Effect of carbohydrate ingested. *J Pediatr Gastroenterol Nutr*. 1994;19:170–174.

31. Keohane PP, Grimble CK, Brown B, et al. Influence of protein composition and hydrolysis method on intestinal absorption of protein in man. *Gut*. 1985;26:907.

32. Hegarty JE, Fairclough PD, Moriarity KJ, et al. Comparison of plasma and intraluminal amino acid profiles in man after meals containing a protein hydrolysate and equivalent amino acid mixture. *Gut*. 1982;23:670.

33. Stocks RJ, Davies DP, Allen F. Loss of breast milk nutrients during tube feeding. *Arch Dis Child*. 1985;60:164.

34. Greer FR, McCormick A, Loker J. Changes in fat concentration of human milk during the delivery by intermittent bolus and continuous mechanical pump infusion. *J Pediatr*. 1984;105:745.

35. Narayan I, Singh B, Harvey D. Fat loss during feeding of human milk. *Arch Dis*. 1984;59:475.

36. Lavin M, Clark RM. The effect of short-term refrigeration of milk and the addition of breast milk fortifier on the delivery of lipids during tube feeding. *J Pediatr Gastroenterol Nutr*. 1989;8:496.

37. International Working Group on Persistent Diarrhoea. Evaluation of an algorithm for the treatment of persistent diarrhoea: A multicenter study. *Bull World Health Organ*. 1996;74:479–489.
38. Kolacek S, Grguric J, Perci M, et al. Home-made modular diet versus semi-elemental formula in the treatment of chronic diarrhoea of infancy: A prospective randomized trial. *Eur J Pediatr*. 1996;155:997–1001.
39. Touhami M, Boudraa G, Mary JY, et al. [Clinical consequences of replacing milk with yoghurt in persistent infantile diarrhea.] [French] *Annales de Padiatrie*. 1992;39:79–86.
40. Fasano. Prevalence of celiac disease in at-risk and not-at-risk groups in the United States: A large multicenter study. *Arch Internal Med*. 2003;163(3):286–292.
41. Thompson T. Do oats belong in a gluten-free diet? *J Am Diet Assoc*. 1997;97:1413–1416.
42. Mora S, Barera G, Ricotta A, et al. Reversal of low bone density with a gluten-free diet in children and adolescents with celiac disease. *Am J Clin Nutr*. 1998; 477–481.
43. Rea F, Polito C, Marotta A, et al. Restoration of body composition in celiac children after 1 year of gluten-free diet. *J Pediatr Gastroenterol Nutr*. 1996;23:408–412.
44. Motil KJ, Grand RJ. Inflammatory bowel disease. In: Walker WA, Watkins JB. *Nutrition in Pediatrics: Basic Science and Clinical Applications*. Hamilton: ON Decker; 1997;516.
45. Bern EM, Calenda KA, Grand R. Inflammatory bowel disease. In: Baker SS, Baker RD Jr, Davis AM. *Pediatric Enteral Nutrition*. New York: Chapman and Hall; 1994;305.
46. Motil KJ, Grand RJ. Nutritional management of inflammatory bowel disease. *Pediatr Clin North Am*. 1985;32:447.
47. O'Morain CA. Does nutritional therapy in inflammatory bowel disease have a primary or an adjunctive role? *Scan J Gastroenterol*. 1990;S172:29–34.
48. Goldschmid S, Graham M. Trace element deficiencies in inflammatory bowel disease. *Gastroenterol Clin North Am*. 1989;18:579.
49. Seidman EG, Lelieko N, Ament M, et al. Nutritional issues in pediatric inflammatory bowel disease. *J Pediatr Gastroenterol Nutr*. 1991;12:424.
50. Elsborg L, Larsen L. Folate deficiency in chronic inflammatory bowel diseases. *Scand J Gastroenterol*. 1979;14:1019.
51. Gerlach K, Morowitz DA, Kirsner JB. Symptomatic hypomagnesemia complicating regional enteritis. *Gastroenterology*. 1970;59:567–574.
52. Hessov I, Haselblad C, Fadth S, et al. Magnesium deficiency after ileal resection for Crohn's disease. *Scand J Gastroenterol*. 1983;18:643.
53. LaSala MA, Lifshitz F, Silverberg M, et al. Magnesium metabolism studies in children with chronic inflammatory disease of the bowel. *J Pediatr Gastroenterol Nutr*. 1985;4:75.
54. Hyams JS. Crohn's disease. In: Hyams WS, Hyams JS, eds., *Pediatric Gastrointestinal Disease: Pathophysiology, Diagnosis, Management*. Philadelphia: WB Saunders, 1993;750–764.
55. Kelts DG, Grand RJ, Shen G, et al. Nutritional basis for growth failure in children and adolescents with Crohn's disease. *Gastroenterology*. 1979;76:720–727.
56. Layden T, Rosenberg J, Nemchausky B, et al. Reversal of growth arrest in adolescents with Crohn's disease after parenteral nutrition. 1976;70:1017–1022.
57. Fleming CR, McGill DB, Berkber S. Home parenteral nutrition as a primary therapy in patients with extensive Crohn's disease of the small bowel and malnutrition. *Gastroenterology*. 1977;73:1077–1081.
58. Strobel CT, Byrne WJ, Ament ME. Home parenteral nutrition in children with Crohn's disease: Effective management alternative. *Gastroenterology*. 1979;77: 272–279.
59. Kirschner BS, Klich JR, Kalman SS, et al. Reversal of growth retardation in Crohn's disease with therapy emphasizing oral nutritional restitution. *Gastroenterology*. 1981;80:10–15.
60. Morin CL, Roulet M, Roy CC, et al. Continuous elemental enteral alimentation in children with Crohn's disease and growth failure. *Gastroenterology*. 1980;79: 1205–1210.
61. Motil KJ, Grand RJ, Maletskos CJ, et al. The effect of disease, drug, and diet on whole body protein metabolism in adolescents with Crohn's disease and growth failure. *J Pediatr*. 1982;101:125–140.
62. Motil KJ, Grand RJ, Matthews DE, et al. Whole body leucine metabolism in adolescents with Crohn's disease and growth failure during nutritional supplementation. *Gastroenterology*. 1982;82:1359–1368.
63. Aiges H, Markowitz J, Rosa V, et al. Home nocturnal supplemental nasogastric feedings in growth retarded adolescents with Crohn's disease. *Gastroenterology*. 1988;97:905–910.
64. Belli DC, Seldman E, Bouthillier L, et al. Chronic intermittent elemental diet improves growth failure in children with Crohn's disease. *Gastroenterology*. 1988; 94:603–610.
65. Polk DB, Hattner JAT, Kerner JA. Improved growth and disease activity after intermittent administration of a defined formula diet in children with Crohn's disease. *J Parent Ent Nutr*. 1992;16:499–504.
66. Morin CL, Roulet M, Roy CC, et al. Continuous elemental and enteral alimentation in the treatment of children and adolescents with Crohn's disease. *J Parent Ent Nutr*. 1982;6:194–199.

67. O'Morain C, Segal AM, Levi AJ, et al. Elemental diet in acute Crohn's disease. *Arch Dis Child*. 1983;53: 44–47.

68. Navarro J, Vargas J, Cezard JP, et al. Prolonged constant rate elemental enteral nutrition in small bowel Crohn's disease. *J Pediatr Gastroenterol Nutr*. 1982;1:541–546.

69. Sanderson IR, Udeen S, Davies PSW, et al. Remission induced by an elemental diet in small bowel Crohn's disease. *Arch Dis Child*. 1987;62:123–127.

70. Thomas AG, Taylor F, Miller V. Dietary intake and nutritional treatment in childhood Crohn's disease. *J Pediatr Gastroenterol Nutr*. 1983;17:75–81.

71. Ruuska T, Avilahti E, Maki M, et al. Exclusive whole protein enteral diet versus prednisolone in the treatment of acute Crohn's disease in children. *J Pediatr Gastroenterol Nutr*. 1993;19:175–180.

72. O'Morain C, Segal AW, Levi AJ. Elemental diet as primary treatment of acute Crohn's disease: A controlled trial. *BMJ*. 1984;288:1859–1862.

73. Saverymuttu S, Hodgson HJF, Chadwick VS. Controlled trial comparing prednisolone with an elemental diet plus nonabsorbable antibiotics in active Crohn's disease. *Gut*. 1985;26:994–998.

74. Okada M, Yao T, Yamamoto T, et al. Controlled trial comparing an elemental diet with prednisolone in the treatment of active Crohn's disease. *Hepatogastroenterology*. 1990;37:72–80.

75. Lochs H, Steinhardt HJ, Klaus-Wentz B, et al. Comparison of enteral nutrition and drug treatment in active Crohn's disease. Results of the European Cooperative Crohn's Disease Study IV. *Gastroenterology*. 1991;11:881–888.

76. Ludvigsson JF, Krantz M, Bodin L, et al. Elemental versus polymeric enteral nutrition in pediatric Crohn's disease: A multicentre randomized controlled trial. *Acta paeditr*. 93:327–335, 2004.

77. Giaffer MH, North G, Holdsworth CD. Controlled trial of polymeric versus elemental diet in treatment of active Crohn's disease. *Lancet*. 1991;335:816.

78. Ikeuchi H, Yammura T, Nakano H, et al. Efficacy of nutritional therapy for perforating and non-perforating Crohn's disease. *Hepatogastroenterology*. 2004;51: 1050–1052.

79. Bamba T, Shimoya T, Saski M, et al. Dietary fat attenuates the benefits of an elemental diet in active Crohn's disease: A randomized, controlled trial. *Eur J Gastroenterol Hapatol*. 2003;15:151–157.

80. Lorenz R, Weber PC, Szimnau P, et al. Supplementation of ulcerative colitis in chronic inflammatory bowel disease—A randomized, placebo-controlled, double-blind cross-over trial. *J Intern Med*. 1989;225(suppl): 225–232.

81. Aslan A, Triadafilopoulos G. Fish oil fatty acid supplementation in active ulcerative colitis: A double blind, placebo-controlled, crossover study. *Am J Gastroenterol*. 1992;87:432–437.

82. Stenson WF, Cort D, Rogers J, et al. Dietary supplementation with fish oil in ulcerative colitis. *Ann Intern Med*. 1992;116:609–614.

83. Hawthorne AB, Daneshmend TK, Hawkey CJ, et al. Treatment of ulcerative colitis with fish oil supplementation: A prospective 12 month randomized trial. *Gut*. 1992;33:922–928.

84. Bannerjee K, Camacho-Hubner C, Babinska K, et al. Anti-inflammatory and growth-stimulating effects precede nutritional restitution during enteral nutrition feeding in Crohn's disease. *J Pediatr Gastroenterol Nutr*. 2004;38:270–275.

85. Zorich NL, Jones NB, Kesler JM, et al. A randomized double-blind study on disease activity in patients with quiescent inflammatory bowel disease. Olestra in IBD Study Group. *Am J Med*. 1997;103:389–399.

86. Seidman EG. Nutritional management of inflammatory bowel disease. *Gastroenterol Clin North Am*. 1989; 17:129.

87. Levenstein S, Prantera C, Luzi C, et al. A low residue or normal diet in Crohn's disease: A prospective controlled trial of Italine patients. *Gut*. 1985;26:989.

88. Levi AJ. Diet in the management of Crohn's disease. *Gut*. 1985;26:985.

89. Mishkin S. Dairy sensitivity, lactose malabsorption, and elimination diets in inflammatory bowel disease. *Am J Clin Nutr*. 1997;65:564–567.

90. Husain A, Korzenik JR. Nutritional issues and therapy in inflammatory bowel disease. *Sem Gastroenterol Dis*. 1998;9:21–30.

91. Ulshen MH. Carbohydrate absorption and malabsorption. In: Walker WA, Watkins JB. *Nutrition in Pediatrics: Basic Science and Clinical Applications*. Hamilton: ON Decker; 1997;649.

92. Lifshitz CH. Breath hydrogen testing in infants with diarrhea. In: Lifshitz F, ed., *Carbohydrate Intolerance in Infancy*. New York: Marcel Dekker; 1982;31–42.

93. Antonowicz C, Chang SK, Grand RJ. Development and distribution of lysosomal enzymes and disaccharidases in human fetal intestine. *Gastroenterology*. 1974;67:51.

94. MacLean WC, Fink BB. Lactose malabsorption by premature infants: Magnitude and clinical significance. *J Pediatr*. 1980;97:383.

95. Sapsford A. Enteral nutrition products. In: Groh Wargo S, Thompson M, Cox JH, eds., *Nutritional Care for High Risk Newborns*. Chicago: Precept Press; 1994;178.

96. MacLean WC, Fink BB. Lactose malabsorption by premature infants: Magnitude and clinical significance. *J Pediatr*. 1980;97:383.

97. Simons FJ, Johnson JD, Kretchmer N. Perspective on milk drinking and malabsorption of lactose. *Pediatrics*. 1977;59:98.

98. Sahi T. Genetics and epidemiology of adult type hypolactasia. *Scand J Gastroenterol.* 1994;29(suppl 202): 7–20.

99. Bayless TM, et al. Lactose and milk intolerance: Clinical implications. *New Eng J Med.* 1975:1156.

100. Huang S, Bayless TM. Lactose intolerance in healthy children. *N Eng J Med.* 1967;276:1283.

101. Hyman JS, et al. Correlation of lactose breath hydrogen test, intestinal morphology, and lactase activity in children. *J Pediatr.* 1980;97:609.

102. Saavedra JM, Perman JA. Current concepts in lactose malabsorption and intolerance. *Annu Rev Nutr.* 1989; 9:475–502.

103. Hyams JS, Krause PJ, Gleason PA. Lactose malabsorption following rotavirus infection in young children. *J Pediatr.* 1981;99:916–918.

104. Davidson GP, Goodwin D, Robb TA. Incidence of lactose malabsorption in children hospitalized with acute enteritis: Study in a well-nourished urban population. *J Pediatr.* 1984;105:587–590.

105. Yelton L, Cox JH. Pediatric human immunodeficiency virus infection. In: Cox JH, ed., *Nutrition Manual for At-Risk Toddlers and Infants.* Chicago: Precept Press; 1997;174.

106. Stoker TW, Castle JL. Special diets. In: Walker WA, Watkins JB. *Nutrition in Pediatrics: Basic Science and Clinical Applications.* Hamilton: ON Decker; 1997;771.

107. Goldberg D. Clinical assessment. In: Cox JH, ed., *Nutrition Manual for At-Risk Toddlers and Infants.* Chicago: Precept Press; 1997;59.

108. Reeves JD, Yip R. Lack of adverse side effects of oral ferrous sulfate therapy in 1 year old infants. *Pediatrics.* 1985;75:352–355.

109. Nelson SE, Ziegler EE, Copeland AM, et al. Lack of adverse reactions to iron fortified formula. *Pediatrics.* 1988;81:360–364.

110. Oski FA. Iron fortified formulas and gastrointestinal symptoms in infants: A controlled study. *Pediatrics.* 1980;66:168–170.

111. Committee on Nutrition American Academy of Pediatrics. Iron fortified formulas. *Pediatrics.* 1989;84: 1114–1115.

112. Oski FA. Iron deficiency in infancy and childhood. *New Eng J Med.* 1993;329:190–193.

113. Benjamin SR. Hepatobiliary dysfunction in infants and children associated with long term parenteral nutrition: A clinico-pathologic study. *Am J Clin Pathol.* 1981;76:276.

114. Farrell MK. Physiologic effects of parenteral nutrition. In: Baker RD Jr, Baker SS, Davis AM. *Pediatric Parenteral Nutrition.* New York: Chapman and Hall; 1997;36.

115. Kleiman R, Warman KY. Nutrition in liver disease. In: Baker SS, Baker RD Jr., Davis AM. *Pediatric Enteral Nutrition.* New York: Chapman and Hall;1994;261.

116. Pettei MJ, et al. Essential fatty acid deficiency associated with the use of a medium chain triglyceride formula in pediatric hepatobiliary disease. *Am J Clin Nutr.* 1991;53:1217–1221.

117. Ziegler MM. Short bowel syndrome in infancy: Etiology and management. *Clin Perinatol.* 1986;13: 167.

118. Taylor SF, Sokol RJ. Infants with short bowel syndrome. In: Hay WW, ed., *Neonatal Nutrition and Metabolism.* St. Louis, MO: Mosby Year Book; 1991;437.

119. Klish WJ. The short gut. In: Walker WA, Watkins JB, eds., *Nutrition in Pediatrics.* Boston: Little, Brown; 1985;561.

120. Vanderhoof JA. Short bowel syndrome. In: Walker WA, Watkins JB. *Nutrition in Pediatrics: Basic Science and Clinical Applications.* Hamilton: ON Decker; 1997;610.

121. Heird WC, Winters RW. Fluid therapy for the pediatric surgical patient. In: Winters RW, ed., *Principles of Pediatric Fluid Therapy.* Boston: Little, Brown; 1985;595.

122. Collier S, Forchielli ML, Lo CW. Parenteral nutrition requirements. In: Baker RD Jr, Baker SS, Davis AM. *Pediatric Parenteral Nutrition.* New York: Chapman and Hall; 1997;78.

123. Buchman AL. Etiology and initial management of short bowel syndrome. *Gastroenterology.* 2004 (in press).

124. Wolman SL, Anderson GH, Marliss EB, et al. Zinc in total parenteral nutrition: Requirements and metabolic effects. *Gastroenterology.* 1979;76:456–467.

125. Prasad AS. Laboratory diagnosis of zinc deficiency. *Am J Coll Nutr.* 1985;4:591–598.

126. Selby PL, Peacock M, Barnbach CP. Hypomagnesemia after small bowel resection. Treatment with vitamin D metabolites. *Br J Surg.* 1984;71:334–337.

127. Fleming CR, George L, Stoner GL, et al. The importance of urinary magnesium values in patients with gut failure. *Mao Clin Proc.* 1996;71:21–24.

128. Anast CS, Winnacker JL, Forte LR, et al. Impaired release of parathyroid hormone in magnesium deficiency. *Clin Endocrinol Metab.* 1976;42:707–717.

129. Hylander E, Ladefioged JL, Madsen S. Calcium balance and bone mineral content following small intestinal resection. *Scand J Gastroenterol.* 1981;16:167–176.

130. Hyman PE, Everett SL, Harada T. Gastric acid hypersecretion in short bowel syndrome in infants: Association with extent of resection and enteral feeding. *J Pediatr Gastroenterol Nutr.* 1987;5:191.

131. Hyman PE, Garvey TQ, Abrams CE. Tolerance to intravenous ranitidine. *J Pediatr.* 1987;110:794.

132. Purdum PP, Kirby DF. Short bowel syndrome: A review of the role of nutrition support. *J Parent Ent Nutr.* 1990;15:93.

133. Vanderhoof JA, Langnas AN, Pinch IW, et al. Short bowel syndrome. *J Pediatr Gastroenterol Nutr.* 1992;14:359.

134. Heird WC, Schwartz SM, Hansen IH. Colostrum induced enteric mucosal growth in beagle puppies. *Pediatr Res.* 1984;18:512A.
135. Bines J, Francis D, Hale D. Reducing parenteral nutrition requirements in children with short bowel syndrome: Impact of α-amino acid based complete infant formula. *J Pediatr Gastroenterol Nutr.* 1998;26:123–128.
136. Lifschitz CH. Enteral feeding in short small bowel. In: Baker SS, Baker RD Jr., Davis AM. *Pediatric Enteral Nutrition.* New York: Chapman and Hall; 1994;280.
137. Christie DL, Ament ME. Dilute elemental diet and continuous infusion technique for management of short bowel syndrome. *J Pediatr.* 1975;87:705.
138. Miller MJ, Carlo WJ, Strohl KP, et al. Determination of oral breathing in premature infants. *Pediatr Res.* 1985; 19:354A.
139. Wong KY, Lan LC, Lin SC, et al. Mucous fistula refeeding in premature neonates with enterostomies. *J Pediatr Gastroenterol Nutr.* 2004;39:43–45.
140. Linsheid TR, Tarnowski KJ, Rasnake LK, et al. Behavioral treatment of food refusal in a child with short gut syndrome. *J Pediatr Psych.* 1987;12:451.
141. Marteau P, Messing B, Arrigoni E, et al. Do patients with short bowel syndrome need a lactose free diet? *Nutrition.* 1997;13:13–16.
142. Mews CF, et al. Topics in neonatal nutrition. Early ileostomy closure to prevent salt and water losses in infants. *J Perinatol.* 1992;12:297–299.
143. Bower TR. Sodium deficit causing decreased weight gain and metabolic acidosis in infants with ileostomy. *J Pediatr Surg.* 1988;23:567–572.
144. Schwartz KB, et al. Sodium needs of infants and children with an ileostomy. *J Pediatr.* 1983;102:509–513.
145. Perimutter DH, Boyle JT, Campos JM, et al. D-lactic acidosis in children: An unusual metabolic complication of small bowel resection. *J Pediatr.* 1983;102:234.
146. Gurevitch J, Sela B, Jonas A, et al. D-lactic acidosis: A treatable encephalopathy in pediatric patients. *Acta Paediatrica.* 1993;82:11.
147. Bryne TA, Morrissey TB, Nattakom TV, et al. Growth hormone, glutamine, and a modified diet enhance nutrient absorption inpatients with severe short bowel syndrome. *J Parent Ent Nutr.* 1995;19:296–302.
148. Szkudlarek J, Jeppesen PB, Mortensen PB. Effect of high dose growth hormone with glutamins and no change in diet on intestinal absorption in short bowel patients: A randomized, double blind, crossover, placebo controlled study. *Gut.* 2000;47:199–205.
149. Scolapio JS. Effect of growth hormone, glutamine, and diet on body composition in short bowel syndrome: A randomized, controlled study. *J Parenter Enteral Nutr.* 1999;23:309–312.
150. Jeppesen PB, Hartmann B, Thulesen J, et al. Glucagon-like peptide 2 improves nutrient absorption and nutritional status in short-bowel patients with no colon. *Gastroenterology.* 2001;120:806–815.
151. Caniano DA, Starr J, Ginn-Pease ME. Extensive short bowel syndrome in neonates: Outcome in the 1980s. *Surgery.* 1998;105:119–124.
152. Galea MH, Holliday H, Carachi R, et al. Short bowel syndrome: A collective review. *J Pediatr Surg.* 1992; 27:592–596.
153. Cooper A, Floyd TF, Ross AJ. Morbidity and mortality of short bowel syndrome acquired in infancy: An update. *J Pediatr Surg.* 1984;19:711–717.
154. Sondheimer JM, Asturias E, Cadnapaphornchai M. Infection and cholestasis in neonates with intestinal resection and long term parenteral nutrition. *J Pediatr Gastroenterol Nutr.* 1998;27:1531–1537.
155. Chaet MS, Warner BW, Farrell MF. Intensive nutritional support and remedial surgical intervention for extreme short bowel syndrome. *J Pediatr Gastroenterol Nutr.* 1994;19:295–298.
156. Thompson JS. Surgical management of short bowel syndrome. *Surgery.* 1993;113:4–7.
157. Warner BW, Chaet MS. Nontransplant surgical options for management of the short bowel syndrome. *J Pediatr Gastroenterol Nutr.* 1997;17:1–12.
158. Goulet O, Jan D, Brousse N. Intestinal transplantation. *J Pediatr Gastroenterol Nutr.* 1997;25:1–11.
159. Horslen S. Optimal management of the post-transplant patient. *Gastroenterology.* 2004 (in press).
160. Hendricks K. Nutrition aspects of chronic liver disease. *Pediatr G-I Nutr News.* (Massachusetts General Hospital) 1988;2.
161. Goulet OJ, deGoyet JDV, Ricour C. Preoperative nutritional evaluation and support for liver transplantation in children. *Transplant Proc.* 1987;14:3249–3255.
162. Weisdorf S, Lysne J, Cerra F. Total parenteral nutrition in hepatic failure and transplantation. In: Lebenthal E, ed., *Total Parenteral Nutrition: Indications, Utilization, Complications, and Pathophysiological Considerations.* New York: Raven Press;1986.
163. Sutton M. Nutritional support in pediatric liver transplantation. *Diet Nutr Support.* 1989;March/April:1–9.
164. Khazal P, Freese D, Sharp H. A pediatric perspective on liver transplantation. *Pediatr Clin North Am.* 1988;35: 409–433.
165. Byers S, Wood RP, Kaufman S, Williams L, Antonson D, Vanderhoof J. Liver transplantation therapy for children: Part I. *J Pediatr Gastroenterol Nutr.* 1988;7: 157–166.
166. Pennington JAT. *Bowes and Church's Food Values of Portions Commonly Used,* 15th ed. Philadelphia: JB Lippincott;1989.

167. U.S. Department of Agriculture. *USDA Provisional Table on the Dietary Fiber Content of Selected Foods;* HNIS/PT-106;1988.

168. Mennella JA, Griffin CE, Beauchamp GK. Flavor programming during infancy. *Pediatrics*. 2004;113: 840–845.

169. Mennella JA, Johnson A, Beauchamp GK. Garlic ingestion by pregnant women alters the odor of amniotic fluid. *Chem Senses*. 1995;20:207–209.

170. Mennella JA, Beauschamp GK. Flavor experience during formula feeding are related to preferences during childhood. *Early Human Dev*. 2002;68:71–82.

171. Liem DG, Mennella JA. Sweet and sour preferences during childhood: Role of early experiences. *Dev Psychobiol*. 2002;41:388–395.

172. Owada M, Anki K, Kitagawa T. Taste preferences and feeding behavior in children with phenylketonuria on a semisynthetic diet. *Eur J Pediatr*. 2000;159:846–850.

Chapter 17

Chronic Renal Disease

Nancy S. Spinozzi

ETIOLOGY AND CONSEQUENCES

Infants and children with chronic renal disease face multiple and frequent dietary manipulations throughout their course of treatment. This occurs at a time when growth and development are at their most dynamic stages and behavioral adaptations to eating and making food choices are greatly influenced. Dietary modifications, along with the physical and emotional effects of chronic illness, can result in outcomes counterproductive to these activities. However, with better understanding of the particular disease and its medical and nutritional management (including the timely initiation of recombinant human growth hormone, rhGH), it is possible to overcome what not too long ago were negative, though tolerated, outcomes: growth retardation and metabolic bone disease.

CHRONIC RENAL FAILURE (CRF)

Chronic renal failure (CRF) in infants and children is almost equally represented by acquired and congenital etiologies.[1] Acquired diseases, such as chronic glomerulonephritis, fortunately have less impact on growth, due to their more insidious onset. Congenital diseases, however, can result in early and severe growth retardation. Therefore, infants and toddlers (ages birth to 4 years) presenting with chronic renal insufficiency (CRI) must be aggressively nourished in order to promote at least a normal growth rate, preferably greater than the fifth percentile of length for age.[2,3] The earlier the age of onset of renal failure (glomerular filtration rate [GFR] less than 30% of normal), the more potentially severe its impact on growth will be.[4–6]

The consequences of chronic renal failure and its treatments for children all potentially influence growth (see Table 17–1). If any of these conditions are left inadequately managed, linear growth of the child will be delayed.[7,8] If properly treated, growth retardation can be arrested; however, catch-up growth is difficult to achieve.

The characteristic symptoms of CRF in children signaling increasing uremia are noted in Table 17–2. Several of those listed, including nausea, growth retardation, swelling, and shortness of breath, may respond favorably to some dietary modification(s). When, despite aggressive attempts at optimizing nutritional intake and preventing renal osteodystrophy, normal growth velocity is unattainable, the initiation of rhGH becomes necessary.[9,10] Of note is that adequate nutrition and control of renal bone disease continue to be significant therapies in the management of children with CRF.

In 1997, the National Kidney Foundation published the *Dialysis Outcomes Quality Initiative (K/DOQI) Clinical Practice Guidelines*, which were updated in 2001. The guidelines include the areas of chronic kidney disease, hemodialysis, peritoneal dialysis, vascular access, nutrition, bone metabolism and disease, and dyslipidemias. Within the nutrition guidelines is a section devoted to the pediatric patient.[11] The guidelines reflect the insufficient quantity of pediatric research and experience currently available; however, an increasing collection of data by the North American Pediatric Renal Transplant Cooperative Study

Table 17–1 Consequences of Chronic Renal Failure

Water/electrolyte imbalance
Accumulation of endogenous/exogenous toxins
Hypertension
Acidosis
Anemia
Renal osteodystrophy
Anorexia/undernutrition
Need for steroid therapy

(NAPRTCS) and several ongoing multicenter studies promises to provide continued expertise for the pediatric practitioner.[12]

To summarize, the impact of CRF on growth in children depends upon the severity and duration of the renal insufficiency, the diagnosis, and the age of onset. The treatments of CRF (dialysis and transplantation) will affect growth as well.

CONSERVATIVE MANAGEMENT

Treating children with CRF without dialysis requires judicious and frequent monitoring of diet intake, biochemical parameters, and growth.[13] Any chronic disease in children requires the historical, accurate recording of growth measurements. In CRF, weight and weight for height are particularly difficult to assess given the often insidious accumulation of extracellular fluid not always apparent in children. Also, the normal ranges for a number of laboratory values are different for children of different ages and should be considered whenever assessing a child's metabolic status.

Table 17–2 Symptoms of Uremia in Children

Nausea
Weakness
Fatigue
Decreased school performance
Loss of attention span
Growth retardation
Changes in urine output
Shortness of breath
Swelling of face/extremities/abdomen
Amenorrhea in adolescent girls

Formula selection in the past favored the use of PM60/40 by Ross Products given its preferred calcium to phosphorus ratio of 2:1 and low content of electrolytes. However, now that normal growth can be obtained in infants with CRI and waste products significantly reduced, formula choice can be limited only to an infant's gastrointestinal tolerance. Although PM60/40 may still be initially considered, the infant should be transitioned to a standard infant formula once growth is evident in order to provide adequate intake of nutrients. This is particularly important to consider in fluid-restricted infants whose volume of formula may need to be reduced.[2]

Calcium and Phosphorus

It has long been recognized that renal osteodystrophy contributes significantly to growth retardation in children with renal insufficiency. [14] Early in the course of renal disease, synthesis of 1,25-dihydroxycholecalciferol (1.25 (OH)2D3) and the excretion of excessive dietary phosphate decrease, leading to the development of renal osteodystrophy and secondary hyperparathyroidism if left untreated. Hyperphosphatemia is considered a late indicator of bone deformities. Current therapy may include any or all of the following: dietary restriction of high-phosphorus foods and fluids (primarily dairy products, chocolate, nuts and colas), supplementation of vitamin D (1,25 $(OH)_2D_3$) and calcium, and the prescription of nonaluminum-, nonmagnesium-containing phosphate binders (calcium carbonate, acetate, glubionate and/or sevelamer hydrochloride) to be taken with meals.[15–19]

In infants, PM60/40 by Ross Products may be the initial formula of choice; however, it contains less phosphorus than the more common infant formulas and it may be inadequate in providing sufficient phosphorus for the growing infant.[2]

Sodium, Potassium, and Fluid

Sodium and fluid restriction might be necessary to prevent or control the incidence of hypertension and edema not uncommonly associated with CRI. Usually, a no-added-salt diet for height age is sufficient. Limitation of fluid should be based on the child's urine output and insensible losses. Hyperkalemia is rarely a problem as long as kidney function is greater than 5% of normal. However, some children may be prescribed medications such as ACE (angiotensin-converting enzyme) inhibitors (used to reduce proteinuria), which cause a reduction in GFR and concomitant reduction in the excretion of potassium ($K+$). Should potassium restriction become necessary, limiting high-potassium foods in the diet is generally adequate. It is necessary to assess and monitor the potassium content of infant formula and nutritional supplements in addition to that of solid foods as blood levels are monitored.

For infants requiring sodium and/or potassium restriction, formulas such as PM60/40 or Carnation Good Start are appropriate. Furthermore, if the volume of formula must be restricted, it is unlikely that any significant contribution of sodium or potassium will come from formula. It should be noted that infants with increased urine losses of sodium and/or potassium will need supplementation to their usual diet.

Protein/Energy

Energy needs are at least 80% of the recommended dietary allowance (RDA) for height age and may be greater than 100%. [20] It is generally accepted that protein restriction much below the RDA for height age is contraindicated in growing children. With dietary phosphate restriction alone, a considerable limitation of protein intake could occur without restriction of protein per se. Routine nutritional assessment including anthropometric measurements and dietary intake will indicate whether the prescribed protein and calorie levels are adequate.[21]

Providing optimal nutrition within the limitations of fluid restriction (voluntary or involuntary) is possible only by caloric supplementation of the formula to as much as 60 kcal/oz. Increasing caloric density by three times normal dilution requires a methodical approach.[2] Attempts should be made to maintain caloric distribution as follows, with the lower intakes of fat calories recommended for children over the age of 2 years:

Carbohydrate	35% to 65%
Protein	16% to 5%
Fat	55% to 30%

Carbohydrate sources such as Polycose (Ross Laboratories) and Moducal (Mead Johnson) are coupled with an oil (canola, corn oil, or medium-chain triglyceride [MCT] oil for premature infants), as illustrated in Figure 17–1. Concentration of the formula with or without the addition of a protein supplement such as Promod (Ross Laboratories) increases protein content. Caloric density can be advanced 2 to 4 calories/day as tolerated.[2] A number of manipulations may be considered in addition to these such as using Duocal, a powdered calorie supplement containing both carbohydrate and fat (SHS North America) or diluting adult products such as Suplena (Ross Laboratories). Ensuring the consistent daily intake of a sufficient volume of formula to meet an infant's nutritional goals for growth most often can be achieved only after the initiation of enteral tube feedings.[21–24] The presence of gastroesophageal reflux in infants with CRI is considered a major factor contributing to feeding problems in this age group.[25] However, continuous nighttime infusions of formula via feeding pump allow maximum tolerance of formula.

Once nutritional goals are realized and a feeding regimen established, additional oral stimulation through nonnutritive sucking can begin.[26] In the author's experience, once children are successfully transplanted they eventually return to normal feeding practices.

Vitamins and Minerals

Because few children with CRI have consistently adequate diets, it is suggested that a multivitamin be routinely recommended. Additionally, 0.5–1 mg folic acid should be included. Iron supplementation may be indicated as well, especially if the child is receiving erythropoietin and ferri-tin and/or transferrin saturation levels are depressed.[27,28]

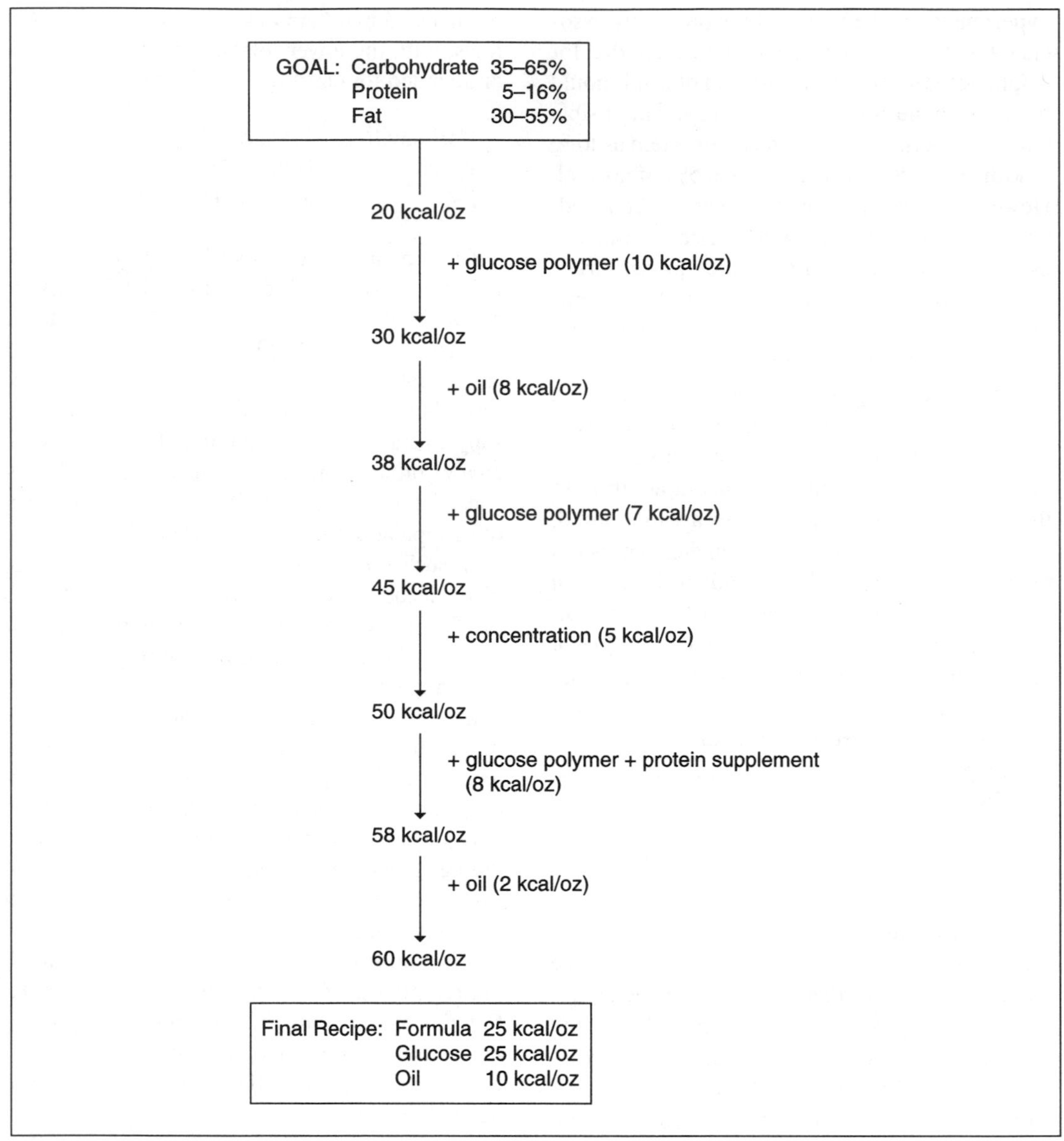

Figure 17–1 Increasing Caloric Density of Formula: An Example. (Editors' note: Very low fat intake in children less than 2 years of age may compromise development of the brain and central nervous system.)

Lipids

Hypertriglyceridemia secondary to decreased hepatic lipase activity is common in CRI. Management with carbohydrate restriction is controversial given the limited caloric intake of many infants and children. Most practitioners currently choose not to restrict carbohydrate at the expense of compromised growth.[29,30]

DIALYSIS

Dialysis is indicated once a child experiences symptoms that significantly interfere with activities of daily living. Peritoneal dialysis (continuous cycling or continuous ambulatory) is the preferred choice of dialytic care for infants and small children. Both hemodialysis and peritoneal dialysis are options for bigger children. Nutritional management is dictated by the type of dialytic therapy chosen; however, the principles are similar to those described for conservative management. Nutrient losses via dialysate (in particular, protein, phosphorus, sodium, and potassium) must be considered when assessing nutritional adequacy of the diet.[31]

Calcium and Phosphorus

Management of calcium and phosphorus balance continues to be necessary even while on dialysis and is the same as that stated previously.

Sodium, Potassium, and Fluid

A child's recommended intake for sodium and potassium is directly related to his or her residual renal function and the type and effectiveness of dialysis. Likewise, the degree of ultrafiltration possible and the child's urine output will dictate an advisable fluid intake. If restriction of sodium and potassium is necessary, which usually happens, the elimination or limitation of the foods containing especially large amounts of sodium and potassium is generally sufficient. Severely restricted diets often encourage noncompliance and dull a child's interest in food. Individualization of diet, taking into consideration the child's food preferences, is essential to successful control of sodium, potassium, and fluid intake.[32]

Protein/Energy

The nutritional requirements for protein and energy for patients undergoing peritoneal dialysis are not clear and the historical reliance on serum albumin levels in the pediatric patient may be in question when assessing adequacy. It is known that some protein is lost to the dialysate, while glucose is absorbed from the dialysate. The degree to which these changes occur can only be determined through measurement of individual patients. Periodic calculations of urinary and dialysate urea nitrogen, dialysate protein and amino acids, and miscellaneous nitrogen losses are necessary.[33] Diets can then be developed and altered when measurements indicate the need, promoting growth while preventing obesity.[34] During periods of peritonitis, there is an increased loss of protein to the dialysate, and the child usually feels ill. Careful attention to dietary intake is important to prevent a potentially significant loss of lean body weight during this time of infection.

Protein and energy requirements for children on hemodialysis have been studied using urea kinetic modeling, as well as actual nitrogen balance techniques.[35,36] It was concluded that a protein intake of 0.3 g/cm/d and an energy intake of 10 kcal/cm/d produced positive nitrogen balance. The protein catabolic and urea generation rates of the children in positive balance were uniformly lower; therefore, there was no increase necessary in dialysis requirements with these levels of intake.

The routine use of urea kinetic modeling is especially helpful in determining dialysis and nutritional adequacy in children.[37,38] Monthly monitoring of protein catabolic rates and urea generation provides insight into subtle changes in dialysis treatment and/or diet intake that otherwise might go unnoticed. Kinetic modeling, usually conducted by the dietitian, allows the dietitian access to the fundamental parameters and concepts of dialysis prescription, ensuring maximum confidence in the nutrition counseling of patients.

Lipids

Hyperlipidemia remains a problem in children on dialysis, particularly peritoneal dialysis.[39] Treatment in growing children remains controversial.[32]

Vitamins

It is advisable that children on both hemodialysis and peritoneal dialysis be provided water-soluble vitamins and folate, which are lost to dialysate.[40] Although studies have not been conducted in children, it is current practice to provide 1 mg folate, 5 to 10 mg vitamin B6, and up to 100 mg ascorbic acid per day.[11] Additional water-soluble vitamins should be given according to the RDAs for height age. There are specially formulated dialysis vitamin preparations on the market such as Nephro-Vite Rx (R&D Laboratories) and Nephrocaps (Fleming & Co.) that fulfill most patients' needs. Infants can be given a standard liquid multivitamin such as Polyvisol (Mead Johnson) and young children can take a flavored chewable multivitamin; however, both should be accompanied by folate.

Carnitine

Secondary carnitine deficiency has been noted in patients receiving dialysis.[41] Treatment remains somewhat controversial, especially in pediatric programs.

TRANSPLANTATION

The ultimate goal of all pediatric end-stage renal disease programs is transplantation. This is the only treatment option thus far that provides children with the opportunity for normal growth and development and potentially for catch-up growth.[42] Clinicians must be constantly vigilant for signs of rejection and infection, especially in the first postoperative year. Immunosuppression and antibiotic therapy result in side effects related to inefficient digestion and metabolism of nutrients, as well as to growth retardation.[43] The advent of new immunosuppressants, while providing increased protection from rejection, also increases the risk of the patient developing hyperglycemia (due to insulin resistance), hyperlipidemia, and hypercholesteremia. Alternate-day steroid therapy has been shown to promote normal and, at times, catch-up growth. The medical course of the patient and the individual transplant program's protocol for immunosuppression will dictate just how quickly a patient can begin tapering to alternate-day dosing.

For small children receiving adult kidneys, parenteral nutrition may be considered immediately postoperatively. Surgically implanting an adult-size kidney in a very small child usually requires significant bowel manipulation to make enough room for the organ and an ileus may result.

Once feedings are resumed, the dietary recommendations are once again individualized. If kidney function is not normal, attention to sodium, potassium, phosphorus, and fluid will be necessary. A rise in blood urea nitrogen (BUN) level and a slow recovery to normal is usual even with normal kidney function due to the catabolic stress of surgery. If it is possible, aggressive nutritional support of the patient should resume soon after transplant.[44]

With the attainment of normal kidney function, a no-added-salt diet is still advisable. Hypertension, now a potential result of high-dose steroid therapy, is frequently seen after transplantation, and sodium restriction, at least during the acute phase (first 6 to 8 months after transplant), is helpful. Also, tubular loss of phosphate is often present, requiring phosphorus supplementation. Dietary phosphorus intake usually is not adequate to maintain blood levels above 3.0 mg/dL.

Perhaps the most important aspect of the diet at this time is instruction in appropriate portion sizes. Most children have never learned to eat nutritionally balanced meals. Additionally, the increased appetite accompanying steroid therapy should be manipulated in a positive, healthy fashion, before a taste develops for high-carbohydrate, high-fat foods. It is common to hear parents describe the mealtimes of their newly transplanted children as lasting all day with one meal overlapping another.

Once steroids are tapered to levels where hypertension and hyperglycemia are no longer problematic, a diet appropriate for height age is indicated. Continued assessment of nutritional adequacy of the diet is necessary even with normal kidney function.

CONCLUSION

The nutritional intake of the child is especially important in order to ensure optimal growth and development during all stages of renal disease. The diet must be adequate and consistent. This is no easy task in light of the symptomatology accompanying the disease. Anorexia and taste changes commonly associated with CRF[45,46] constantly challenge attempts to promote optimal nutritional care. Additionally, dietary modification (see Table 17–3) and implementation must be individualized for all age groups, taking into account developmental levels, growth potentials, and renal functional limitations. Input from the entire renal team at all times is critical to ensuring successful nutritional management of this population. Frequent evaluation of food intake, growth, kidney function, and developmental stages is essential to adequate care.

Table 17–3 Major Nutritional Considerations

Nutrient	*Indication for Treatment*	*Modification*
Phosphorus	CRI, elevated parathyroidhormone level, with or without hyperphosphatemia	Phosphate binders; low-phosphate diet; calcium and vitamin D supplement
	Posttransplant tubular loss; hypophosphatemia	Add supplement
Sodium	Hypertension; fluid retention	No Added Salt
	Daily steroid therapy	No Added Salt
	Increased urine losses	Add supplement
	Increased peritoneal dialysate losses	Add supplement
Potassium	$< 5\%$ GFR; hyperkalemia	Restrict diet
	Diuretic therapy; hypokalemia; diarrhea)	Add supplement
Protein	Infants with CRI (no dialysis)	RDA
	Children with CRI (no dialysis)	Limit to RDA
	Children on hemodialysis	RDA
	Infants/children on peritoneal dialysis	$>$ RDA
	Posttransplant	
Energy	Undernutrition/anorexia	$\geq$ RDA
	Infants with CRI (no dialysis)	$\geq$ RDA
	Children on hemodialysis	$\geq$ RDA
	Dextrose absorption from peritoneal dialysate	$\leq$ RDA
	Posttransplant steroid therapy	Varies
	Steroid-induced hyperglycemia	No concentrated sweets

REFERENCES

1. Fine RN. Growth in children with renal insufficiency. In: Nissenson A, Fine RN, Gentile D, eds., *Clinical Dialysis*. New York: Appleton-Century Crofts; 1984:661.
2. Spinozzi NS, Nelson P. Nutrition support in the newborn intensive care unit. *J Renal Nutr.* 1996;6:188–197.
3. Ellis EN, Yiu V, Harley F, et al. The impact of supplemental feeding in young children on dialysis: A report of the North American Pediatric Renal Transplant Cooperative Study. *Pediatr Nephrol.* 2000;16:404–408.
4. Betts PR, White RHR. Growth potential and skeletal maturity in children with chronic renal insufficiency. *Nephron.* 1976;16:325–332.
5. Broyer M. Growth in children with renal insufficiency. *Pediatr Clin North Am.* 1982;29:991–1003.
6. Rizzoni G, Broyer M, Guest G, et al. Growth retardation in children with chronic renal disease: Scope of the problem. *Am J Kidney Dis.* 1986;7:256–261.

7. Rizzoni G, Basso T, Setari M. Growth in children with chronic renal failure on conservative treatment. *Kidney Int.* 1984;26:52–58.

8. Kleinknecht C, Broyer M, Hout D, et al. Growth and development of nondialyzed children with chronic renal failure. *Kidney Int.* 1983;24(S15):40–47.

9. Fine RN, Kohout EC, Brown D, Perlman AJ. Growth after recombinant human growth hormone treatment in children with chronic renal failure: Report of a multicenter randomized double-blind placebo-controlled study. *J Pediatr.* 1994;124:374–382.

10. Berard E, Crosnier H, Six-Beneton A, et al. Recombinant human growth hormone treatment of children on hemodialysis. *Pediatr Nephrol.* 1998;12:304–310.

11. National Kidney Foundation. K/DOQI Clinical Practice Guidelines for Nutrition in Chronic Renal Failure. *Am J Kidney Dis.* 2000;35(6):S105–S136.

12. Neu AM, Ho PL, McDonald RA, Warady BA. Chronic dialysis in children and adolescents. The 2001 NAPRTCS Annual Report. *Pediatr Nephrol.* 2002;17:656–663.

13. Hellerstein S, Holliday MA, Grupe WE, et al. Nutritional management of children with chronic renal failure. *Pediatr Nephrol.* 1987;1:195–211.

14. Salusky IB, Goodman WG. The management of renal osteodystrophy. *Pediatr Nephrol.* 1996;10:651–653.

15. Brookhyser J, Pahre SN. Dietary and pharmacotherapeutic considerations in the management of renal osteodystrophy. *Adv Renal Replacement Therapy.* 1995;2:5–13.

16. Tamanah K, Mak RH, Rigden SP, Turner C, et al. Long-term suppression of hyperparathyroidism by phosphate binders in uremic children. *Pediatr Nephrol.* 1987;1:145–149.

17. Schiller LR, Sheikh MS, et al. Effect of the time of administration of calcium acetate on phosphorus binding. *New Engl J Med.* 1989;320:1110–1113.

18. Schmitt, J. Selecting an appropriate phosphate binder. *J Renal Nutr.* 1990;1:38–40.

19. Bleyer AJ, Burke SK, Dillon M, et al. A comparison of the calcium-free phosphate binder sevelamer hydrochloride with calcium acetate in the treatment of hyperphosphatemia in hemodialysis patients. *Am J Kidney Dis.* 1999;33:694–701.

20. Betts PR, Macgrath G. Growth pattern and dietary intake of children with chronic renal insufficiency. *Br Med J.* 1974;2:189.

21. Nelson P, Stover J. Nutritional recommendations for infants, children and adolescents with ESRD. In: *A Clinical Guide to Nutrition Care in End-Stage Renal Disease*, 2nd ed. Chicago, Ill: American Dietetic Association; 1994:79–97.

22. Yiu VWY, Harmon WE, Spinozzi NS, et al. High-calorie nutrition for infants with chronic renal disease. *J Renal Nutr.* 1996;6:203–206.

23. Ledermann SE, Spitz L, Malony J, et al. Gastrostomy feeding in infants and children on peritoneal dialysis. *Pediatr Nephrol.* 2002;17:246–250.

24. Reed EE, Roy LP, Gaskin KJ, Knight JF. Nutritional intervention and growth in children with chronic renal failure. *J Renal Nutr.* 1998;8:122–126.

25. Ruley EJ, Boch GH, Kerzner B, Abbott AW. Feeding disorders and gastroesophageal reflux in infants with chronic renal failure. *Pediatr Nephrol.* 1989;3:424–429.

26. Bebaum JC, Pererra GR, Watkins JB, et al. Non-nutritive sucking during gavage feeding enhances growth and maturation in premature infants. *Pediatrics.* 1983;71:41–45.

27. Eschbach MD, Egrie JC, Downing MR, et al. Correction of the anemia of end-stage renal disease with recombinant human erythropoietin. *N Engl J Med.* 1987;310:73–78.

28. Van Wyck DB, Stivelman JC, Ruiz J. Iron status in patients receiving erythropoietin for dialysis-associated anemia. *Kidney Int.* 1989;35:712–716.

29. Arnold WC, Danford D, Holliday MC. Effects of calorie supplementation on growth in children with uremia. *Kidney Int.* 1983;24:205.

30. Betts PR, Magrath G, White RHR. Role of dietary energy supplementation in growth of children with chronic renal insufficiency. *Br Med J.* 1977;1:416.

31. Wolfson M. Nutritional management of the continuous ambulatory peritoneal patient. *Am J Kidney Dis.* 1996;27:744–749.

32. Secker D, Pencharz MB: Nutritional therapy for children on CAPD/CCPD: Theory and practice. In: Fine RN, Alexander SR, Warady BA, eds., *CAPD/CCPD in Children.* Boston, MA: Kluwer Academic; 1998:567–603.

33. Schleifer CR, Teehan BP, Brown JM, Raimondo J. The application of urea kinetic modeling to peritoneal dialysis: A review of methodology and outcome. *J Renal Nutr.* 1993;3:2–9.

34. Harvey E, Secker D, Braj B, Picone G, Balfe JW. The team approach to the management of children on chronic peritoneal dialysis. *Adv Renal Replacement Ther.* 1996;3:3–13.

35. Spinozzi NS, Grupe WE. Nutritional implications of renal disease. *J Am Diet Assoc.* 1977;70:493–497.

36. Grupe WE, Harmon WE, Spinozzi NS. Protein and energy requirements in children receiving chronic hemodialysis. *Kidney Int.* 1983;24:S6–S10.

37. Harmon WE, Spinozzi NS, Meyer A, Grupe WE. The use of protein catabolic rate to monitor pediatric hemodialysis. *Dial Transplant.* 1981;10:324.

38. Goldstein SL, Sorof JM, Brewer ED. Natural logarithmic estimates of Kt/V in the pediatric hemodialysis population. *Am J Kidney Dis.* 1999;33:518–522.
39. Querfeld U, Salusky IB, Nelson P, et al. Hyperlipidemia in pediatric patients undergoing peritoneal dialysis. *Pediatr Nephrol.* 1988;2:447–452.
40. Warady BA, Kriley M, Alon U, Hellerstein S. Vitamin status of infants receiving long-term peritoneal dialysis. *Pediatr Nephrol.* 1994;8:354–356.
41. Matera M, Bellinghieri G, Costantino G, et al. History of L-carnitine: Implications for renal disease. *J Renal Nutr.* 2003;13:2–14.
42. Fine RN. Renal transplantation for children—The only realistic choice. *Kidney Int Suppl.* 1985;17:515–517.
43. Neu AM, Warady BA. Dialysis and renal transplantation in infants with irreversible renal failure. *Adv in Renal Replacement Ther.* 1996;3:48–59.
44. Seagraves A, Moore EE, Moore FA, et al. Net protein catabolic rate after kidney transplantation: Impact of corticosteroid immunosuppression. *J Parenter Enteral Nutr.* 1986;10:453–455.
45. Spinozzi NS, Murray CL, Grupe WE. Altered taste acuity in children with ESRD. *Pediatr Res.* 1978;12:442. Abstract.
46. Shapera MR, Moel DI, Kamath SK, et al. Taste perception of children with chronic renal failure. *J Am Diet Assoc.* 1986;86:1359–1365.

CHAPTER 18

Growth Failure

Kattia M. Corrales and Sherri L. Utter

INTRODUCTION

Growth failure (also known as failure to thrive) is a serious condition of undernutrition and poor growth usually identified in the first 3 years of life. Nutritional inadequacy is central to the pathogenesis of growth failure because poor growth in a child is essentially the result of not taking, not being offered, or not retaining adequate calories.[1] The etiology of growth failure has historically been classified as either organic or nonorganic in nature. Organic growth failure indicates malnutrition due to an underlying medical condition causing inadequate intake, absorption, or utilization of nutrients. Nonorganic growth failure suggests a social or behavioral dysfunction leading to inadequate oral intake (Exhibit 18–1). However, a dichotomous classification is often inappropriate, because many children with growth failure will present with both physiologic and psychosocial conditions that inhibit their growth. The development and progression of growth failure involves a complex and multifactorial process influenced by several factors, including medical status and temperament, as well as familial, economic, and psychosocial conditions. A multidisciplinary team, including a pediatrician, child psychologist or behaviorist, dietitian, nurse clinician, and social worker is often most effective in the treatment of growth failure.[2–4]

DIAGNOSTIC CRITERIA AND EVALUATION OF GROWTH

Despite the common use of the term, an exact and consistent method for identifying growth failure has not been established.[5] Growth failure is defined by both anthropometry and by diagnostic criteria related to the etiology of undernutrition. Anthropometric definitions of growth failure are typically based on growth that deviates from the norms established by the 2000 Centers for Disease Control (CDC) growth charts. These charts are recommended for use, regardless of race or ethnic origin.[6] Weight, length/height, and head circumference are plotted to obtain percentiles for weight for age, length/height for age, head circumference for age, weight for length/height, and body mass index (BMI). The following criteria are commonly used to identify growth failure:

Growth below a specified percentile on the growth chart:
- Weight for age plotting less than the 3rd or 5th percentile on the CDC growth charts
- Weight for length/height plotting less than the 3rd or 5th percentile

Poor growth velocity
- Decreased growth velocity where weight falls more than two major percentiles over 3 to 6 months
- Decrease of more than 2 standard deviations on the growth chart over a 3- to 6-month period

Evaluation of Growth

It is best to assess the progression of growth longitudinally when evaluating for growth failure. A single point on the growth chart does not provide information about a child's growth pattern or

Exhibit 18–1 Risk Factors for Failure to Thrive

Organic Factors

Inability to take in adequate calories

- Difficulty with sucking, mastication, swallowing
- Neurologic disease
- Systemic disease resulting in anorexia/food refusal

Inability to retain/utilize adequate calories

- Persistent vomiting
- Gastroesophageal reflux
- Rumination syndrome
- Malabsorption/maldigestion
  - Inflammatory bowel disease, celiac disease, short gut syndrome, cystic fibrosis, HIV
- Poor nutrient utilization
  - Renal tubular acidosis, inborn errors of metabolism

Increased calorie requirements

- Congenital heart disease
- Brochopulmonary dysplasia
- Fevers
- Hyperthyroidism

Altered growth potential

- Perinatal complications
  - Prematurity, intrauterine growth retardation, exposure to drugs/toxins
- Congenital anomalies
- Chromosomal abnormalities
- Endocrinopathies
  - Growth hormone deficiency, hypothyroidism, hypercortisolism

Nonorganic Factors

Inability to provide adequate calories

- Poverty
- Inadequate breast milk production

Psychosocial issues

- Disordered feeding environment
- Dysfunctional parent-child interaction
  - Behavioral feeding problem, neglect, abuse, sickly/difficult child, isolated/overwhelmed mother, emotionally/physically unavailable father
- Stress and loss in the social environment
  - Marital stress, family history of death and loss, chronic illness, poverty

Lack of knowledge/misinformation regarding feeding practices

- Errors in formula preparation
- Excessive juice consumption
- Misperceptions about diet and feeding practices
- Unusual health and nutrition beliefs

Source: Data from endnote references 15, 68, 69, 73, 74, and 75

deviation from previously established growth channels. Although normal shifting of percentiles for linear growth may occur during the first 2 years of life,[7] a weight decrease of more than two major percentiles from a previously established growth channel should be considered evidence of growth failure.[8,9] Edwards and associates[10] found that the maximum weight percentile achieved by a child between 4 and 8 weeks of age is a better predictor of the percentile at 12 months than is the birth weight percentile. They propose that growth failure be defined as a weight deviation of two or more major percentiles below the maximum weight percentile achieved by 4 to 8 weeks for a period of a month or more.

Weight for age should not be used as the single measure for identifying growth failure because some children are both underweight and short, relative to reference standards (weight for age and length/height for age less than the 3rd or 5th percentile), but have weight for length/height ratios within the normal range. These children may be genetically small, be demonstrating constitutional growth delay, or have suffered a nutritional insult earlier in life, yet not be acutely malnourished or showing a weight for length/height deficit.[11–13]

When evaluating delays in linear growth, genetic growth potential based on parental height and the possibility of constitutional growth delay should be taken into consideration. Constitutional growth delay (CGD) is a normal variation of growth where linear growth velocity and weight gain slows beginning as early as 3 to 6 months of age, resulting in downward crossing of growth percentiles. This pattern of growth may continue until 2 or 3 years of age with subsequent establishment of a growth channel and normal growth velocity parallel to the growth curve for the remainder of the prepubertal years.[12] Bone age can be determined to help differentiate stunting from genetic short stature.[14,15] If bone age lags behind chronologic age and equals length/height age, this suggests the child has room to make additional gains in length/height. In genetic short stature bone age typically is the same as chronologic age.

Special consideration should be used when evaluating premature and small-for-gestational-age (SGA) infants as they are generally small at birth relative to reference standards, but exhibit different patterns of growth in infancy and early childhood.[12,16] Guidelines for the assessment and nutritional management of premature and SGA infants appear in Chapter 4.

CLASSIFICATION OF SEVERITY OF UNDERNUTRITION

Gomez and Waterlow Criteria

Percentile values on the growth chart can help identify a growth problem but do not relate the severity of undernutrition. The Gomez and Waterlow criteria[17,18] were developed to determine the degree of malnutrition in children in developing countries and have been used in clinical practice in the United States. These categorization systems compare actual weight and/or length/height with the expected standards (for example, the 50th percentile on the 2000 CDC growth chart) (Table 18–1). Degree of undernutrition is divided into four levels: normal, mild, moderate, and severe. The Waterlow[18] criteria take into account both weight and length/height. Weight for length/height is evaluated as an index of wasting due to acute undernutrition. Length/height for age is evaluated as an index of stunting due to chronic undernutrition. The Gomez[17] criteria evaluate weight for age but do not account for stature, thereby increasing the risk for inappropriate labeling of malnutrition For example, a child who is short in stature but at an appropriate weight for length/height may appear underweight using the Gomez criteria but of normal weight using the Waterlow criteria. Ultimately, categorization systems for assessing the degree of undernutrition should be used to identify children at risk for malnutrition in the context of an assessment of developmental, dietary, and psychosocial factors.[19]

Standard Deviation

The standard deviation (SD) score, also called the Z score, is useful in expressing how far a

Table 18–1 Classification of Severity of Undernutrition

	Gomez Criteria	*Waterlow Criteria*	
Grade of Malnutrition	*Percent of Median Weight for Age (Underweight)*	*Percent of Median Weight for Height (Wasting)*	*Percent of Median Height for Age (Stunting)*
Normal	90–110	90–110	>95
I. Mild	75–89	80–89	90–94
II. Moderate	60–74	70–79	85–89
III. Severe	<60	<70	<85

Source: Data from endnote references 17 and 18.

child's weight and length/height fall from the median, or 50th percentile, on the reference growth charts for children of the same age and sex.[20]

$$\text{Z score} = \frac{\text{measurement value} - \text{median for age value of reference population}}{\text{standard deviation for age of reference population}}$$

Categorizing growth according to progressive decrements in SD scores (−2.0, −3.0, −4.0) can be used to describe the relative severity of undernutrition. Percentiles and equivalent SD scores for weight for age, length/height for age, and weight for length/height can be easily calculated using computer software developed by the CDC and the World Health Organization (WHO).[21] A SD of zero is equivalent to the 50th percentile; −1.65 SD corresponds to the 5th percentile cut-off used in the National Nutrition Surveillance System. The WHO recommends that a cut-off point of −2.0 SD below the 2000 CDC growth chart median weight for age, length/height for age, and weight for length/height be used to discriminate between well-nourished and poorly nourished children.[22] When compared over time, a positive change in SD indicates growth, whereas a negative change indicates a slowing of the growth rate. Categorizing growth in this manner is the most accurate technique for classifying growth deficits in children and is the method preferred by the WHO[23] but proves more difficult in the clinical setting without the necessary software.

Anthropometry

Essentially, growth is the desired final outcome in the treatment of growth failure. Consistent and accurate technique in measuring growth parameters is imperative. Routine use of upper arm measurements may not be indicated but may be useful, especially in the malnourished child with edema. Triceps skinfolds and midarm muscle circumference may provide a better index of nutritional status than does the weight for length/height measurement because the arm is relatively free of edema.[24] Techniques for obtaining accurate anthropometric data are covered in Chapter 2.

MEDICAL EVALUATION

A complete medical history and physical examination are necessary to assess possible organic causes leading to growth failure. Exhibit 18–2 provides guidelines for obtaining information needed to assess the patient with growth failure.

A variety of medical conditions, especially those chronic in nature, can result in poor weight gain. A child should be evaluated for possible gastrointestinal symptoms, such as vomiting and diarrhea, recurrent infections, medication use, and previous hospitalizations. The child's perinatal history should be investigated because perinatal factors exert a powerful influence on patterns of postnatal growth. A family history should also be obtained to evaluate for chronic

Exhibit 18–2 Guidelines for the Assessment of Failure to Thrive

Health History

Individual:
- Gestational age
- Birth weight
- Type of delivery/APGAR scores/complications
- Prenatal history
- Growth history/pattern
- Activity level/energy
- Developmental milestones
- Illness (including acute/recurring/chronic)
- Hospitalizations (accidents/injuries/surgeries)
- Medications

Family:
- Mental illness
- Alcohol/drug abuse
- Genetic disorder
- Chronic or metabolic disorder
- Eating disorder
- Parental height
- Growth and development of siblings
- Maternal age

Clinical Exam

- Nausea, vomiting
- Diarrhea, steatorrhea, or constipation
- Stool size, frequency, consistency, color, odor
- Clinical manifestations of malnutrition
- Rumination
- Signs of abuse or neglect
- Poor oral health, diaper rash, general hygiene
- Accurate anthropometrics
- Dysmorphic features
- Gross motor skills and tone
- Developmental assessment

*Biochemical Data**

- Hematocrit (Hct)
- Hemaglobin (Hgb)
- Urinalysis (SG, pH)
- Erythrocytes sedimentation rate
- Electrolytes
- Albumin
- Prealbumin
- Blood urea nitrogen/creatinine
- Lead (Pb)
- Alkaline phosphatase
- Urine culture
- Stool for pH, reducing substances, ova, parasites, occult blood
- Sweat test
- TB test

*Laboratory testing should be limited to screening tests or those indicated by findings on the history and physical

Social History

- Multiple caregivers
- Support systems available to caregiver
- Maturity of caregiver
- Social environment (marital dissatisfaction, financial issues, disorganized lifestyle)
- History of abuse or neglect of child, sibling, or caregivers
- Socioeconomic status
- Perception of problem by caregivers
- Involvement in public programs (EIP, WIC, Food Stamps)
- History of loss

Nutrition History

- 24-hour recall/3–5 day food record
- Formula/Breastfeeding history
- Formula preparation
- History of food allergies/intolerances
- Food restrictions/special diets
- Age at introduction of solids/acceptance
- Amount of juice, soda, water and/or milk consumed
- Meal time/snacks (who feeds, where, duration)
- Self-feeding skill
- Difficulty chewing/swallowing/sucking
- Cues for hunger/satiety
- Rewards/punishments
- Feeding behavior/environment

Caregiver-Child Interaction

- Evidence of bonding (richness of interaction, eye and physical contact, sense of mutual pleasure, warmth and affection, consistency of response)
- Caregiver's attentiveness to child's cues
- Appropriateness of caregiver's expectations
- Clarity of child's cues to caregiver
- Caregiver's tolerance level

Source: Data from endnote references 68, 69, 74, and 75.

illnesses, mental illness, parental height, and the growth patterns of siblings. The physical examination should evaluate for dysmorphic features to identify syndromes that may be associated with poor growth, gross motor skills and tone, as well as signs of neglect or abuse.

Because poor nutrition and psychosocial factors are the most frequent causes of growth failure, laboratory testing is rarely warranted unless findings on the history and physical examination indicate a need.[25,26] A few screening tests may be useful. Screening for lead toxicity and anemia should be considered because approximately 50% of children with growth failure present with iron deficiency, and lead intoxication can result in poor growth.[27] Nutritional status can be further evaluated with serum protein tests, such as those for albumin and prealbumin. Alkaline phosphatase can be checked to evaluate for rickets (elevated) or zinc deficiency (depressed). Zinc deficiency has been implicated in poor growth.[28] Urinalysis, serum electrolytes, blood urea nitrogen, and creatinine levels can help evaluate for infection or renal dysfunction. If stool patterns are abnormal, the stool can be checked for pH, reducing substances, fat, ova, parasites, or occult blood to evaluate for possible infection, malabsorption, or allergy.

PSYCHOSOCIAL EVALUATION

Poverty and Familial Stress

Although growth failure can occur in any socioeconomic group,[29] incidence is especially high in urban and rural families living in poverty.[30–32] Rates of poverty have not decreased significantly since the late 1970s and appear to be more prevalent in African-American and Latino children and in children of single-parent families.[33] Poverty has been and continues to be a significant contributor to growth failure because it not only limits resources, such as food, shelter, and access to medical care, but also can compound already existing familial stress.

Parental stress and marital discord have been significantly correlated with growth failure.[34] Parental depression or intellectual impairment, drug abuse, and social isolation, especially in regard to a mother with poor social support,[35] have also been associated with growth failure.[31,36–39] Familial stress is a risk factor in growth failure because it can impair a parent's ability to perceive and provide for a child's emotional and physiologic needs. A parent who is in ill health, depressed, experiencing economic problems, or abusing drugs may not be able to respond to a child's hunger cues or to provide a stable home environment.[30] A history of neglect and abuse in the parent's own childhood—as well as signs of present abuse in the child—should always be explored in the evaluation of these cases. Whereas child abuse may not make up a significant number of growth failure cases,[40,41] one study found that a surprising 80% of mothers of children with growth failure had experienced child abuse in their own childhood. Withholding of food[42] and death by suspicious circumstances[39] have been reported in the growth failure literature.

PARENT-CHILD INTERACTIONS

Children with growth failure have been described as temperamental, lethargic, passive, and developmentally and physically immature.[1,37] They may be apathetic and hypervigilant and may demonstrate delays in cognitive and motor development.[43] They may have sleeping and elimination difficulties; be overly sensitive to stimulation; and exhibit oppositional behavior, defiance, and clingingness.[35,44] Feeding difficulties, which are prevalent in this population, may present in the form of abnormal duration of feeding time, poor appetite, delayed tolerance to different food textures, and deviant food behavior.[45,46] The child, as a result, may be viewed as difficult and sickly, and the caretaker may feel incompetent in parenting. The end result is a breakdown in the parent-child relationship. Parental perception that the child is vulnerable or at risk for death, whether from acute or chronic illness or from imagined problems, may alter the parent's ability to support age and culturally appropriate separation and individualization.[47] This condition, known as the vulnerable child syndrome, may result in a similar breakdown in the parent-child relationship and eventual feeding and growth issues in the child.

Whether aberrant behavior is inherent in the child or is the child's reaction to familial stress is not entirely clear. Ramsay and colleagues[45] found that many feeding skill disorders in children with growth failure were present at birth. They argued that these could be the result of a neurophysiologic process manifested by oral sensorimotor impairment of varying degrees, ranging from mild in the case of the healthy-looking child with nonorganic causes of growth failure, to severe in the case of the child with cerebral palsy.[45] However, the role of parent-infant interactions in the development of feeding disorders has also been extensively explored.[35,42,48,49] Chatoor and associates describe a developmental model that can help explain the complex interrelationship between parent and child resulting in feeding disorders.[49] They describe three stages of child development at which adaptive and maladaptive feeding behaviors can occur:

1. Disorders of homeostasis are thought to develop during the first 2 months of life when the child attempts to reach a balance between internal and external states and to form the basic rhythms of sleep, wakefulness, feeding, and elimination. For example, a child with congenital abnormalities, who may have delayed introduction and advancement of feedings or limited interaction with caregivers, may not achieve a balance between internal state and environmental limits. A parent who is unable to offer a stable environment for the child or to attend to the infant's cues on hunger, satiety, and emotional needs can contribute to disorders of homeostasis.
2. During the attachment phase, which begins between 2 and 6 months of age, the infant begins to interact with his or her environment in a more complex manner. At this stage of mutual interaction, a variety of factors can contribute to attachment disorders, including poor parenting skills, social isolation, and economic hardship, as well as a temperamental or overly sensitive infant who has difficulties in establishing normal patterns of sleep and eating. Because most interactions between infant and caregiver at this stage revolve around feeding, it is not surprising that a history of vomiting, diarrhea, and poor weight gain are common presenting features in poorly attached children. Fleisher and associates go on to argue that vomiting and rumination disorders in children may often be directly related to psychosocial issues. If these issues are missed, invasive and unnecessary medical intervention may occur.[50]
3. During the separation and individuation stage, which typically occurs between 6 months and 3 years of age, the child begins to deal with issues of autonomy and independence.[43] The child also begins to differentiate between somatophysiologic states (such as hunger, satiety, anger, frustration) and the need for affection. Separation disorders are thought to be related to the child's need for autonomy and the parent's inability to "let go." As the parent becomes more anxious about the child's eating, the child becomes more willful about gaining independence. Specific problems include a child who refuses to sit for meals, displays excessive aversion to different food textures or mixed foods, or is actively resistant to being fed.[43,48] A parent who force-feeds, coaxes with toys or other distractions to get the child to eat, or does not accept messes at meals contributes to the poor feeding situation.

NUTRITION EVALUATION

A complete diet history should be obtained to identify both nutritional and behavioral problems in feeding. Information about amounts and types of food eaten, food textures, portion sizes, and timing of feedings should be obtained. A 24-hour-diet recall or, if possible, a 3- to 7-day food record can be used to gather this information. Questions during the diet history should also address the child's feeding capacities, including the preferred duration and pace of feeding, the child's ability to remain focused on feeding, and the child's readiness or ability to self-feed. Guidelines for general nutrition assessment are described in Chapter 2. Exhibit 18–2 provides guidelines for the assessment of failure to thrive.

The most common mistake in formula preparation is improper dilution of formula, usually either secondary to a poor understanding of proper preparation or a parent's attempt to preserve formula due to financial concerns.[1] Polydipsia, polyuria, and a voracious appetite have been described as indications of an overly diluted formula.[40] Overly concentrated formula, on the other hand, can lead to early satiety, vomiting or diarrhea, and a subsequent net loss in nutrients. Another commonly identified problem in formula preparation is the addition of large quantities of cereal or baby food to the bottle, which displaces nutrients such as protein and fat.

In the breast-fed child, poor weight gain may result from an insufficient milk supply, poor maternal diet, inadequate let-down reflex, infrequent or short feedings, milk-suppressing medications, a sick baby, or a baby with difficulty latching or weak, unsustained suck.[51] Exclusive breastfeeding beyond 6 months of age, without the introduction of solids, can limit nutrient intake and inhibit the development of feeding milestones.[52,53]

Large amounts of juice, as well as other sugary beverages or water, can displace consumption of more nutrient-dense foods and be detrimental to growth.[54–56] Excessive juice consumption (over 12 to 16 oz per day) has also been associated with malabsorption and diarrhea in children.[57] A reduction or complete removal of juice from the child's diet may result in weight gain.

Finally, parental health beliefs and misconceptions about what constitutes a healthy diet for infants and children should be explored in the diet history. For example, a history of heart disease or obesity in the family or simply the pursuit of a "healthy diet" may induce parents to limit sweets, carbohydrates, fats, and food portions in their children's diets, even when children are not growing properly.[52,58] Vegetarian diets may not provide adequate amounts of several nutrients required for growth, such as protein, calcium, iron, vitamin B12, riboflavin, and zinc.[59,60]

Caregivers should be instructed on ways to make these diets more appropriate. Chapter 8 provides more information regarding vegetarian diets in children.

ASSESSMENT OF THE DIET

The caloric content of the diet must be compared with the child's specific needs for growth to evaluate whether the usual intake is inadequate. Protein, calcium, zinc, and iron intake should also be evaluated. The RDAs and the Recommended Daily Intakes (RDIs) can be used for this assessment (see Chapter 2 and Appendix I). Children with increased metabolic needs from chronic illness or increased losses from vomiting, diarrhea, or malabsorption may have nutritional needs different from the RDAs or RDIs.

Feeding Observation

Particular attention should be paid to behavioral factors that may lead to inadequate caloric intake. A feeding observation can be extremely helpful in identifying parent-infant interactions, as well as particular problems with feeding. Feeding observations can be done in the clinic or hospital setting but are more informative if done in the home. Particular points to note during a feeding observation are detailed in Exhibit 18–3. Several practical checklists have been developed specifically to assist in the observation of feeding interactions in nonorganic growth failure.[61,62]

Nutritional Therapy

Nutritional therapy of the child with growth failure has three principal goals:

1. Achievement of appropriate weight for length/height

Exhibit 18–3 Feeding Observation

General observations

- Does the child eat alone? Who feeds the child or sits with the child during meals? How many people are involved in the feeding?
- Note the location of feeding (kitchen, living room, day care, car), mealtime atmosphere, size and preparation of meals.
- Is the food offered on schedule or is the child allowed to "graze" all day?

Child behaviors

- Is the child interested in eating (reaches for bottle or spoon; opens mouth eagerly) or easily distracted (plays with food/toys; talks instead of eating) or uninvolved (looks around; opens mouth only when food touches lips)?
- Does the child:
  1. Have a poor suck, tire easily, and fall asleep after short feeding?
  2. Throw food, cry, vomit or ruminate, spit up, gag, turn head, arch, hold food in mouth, play with food?
  3. Make eye contact with the caregiver?
  4. Take greater than 30 minutes to eat?
  5. Refuse to stay seated?
  6. Express hunger or satiety? Request or refuse particular foods? How does the child communicate his/her likes/dislikes?

Caregiver behaviors

Does the caregiver:

- Position or sit the child so that eye contact is possible or is there little interaction between caregiver and child during feeding?
- Feed mechanically or prop bottle?
- Fail to establish a consistent feeding pattern?
- Ignore or seem unaware of the child's feeding cues?
- Appear bothered by messiness? Clean the child excessively during feeding?
- Appear anxious, depressed, overwhelmed, easily distressed, uninterested, hostile?
- Encourage self-feeding? Distract the child with toys? Offer rewards for eating?
- Terminate or interrupt feeding inappropriately, causing distress in the infant?
- What is the caregiver's reaction when the child does not eat? Does the caregiver become frustrated and angry? Force feed?

Source: Adapted with permission from MacPhee M, Schneider J. A clinical tool for nonorganic failure-to-thrive feeding interactions, *Journal of Pediatric Nursing*, vol. 11, no. 1, pp. 29–39, © 1996, W.B. Saunders Company; Satter E. The feeding relationship: Problems and interventions, *Journal of Pediatrics*, vol. 117, pp. 182–183, © Mosby-Yearbook.

2. Provision of macro- and micronutrient needs necessary for growth
3. Concrete and individualized nutrition instruction to caregivers

Catch-up growth is a period of accelerated growth achieved by providing calories in excess of the RDAs. Approximately 20–30% more energy may be needed for a child to achieve catch-up growth. Protein requirements will also increase.[63] Guidelines for estimating catch-up growth requirements are detailed in Exhibit 18–4. The Schofield equation[64], which has been found to more closely estimate resting energy

Exhibit 18–4 Estimating Catch-Up Growth Requirements

1. Plot the child's height and weight on the NCHS growth chart.
2. Determine the child's recommended calories for age (RDA or RDI).
3. Determine the ideal weight (50th percentile) for the child's height.
4. Multiply the RDA calories by ideal body weight for height (kg)*.
5. Divide this value by the child's actual weight.

Catch-up growth requirement:

$$\frac{\text{RDA calories for age** } \times \text{ ideal weight for height (kg)}}{\text{Actual weight}}$$

Protein requirements:

$$\frac{\text{RDA for protein for age } \times \text{ ideal weight for height}}{\text{Actual weight}}$$

* Ideal weight for age can be used in this part of the equation.

** Catch-up growth equations for children with developmental delay may utilize RDA for height age. (Determine at what age present height would be at 50th percentile. Use RDA for that age.)

expenditure in children with growth failure under 3 years of age, can be used in conjunction with an activity factor in place of RDA in the catch-up growth equation.[65] However, calculation of catch-up needs is simply an estimate. Weight gain at or above an expected rate for age is a better determinant of whether the child is receiving sufficient calories and protein (Table 18–2).

Aggressiveness of refeeding should be determined by the degree of malnutrition. Refeeding the severely malnourished child too quickly can result in vomiting, diarrhea, circulatory decompensation, and metabolic alterations (Exhibit 18–5). In these instances, the diet may require restriction to normal calories for age for the first 7 to 10 days, then gradually be increased toward catch-up growth requirements.[30] A multivitamin with minerals, including zinc and iron, is recommended to ensure that micronutrient needs are met.[13,14,30] Efforts to promote catch-up growth should continue until the child regains previous growth percentiles. Intake and rate of growth will spontaneously decelerate toward the normal level for age as deficits in weight for

Table 18–2 Average Gains in Weight and Height for Age

Age	*Weight (grams/day)*	*Height (mm/day)*
Premie	15–30	0.17
0–3 months	20–30	1.03
3–6 months	15–21	0.68
6–12 months	10–13	0.47
1–6 years	5–8	0.23
7–10 years	5–11	0.15

Source: Data from Fomon, SJ et al., Body composition of reference children from birth to age 10 years, *American Journal of Clinical Nutrition*, vol. 35, p. 1169, © 1982, American Society for Clinical Nutrition.

Exhibit 18–5 Metabolic Alterations Associated with Refeeding Syndrome

Severe hypophosphatemia
Hypokalemia
Hypomagnesemia
Glucose intolerance
Fluid intolerance

Source: Reprinted with permission from Solomon SM, Kirby DF. The refeeding syndrome: A review. *Journal of Parenteral and Enteral Nutrition*, vol. 14, pp. 90–96, © 1990, American Society for Parenteral and Enteral Nutrition.

length/height are repleted.[13] Catch-up growth in length may lag several months behind that in weight.[30]

It is often difficult to meet catch-up growth needs without increasing the caloric density of the diet via high-calorie foods or additives (Exhibit 18–6). Because nutritional intervention is often more effective if accompanied by techniques for behavioral change, it is important that any problematic behaviors identified during the feeding observation or diet history be addressed early. Concrete nutritional and behavioral guidelines should be developed. All individuals involved in caring for the child, including day care workers, babysitters, and grandparents, need to be included in the treatment plan.

Community-based management of growth failure must be coordinated, interdisciplinary, and family focused. Periodic home visits by public health nurses (or dietitians, if available in the community) can be incorporated as part of the treatment plan. Visiting nurses can reinforce care plans in the home environment and also get a firsthand view of specific family dynamics that may be contributing to the child's poor growth. Intervention by a social worker can be instrumental in helping a family to find resources for food and shelter and to apply to such programs as the Supplemental Nutrition Program for Women, Infants and Children (WIC), Food Stamps, medical assistance, and Aid to Families with Dependent Children (AFDC). See also Chapter 12 for other useful community resources.

When nutritional and behavioral approaches fail to promote weight gain, additional therapies may include appetite stimulation, tube feedings, and hospitalization. Cyproheptadine hydrochloride (Periactin), typically used as an antihistamine, has been prescribed in persistent growth failure due to its appetite-stimulating activity.[66] However, both the American Academy of Pediatrics and the Food and Drug Administration believe that the potential side effects (central nervous system effects) of this drug outweigh any perceived benefits.[67] Tube feedings are rarely indicated but may prove helpful as a temporary measure to allow for focus on behavioral modification.[13,67] Parenteral nutrition is seldom indicated. Considerations for hospitalization include failed outpatient management, evidence of physical abuse and severe neglect, poor parental functioning, severe malnutrition, and medical instability.[68,69] Interventions such as physical therapy, speech therapy, or day care can benefit both the child and parent. These can offer stimulation and supervision to the child and can alleviate stress in the parent, allowing the parent to return to work or focus on his or her own psychosocial treatment.[70]

PROGNOSIS

Outcomes are variable due to the many possible factors that can contribute to growth failure. Deficiencies in growth during infancy and childhood harbor potential risk for subsequent lasting deficits in growth, development, and social and emotional functioning.[71,72] Therefore, growth failure should be identified as early as possible and treated by a multidisciplinary team. Focus should be on the achievement of appropriate weight for length/height and on maintaining growth velocity. In many situations, the prognosis can be excellent if medical, nutritional, and psychosocial needs of these children and families are met.[1,13]

Exhibit 18–6 Caloric Supplementation and Feeding Suggestions

	Method	*Considerations*
Infants		
• Formula:	Increase caloric density by 2 kcal/oz every 2–3 days.	• Caloric density should not be increased over 24 kcal/oz by concentration. High formula osmolality and renal solute load can result in vomiting and dehydration in the child. • Monitor for weight gain and signs of intolerance (vomiting, diarrhea, stool-reducing substances). • If not tolerating caloric increase, return to previous step for 2 to 3 more days. • Consult lactation specialist for additional suggestions on breastfeeding.
20 kcal/oz	Normal dilution	
24 kcal/oz	Increased concentration Example: 13 oz liquid concentrate to 8 oz of water	
26-30 kcal/oz	Add fortifiers to 24 kcal/oz formula: carbohydrate additive (8 kcal/tsp), vegetable oil (45 kcal/tsp), protein additive, MCT oil (only if medically indicated)	
• Breast milk:	Increase caloric density by 2 kcal/oz every 2–3 days	
24 kcal/oz:	1 tsp formula to 3 oz breast milk	
26-30 kcal/oz:	Add fortifiers to 24 kcal/oz breast milk to increase caloric density	

- Food: Use high calorie baby foods. Read labels to determine caloric content.
  Example: plain meats, high-meat dinners; bananas, peaches, apricots; mixed vegetables, sweet potatoes, custards/puddings; cereals prepared with concentrated formula.
  Baby foods can be fortified with moderate amounts of infant cereal, dry milk powder, carbohydrate additive, oil, margarine.

- Juices: Avoid

	Method	Considerations
Toddlers		
• Beverages:	25–30 kcal/oz	Feeding Suggestions • Establish a regular feeding schedule. (example: three meals, three snacks) • Restrict food or liquids, except water, to meals/snacks only. • Offer solids first, then liquids. • Offer small portions and allow the child to ask for seconds. • Reinforce positive behaviors. Ignore the negative. • Limit meals and snacks to 20 to 30 minutes. • Decrease distractions during feeding. • No force feeding.
Milk drinks:	Add dry milk powder (15 kcal/tbsp), cream (30-50 kcal/tbsp), instant breakfast powder (30 kcal/oz); nutritional supplements, frappes, milkshakes.	
• Foods:		
Solids	Increase caloric density of foods preferred by child.	
Semisolids	Add carbohydrate additives, vegetable oil/butter/margarine (45 calories/tsp).	
Entrees	Add gravies, sauces, cheese (100 kcal/oz), mayonnaise (100 kcal/tbsp), cooked meats (50–75 kcal/oz).	
Finger foods	String cheese, luncheon meats, chicken nuggets, eggs, small sandwiches, French fries, muffins, waffles, vegetables or pasta with added fat. Use cream cheese (50 kcal/tbsp), peanut butter (100 kcal/tbsp) on crackers/bread.	
• Juice: Limit to 4 oz/day or remove from diet completely		

Source: Adapted with permission from Rathbun JM, Peterson KE. Nutrition in failure to thrive. In: Grand FJ, Sutphen JL, Dietz WH, eds., *Pediatric Nutrition: Theory and Practice*; 1987; 627-643, Newton, MA: Butterworth-Heinemann Publishers.

REFERENCES

1. Bithoney WG, Dubowitz H, Egan H. Failure to thrive/growth deficiency. *Pediatr Rev.* 1992;13:453–459.
2. Bithoney WG, McJunkin J, Michalek J, Egan H, Snyder, J, Munier A. Prospective evaluation of weight gain in both nonorganic and organic failure to thrive children: An outpatient trial of a multidisciplinary team intervention strategy. *Dev Behav Pediatr.* 1989;10:27–31.
3. Bithoney WG, McJunkin J, Michalek J, Snyder J, Egan H, Epstein D. The effect of a multidisciplinary team approach on weight gain in nonorganic failure to thrive children. *Dev Behav Pediatr.* 1991;12:254–258.
4. Hobbs C, Hanks HGI. A multidisciplinary approach for the treatment of children with failure to thrive. *Child Care Health Dev.* 1996;22:273–284.
5. Wilcox WD, Nieburg P, Miller DS. Failure to thrive: A continuing problem of definition. *Clin Pediatr.* 1989;28: 391–394.
6. Centers for Disease Control and Prevention, National Center for Health Statistics. CDC growth charts: United States. www.cdc.gov/growthcharts/, May 30, 2000.
7. Smith DW, Truog W, Rogers FE, et al. Shifting linear growth during infancy: Illustration of genetic factors in growth from fetal life through infancy. *J Pediatr.* 1976; 89:225–230.
8. Fomon SJ. Normal growth, failure to thrive and obesity. In: *Infant Nutrition.* Philadelphia: WB Saunders Co.; 1974.
9. Karlberg P, Angstrom I, Karlberg J, Kristiansson B. Evaluation of growth during the first two years of life. In: Kristiansson B, ed., *Low Rate of Weight Gain in Infancy and Early Childhood.* Goteborg, Sweden: Department of Paediatrics, University of Goteborg; 1980.
10. Edwards AGK, Halse PC, Waterston AJR. Recognizing failure to thrive in early childhood. *Arch Dis Child.* 1990; 65:1263–1265.
11. Horner JM, Thorsson AV, Hintz RL. Growth deceleration patterns in children with constitutional short stature: An aid to diagnosis. *Pediatrics.* 1978;62:529–534.
12. Lifshitz F, Tarim O. Worrisome growth patterns in children. *Int Pediatr.* 1994;9:181–188.
13. Maggioni A, Lifshitz F. Nutritional management of failure to thrive. *Pediatr Clin North Am.* 1995;42:791–810.
14. Frank DA, Silva M, Needlman R. Failure to thrive: Mystery, myth, and method. *Contemp Pediatr.* 1993;10: 114–133.
15. Avery ME, First LR, eds. *Pediatric Medicine.* Baltimore, MD: Williams & Wilkins; 1989.
16. Binkin, NJ, Yip R, Fleshood L, Trowbridge FL. Birth weight and childhood growth. *Pediatrics.* 1988;82: 828–834.
17. Gomez F, Galvan R, Frenk S, Munoz JC, Chavez R, Vasquez J. Mortality in second and third degree malnutrition. *J Trop Pediatr.* 1956;2:77.
18. Waterlow, JC. Classification and definition of protein-calorie malnutrition. *BMJ.* 1972;3:566–569.
19. Raynor P, Rudolf MC. Anthropometric indices of failure to thrive. *Arch Dis Child.* 2000;82:364–365.
20. Waterlow JC, Buzina R, Keller W, Lane JM, Nichaman MZ, Tanner JM. The presentation and use of height and weight data for comparing the nutritional status of groups of children under the age of ten years. *Bull WHO.* 1977;55:486–498.
21. Epi Info, Version 3.2.2, www.cdc.gov/epiinfo, April 14, 2004.
22. WHO Working Group. Use and interpretation of anthropometric indicators of nutritional status. *Bull WHO.* 1986;64:929–941.
23. *World Health Organization: Measuring Changes in Nutritional Status.* Geneva, Switzerland: World Health Organization; 1983.
24. Blackburn GL, Thornton PA. Nutritional assessment of the hospitalized patient. *Med Clin North Am.* 1979;63: 1103–1115.
25. Berwick DM, Levy JC, Kleinerman R. Failure to thrive: Diagnostic yield of hospitalization. *Arch Dis Child.* 1982;57:347–351.
26. Sills RH. Failure to thrive. The role of clinical and laboratory evaluation. *Am J Dis Child.* 1978;132:967–969.
27. Bithoney WG. Elevated lead levels in children with nonorganic failure to thrive. *Pediatrics.* 1986;78:5.
28. Walravens PA, Hambidge KM, Koepfer DM. Zinc supplementation in infants with a nutritional pattern of failure to thrive: A double-blind, controlled study. *Pediatrics.* 1989;83:532–538.
29. Wright CM, Waterston A, Aynsley-Green A. The effect of deprivation on weight gain in infancy. *Acta Paediatr Scand.* 1994(a);83:357–359.
30. Frank DA, Zeisel SH. Failure to thrive. *Pediatr Clin North Am.* 1988;35:1187–1206.
31. Hufton IW, Oates RK. Nonorganic failure to thrive: A long-term follow-up. *Pediatrics.* 1977;59:73–77.
32. Raynor P, Rudolf MC. What do we know about children who fail to thrive? *Child Care Health Dev.* 1996;22: 241–250.
33. Federal Interagency Forum on Child and Family Statistics. *America's Children: Key National Indicators of Well-Being 2003.* Washington, DC: Federal Interagency Forum on Child and Family Statistics, U.S. Government Printing Office; July 2003.
34. Altemeier WA, O'Connor SM, Sherrod KB, Vietze PM. Prospective study of antecedents for nonorganic failure to thrive. *J Pediatr.* 1985;106:360–365.

35. Dahl M. Early feeding problems in an affluent society. III. Follow-up at two years: Natural course, health, behaviour and development. *Acta Paediatr Scand.* 1987;76: 872–880.
36. Lobo ML, Barnard KE, Coombs JB. Failure to thrive: A parent-infant interaction perspective. *J Pediatr Nurs.* 1992;7:251–260.
37. Bithoney WG, Newberger EH. Child and family attributes of failure-to-thrive. *Dev Behav Pediatr.* 1987;8:32–38.
38. Pollitt E, Eichler AW, Chon C. Psychosocial development and behavior of mothers of failure to thrive children. *Am J Orthopsychiatr.* 1975;45:525–537.
39. Weston JA, Colloton M. A legacy of violence in nonorganic failure to thrive. *Child Abuse Negl.* 1993;17:709–714.
40. Schmitt BD, Mauro RD. Nonorganic failure to thrive: An outpatient approach. *Child Abuse Negl.* 1989;13:235–248.
41. Wright CM, Talbot E. Screening for failure to thrive: What are we looking for? *Child Care Health Dev.* 1996;22:223–234.
42. Krieger I. Food restriction as a form of child abuse in ten cases of psychological deprivation dwarfism. *Clin Pediatr.* 1974;13:127–133.
43. Chatoor I, Egan J. Nonorganic failure to thrive and dwarfism due to food refusal: A separation disorder. *J Am Acad Child Psychiatr.* 1983;22:294–301.
44. Rathbun JM, Peterson KE. Nutrition in failure to thrive. In: Grand RJ, Sutphen JL, Dietz WH, eds., *Pediatric Nutrition: Theory and Practice.* Boston: Butterworth; 1987:627–643.
45. Ramsay M, Gisel EG, Boutry M. Non-organic failure to thrive: Growth failure secondary to feeding skill disorder. *Dev Med Child Neurol.* 1993;35:285–297.
46. Glaser HH, Heagarty MC, Bullard DM, Pivchik EC. Physical and psychological development in children with early failure to thrive. *J Pediatr.* 1968;73:690–698.
47. Thomasgard M, Metz WP. The vulnerable child syndrome revisited. *J Dev Behav Pediatr.* 1995;16:47–53.
48. Satter E. The feeding relationship: Problems and interventions. *J Pediatr.* 1990;117:S181–S189.
49. Chatoor I, Schaeffer S, Dickson L, Egan J. Non-organic failure to thrive: A developmental perspective. *Pediatr Ann.* 1984:123:832–843.
50. Fleisher DR. Functional vomiting disorders in infancy: Innocent vomiting, nervous vomiting, and infant rumination syndrome. *J Pediatr.* 1994;125:S84–S94.
51. Neifert MR. Prevention of breastfeeding tragedies. *Pediatr Clin North Am.* 2001;48(2):273–297.
52. Pugliese MT, Weyman-Daum M, Moses N, Lifshitz F. Parental health beliefs as a cause of nonorganic failure to thrive. *Pediatrics.* 1987;80:175–182.
53. Weston JA, Stage JA, Hathaway P, et al. Prolonged breastfeeding and nonorganic failure to thrive. *Am J Dis Child.* 1987;141:242–243.
54. Dennison BA, Rockwell HL, Baker SL. Excess fruit juice consumption by preschool-aged children is associated with short stature and obesity. *Pediatrics.* 1997;99: 15–22.
55. Smith MM, Lifshitz F. Excess fruit juice consumption as a contributing factor in nonorganic failure to thrive. *Pediatrics.* 1994;93:438–443.
56. Dennison BA, Rockwell HL, Nichols MJ, Jenkins P. Children's growth parameters vary by type of fruit juice consumed. *J Am Coll Nutr.* 1999;18:346–352.
57. Hyams JS, Etienne NL, Leichtner AM, Theuer RC. Carbohydrate malabsorption following fruit juice ingestion in young children. *Pediatrics.* 1988;82:64–68.
58. McCann JB, Stein A, Fairburn CG, Dunger DB. Eating habits and attitudes of mothers of children with nonorganic failure to thrive. *Arch Dis Child.* 1994;70:234–236.
59. Truesdell DD, Acosta PB. Feeding the vegan infant and child. *J Am Diet Assoc.* 1985;85:837–840.
60. Zmora E, Corodicher R, Bar-Ziv J. Multiple nutritional deficiencies in infants from a strict vegetarian community. *Am J Dis Child.* 1979;133:141.
61. MacPhee M, Schneider J. A clinical tool for nonorganic failure-to-thrive feeding interactions. *J Pediatr Nurs.* 1996;11:29–39.
62. Chatoor I, Schaeffer S, Dickson L, Egan J, Conners K, Leong N. Pediatric assessment of non-organic failure to thrive. *Pediatr Ann.* 1984;123:844–850.
63. Whitehead RG. Protein and energy requirements of young children living in developing countries to allow catch-up growth after infections. *Am J Clin Nutr.* 1977; 30:1545.
64. Schofield WN. Predicting basal metabolic rate, new standards and review of previous work. *Hum Nutr Clin Nutr.* 1985;39: 5–41.
65. Sentongo TA, Tershakovec AM, Mascarenhas MR, Watson MH, Stallings VA. Resting energy expenditure and prediction equations in young children with failure to thrive. *J Pediatr.* 2000;136:345–50.
66. Lemons PK, Dodge NN. Persistent failure-to-thrive: A case study. *J Pediatr Health Care.* 1998;12:27–32.
67. Tolia V. Very early onset nonorganic failure to thrive in infants. *J Pediatr Gastroenterol Nutr.* 1995;20:73–80.
68. Duggan C. Failure to thrive: Malnutrition in the pediatric outpatient setting. In: Walker WA, Watkins JB, eds., *Nutrition in Pediatrics: Basic Science and Clinical Applications.* Boston: Decker Publishers; 1996:705–714
69. Yetman RJ, Coody DK. Failure to thrive: A clinical guideline. *J Pediatric Health Care.* 1997;11:134–137.
70. Hathaway P. Failure to thrive: Knowledge for social workers. *Health Social Work.* 1989;14:122–126.
71. Corbett SS, Drewett RF, Wright CM. Does a fall down a centile chart matter? The growth and developmental sequelae of mild failure to thrive. *Acta Paediatr.* 1996;85: 1278–1283.

72. Grantham-McGregor SM, Powell CA, Walker SP, Himes JA. Nutritional supplementation, psychosocial stimulation and mental development of stunted children: The Jamaican study. *Lancet.* 1991;338:1–5.

73. Berhrman RE, Kliegman RM. Failure to thrive. In: *Nelson Essential of Pediatrics.* Philadelphia: WB Saunders Co; 1998:37–39.

74. Gahagan S, Holmes R. A stepwise approach to evaluation of undernutrition and failure to thrive. *Pediatr Clin North Am.* 1998;45:169–187.

75. Rathbun JM, Peterson KE. Nutrition in failure to thrive. In: Grand RJ, Sutphen JL, Dietz WH, eds., *Pediatric Nutrition: Theory and Practice.* Newton, MA: Butterworth-Heinemann; 1987:627–643.

Chapter 19

Cardiology

Jacqueline Jones Wessel and Patricia Queen Samour

Nutrition issues for pediatric cardiology range from specific medical nutrition therapy for infants and children with congenital heart disease (CHD), chylothorax, and guidelines for nutrition during extracorporal life support (ECLS or ECMO) to population screening guidelines for cholesterol education. These issues will be discussed in this chapter.

CONGENITAL HEART DISEASE

Nutrition support for infants and children with CHD covers a wide range of topics from acute care in infancy to chronic care in childhood. The magnitude of the effect of the cardiac defect on growth, development, and nutritional status depends on the particular lesion and its severity.[1] Malnutrition and growth retardation are common worldwide in infants and children with CHD.[2–13]

A study by Mitchell and associates[13] evaluated the nutritional status of 48 children admitted for surgical repair of CHD. All of the children were markedly malnourished; 83% had at least five biochemical or hematologic indices of malnutrition and 52% had weights below the third percentile. Controversy exists concerning the etiology of growth failure and the role of inadequate energy intake, hypermetabolism, malabsorption, and cardiac anomaly (see Table 19–1).

Inadequate energy intake has been cited as a component of the growth failure in infants and children with CHD.[14–18] Energy intake of children with CHD was 76% of the intake of unaffected children of the same age; eight infants with CHD had an intake of 82% of the estimated average requirements in a study by Barton and colleagues.[18]

Hypermetabolism has been described in CHD.[18] Total daily energy expenditure (TDEE) was measured in infants with CHD by the doubly labeled water method. TDEE includes basal metabolism as well as the energy of activity, sweating, and the mechanical labor of the heart and lungs.[19] A significantly higher TDEE was found for infants with CHD (101 +/− 3 kcal/kg/ day), as compared with the TDEE for healthy infants (67 +/− 14 kcal/kg/ day).[18] The calculated increase in total daily energy expenditure was 36% above that of healthy infants, except for one infant who had a very high TDEE.[19] Another study did not find significantly higher resting energy expenditure (REE), measured by respiratory gas exchange method, in infants with CHD, except in a subgroup of infants with pulmonary hypertension and cardiac failure.[20] Leitch and associates[21] found increased TDEE but not increased REE as a primary factor in reduced growth of infants with CHD as compared to age-matched controls.[21] Energy expenditure before and after cardiac surgery was measured in a doubly labeled water technique in 18 children with CHD, ages 4 to 33 months. Preoperative energy expenditures were clearly elevated in a third of the children. This suggests that in a proportion of infants and children with CHD, increased basal metabolic rate is a factor in the failure to thrive that is observed. Postoperative energy expenditures were measured 6 hours after operation and values fell to below normal for healthy children who did not have surgery.[22] This indicates that surgical stress leads to a smaller energy requirement in this phase of recovery.

Malabsorption has been suggested as a cause for growth failure. Mild protein malabsorption and more significant fat malabsorption were found in infants with congestive heart failure (CHF) and cyanosis.[23] Fat malabsorption with steatorrhea, bile salt loss, and delayed gastric emptying was found by Yahav and colleagues[16] but malabsorption was not felt to be sufficient to cause growth failure. Vaisman and associates[24] noted increased fat malabsorption in sicker infants, with total body water 120% of predicted, but infants regularly receiving diuretics did not significantly malabsorb.[24]

Delayed gastric emptying has been found in infants with CHD.[25] This may predispose an infant to gastroesophageal reflux and increase the potential for aspiration.[26] Premature satiety may be a result of delayed emptying,[1] as well as further compromising energy and nutrient intake.

The type of cardiac lesion affects the pattern of growth failure. Cardiac lesions are designated as cyanotic and acyanotic, depending on the hemodynamic effect. Patients with cyanotic heart lesions (Table 19–1) usually exhibit reduced height and weight.[4–6,12,26] Acyanotic lesions with a large degree of left-to-right shunting typically affect weight rather than height in the early stages.[2,26,27] One study that found acyanotic children were more affected in growth than cyanotic children attributed some of the difference to the time of operative repair; acyanotic children were operated on at an older age than those with a cyanotic heart lesion.[11] The occurrence of pulmonary hypertension in children with left-to-right shunts affects growth; these children tend to weigh less than do children with cyanotic heart lesions.[26,28] One study found that growth retardation was proportional to the size of the shunt.[12] Another study using Waterlow's criteria for failure to thrive found the prevalence of malnutrition in children with left-to-right intracardial shunting to be 83%; children with pulmonary hypertension as well had even greater nutritional problems.[9] Obstructive malformations, such as pulmonary stenosis and coarctation of the aorta, typically result in impaired linear growth, with linear growth more affected than weight[2,29] (Table 19–2). Strategies to nourish these challenging infants and children in the acute and chronic aspects of care will be discussed.

ACUTE CARE

In infancy, nutrition support is essential during the diagnosis, corrective surgeries, and postoperative rehabilitation period. Parenteral nutrition is often used in the acute phase, then enteral nutrition through tube feedings, and a transition to breast- or bottle-feeding.

Some infants with cardiac problems are admitted to the newborn intensive care unit in an acutely ill state within the first days of life. Some can be stabilized and surgery deferred for weeks; others may need immediate surgery. Depending

Table 19–1 Types of Cardiac Lesions

Acyanotic		*Cyanotic*
Obstructive Malformations	*Left-to-right Shunt Malformations*	
Pulmonary stenosis	Patent ductus arteriosis (PDA)	Transportation of great arteries (TGA)
Aortic stenosis	Ventricular septal defect (VSD)	Tetralogy of Fallot
	Atrial septal defect (ASD)	

Source: Data from endnote references 1 and 16.

Table 19–2 Factors Affecting Growth Failure in Infants and Children with Congenital Heart Disease

Factor	*Effect*
1. Type of cardiac lesion	
Cyanotic	Reduced height and weight
Acyanotic	
Obstructive	Linear growth affected more than weight
Left-to-right shunt	Reduced weight more than height in early stages Weigh less than cyanotic children Large shunts affect body fluid compartments
2. Inadequate energy intake	Energy intake may average only 80–90% of an infant/child without CHD
Decreased energy for feeding	May approach feeding eagerly but tires quickly and cannot finish the feeding
Anorexia, early satiety seen in children	Poor intake
3. Increased metabolic rate	Increased energy cost for infants and 36% increase in metabolic rate observed in children with CHD
4. Dysmotility and malabsorption	
Delayed gastric emptying	Premature satiety; increased potential for gastroesophageal reflux
CHF may cause compressive hepatomegaly, reducing gastric capacity	Increased potential for gastroesophageal reflux and aspiration
Mild abnormalities in absorption of nutrients; tendency toward fat malabsorption with increased total body water	Mild steatorrhea, bile salt loss Sicker infants with elevated body water may have lower intake and mild fat malabsorption
5. Prenatal factors	
Trisomy 21 (Down syndrome)	Postnatal growth delay may be characteristic of syndrome

Source: Data from references 16, 19, 23, 29.

on the type of cardiac defect, multiple surgeries may be planned for a staged repair. As in any surgery, the best outcome is achieved in the patient who is in good nutritional status and positive nitrogen balance. The immediate goal for nutrition support in infants is to achieve the best nutritional status possible in preparation for surgery. Other, less immediate nutrition support goals are to encourage normal growth and support normal feeding skill development. Optimal nutrition support may be impossible, due to the many complicating factors in these patients. Also, providing for normal growth and development may not be possible or realistic in the short-term future of the acute care setting.

The nutrition support plan may be viewed as having four phases. The immediate goals of the acute phase are to minimize catabolism, preserve lean body mass, and correct abnormal laboratory values as possible. It is usually not possible for calories to be provided for growth at this time and may well be inappropriate. This phase typically involves the use of parenteral nutrition and intravenous (IV) fluids. The second phase goal is to begin enteral nutrition. Parenteral and enteral nutrition are used simultaneously in the gradual transition to full enteral feedings. The third phase is to provide for optimal growth. Calories are increased gradually, as tolerated, to provide sufficient calories for growth. Because of higher calorie needs and limited fluid tolerance, higher calorie formulas are often used. Formulas can be gradually increased in density using less water until the protein needs are reached; then additional calories can be added from fat and/or carbohydrate. The fourth phase is to provide for feeding skill development. After calorie needs are determined, ways of providing this intake are investigated. Whereas feedings by mouth may be used, they may not be relied upon totally to provide sufficient consistent intake for appropriate growth in many circumstances. Strategies for encouraging age-appropriate feeding skills are used.

Nutrition support in the acutely ill infant, however, requires careful attention. The infant may be fluid restricted; there may be arterial lines needing at least 1 cc/hour/line to keep patent; and medications may use significant amounts of fluid for dilution and administration. It is not uncommon to have only 60–80 cc/kg of fluid allotted for nutrition in the first phase of nutrition support.

Laboratory values may not be normal. The use of diuretics may deplete total body potassium; calcium, phosphorus, and magnesium levels may also be abnormal.[30] Due to the need for fluid restriction, the renal lab values may reflect some degree of dehydration, with elevated sodium and blood urea nitrogen (BUN). Acid base status may also be altered, further complicating potassium management.

Some infants may develop other problems. Renal problems may develop, such as acute tubular necrosis. Some infants may temporarily need peritoneal dialysis, further complicating nutrition support (see Chapter 17). For infants and children needing support prior to surgery or those unable to be weaned from the bypass pump after surgery, ECLS or ECMO may be used.[31,32]

EXTRACORPOREAL LIFE SUPPORT

Extracorporeal life support offers its own unique nutrition problems.[33] Some strategies are to fluid restrict while on bypass, with as little as 60 cc/kg allotted for nutrition. Total parenteral nutrition (TPN) can be infused as part of the ECLS circuitry, and hyperosmolar central line-type solutions can be used as tolerated for calories. Due to the fluid restriction, glucose infusion rate (GIR) should be calculated with each fluid change. A low-volume amount of D25% (25% dextrose) may yield a modest GIR; care should be taken if fluids are liberalized with altering dextrose percent. Although there has been concern about the effect of IV lipid on the membrane,[34] many centers have found that the use of IV lipid has not been associated with increased problems. Some centers infuse IV lipid through a peripheral line. Research is being conducted to provide clarification on this issue.[34]

Problems have been noted with potassium, calcium, and direct bilirubin for patients using ECLS. There is an increased need for potassium in most infants undergoing ECLS, and TPN is often written for low sodium and higher potassium. Ionized hypocalcemia can be a problem in infants and children after ECMO initiation.[35] Later in the course of the ECLS run, hypercalcemia can be a concern.[36] The elevation of direct bilirubin has been noted in neonates treated with ECLS.[37–40] A study reviewing outcomes found 39% of ECLS neonates had direct hyperbilirubinemia; 46% of these infants had severe elevations. However, 9 weeks after ECLS treatment, all cases were resolved.[39] Cholestasis has been associated with a plasticizer, di-(2 ethylhexyl) phthlate (DEHP), used in the ECLS circuitry tubing and hemolysis that occurs during ECLS.[38–40] Another study did not find plasma DEHP levels to correlate with short-term toxicity.[40] Heparin bonding of the tubing used in the circuit resulted in very little leaching of DEHP, as compared with standard tubing.[40] An FDA advisory was issued in 2002[41]and the American Academy of Pediatrics raised concern in 2003 about DEHP.[42] ECLS tubing is considered to be in the high exposure category DEHP by the FDA.[41] Tubing and other medical items without DEHP are now commercially available.

The use of enteral feeding while patients are on ECLS has been controversial. Continuation of transpyloric feedings after the initiation of ECLS has been successful in pediatric burn patients[43]; others have used enteral nutrition successfully in other pediatric ECLS patients.[44] A small study has shown that minimal enteral or trophic feedings for neonates during the third to ninth days of ECLS can be successful. Assessment of intestinal integrity, however, showed intestinal integrity of ECLS patients to be compromised.[45] Although minimal enteral feeding did not result in further deterioration, this finding should suggest caution with enteral feedings. The risk/benefit ratio of initiating feedings on ECLS should be assessed on an individual basis. Neonates are at a greater risk of feeding hazards on ECLS, due to the possibility of acquiring necrotizing enterocolitis. Many ECLS runs are short, and the risks of feeding a neonate may not be worth the benefit of enteral nutrition. For the longer ECLS neonatal run, such as a bridge to cardiac transplantation, the benefits of enteral nutrition may outweigh the risks.

PARENTERAL NUTRITION SUPPORT

To plan the nutrition support for an acutely ill infant, the multidisciplinary team should review all fluids objectively. Laboratory tests, including renal panel, glucose, and ionized calcium should be monitored daily. Phosphorus and magnesium should be monitored daily until stable and liver function and triglycerides checked weekly or as indicated. A bed scale can be helpful for the nursing staff to obtain daily weights used to evaluate fluid status. The pharmacist can determine whether the medications are appropriate and are concentrated appropriately. Any dextrose used in fluid administration should be counted toward the overall glucose infusion rate and carbohydrate and calorie intake. Sodium used in these fluids also should be calculated because it can represent a significant and unexpected intake. Line patency fluids should be counted toward electrolyte, carbohydrate, calorie (if dextrose is a component), and fluid intake. Parenteral nutrition fluids should be written last, accounting for the content of the other fluids. Because fluid is such an issue and may require altering in the course of the day, it may be helpful if total nutrient admixtures are not used and lipids run separately. Parenteral nutrition is usually very concentrated in the cardiac infant, due to fluid restrictions. Central lines are generally used because peripheral parenteral nutrition lines should not contain more than 12.5% dextrose. With increasing dextrose concentrations, the osmolality of solutions increases dramatically. Typically, the maximum dextrose concentration used in central lines is 25%. Higher dextrose percentages increase the risk of thrombosis. The risks and benefits of providing higher calories through a higher percentage of glucose should be considered carefully. Glucose infusion rates should be calculated daily or with every dextrose-containing fluid change. Postoperative infants may tolerate only a GIR of 10–12 mg glucose/kg/minute.

Intravenous lipids are a concentrated source of calories and a source of essential fatty acids. Twenty percent lipids are typically used (see Chapter 25). A 30% lipid solution is available for three in one mixtures but pediatric applications for this product have not been seen in the literature. Lipids should be used over the greatest amount of time possible—24-hour infusion, if not contraindicated by a lipid incompatible medication. Triglyceride levels may be monitored to assess tolerance to this therapy.

Protein needs are important to consider in this stressed population. Chaloupecky and colleagues[46] found that the provision of a small amount of IV protein, 0.8 g/kg/day, blunted the muscle proteolysis hypercatabolic response in infants after cardiac surgery, in contrast to an isocaloric maintenance dextrose solution. Starting parenteral nutrition with protein immediately postoperatively would seem to be warranted, even if only half of maintenance fluids can be used for this endeavor, due to electrolyte fluctuations.

It may not be possible for mineral needs for bone development to be met in the short term, due to the use of IV nutrition and fluid restriction. Diuretic use may alter calcium status. Premature and term infant calcium and phosphorus requirements for bone mineralization often cannot be realized until later. The use of premature infant or premature follow-up formulas may be considered as a component of the nutrition support for a fluid-restricted infant with higher mineral needs.

ENTERAL NUTRITION SUPPORT

Gut perfusion may not be optimal in some infants with cardiac anomalies. They also may have had a period of asphyxia, further complicating the question of gut integrity. Because the risk of necrotizing enterocolitis is higher in infants with cardiac disease[47] or compromised intestine,[48,49] a slow, cautious approach to enteral feeding, such as the protocol used for feeding premature infants, is reasonable.[50] Parenteral nutrition can be the backup nutrition source until full-volume enteral feedings have been established. Trophic feedings, a method of using 10 cc/kg or less of breast milk or formula and keeping feedings at this level for 5 to 7 days,[51] may also be indicated for premature cardiac infants or term infants with a compromised gut. Breast milk use would be preferable for these infants, if possible, due to the lower association with necrotizing enterocolitis (NEC)[52] and other positive benefits—ease of digestion and absorption, immunochemical and cellular component protection,[53] and promotion of mother-infant interaction.[54]

In the transition from parenteral to enteral nutrition, caution should be used with the addition of hyperosmolar medications. NEC has also been associated with hyperosmolar formula, and the addition of medications can make an isotonic feeding hypertonic.[54,55] Hyperosmolar medications have also been known to cause osmotic diarrhea.[56] Many infants with CHD will need additional calories.[57] Increased calorie density of infant formulas from 20 kcal/oz to 30 kcal/oz may be necessary. Once at or close to the full amount of the allowed volume, density can be gradually increased. The volume of enteral fluid tolerated by each patient should be determined by the multidisciplinary team. However, the amount of fluid used is often related to the amount of diuretic therapy. Diuretics may be used to lessen the effects of high-volume feedings but side effects of potassium wasting, acid base problems,[25] and potential for calcium and magnesium problems exist. Usually if the calorie increase is done slowly, increasing by 1 to 2 kcal/oz at a time, infants tolerate this change.[54] To increase the caloric density of formulas, they can be made using less water with powdered or concentrated formula, which keeps the original proportion of carbohydrate, protein, and fat the same. Although this change does increase the osmolality of the formula, in practice, the medications added to formulas alter the osmolality to a much greater extent than the formula alone.[54] Osmolality of products commonly used in intensive care nurseries is discussed elsewhere.[56,58,59] In practice, some clinicians use an IV preparation of a medicine, such as IV potassium chloride instead of the oral form, which has a greater osmolality due to the syrup suspension of the medication.[54]

The enteral formulas used for infants and children with CHD are the same as for other children. Although a moderate sodium restriction (2.2–3.0 mEq/day) for children has been suggested,[25] there is not a great deal of difference (0.1 mEq/dl) between standard-term infant formulas such as Similac (Ross Laboratories) and Enfamil (Mead Johnson), and the electrolyte- and mineral-restricted formula Similac PM60/40 (Ross Laboratories) used for infants with renal disease. Mineral and potassium restriction is not needed in CHD, and the lower potassium in the special formula, 0.31–0.39 mEq/dL less than standard-infant formulas, may increase the amount of supplementation needed.[60] However, when the caloric density of formulas is increased, the amount of electrolytes and minerals is also increased and should be calculated as well.

Calorie needs of infants and children with CHD are greater than those without cardiac problems. Studies using nutrition intervention in either the in- or outpatient setting have shown that normal growth can be achieved using higher calorie intakes. Continuous intragastric infusion of an average of 137 kcal/kg/day in 146 ml/kg/day of formula was used with a small group of 2- to 24-week-old infants with normal growth in weight and length.[61] Partial (12-hour) and total (24-hour) continuous nasogastric tube feedings of 31.8-kcal/oz formula were compared with oral feedings in a group of young infants over a 5-month period. The formulas were made using a cow's milk- or soy protein-based formula with added rice cereal and glucose polysaccharides. Approximately 147 kcal/kg and 167 ml/kg were given in the 24-hour infusion group and 70 kcal/kg from tube feeding plus oral intake, for a total of 122 kcal/kg in the 12-hour infusion group; the oral feeding control group averaged 95 kcal/kg. Comparing Z scores, only the 24-hour infusion group had improvement in length and weight.[62] Another study using 24-hour continuous infusion with infants at ages from 1 week to 9 months who had previously displayed poor growth showed a growth improvement of 198%. The calorie range used was 120 to 150 kcal/kg with a 24- to 30-kcal/oz range in calorie densities of the formulas.[63] Infants with mild CHD were given higher-calorie formula recipes to increase calorie intake by 20% in oral feedings. Favorable growth was seen in 60% of the group with the higher calorie intake.[64] Higher-calorie formulas were used in a study with oral feedings and infants with CHD. Calories were increased by 32%, and weight gain improved significantly. The author's recommendation is to begin supplementation from the time of diagnosis to optimize growth.[65] A study using nutritional counseling in underweight infants and children with CHD showed increased oral calorie intake and improved anthropometric studies over a 6-month period of counseling.[66] Interestingly, a small study reviewing feeding and growth of breast-fed versus bottle-fed infants with CHD showed better growth in the breast-fed infants.[67] A naturalistic study reviewing the behavioral and physiologic response of infants during feeding did not show a pattern in infants with CHD, as compared with healthy controls, but there was a wide range of individual differences among the 20 infants studied.[68]

The exact energy intake amount is difficult to estimate, but many infants will need 135 to 155 kcal/kg in enteral nutrition. Toddlers and children may need 20–33% more than normal estimated needs. Postrepair, the calorie needs will usually decrease,[22] but may still stay 10 to 15 kcal/kg above the average for some infants or children. Calorie needs may be estimated using indirect calorimetry while in the hospital; many nurseries, however, do not have the equipment to accurately assess infants under 5.0 kg. The best method is to set an estimated goal, assess growth parameters, and make adjustments as needed until appropriate growth is achieved.

CHRONIC CARE

Feeding methodology often becomes an issue in the follow-up care of infants and children with cardiac problems. In infancy, when caloric needs are very high, a typical infant will eat eagerly for a set time, then quit. Parents and caregivers may assume the infant is full, but it may be that the infant has just used the energy it has available for eating and cannot be cajoled or stimulated into taking more. Other infants and children may refuse to eat or eat very poorly. Thommessen and associates found 65% of parents of infants and children with CHD document feeding problems. The reported feeding problems were a good predictor for low voluntary food intake and low growth outcome.[69]

Some options are to use higher calorie formulas or supplements to decrease the volume needed for optimal caloric intake. Other options include using an indwelling nasogastric tube and finishing the feed by a bolus tube feeding. If an infant is close to the goal, the infant may be able to feed by mouth all day and get tube feedings overnight to make up the daytime deficit. This is usually calculated daily by parents or caregivers and given either by bolus feedings or continuous infusion at night. In situations where caregivers are unable to make these calculations, estimations can be used, with frequent checks to make sure that the estimates are still appropriate. For some infants, 24-hour infusions may be needed. Attempts can be made to compress feedings into a shorter infusion time, giving a few hours off of infusion for social and developmental needs. For infants and children not able to take feedings by mouth, an oral stimulation program should be initiated, and oral motor follow-up care can be instituted by an experienced occupational therapist or speech pathologist.

For infants and children who are thought to need tube feeding assistance for greater than 3 months, a gastric tube (G-tube) is a positive step toward simplifying the care. G-tubes can be inserted in surgery or by endoscopy (percutaneous endoscopic gastrostomy). G-tubes and tube feedings should be viewed as tools to improve the quality of life. Without the pressure of forced or unpleasant mealtimes or around-the-clock marathons, feedings can be pleasurable, with the best possible behavioral and developmental outcome. Feedings should typically not exceed 30 minutes in length and should be a pleasant time for both caregiver and the infant or child.

Growth must be monitored carefully. Preventive measures and early nutritional intervention is the best approach to correcting growth problems in childhood. Multidisciplinary teamwork is again important; growth or appetite problems can be caused by a change in clinical course or by a change in medications. Celiac disease has been found in children with CHD and poor growth.[70] It is necessary to consider all possibilities for failure to thrive when cardiac status is stable and calorie intake appears sufficient for good growth. Reevaluation of all parameters on an ongoing basis provides the best outcome.

NUTRITION MANAGEMENT OF CHYLOTHORAX

Chylothorax is the presence of lymphatic fluid in the pleural space caused by a leak or tear in the thoracic duct. In children this may be a complication of cardiac or thoracic surgery, trauma, malignant infiltration or it may occur spontaneously.[71] It has been described in children with Trisomy 21, Noonan's, and Turner's Hennekam, and cardio-facio-cutaneous syndromes.[72–79]

Chyle is lymphatic fluid that contains about 30 g/L of protein, 4–40 g/L of lipid and cells predominately lymphocytes.[80] A description of the cellular components of chyle and serum is available elsewhere.[81] Chyle provides about 200 kcal/L.[80] It appears clear and light yellow if a person is not being fed.[82] The fluid typically has a milky turbid appearance[83] from the presence of chylomicrons after being fed with a diet containing fat.[84] Milky effusions have also been noted that were not chylous[84]; further investigations such as triglyceride level are warranted before a definitive diagnosis is made.[85] Büttiker and colleagues have suggested for pediatrics that the diagnosis of chylothorax be made when the analysis of the pleural fluid contains a triglyceride level over 1.1 mmol/L, an absolute cell count of over 1,000 cells/μL, with a lymphocyte fraction of over 80% on a minimal enteral intake of fat.[85] Some patients who were NPO (ate nothing by mouth) but had an enteral diet before surgery, however, were found to still generate high triglyceride levels in chyle.[85] For a patient who was NPO prior to surgery for some time, or a newborn, minimal enteral intake would be needed.

The flow of chyle may be affected by many factors: elevated capillary pressure, decreased plasma colloid osmotic pressure, and increased interstitial fluid colloid osmotic pressure,[80] as well as enteral water intake.[86] In the 1970s, it was noted that some patients have a reduction in chyle production when using a diet containing fat as medium-chain triglycerides (MCTs).[87,88] Long-chain (LCT) fats utilize lymphatic transport as chylomicrons whereas MCTs primarily utilize portal transport bound to albumin. However, as the LCT intake increases along with MCT intake, a higher percentage of MCT will also be transported by the lymphatic circulation.[80] Some studies have shown no difference in duration or amount of drainage when TPN is compared to an MCT diet.[89] Others have not found that to be uniformly true[85] and some have found significant increases in triglyceride content in pleural effusion when a formula with high MCT (87½% of total fat) was given.[90,91] MCTs have been found in chyle by several investigators. Jensen and associates found 20% of the chyle triglyceride to be MCT when an enteral product containing all MCT oil as the fat source was given.[92] Decanoic acid, C10:0, was present in quantities three times that of octanoic acid, C 8:0, despite the fact that MCT is made up of approximately 29% decanoic and 67% octanoic acid.[92]

A conservative method of treatment starts with nutrition therapy as TPN with intravenous lipid transitioning to a high MCT formula. Beghetti and colleagues found that 80% of children with chylothorax responded to conservative treatment. Most responded in less than 30 days.[71] In an attempt to determine which patients would be successful at conservative treatment and which would need surgery, the effusion output of 15 ml/kg/day at 7 days was examined as a cutoff value. In their study, however, it would have led to unnecessary surgery in 10 patients.[71]

Somatostatin and octreotide have been used for treatment of chylothorax. Somatostatin is short acting and is infused continuously; it also has been shown to reduce splanchnic, hepatic, and portal blood flow and inhibits gastrointestinal motility.[93] In one case report, 2 weeks of therapy was needed on a 4-month-old infant post cardiac surgery.[94] Octreotide, a long-acting synthetic analogue of somatostatin, can be given subcutaneously in two to three divided doses and has been shown to reduce chyle output and triglyceride content in the chyle.[95,96]

Nutrition Management Issues

MCT does not include significant amounts of essential fatty acids; essential fatty acid (EFA) needs can be met by providing 2–4% of the total calories. Most formulas have some long-chain fat. Essential fatty acid deficiency has been seen with infants with hepatobiliary disease and a high MCT formula, thought to be due to impaired fat absorption.[97] There is currently not an infant formula available with very high MCT content. Portagen is now not recommended for use as an infant formula by the manufacturer. It is also available as a powder which is not commercially sterile. Some nutritionists are adapting adult formulas for use in infants, using them diluted to 20 to 24 cal/oz. In general, the protein content tends to be higher which for some patients may be suitable, and the calcium and phosphorus are in a 1:1 ratio instead of the 1.4:1 higher calcium to phosphorus ratio of infant formulas. A fat-free formula (also carbohydrate-free) such as ProViMin can be used with MCT. A source of EFA is needed from either enteral or as an IV source. Carbohydrate would also need to be added for this formula. Pediatric Vivonex is a lower fat

Table 19–3 Selected Formulas with High MCT Content

Formula	*Type*	*Calories/ml*	*Total fat g/L*	*MCT g/L*	*Fat % of calories*	*MCT % of fat*	*Protein grams/L*
Portagen (Mead Johnson)*	Powder, non infant	1.01 cal/ml	48	41.8	40	87	36
Lipisorb (Mead Johnson)	Liquid	1.35 cal/ml	57	48.5	35	85	57
ProViMin (Ross)	Powder	Casein-based, fat-free, carbohydrate-free. Meets nutrition recommendations for vitamin and mineral intake for infants when fed at dilution of 3.25g protein/100 kcal. Ca to P in a 1.4:1 ratio. Allows flexibility in adding amount and type of fat and/or carbohydrate.					
Pediatric Vivonex (Novartis)**	Powder	0.8 cal/ml	24	16.3	25	68	24

*Not intended as a sole source of nutrition. For chronic (long-term) use: supplementation of essential fatty acids and other nutrients should be considered [manufacturer's notation].

**Although the percentage of fat as MCT is not as high as it is low fat, the amount of LCT is reasonable.

Source: Manufacturer's product labels.

elemental formula that has a lower amount of LCT and might be considered. Nutritional comparisons of formulas should be done for each patient looking at their specific needs. See Table 19–3 for some selected formulas available for patients needing a high MCT oil formulation.

NUTRITION MANAGEMENT OF PEDIATRIC HYPERLIPIDEMIA

The aim of nutrition support in pediatric hyperlipidemia is to provide nutrition for normal growth and development, as well as to normalize lipid levels as much as possible to decrease the risk of cardiovascular disease.[98] The guidelines for diet modification are for children over 2 years of age. Before that, age restriction of fat intake may result in altered growth.[99] The National Cholesterol Education Program (NCEP) and the American Heart Association (AHA) advocate dietary changes for all healthy children over 2 years of age and for adolescents.[99,100] The dietary changes suggested for all are actually very similar to the Step I guidelines and can be incorporated into the use of the food pyramid (see Appendix L) with low-fat dairy products. The American Academy of Pediatrics recommends that total fat intake should not fall below 20% of total calories for children and adolescents.[99]

The NCEP has guidelines for cholesterol and lipoprotein screening in children and adolescents with positive family histories of cardiovascular disease or hypercholesterolemia (over 240 mg/dl)[99] (see Table 19–4).

The Step I diet is used for children and adolescents with elevated total or low-density (LDL) cholesterol and is used initially for 3 months. If the serum levels do not decrease to acceptable levels after 3 months, the Step II diet is used for 6 to 12 months. There is further reduction in cholesterol intake and saturated fatty acid percentage in the diet. Step I and II diets have been shown to decrease total and LDL cholesterol by 10–15% within 3 weeks, with children with higher lipid levels having the greater response.[101,102] If serum levels are still not down to acceptable levels, medication may be considered for children over 10 years of age.[99] Details on the foods that constitute the Step I and II diet are described elsewhere.[103]

Increasing the fiber intake of the diet to the patient's age plus 5 g of dietary fiber is advocated for all children.[104] Fiber may be helpful in reducing cholesterol. However, studies on the effect of the lipid-lowering effect of fiber in children are inconclusive.[105] An dietary intervention program designed for preschoolers, Healthy Start has been shown to reduce serum cholesterol when measured over the course of the school year. This

Table 19–4 Steps I and II Dietary Modifications

Nutrient	*Step I Diet*	*Step II Diet*
Total fat	No more than 30% on average of total calories	Same
Saturated fatty acids	Less than 10% of total	Less than 7% of total calories
Polyunsaturated fatty acids	Up to 10% of total calories	Same
Monounsaturated fatty acids	Remaining fat calories	Same
Cholesterol	Less than 300 mg/day	Less than 200 mg/day
Protein	About 15–20% of total calories	Same
Calories	To achieve normal weight and promote normal growth and development	Same

Source: Reproduced with permission from *Pediatrics*, Vol. 89, pages 525–527, 1992.

program in a largely minority Head Start preschool population reduced the total and saturated fat content of snacks and meals.[106]

A few studies indicate that reducing obesity in children reduces obesity-related health risks.[107,108] In a study by Reinehr and Andler, weight loss, a reduction in body mass index (BMI) was shown to improve the atherogenic profile and insulin resistance in children 4 to 15 years.[109] Activity is important in reducing the likelihood of childhood obesity, and it is also an important facet of promoting cardiovascular health.[103] Playing outdoors and high-activity playing have been shown to have positive effect on risk factors for CHD in 4- to 7-year-old children.[110] The activity level of the family influences the activity of the children. A family commitment to a healthy lifestyle, including diet and activity level, is essential.

REFERENCES

1. Greecher CP. Congenital heart disease. In: Groh-Wargo S, Thompson M, Cox J, eds., *Nutritional Care for High Risk Newborns*. Revised ed. Chicago: Precept Press; 2002.
2. Mehrizi A, Drash A. Growth disturbance in congenital heart disease. *J Pediatr*. 1962;61:418–429.
3. Glassman MS, Woolf PK, Schwarz SM. Nutritional considerations in children with congenital heart disease. In: Baker SB, Baker RD Jr, Davis A, eds., *Pediatric Enteral Nutrition*. New York: Chapman & Hall; 1994;340.
4. Venogopalan P, Akinbami FO, Al-Minai KM, et al. Malnutrition in children with congenital heart disease. *J Saudi Med J*. 2001;22:1964–1967.
5. Cameron JW, Rosenthal A, Olson AD. Malnutrition in hospitalized children with congenital heart disease. *Arch Pediatr Adolesc Med*. 1995;149:1098–1102.
6. Villasis-Keever MA, Aquiles Pineda-Cruz R, Halley-Castillo E, et al. Frequency and risk factors associated with malnutrition in children with congenital cardiopathy. *Saluda Publica Mex*. 2001;43:313–323.
7. Thompson Chagoyan OC, Reyes Tsubaki N, Rubiela Barrios OL, et al. The nutritional status of the child with congenital cardiopathy. *Arch Inst Cardiol Mex*. 1998;68: 119–123.
8. Dimiti AI, Anabwani GM. Anthropometric measurements in children with congenital heart disease at Kenyatta National Hospital (1985–1986). *East Afr Med J*. 1991;68:757–764.
9. Leite HP, de Camargo Carvalho AC, Fisberg M. Nutritional status of children with congenital heart disease and left-to-right shunt. The importance of the presence of pulmonary hypertension. *Arq Bras Cardiol*. 1995;65:403–407.
10. Miyague NI, Cardoso SM, Meyer F, et al. Epidemiological study of congenital heart defects in children and adolescents. Analysis of 4,538 cases. *Arq Bras Cardiol*. 2003;80:269–278.
11. Jacobs EG, Leung ML, Karlberg JP. Postnatal growth in southern Chinese children with symptomatic congenital heart disease. *J Pediatr Endocrinol Metab*. 2000;3:387–401.
12. Tambic-Bukovac L, Malcic I. Growth and development in children with congenital heart disease. *Lijec Vjesh*. 1993;115:79–84.
13. Mitchell IM, Logan RW, Pollock JCS, et al. Nutritional status of children with congenital heart disease. *Br Heart J*. 1995;73:277.
14. Krieger I. Growth failure and congenital heart disease. Energy and nitrogen balance in infants. *Am J Dis Child*. 1970;120:497–502.
15. Huse DM, Feldt RH, Nelson RA, et al. Infants with congenital heart disease. *Am J Dis Child*. 1975;129: 65–69.
16. Yahav J, Avigad S, Frand M, et al. Assessment of intestinal and cardiorespiratory function in children with congenital heart disease on high calorie formulas. *J Pediatr Gastroenterol Nutr*. 1985;4:778–785.
17. Hansen SR, Dorup I. Energy and nutrient intakes in congenital heart disease. *Acta Paediatr*. 1993;82: 166–172.
18. Barton JS, Hindmarsh PC, Scrimgeour CM, et al. Energy expenditure in congenital heart disease. *Arch Dis Child*. 1994;70:5–9.
19. Broekhoff C, Houwen RHJ, de Meer K. Energy expenditure in congenital heart disease. (Commentary) *J Pediatr Gastroenterol Nutr*. 1995;21:322–323.
20. Menon G, Poskitt EME. Why does congenital heart disease cause failure to thrive? *Arch Dis Child*. 1985;60: 1134–1139.
21. Leitch CA, Karn CA, Peppard RJ, et al. Increased energy expenditure in infants with cyanotic congenital heart disease. *J Pediatr*. 1998;133:755–760.
22. Mitchell IM, Davies PS, Day JM, et al. Energy expenditure in children with congenital heart disease, before and after cardiac surgery. *J Thorac Cardiovasc Surg*. 1994;107:374–380.
23. Sondheimer JM, Hamilton JR. Intestinal function in infants with severe congenital heart disease. *J Pediatr*. 1978;92:572–578.
24. Vaisman N, Leigh T, Voet H, et al. Malabsorption in infants with congenital heart disease with diuretic treatment. *Pediatr Res*. 1994;36:545–549.

25. Cavell B. Gastric emptying in infants with congenital heart disease. *Acta Paediatr Scand.* 1981;70:517–520.

26. Forchielli ML, McColl R, Walker WA, et al. Children with congenital heart disease: A nutrition challenge. *Nutr Rev.* 1994;52:348–353.

27. Umansky R, Hauck AJ. Factors in the growth of children with patent ductus arteriosis. *Pediatrics.* 1992;146: 1078–1084.

28. Salzer JR, Haschke M, Wimmer M, et al. Growth and nutritional intake of infants with congenital heart disease. *Pediatr Cardiol.* 1989;10:17–23.

29. Stranway A, Fowler R, Cunningkam K, et al. Diet and growth in congenital heart disease. *Pediatrics.* 1976;57: 75–86.

30. Pronsky ZM, Solomon E, Crowe JP, Young V, Smith C. *Food-medication interactions.* Revised ed. Pottstown, PA: Food Medication Interactions; 2003.

31. Walters HL III, Hakimi M, Rice MD, et al. Pediatric cardiac surgical ECMO: Multivariate analysis of risk factors for hospital death. *Am Thorac Surg.* 1995; 60:329–336.

32. Ishino K, Wong Y, Alexi-Meskishvili V, et al. Extracorporeal membrane oxygenation as a bridge to cardiac transplantation. *Artif Organs.* 1996;30:728–732.

33. Brown RL, Wessel J, Warner BW. Nutritional considerations in the extracorporeal life support patient. *Nutr Clin Prac.* 1994;9:22–27.

34. Buck ML, Ksenich RA, Wooldridge P. Effect of infusing fat emulsion into extracorporeal membrane oxygenation circuits. *Pharmacotherapy.* 1997;17:1292–1295.

35. Meliones JN, Moler FW, Custer JR, et al. Hemodynamic instability after the initiation of extracorporeal membrane oxygenation: Role of ionized calcium. *Crit Care Med.* 1991;19:1247–1251.

36. Fridricksson J, Wessel JJ, Warner BW, et al. Hypercalcemia associated with extracorporeal life support ECLS. ECMO Conference, 1997. Abstract.

37. Walsh-Sukys MC, Cornell DJ, Stork EK. The natural history of direct hyperbilirubinemia associated with extracorporeal membrane oxygenation. *Am J Dis Child.* 1992;146:1176–1180.

38. Shneider B, Maller E, VanMarter L, et al. Cholestasis in infants supported with extracorporeal membrane oxygenation. *J Pediatr.* 1989;115:462–465.

39. Shneider B, Cronin J, VanMarter L, et al. A prospective analysis of cholestasis in infants supported with extracorporeal membrane oxygenation. *J Pediatr Gastroenterol Nutr.* 1991;13:285–289.

40. Karle VA, Short BL, Martin GR, et al. Extracorporeal membrane oxygenation exposes infants to the plasticizer di(ethylhexyl) phthalate. *Crit Care Med.* 1997;25: 606–703.

41. FDA. FDA Public Health Notification. *PVC Devices Containing the Plasticizer DEHP.* Retrieved May 2004 from www.fda.gov/safety.

42. Shea KM. American Academy of Pediatrics Committee on Environmental Health. Pediatric exposure and potential toxicity of pthalate plasticizers. *Pediatrics.* 2003;111:1467–1474.

43. Wessel JJ, Wieman RW, Gottschlich MM. Enteral feeding during pediatric extracorporeal membrane oxygenation (ECMO) patients. ASPEN 20th Clinical Congress; 1996:389. Abstract.

44. Pettigano B, Heard M, Davis B, et al. Total enteral nutrition versus total parenteral nutrition during pediatric extracorporeal membrane oxygenation. *Crit Care Med.* 1998;26:358–363.

45. Piena M, Albers MJ, VanHaard PM, Gischler SJ, Tibboel D. Safety of enteral feeding in neonates during extracorporeal membrane oxygenation treatment after evaluation of intestinal permeability changes. *J Pediatr Surg.* 1998;33:30–34.

46. Chaloupecky V, Hucin B, Tlaskal T, et al. Nitrogen balance, 3-methylhistidine excretion, and plasma amino acid profile in infants after cardiac operations for congenital heart defects: The effect of early nutritional support. *J Thorac Cardiovasc Surg.* 1997;14:1053.

47. Ostlie DJ, Spilde TL, St. Peter SD, et al. Necrotizing enterocolitis in full-term infants. *J Pediatr Surg.* 2003;38: 1039–1042.

48. Anderson DM, Kliegman RM. The relationship of neonatal alimentation practices to the occurrence of endemic necrotizing enterocolitis. *Am J Perinatol.* 1991;8:62.

49. Kliegman RM, Walsh MC. Necrotizing enterocolitis: Pathogenesis, classification, and spectrum of illness. *Curr Probl Pediatr.* 1987;17:213.

50. Book LS, Herbst JJ, Jung AL. Comparison of fast- and slow-feeding rate schedules to the development of necrotizing enterocolitis. *J Pediatr.* 1976;89:463.

51. Meetze W, Valentine C, McGuigan JE, et al. Gastrointestinal priming prior to full enteral nutrition in very low birth weight infants. *J Pediatr Gastroenterol Nutr.* 1992;15:163.

52. Lucas A, Cole TJ. Breast milk and neonatal necrotizing enterocolitis. *Lancet.* 1990;336:1519.

53. American Academy of *Pediatrics. Pediatric Nutrition Handbook.* Elk Grove Village, IL: American Academy of Pediatrics; 1985:9.

54. Sapsford A. Enteral nutrition products. In: Groh-Wargo S, Thompson M, Cox J, eds., *Nutritional Care for High Risk Newborns.* Revised ed. Chicago: Precept Press, 1994:176.

55. White KC, Harkavy KL. Hypertonic formula resulting from added oral medications. *Am J Dis Child.* 1982; 136: 931.

56. Zenk L, Hutzable R. Osmolality of infant formulas, tube feedings, and total parenteral solutions. *Hosp Form*. 1978;577:8.
57. Salzer HR, Haschke F, Wimmer M, et al. Growth and nutritional intake of infants with congenital heart disease. *Pediatr Cardiol*. 1989;10:17.
58. Ernst JA, Williams JM, Glick MR, et al. Osmolality of substances used in the intensive care nursery. *Pediatrics*. 1983;72:347.
59. Jew R. Osmolality of medications and formulas used in the newborn intensive care nursery. *Nutr Clin Prac*. 1997;12:158–163.
60. Sapsford A. Composition of human milk, selected infant formulas, and modular supplements. In: Groh-Wargo S, Thompson M, Cox J, eds., *Nutritional Care for High Risk Newborns*. Revised ed. Chicago: Precept Press; 1994:421–429.
61. Bougle D, Iselin M, Kahyat A, et al. Nutritional treatment of congenital heart disease. *Arch Dis Child*. 1986; 61:799–801.
62. Schwarz SM, Gewitz MH, See CC, et al. Enteral nutrition in infants with congenital heart disease and growth failure. *Pediatrics*. 1990;86:368–373.
63. Vanderhoof JA, Hofshire PJ, Baluff MA, et al. Continuous enteral feedings. An important adjunct in the management of complex congenital heart disease. *Am J Dis Child*. 1982;136:825–827.
64. Khajuria R, Grover A, Bidwai PS. Effect of nutritional supplementation on growth of infants with congenital heart diseases. *Indian Pediatr*. 1989;26:76–79.
65. Jackson M, Poskitt EM. The effects of high energy feeding on energy balance and growth in infants with congenital heart disease and failure to thrive. *Br J Nutr*. 1991;65:131–143.
66. Unger R, et al. Calories count. Improved weight gain with dietary intervention after cardiac surgery in children. *Am J Dis Child*. 1992;146:1078–1084.
67. Combs VL, et al. A comparison of growth patterns in breast and bottle-fed infants with congenital heart disease. *Pediatr Nurs*. 1993;19:175–179.
68. Lobo ML, Michel Y. Behavioral and physiological response during feeding in infants with congenital heart disease: A naturalistic study. *Prog Cardiovasc Nurs*. 1995;10:26–34.
69. Thommessen M, Heiberg A, Kase BF. Feeding problems with children with congenital heart disease: The impact on energy intake and growth outcomes. *Eur J Clin Nutr*. 1992;46:457–464.
70. Congdon PJ, Fiddler GI, Littlewood JM, et al. Coeliac disease associated with congenital heart disease. *Arch Dis Child*. 1982;57:78–79.
71. Beghetti M, La Scala G, Belli D, et al. Etiology and management of pediatric chylothax. *J Pediatr*. 2000; 136:653–658.
72. Prasad R, Singh K, Singh R. Bilateral congenital chylothorax with Nona syndrome. *Indian Pediatr*. 2002;39: 975–976.
73. Mire O, Mildenberger E, van Baalen A, et al. Neonatal chylothorax with Trisomy 21 Z Geburtshilfe. *Neonat*. 2004;208:29–31.
74. Lanning P, Simia S, Saramo I, et al. Lymphatic abnormalities in Noonan's syndrome. *Pediatr Radiol*. 1978; 7:106–109.
75. Munoz Conde J, Gomez de Terroros I, Sanchez Ruiz F. Chylothorax associated with Turner's Syndrome in a child. *An Esp Pediatr*. 1975;8:449–454.
76. Goens MB, Campbell D, Wiggins JW. Spontaneous chylothorax in Noonan syndrome. *Am J Dis Child*. 1992;146:1453–1456.
77. Hamada H, Fujita K, Kubo T, et al. Congenital chylothorax in a trisomy 21 newborn. *Arch Gynecol Obstet*. 1992;252:55–58.
78. Chan PC, Chiu HC, Hwu WL. Spontaneous chylothorax in a case of cardio-facio-cutaneous syndrome. *Clin Dysmorph*. 2002;11:297–298.
79. Bellini C, Mazzella M, Arioni C, et al. Hennekam syndrome presenting as non immune hydrops fetalis, congenital chylothorax, and congenital lymphangiectasis. *Am J Med Genetics*. 2003;120A:92–96.
80. McCray S, Parrish CR. When chyle leaks: Nutrition management options. *Practical Gastroenterology*. 2004;17:60–76.
81. Orange JS, Geha RS, Bonilla FA. Acute chylothorax in children: Selective retention of memory T cells and natural killer cells. *J Pediatr*. 2003;143:243–249.
82. Valentine VG, Raffin TA. The management of chylothorax. *Chest*. 1992;102:586–591.
83. Wallis RLM, Schölberg HA. On chylous and pseudochlylous ascites. *Q J Med*. 1911; 4:153–204.
84. Staats BA, Ellefson RD, Budahn LL, et al. The lipoprotein profile of chylous and nonchylous effusions. *Mayo Clin Proc*. 1980;55:700–704.
85. Büttiker V, Fanconi S, Burger R. Chylothorax in children: Guidelines for diagnosis and management. *Chest*. 1999;116:662–687.
86. Robinson CLN. The management of chylothorax. *Ann Thorac Surg*. 1985; 85:835–840.
87. Gershanik JJ, Jonsson HT, Riopel DA, et al. Dietary management of neonatal chylothorax. *Pediatrics*. 1974; 53:400–403.
88. Kosloske AM, Martin LW, Schubert WK. Management of chylothorax in children by thorancentesis and medium chain triglyceride feedings. *J Pediatr Surg*. 1974; 9: 365–371.
89. Allen EM, van Heeckeren DW, Spector RL, et al. Management of nutritional and infectious complications of postoperative chylothorax in children. *J Pediatric Surg*. 1991;26:1169–1174.

90. Peitersen B, Jacobsen B. Medium chain triglycerides for treatment of spontaneous, neonatal chylothorax. Lipid analysis of the chyle. *Acta Paediatr Scan*. 1977;66: 121–125.

91. Fernandez Alvarez JR, Kalache KD, Grauel EL. Management of spontaneous congenital chylothorax: Oral medium chain triglycerides versus total parenteral nutrition. *Am J Perinatol*. 1999;16:415–420.

92. Jensen GL, Mascioli EA, Meyer LP, et al. Dietary modification of chyle composition in chylothorax. *Gastroenterology*. 1989;97:761–765.

93. Grosman I, Simon D. Potential gastrointestinal uses of somatostatin and its synthetic analogue octreotide. *Am J Gastroenterol*. 1990;85:1061–1072.

94. Rimensberger PC, Muller B, Challenges A, et al. Treatment of a persistent postoperative chylothorax with somatostatin. *Ann Thorac Surg*. 1998;66:253–254.

95. Cheung Y, Leung MP, Yip M. Octreotide for treatment of postoperative chylothorax. *J Pediatr*. 2001; 39:157–159.

96. Goyal A, Smith NP, Jesudasson EC, et al. Octreotide for treatment of chylothorax after repair of congenital diaphragmatic hernia. *J Pediatr Surg*. 2003;38:E32–33.

97. Pettei MJ, Dafary S, Levine JJ. Essential fatty acid deficiency associated with the use of a medium-chain-triglyceride infant formula in pediatric hepatobiliary disease. *Am J Clin Nutr*. 1991;53:1217–1221.

98. American Academy of Pediatrics Committee on Nutrition. Statement on cholesterol. *Pediatrics*. 1992;90: 469–473.

99. NCEP Expert Panel on Blood Cholesterol Levels in Children and Adolescents. National Cholesterol Education Program (NCEP). Highlights of the report of the expert panel on blood cholesterol levels in children and adolescents. *Pediatrics*. 1992;89:525–527.

100. American Heart Association Nutrition Committee. Nutrition and children: A statement for healthcare professionals from the nutrition committee. *Circulation*. 1997;95:2332–2333.

101. Kris-Etherton PM, Krammel D, Russell ME, et al. The effect of diet on plasma lipids, lipoproteins, and coronary heart disease. *J Am Diet Assoc*. 1988;88:1373–1400.

102. DISC Collaborative Research Group: Efficacy and safety of lowering dietary intake of fat and cholesterol among school children in The Woodlands, Texas. *Pediatrics*. 1990;86:520–526.

103. Nutrition management of hyperlipidemia. In: William CP, ed., *Pediatric Manual of Clinical Dietetics*. Chicago: American Dietetic Association; 1998:265–283.

104. Williams CL, Bolella M, Wynder EL. A new recommendation for dietary fiber in childhood. *Pediatrics*. 1995;96:985–988.

105. Kwiterovitch PO. The role of fiber in the treatment of hypercholesterolemia in children and adolescents. *J Pediatr*. 1995;S1005–S1009.

106. Williams CL, Stobino BA, Bollella M, et al. Cardiovascular risk reduction in preschool children: the "Healthy Start" project. *J Am Coll Nutr*. 2004;23: 117–123.

107. Wabitsch M, Hauner H, Heinze E, et al. Body fat distribution and changes in atherogenic risk factor profile in obese adolescent girls during weight loss. *Am J Clin Nutr*. 1994;60:54–60.

108. Sung RYT, Yu CW, Chang SKY, et al. Effects of dietary intervention and strength training on blood lipid levels in obese children. *Arch Dis Child*. 2002;86: 407–410.

109. Reinehr T, Andler W. Changes in the atherogenic risk factor profile according to degree of weight loss. *Arch Dis Child*. 2004;89:419–422.

110. Saakslahti A, Numminen P, Varstala V, et al. Physical activity as a preventive measure for coronary heart disease risk factors in early childhood. *Scand J Med Sci Sports*. 2004;14:143–149.

Chapter 20

Diabetes

Laurie Anne Higgins and Karen Hanson Chalmers

MEDICAL NUTRITION THERAPY FOR THE CHILD WITH DIABETES

Through considerable research and new technologies during the last 20 years, the knowledge base of childhood diabetes has been extended, giving health care professionals new tools to help this population balance and improve their diabetes management. These tools include intensive insulin therapy, new medications, self-blood glucose monitoring devices, psychological intervention, inclusion and education for family and support persons, insulin/food adjustment for exercise, and state-of-the-art medical nutrition therapy. The challenge to the dietitian on the diabetes team is to support the family's efforts and to help promote healthy eating habits by using information gained from current research coupled with insight into family dynamics.

Empowering parents to care for their child with insulin-dependent diabetes (type 1) is the ultimate challenge for many health care professionals dealing with pediatric patients. Families already faced with altering their lifestyle to include insulin injections, blood glucose monitoring, and scheduled meals must face these challenges in combination with feelings of anger, fear, denial, and guilt.

Meal planning is one of the most important tools of diabetes self-management. However, studies have shown that "diet" is overwhelmingly the number one problem in diabetes care.[1] Many factors associated with poor adherence to diabetes-related meal planning are psychosocial in nature (e.g., anger, denial, frustration, poor understanding, social pressures, and restriction of favorite foods).[1] The revised American Diabetes Association Principles and Nutrition Recommendations: 2004[2] provide a positive approach to this potentially overwhelming topic. Health educators on the diabetes team must not lose sight of the fact that food provides more than nutrients, especially for children. Changes in eating should not be viewed as restrictions and losses, but rather as a healthful way for the whole family to eat. To be successful, the meal plan must not only meet nutritional requirements but must be realistic and workable, without making major routine changes to those involved. Every attempt should be made to establish a meal plan that reflects the child's food preferences and the family's social and cultural attitudes. Flexibility and graduated goal setting are important keys to success, increasing the chances of the child's achieving optimal management, and decreasing the development of complications. The goals for medical nutrition therapy are listed in Table 20–1.

THE DIABETES TEAM

Diabetes requires teamwork. This was clearly demonstrated in the 1993 published results of the landmark Diabetes Control and Complications Trial (DCCT).[3] The DCCT supported the importance of a coordinated team approach to achieve nutrition goals. The ultimate therapeutic diabetes team utilized in the DCCT consisted of the patient and family as the primary players, along

Table 20–1 Goals of Medical Nutrition Therapy for Children and Adolescents

1. To provide adequate nutrition to maintain normal growth and development based on a child's appetite, food preferences, and family lifestyle
2. To maintain near-normal blood glucose levels and reduce or prevent the risks of short- and long-term diabetes
3. To achieve optimal serum lipid levels
4. To preserve social and psychological well-being
5. To improve the child's overall health through optimal nutrition
6. To provide a level of information that meets the interest and ability of the family
7. To provide information on current research to help the family make appropriate nutrition decisions

with the diabetes nurse educator, dietitian, behaviorist, and the diabetologist.[4] The DCCT also provided important information specific to successful nutrition intervention strategies firmly based on scientific evidence. In 1994, shortly after the DCCT clinical findings were published, the American Diabetes Association (ADA) published a revised set of nutrition guidelines refocusing on an "individualized approach to nutrition self-management that is appropriate for the personal lifestyle and diabetes management goals of the individual with diabetes."[5]

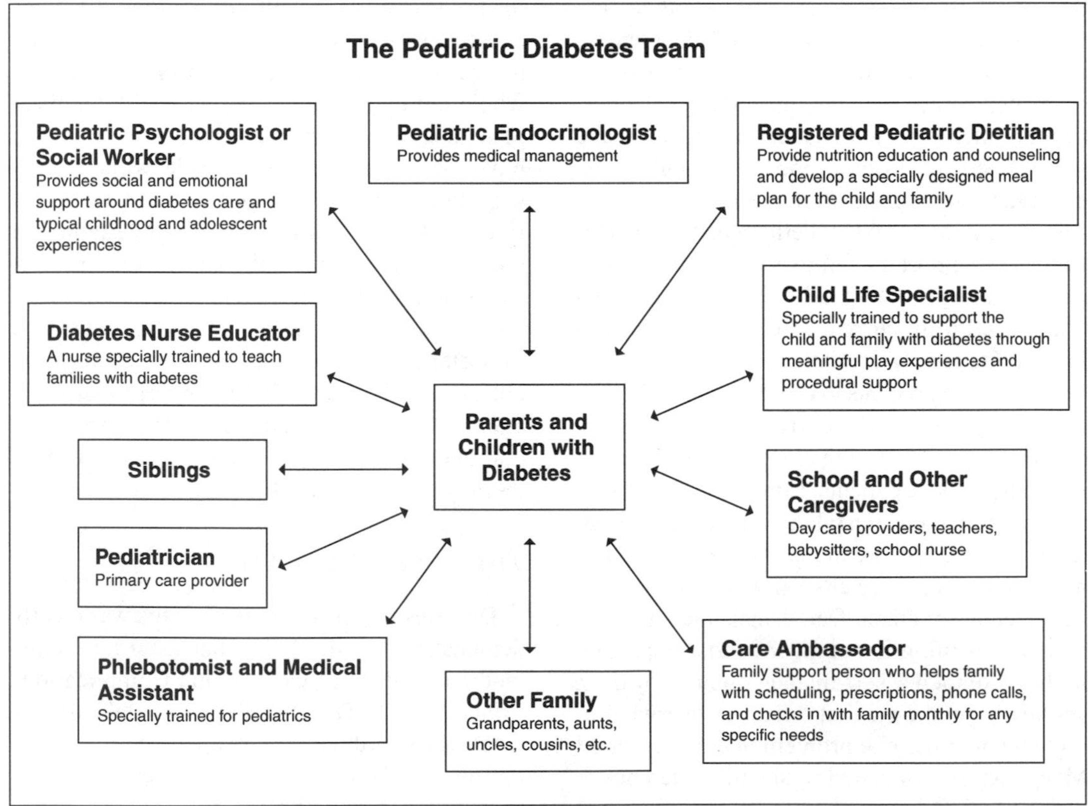

Figure 20–1 Source: Reprinted with permission.

Pediatric diabetes centers have built on the model of the DCCT to also include pediatric phlebotomists, child-life specialists, and care ambassadors (see Figure 20–1). Often the last part of an office visit is having the blood drawn because that leaves the child very upset. The pediatric phlebotomist and child-life specialist can work with the family to reduce a child's anxiety, which can make this part of the visit much less traumatic. A child-life specialist can be instrumental in providing the family with therapeutic play and techniques to help them with the often-difficult task of blood sugar checks and insulin injections. The care ambassador is usually a college graduate who is assigned to a family to help them navigate the health care system. The care ambassador will make sure that the family has regular scheduled appointments and contacts the families between visits to assist them with whatever they need for their child's care,[6] such as changing or making their appointments with members of the diabetes team and renewing a prescription. Research has shown that patients with a care ambassador attend more clinic visits and have fewer severe hypoglycemic episodes and less visits to the emergency room.[7]

NUTRITION PRINCIPLES FOR THE MANAGEMENT OF DIABETES AND RELATED COMPLICATIONS

A positive approach to meal planning is to encourage family members and other support persons to follow the same lifestyle recommendations as the child with diabetes. In our attempt to maintain the "pleasures of the table," it is essential that the nutrition recommendations promote "normal" healthy eating and prevent isolating and dividing the child and family in their food choices. Today, there is no one "diabetic" or "ADA" diet and the recommended USDA/DHHS Dietary Guidelines for Americans, 2000[8] and the newer 2005 Dietary Guidelines (Appendix J) apply to all healthy individuals, including those with diabetes. (See Table 20–2 on macronutrient recommendations.) The current nutrition recommendations can only be defined as a nutrition prescription based on assessment and treatment goals and outcomes.[2]

Calories

The meal plan should include enough calories (kcals) to maintain a consistent growth pattern and to achieve and/or maintain a desirable body

Table 20–2 The DRI's 2001: Nutrition Recommendations

The Current Recommended Goals Are:

Calories	Requirements for growth, based on nutrition assessment	
Protein	10–20% of daily calories (recommendations are no different than those for a child without diabetes)	
Carbohydrate	Distribution based on nutritional assessment, blood glucose, and lipid goals	
Fat	Distribution based on nutritional assessment, weight, and lipid goals, with less than 10% of calories from saturated fat	
Fiber	1–3 years of age	19 grams/day
	4–8 years of age	25 grams/day
	9–13 years of age	
	Males	31 grams/day
	Females	26 grams/day
	14–18 years of age	
	Males	38 grams/day
	Female	26 grams/day

Source: Data from endnote reference 8.

weight. In growing children, caloric intake should not be restricted and should be the same as for children without diabetes. Because energy needs vary during periods of growth, comparing and validating calorie needs based on age, height, ideal body weight (IBW), activity, and average energy allowance per day (see Table 20–3 and Appendix I) will provide the best method to estimate energy needs for an individual child.[9]

Table 20–3 Estimating Caloric Requirements for Children

1. Based on nutrition assessment and typical day recall
2. Validate caloric needs

Method 1	National Academy of Sciences Recommended Dietary Allowances (see Appendix K)	
Method 2	1,000 kcal per first year	
	All children under 11 years, add 100 kcal per year up to age 11 years	
	Girls 11–15 years, add 100 kcal or less per year after age 10 years	
	Girls >15 years, calculate as adult	
	Boys 11–15 years, add 200 kcal per year after age of 10 years	
	Boys >15 years, add	
	23 kcal/lb if very active	
	18 kcal/lb if usual activity level	
	16 kcal/lb if sedentary	
Method 3	1,000 kcal for first year, add	
	125 kcal × age for boys	
	100 kcal × age for girls	
	Up to 20% more kcal for activity	
	For toddlers 1–3 years, add 40 kcal per inch of length	
Method 4*	Ages 11 to 22 years	
	Boys 16 to 17 kcal/cm	
	Girls 13 to 14 kcal/cm	
Method 5	Schofield Equation for Calculation Basal Metabolic Rate in Children	
	Males**	
	0–3 years	REE = 0.167W + 15.174H − 617.6
	3–10 years	REE = 19.59W + 1.303H + 414.9
	10–18 years	REE = 16.25W + 1.372H + 515.5
	> 18 years	REE = 15.057W + 1.0004H + 705.8
	Females	
	0–3 years	REE = 16.252W + 10.232H − 413.5
	3–10 years	REE = 16.969W + 1.618H + 371.2
	10–18 years	REE = 8.365W + 4.65H + 200
	>18 years	REE = 13.623W + 23.8H + 98.2
	REE × activity	

Sources: Modified and reprinted with permission. American Diabetes Association. *Maximizing the Role of Nutrition in Diabetes Management*, © 1994 ADA; *Mahan LK, Rosebrough RH. Nutritional requirements and nutrition status assessment in adolescence. In: Mahan LK, Rees JM, eds., *Nutrition in Adolescence.* St. Louis, MO: Mosby; 1984; and **Adapted from Schofield W. Predicting basal metabolic rate, new standards and review of previous work. *Hum Nutr Clin Nutr.* 1985;39C Suppl 1:5–41.

Other guidelines for determining calorie needs of infants and children are found in Chapters 2, 5, and 6.

Carbohydrate and Sweeteners

The percentage of calories from carbohydrate will vary and is individualized based on nutritional assessment and treatment goals. Many factors influence the glycemic response to foods, including the total amount of carbohydrate, type of carbohydrate (glucose, sucrose, fructose, lactose, starch), degree of processing, and combination with other foods and ingredients. One of the most common misconceptions about carbohydrate is the belief that sugars are more rapidly digested and absorbed than are starches and thereby sugar contributes significantly to hyperglycemia. However, research published in the past 10 to 15 years has found little or no scientific evidence that supports this theory. Studies show a strong relationship with the total carbohydrate and the premeal insulin dose;[2] therefore, adjustment of the premeal insulin can allow a child to incorporate most carbohydrates into the meal plan and still maintain appropriate blood sugar control.

Glycemic Index

The glycemic index is the blood glucose response area above the fasting glucose concentration following the ingestion of a 50-gram carbohydrate portion of food that is compared to the glucose response area of an index food in the same subjects.[10] The glycemic index is not a precise tool because the exact effect of foods on blood glucose differs significantly among individuals and is affected by many factors such as processing, preparation, and digestion.[5] On the other hand, the glycemic index can be used as an indicator of the general glucose response of an individual food. This can also be a helpful tool when encouraging a child or adolescent to increase the amount of whole-grain products and fresh fruits and vegetables into their meal plan because these foods tend to demonstrate a slower glucose response.

Sucrose

Flexibility in allowing some sucrose into the diet may lead to better adherence to the meal plan. Sucrose may be incorporated into the diet of a child or adolescent on a regular basis assuming an adequate, consistent intake of food from all of the essential food groups. To moderate the impact of many new food choices on the blood glucose levels, it is advisable to substitute sucrose and sucrose-containing foods for other carbohydrates in the diet and not simply to add these foods to the meal plan.[11] Because most sources of sugar for children under 10 years are from milk and milk products, fruit drinks, and carbonated soft drinks, it is important to promote overall healthy eating and optimal dental health by limiting empty calorie foods. Added sucrose-containing foods should be related to extra activity and special occasions. These foods should be promoted as special "treat" or "once in a while" foods.

Nutritive Sweeteners

Sweeteners other than sucrose also contain large amounts of carbohydrate and calories and can impact glycemic control. Common sweeteners such as fructose, corn syrup, honey, molasses, carob, dextrose, lactose, and maltose do not decrease calories or carbohydrate and offer no significant advantage over foods sweetened with sucrose.[2] Although fructose has been shown to produce a somewhat smaller rise in blood glucose compared to the other sweeteners just listed, research evidence suggests potential negative effects of large amounts of fructose (double the amount usually consumed or 20% of daily calories) on cholesterol and LDL cholesterol.[12]

Commonly used sugar alcohols such as sorbitol, mannitol, xylitol, erthritol, lactitil, isomalt, maltitol, and hydrogenated starch hydrolysate may produce less of a glycemic response and average about 2.4 to 3.0 kcals/gm compared with 4 kcals/gm from other carbohydrates.[13] However, gastrointestinal side effects such as stomach distress or diarrhea are noted when sugar alcohols are ingested in large amounts (50 gms/day for sorbitol, 20 gms/day for mannitol). Children may be more sensitive and have been shown to have diarrhea with intake as low as 0.5 or less g/kg body wt.[14]

Table 20–4 These recommendations are set by the FDA for ADI and include a 100-fold safety factor. The World Health Organization's Joint Expert Committee of Food Additives set the ADI for saccharin.

	ADI (mg/kg body wt)	*Average amount (mg) in 12-oz. can of soda**	*Cans of soda to reach ADI for 45 kg (100 lb.) child*	*Amount (mg) in a packet of sweetener*	*Packets to reach ADI for a 45 kg (100 lb.) child*
Acesulfame K	15	40**	17	50	13
Aspartame	50	200	11	35	63
Saccharin	5*	140	1.6	36	6.25
Sucralose	5	70	3.2	5	45

*This number represents an average; different brand names and fountain drinks may have varied amounts of sweeteners.
**Based on the most common blend with 90-mg aspartame.

Source: Copyright ©1999 American Diabetes Association, Inc. *American Diabetes Association Guide to Medical Nutrition Therapy for Diabetes, 1999.* Reprinted and adapted with permission from The American Diabetes Association.

Nonnutritive Sweeteners

Aspartame, acesulfame K, saccharin, and sucralose are the most common noncaloric sweeteners used in the United States today and have been approved by the Food and Drug Administration (FDA). The FDA also determines an acceptable daily intake (ADI) for these intense sweeteners. ADI is defined as the amount of a food additive that can be safely consumed on a daily basis over a person's lifetime without any adverse effects and includes a 100-fold safety factor (Table 20–4).

Aspartame contains 4 kcals/gm but is 160 to 220 times sweeter than sucrose; therefore, aspartame provides negligible calories. Aspartame is rapidly metabolized in the gastrointestinal tract and does not accumulate in the system at recommended intakes. Aspartame is not heat stable and may decompose on long exposure to high temperatures. Aspartame safety data has been evaluated by regulatory agencies and expert committees, including the FDA, the EU Scientific Committee for Food (SCF), and the Joint FAO/WHO Expert Committee on Food Additives (JECFA), which have deemed it safe for its intended use. It has been 30 years since the foundations of the aspartame safety database was started and there are over 700 citations regarding aspartame in the U.S. National Library of Medicine's MEDLINE, many of these addressing the safety of aspartame. Aspartame is presently approved in more than 100 countries and has been widely used by hundreds of millions of people over the last 20 years with no adverse effects.[15] However, because aspartame is composed of phenylalanine and aspartic acid, it should be restricted in those with phenylketonuria, a homozygous recessive inborn error of metabolism in which persons are unable to metabolize the amino acid phenylalanine.

Acesulfame K has no caloric value and is 200 times sweeter than sucrose. Also, it is not metabolized by the body and is eliminated unchanged in the urine. Acesulfame K is heat stable and blends well with other sweeteners. The amount of potassium (K) in this sweetener is minimal with only 10 mg of potassium in one packet. No safety concerns have been raised about acesulfame K and it has been reported safe for all individuals.[5,13]

Saccharin is 200 to 700 times sweeter than sucrose and has no caloric value. Saccharin is heat stable, is not metabolized by the body, and is excreted unchanged in the urine. Parents often question their child's safety based on highly publicized research results in the 1970s suggesting a possible causal relationship between saccharin and bladder tumors in laboratory rats. It has been documented that the saccharin samples used in the studies were impure and the results were incorrectly interpreted.[13,16]

Sucralose is the most recent noncaloric sweetener to be approved by the FDA and confirmed by many regulatory agencies throughout the world. Sucralose, which is 600 times sweeter than sugar, is the only low-calorie sweetener made from sugar and is excreted in the urine essentially unchanged.[13] Sucralose is not recognized by the body as either sugar or carbohydrate because it is not broken down or metabolized by the body. Furthermore, it does not affect blood glucose levels. Sucralose is marketed as Splenda Granular, which contains maltodextrin or dextrose and does provide some carbohydrate and calories. One cup of Splenda granular contains 96 calories and 24 grams of carbohydrates. Sucralose is heat stable and may be used during cooking and baking. The FDA states that no adverse or carcinogenic effects are associated with sucralose consumption.

Fiber

Total dietary fiber consists of structural and storage polysaccharides and lignin in plants that are not well digested in humans.[17] Soluble fiber is made up of pectins, gums, mucilages, and some hemicelluloses. Insoluble fiber is made up of noncarbohydrate components, which include cellulose, lignin, and many hemicelluloses.

Increased intake of soluble fiber has been positively linked to improved glycemic control; however, interpretation of recent data collected in carefully controlled studies indicates that the effect of soluble fiber on blood glucose absorption, in the amounts consumed from foods, is probably clinically insignificant. Therefore, fiber recommendations for children with diabetes are the same as for children without diabetes: increase both types of fiber from a wide variety of food sources and base this increase upon the child's usual eating habits, glucose, and lipid goals.

Dietary fiber may be useful in the treatment or prevention of constipation, gastrointestinal disorders, and colon cancer. Furthermore, large amounts of soluble fiber (20 gm/day) have been shown to have a beneficial effect on fasting total and LDL cholesterol levels, with maintenance of fasting HDL cholesterol concentration.[5] However, a high-fiber diet for some very young children may result in an insufficient caloric intake necessary for growth due to the satiety value provided by fiber, as well as possible impairment of mineral absorption. Therefore, the amount of dietary fiber recommended for children should be based upon individual eating habits and lipid goals.

Protein

Current nutrition recommendations for children with diabetes encourage protein from both animal and vegetable sources comprising 10–20% of calories per day. Protein intake in children and adolescents should be sufficient to ensure adequate growth and development, and maintenance of body protein stores. At this time, there are no data to support a higher or lower protein intake than the recommended dietary allowances for children with diabetes; see Appendix I. It is estimated that the average protein intake in the United States for all ages is about 15–20% of the total daily calories, with the majority of protein intake coming from animal products. In a study assessing the macro- and micronutrient intake of children with insulin-dependent diabetes, it was noted that protein intake was within recommended levels. The majority of the children, however, were consuming levels at the upper limit of the RDA,[18] which may be a concern. It is estimated that about 20–30% of patients with type 1 or type 2 diabetes will develop evidence of nephropathy. Approximately 50% of the type 1 patients will go on to develop end stage renal disease (ESRD) within 10 years and 75% within 20 years.[19] Therefore, protein intake should be carefully assessed, with a focus on the family's overall protein intake. Children engaging in consistent competitive exercise may need some additional protein due to increased energy needs, which can be met by increasing consumption of low-fat protein-rich foods rather than intake of liquid or powdered protein supplements.

Total Fat

The primary dietary fat goal in children with diabetes is a healthy fat diet, sufficient to optimize growth and development. In 1991 the National Cholesterol Education Program (NCEP) developed the guidelines for fat intake for children over 2 years of age to decrease risk of cardiovascular disease.[20] Type 1 diabetes has been associated with an increased risk of cardiovascular disease, but evidence suggests that blood glucose control may directly influence the levels of several plasma lipid components.[5]

The American Heart Association recommends that intervention occur if the average of three fasting lipid profiles is above the cutoff points (see Chapter 19). Studies have shown intake levels for cholesterol, fat, and saturated fat in children with Insulin Dependent Diabetes Mellitus (IDDM) are close to the recommendations for children without diabetes.[21] This is likely supported by the fact that the national trend has been leaning toward decreasing overall fat intake, but saturated fat intake is still high.[8] Unfortunately, some children and adolescents with diabetes consume fat levels well above what is recommended and these individuals may be at an even greater risk than children without diabetes. In 2004, the American Diabetes Association published guidelines for the management of dyslipidemia in children with diabetes (see Table 20–5).[22] Careful consideration should be given to strict fat re-

Table 20–5 Management of Dyslipidemia in Children and Adolescents with Diabetes

Screening
- After glycemic control is achieved:
- Type 1
  - Obtain lipid profile at diagnosis and then, if normal, every 5 years
  - Begin at age 12 years (or onset of puberty, if earlier)
  - Begin prior than 12 years (if prepubertal) only if positive family history
- Type 2
  - Obtain lipids profile at diagnosis and then every 2 years
- Goals
  - LDL <100 mg/dl
  - HDL >35 mg/dl
  - Triglycerides <150 mg/dl

Treatment Strategies
- Maximize glycemic control
- Weight reduction, if necessary
  - Diet
    - <7% of calories from saturated fat
    - <200 mg cholesterol per day
    - Consider LDL-lowering dietary options
    - Increase soluble fiber
    - Limit intake of trans fatty acids
  - Emphasize weight management and physical activity
  - Medication in collaboration with a physician
- Manage other cardiac disease risk factors
  - Blood pressure
  - Smoking
  - Obesity
  - Inactivity

Source: American Diabetes Association. *Diabetes Care,* 2003;26:2194–2197. Copyright © 2003. Reprinted and adapted with permission from the American Diabetes Association.

striction for children less than 2 years of age, because the development of the brain and central nervous system are dependent in part on adequate intake of fats.

Vitamins and Minerals

There is often no need for additional vitamin and mineral supplements for the majority of people with diabetes as long as the dietary intake is balanced and adequate. However, a child's normal eating habits throughout the growth cycle may exclude or severely limit foods or food groups and thus nutrient supplementation may be needed. The response to vitamin and mineral supplements will be favorable only when deficiencies are present; therefore, micronutrient adequacy should be evaluated periodically as children's food preferences change. Supplementation with certain vitamins and minerals, such as chromium, magnesium, zinc, and antioxidants, has been suggested as treatments for diabetes and other health issues. Sodium recommendations are addressed below.

Chromium

Chromium deficiency in both animal and human studies is associated with elevated blood glucose, cholesterol, and triglyceride levels, and with reduction in body growth and longevity. Populations at risk for chromium deficiency include the elderly and those on long-term total parenteral alimentation. Fortunately, most people with diabetes are not chromium deficient. The American Diabetes Association does not recommend chromium supplementation unless a deficiency is clearly documented.

Magnesium

Magnesium deficiency has been associated with insulin resistance, carbohydrate intolerance, and hypertension, among other disorders. Only those patients at high risk should routinely be evaluated, such as those in poor glycemic control (diabetic ketoacidosis and prolonged glycosuria), those on diuretics, or those with intestinal malabsorption.

Sodium

Sodium recommendations for children and adolescents with diabetes are the same as for the general population (see Chapters 5 and 6). The effect of sodium on blood pressure varies greatly between people depending on their level of sodium sensitivity. Research has not shown that those with diabetes are at a greater risk of developing hypertension if consuming a high-sodium diet. Routine monitoring of blood pressure is important and will help identify children and adolescents who may benefit from a reduction in sodium intake. Because sodium intake recommendations are the same as for the general population, guidelines should be directed toward the entire family.

Zinc

Although insulin is stored as inactive zinc crystals in the beta cells and zinc is involved in insulin action, supplementation is only suggested to benefit those children with a zinc deficiency. When the dietary intake of children with type 1 diabetes was investigated, low intakes of zinc were noted in many 4- to 6-year-old children; however, a nationwide sample of all children also indicated inadequate zinc intake.[23] Low zinc intake may be attributed to limited consumption of animal products, particularly meat in this age group. Poor growth has also been attributed to zinc deficiency in children with type 1 diabetes. Zinc supplementation in children with low zinc levels increased the rate of linear growth.[24]

Antioxidants

In a sample of 66 children with type 1 diabetes who were less than 10 years of age, most exceeded the RDAs for most vitamins and minerals, with the exception of vitamin E and C. However, supplementation with these antioxidants is not recommended.[23]

Recommendations

Vitamin and mineral supplements should not be used in place of a varied, balanced diet to ensure that children and adolescents receive adequate nutrients. Inadequate nutrient intake is rare in children with diabetes as long as the child is growing, gaining weight, and staying active, so there is no evidence or justification for routine supplementation. Those children at risk for nutrient deficiencies and who may benefit from a multivitamin supplement with antioxidants include those who are not consuming a variety of foods, are strict vegetarians, are taking medications known to alter certain micronutrients, or who have consistently poor glycemic control, which can result in excess excretion of water soluble vitamins.

Alcohol

Alcohol use and abuse should be discussed with the adolescent in an objective manner. Although the consumption of alcohol is illegal and is always discouraged for teens, facts about how alcohol affects blood glucose levels should be available to teens who express an interest in drinking. It should be made clear that alcohol lowers the blood glucose level and blocks gluconeogenesis, possibly leading to erratic behavior, loss of consciousness, or seizures, particularly if food is not consumed with the alcohol.[25] In addition, the teen should understand that glucagon is not effective in the treatment of alcohol-induced hypoglycemia because alcohol depletes glycogen stores.

Pointing out that alcohol alters the ability to think clearly may help the teen be more cautious about drinking alcohol or avoiding it altogether. It is important that those who choose to drink make sure that they wear diabetes identification because intoxication and symptoms of hypoglycemia can often be confused for one another. Drinking alone should always be discouraged.

If alcohol is consumed, it should be consumed in moderate amounts (no more than one drink per day for most females and no more than two drinks a day for most males) and only if diabetes is under good control. One drink or alcohol portion is defined as 12 oz. of beer, 5 oz. of wine, or 1.5 oz. of 80-proof distilled spirits. Each of these portions provides about 0.5 oz. of alcohol. As a general rule, it takes about 2 hours for the average 150-pound male to metabolize 1 oz. of alcohol.[2]

DESIGNING THE MEAL PLAN

The ultimate goals when designing a meal plan for a child who has been recently diagnosed with type 1 diabetes are to:

- Provide healthy eating guidelines for the child and family
- Promote positive behavioral changes
- Provide healthy meals and snacks
- Focus on healthy eating habits of the entire family

The amount of time required by the family to learn meal planning depends on multiple factors such as family dynamics, emotional status, extended support system, preconceived ideas about the "diabetic diet," and the family's social and cultural attitudes. The child should participate in the initial visit and be reassured that he or she will not be put on a "diet" or have many favorite foods taken away. Rather, healthy guidelines (a meal plan) will be provided based on the child's usual eating pattern to help promote healthy food choices. To avoid isolating the child and dividing the family, it should be emphasized that meal planning is simply a healthy eating plan for both the child and the entire family. Eating the same foods provides a sense of unity within the family.

Nutrition Counseling

At the time of diagnosis, the parent and/or child may be asked to keep a record of what is eaten at each meal and snack. This helps establish the amount of food that is currently needed to satisfy the child's appetite. An accurate measurement of weight and height (or length), information on recent weight loss, and a calculation of IBW are needed to estimate the child's current nutrient and caloric needs. Determining the percentile of the height (length), weight, weight for height, and the range for IBW will identify the child's initial nutrition status and help guide the development of the meal plan. A newly diagnosed child is more likely to experience increased hunger due to glycosuria. It is important to respond to this stimulated appetite by providing sufficient food so that hunger and restriction are not associated with having diabetes. Appetite of most children will stabilize within the first few weeks after diagnosis, though it could take longer. If children have lost weight or not grown to their potential, their appetite may be higher than estimated needs. Within reason, the meal plan should reflect the amount of food the child desires and be readjusted once the appetite decreases. The family should be educated that the meal plan might need to be adjusted 2 or 3 weeks after diagnosis once the child has gained back the weight.

Nutrition intervention in the hospital setting should be based on the family's ability, interest, and readiness to learn. Attempts to present all concepts upon initial diagnosis may result in confusion and the family members' loss of confidence in their ability as caretakers. Provide only general guidelines such as consistency with timing, amount and types of foods, and the relationship between food, insulin, and exercise, and their effect on blood glucose. Routine follow-up by phone is beneficial because many questions arise when the child returns home and normal activity resumes. Above all, it should be stressed that:

- Parents should not promote distorted eating to maintain blood glucose control.
- Any changes associated with food choices should be made slowly.
- Ranges for food choices should be used with young children (i.e., 1–2 oz. protein, 1/2–1 fruit), offering smaller amounts first and using the larger end of the range if more food is requested.
- During hospitalization, the length of time required to achieve *initial* nutrition management survival skills varies considerably between families and may require 2 to 4 hours of education not including time for menu writing and food selection using the meal plan.
- After leaving the hospital, actual teaching may require from two to four outpatient visits to achieve *ultimate* nutrition education goals.

The initial visit in the outpatient setting should lay the groundwork in nutrition basics and serve to develop a sound and trusting relationship with the child and family. The Children's Checklist (Exhibit 20–1) offers a detailed analysis of the child's and family's eating habits and behaviors, food preferences, and family lifestyle, and will assist the registered dietitian in producing a realistic and workable meal plan for this very important population.

General guidelines to help develop a positive working relationship with the child and their caretakers include:

- Include the child in the interview to allow him or her to be part of the decision-making process. The child will dictate the amount of food based on hunger and the parent will dictate the food choices.
- Do not refer to or label a child as a diabetic but as a child with diabetes.
- Interview the prepubertal child separately and then together with family to stimulate self-management.
- Provide reassurance that many of the child's usual foods can be included in his or her meal plan.
- Describe the meal plan as a guideline for healthy eating rather than a diet.
- Stress healthy eating practices for the entire family rather than just focusing on the child with diabetes.
- Avoid negative words when explaining meal planning such as "cannot", "do not", "never", "should not", "bad", "restrict", and especially the word "diet". In a child's mind, "diet" connotes deprivation or a short-term process, rather than an ongoing process.
- Avoid using the terms "good" or "bad" for foods. Instead, use "healthy" and "not as healthy" to describe individual foods.
- Ask about favorite foods and avoid eliminating these foods. Instead, stress balance, moderation, and variety.
- Review the reality of special treats for birthday parties, holidays, and special occasions and relate "treat" foods with extra exercise and active days.
- Encourage the caregiver to include the child in shopping and meal preparation.

Exhibit 20–1 Children's Checklist: Assessing the Child Newly Diagnosed with Diabetes

Growth (Anthropometrics)
- Height
- Weight
- BMI or weight for height
- History of growth pattern
- Recent weight changes

Biochemical Indices
- Blood glucose
- Glycosylated hemoglobin
- Lipid profile
- Microalbumin
- Ketones

Psychosocial Information
- Identify the family unit at home (two parents, separated parents, single parent, divorced, siblings, other family, friends, or caretakers)
- Evaluate the emotional state of the parents, child, and siblings (anger, fear, guilt, denial, anxiety)
- Assess the child's interactions with parents and siblings
- Identify the person(s) responsible for shopping and cooking
- Evaluate the knowledge, comprehension, and literacy levels
- Identify cultural/religious systems that influence attitudes
- Identify family members or friends with diabetes
- Assess parental and family beliefs about the "diabetic diet"

Child's Usual Food Intake Prior to Symptoms of Diabetes

Home:
- Eats scheduled meal/snacks
- Includes staple foods, such as milk, cheese, yogurt, bread
- Eats meats, fruit, and vegetables on a regular basis
- Consumes beverages at meals/snacks other than milk
- Drinks soda/juice/water for thirst
- Includes foods with most meals/snacks
- Follows a special diet

School:
- Brings lunch from home or has a school lunch
- Drinks beverage at lunch/snacks
- Scheduled snacks are part of regular class activities
- Obtains snack at school or has snack sent from home
- Consider the frequency, length, and time of day of the gym class
- Participates in school sports or activities after school

Weekends:
- Evaluate the meals prepared or eaten with others on weekends
- Identify the meal schedule if different from weekdays
- Determine the restaurant-eating habits on weekends
- Assess the sports/activities scheduled on weekends

Eating Behaviors

Child:
- Overeats or undereats
- Relies on convenience and fast foods

continues

Exhibit 20–1 continued

- Experiences food jags often
- Refuses many of the family foods offered
- Determine the location where meals and snacks are consumed
- Finishes meals in reasonable amount of time
- Respects the limits set for acceptable eating behavior at the table
- Has food allergies or intolerances

Family:

- Evaluate the parents as role models:
  Healthy eaters, structured meals, planned meals, limit junk food in homes?
  Unhealthy eaters, overweight, chronic dieters?
- Identify the supervision at meals/snacks
- Evaluate the limit setting around food choices
- Assess any cultural/religious eating behaviors
- Identify whether food is used as a reward

- Revise or draft a realistic and workable meal plan with input from the parent and/or child.
- Encourage the parents to always keep the lines of communication open so the child can request special foods that he or she wants to eat and that can be worked into the meal plan. Avoid being the "food police." If the child is always told "no", he or she may start to sneak food, which will cause unexplained high blood glucose levels.
- Advise the caregivers that it is not advisable to omit foods from the meal plan because of a single high blood glucose reading. An elevated blood glucose level caused by stress may decrease rapidly when the stress is reduced, and hypoglycemia may occur if food is omitted.
- Continued nutrition follow-up and education are required every 6 months to 1 year as the child grows and develops and as the family works to gain expertise in the nutrition management of diabetes.

Meal-Planning Approaches

One of the primary reasons patients with diabetes have such a difficult time understanding food issues is due to a lack of nutrition education and counseling by a registered dietitian. Instead, patients may simply be told to restrict sugar or may be given a basic sample menu to follow without an adequate educational foundation. The DCCT provided important insight into the role of nutrition intervention in intensive diabetes treatment and stated that registered dietitians are best qualified to match appropriate meal-planning approaches to the needs of the patient. Today, there are several effective methods for teaching patients about food. Any method can be equally effective when "geared to the patient's intellectual level, repeated frequently, and evaluated."[26]

The two most common approaches used with children are (1) carbohydrate counting and (2) an exchange list system for meal planning. These methods give structure to meal planning and provide the right balance between food, insulin, and exercise.

Carbohydrate Counting

A growing number of children are maintaining glucose levels on multiple daily injections (MDI) or continuous subcutaneous insulin infusion (CSII) using pump therapy. The carbohydrate (CHO) counting system allows the users greater flexibility in the timing of meals, the amount of food eaten at each meal, and the selection of specific foods. The meal-planning objective is to coordinate food intake (carbohydrate) by matching the peak activity of insulin with the peak levels of glucose resulting from the digestion and absorption of food. With this system, only the carbohydrate value of the food is counted, which allows more precise adjustment of premeal, short-acting insulin (Humalog or Novolog) using an insulin-to-CHO ratio. The insulin-to-CHO ratio is based on the assumption that carbohydrate intake is the main consideration in determining meal-related insulin requirements together with self-monitored blood glucose (SMBG) values. Targeted blood glucose values are set by the MD and the patient. The general rule is that approximately 1 unit of short-acting insulin will be needed for every 10 to 15 grams of carbohydrate.[27] The child's insulin-to-CHO ratio should be individually determined by the certified diabetes educator (CDE) based on the child's present insulin needs and meal plan. A child's ratio can range from 1 unit of insulin for every 5 to 40 grams of carbohydrate depending on age, activity, and insulin needs. Care must be taken not to overeat because increased availability of insulin and food may promote unwanted weight gain. A good understanding of how carbohydrate affects blood glucose, what food groups contain carbohydrate, and the importance of portion control is necessary for carbohydrate counting to be effective. Reference books providing carbohydrate content of specific foods are also helpful. Continuous reinforcement of healthy eating habits is advisable, because many young people tend to omit food groups as well as meals to accommodate busy schedules or to control weight.

The Exchange System

The lists of food choices (exchange lists) are based on three main food groups—the carbohydrate group (starch, fruit, milk, vegetables, and other carbohydrates), the meat and meat substitute group (protein), and the fat group. Examples of the specific amount of carbohydrate, protein, fat, or combination of these nutrients in each food group are found in Table 20–6. Foods with similar nutrient values are listed together and may be exchanged or traded for any other food on the same list. Exchange lists are used to achieve a consistent timing and intake of carbohydrate, protein, and fat and provide needed variety when planning meals. Exchange lists and a meal plan can be a

Table 20–6 Nutrient Content of Exchanges

Groups/List	*Carbohydrates (grams)*	*Protein (grams)*	*Fat (grams)*	*Calories*
Carbohydrate Group				
Starch	15	3	0–1	80
Fruit	15	—	—	60
Milk				
Fat-free, low-fat	12	8	0–3	90
Reduced-fat	12	8	5	120
Whole	12	8	8	150
Other carbohydrates	15	Varies	Varies	Varies
Nonstarchy vegetables	5	2	—	25
Meat and Meat Substitutes Group				
Very lean	—	7	0–1	35
Lean	—	7	3	55
Medium fat	—	7	5	75
High fat	—	7	8	100
Fat Group	—	—	5	45

Source: Reprinted by permission from the American Dietetic Association. *Exchange Lists for Meal Planning,* © 2003. American Diabetes Association, Inc.

starting point for those patients on intensive insulin management and can help them to understand and learn the carbohydrate content of foods.

INSULIN THERAPY

Insulin regimens for children vary. *Conventional insulin therapy* may include one to two daily injections of intermediate-acting insulin (NPH or Lente) or long acting/basal insulin (Ultralente/Lantus), possibly combined with a small amount of short-acting insulin (Regular, Humalog, or Novolog). *Intensive insulin therapy* can include four or more daily injections (MDI) using a short-acting insulin with either an intermediate or long-acting insulin or CSII pump therapy. A multiple daily injection regimen allows more freedom in the scheduling of meals and may eliminate the need for many snacks; however, intensive insulin therapy does increase the risk of hypoglycemia. The onset, peak, and duration of the common types of insulin are listed in Table 20–7.

Many circumstances require that permanent or temporary insulin adjustments be made. As a child grows and food intake increases, the insulin dose also increases. During brief periods of illness or times of stress or decreased activity, insulin needs may also increase. A change in the child's level of activity, which may be especially dramatic at the beginning and end of the school year, usually requires an adjustment in the insulin dosage. When a problem or behavior that affects insulin dosage resolves or changes, the child's insulin dose will need to be readjusted. Otherwise, an increase of food in response to the higher insulin levels may result in inappropriate weight gain or hypoglycemia, while too little insulin may result in hyperglycemia.

Snacks

In conventional insulin therapy, the intermediate or long-acting insulin has a peaking action. To prevent hypoglycemia, patients are encouraged to eat snacks between each meal and at bedtime. Typically, a snack of 15 to 20 g of carbohydrate is recommended for young children and a snack of 20 to 30 g of carbohydrate or higher is recommended for adolescents. The length of time at recess and in physical education (PE) classes and the type and length of after-school activities will influence the kind and amount of food needed for snacks. For example, if PE is offered only on Monday and Wednesday at 10:00 A.M., the child may need a larger snack on those days, preferably

Table 20–7 Activity of Insulin Types*

Insulin	*Onset*	*Peak*	*Effective Duration*
Very Rapid Acting			
Lispro (Humalog) Aspart (Novolog)	10–30 minutes	30 minutes–3 hours	3–5 hours
Rapid Acting			
Regular	30 minutes	1–5 hours	8 hours
Intermediate Acting			
NPH	1–4 hours	4–15 hours	14–26 hours
Lente	1–4 hours	4–12 hours	16–26 hours
Long Acting			
Ultralente	4–6 hours	8–30 hours	24–36 hours
Lantus (Glargine)	1–2 hours	Without	24 hours

*The peak and duration of insulin action may vary in the pediatric population.

Source: Adapted from *The Joslin Guide to Diabetes.*

a snack with 20 to 30 g of carbohydrate and 1 to 2 oz. of protein. For very active days and extended appetite control, a long-lasting snack (2 to 3 hours), containing carbohydrate, protein, and fat can be given. For inactive children, whose main activity is not likely to increase beyond watching television and studying, snacks may only contain 15 to 20 g of carbohydrate.

CSII/PUMP THERAPY

Since the introduction of CSII in the 1970s, the benefits of pump therapy have become very popular in patients with type 1 diabetes. Diabetes centers around the country started using the pump on pediatric patients in the 1980s. Pump therapy demonstrated the benefits of improved glycemic control,[28,29] reduced episodes of hypoglycemia, improved linear growth, and decreased episodes of recurrent diabetic ketoacidosis (DKA).[30] Pumps are becoming more widely used even in children as young as 1 to 2 years of age. The advantage of the pump for the small child is that it offers the parents the ability to dose a very small amount of insulin and provide multiple doses throughout the day without having to give the child shots by syringe or pen.

Pump therapy provides only a fast-acting insulin (Humalog or Novolog), which eliminates the unpredictable action of the longer-acting insulin. The pump delivers a small amount of insulin continuously (basal) and can be programmed to deliver boluses when eating a meal or snack or for correcting high blood glucoses. There are pros and cons of pump therapy, which should be considered very closely prior to putting any child on an insulin pump.

LANTUS (GLARGINE)

Lantus is becoming more popular in school-age children, adolescents, and young adults. It allows the child the flexibility of the pump but without the additional equipment that comes with the pump. Lantus is approved for children over 6 years of age. Lantus is a 24-hour basal insulin that is usually given once a day by syringe, usually in the evening at bedtime or at a time that it can be given consistently. Some children have benefited from splitting the dose, due to Lantus possibly not lasting a full 24 hours. This allows for complete 24-hour coverage. Lantus cannot be mixed with other insulins so it is injected separately. When using Lantus, the child or adolescent must use a rapid-acting insulin (Humalog or Novolog) each time carbohydrate is eaten, or when blood glucose levels are outside of target range and need to be corrected. This may be translated into at least four to five shots in an older child and as many as five to six shots in a younger child. To avoid additional insulin injections at school, NPH insulin can be added at breakfast with the rapid insulin to cover the morning snack and lunch. Lantus has also been used at bedtime in place of NPH if there is apprehension regarding hypoglycemia in the middle of the night.

Before a family or child starts pump therapy or multiple daily injections using Lantus and a rapid-acting insulin, it is necessary that the child and the family master more advanced skills. These skills include having a good understanding of advanced carbohydrate counting, which includes using insulin-to-carbohydrate ratios, the sensitivity or correction factors to determine each insulin dose, and the necessary math skills needed to calculate dosage.

AGE-SPECIFIC DEVELOPMENTAL CONSIDERATIONS

The most important psychosocial issues facing families with children with diabetes are:

- Defining responsibilities and support for diabetes management within the family
- Sharing treatment responsibilities among family members
- How and when these responsibilities are transferred from parent to child as the child develops[31]

As the child with diabetes progresses through the different stages of development, it is important to address how these changes affect the parents and/or the child and focus on the normal

Table 20–8 Challenges Facing Parents and/or Children with Diabetes

(0–3 yr old) Parents of infants and toddlers
- Monitoring diabetes control and avoiding hypoglycemia
- Establishing a meal schedule despite the child's normally irregular eating patterns
- Coping with the very young child's inability to understanding the need for injections
- Managing the conflicts with older siblings that result from unequal sharing of parental attention

(4–7 yr old) Preschoolers and early elementary school children
- Mastering separation from the family and adapting to the expectations of teachers
- Blaming self for having diabetes; regarding injections and restrictions as punishments
- Educating school personnel, coaches, and scout leaders about diabetes (parents)

(8–11 yr old) Later elementary school children
- Engaging in a wide range of activities with peers
- Understanding long-term benefits of diabetes care
- Becoming involved in diabetes self-care tasks (selecting snacks, selecting and cleaning injection sites, and identifying symptoms of low blood glucose)

(12–15 yr old) Early adolescents
- Integrating physical changes into self-image
- Acknowledgment from parents that the young teenager is on the threshold of becoming an adult
- Assuming increased responsibility for diabetes management in the face of physiologic changes caused by puberty that lead to insulin resistance and sensitivity
- Fitting in with the peer group
- Maintaining good glycemic control despite concerns about possible weight gain

(16–19 yr old) Late adolescents
- Making decisions regarding plans after high school
- Living more independently of parents
- Strengthening relationships with fewer friends
- Assuming more independent responsibility for health and health care

Source: Reprinted with permission from Lebovitz, HE. Psychosocial adjustment in children with type 1 diabetes. In: Lebovitz HE, ed., *Therapy for Diabetes Mellitus and Related Disorders*, 3rd ed., p. 72. ©1998, American Diabetes Association.

developmental issues of each stage. Table 20–8 outlines the psychosocial and developmental adjustments children, adolescents, and families must face and consider in managing diabetes.

AGE-SPECIFIC FOOD CONSIDERATIONS

Birth to 12 Months

Initially, most infants consume 100% of their calories as breast milk or formula, eating every 3 to 4 hours. The American Academy of Pediatrics recommends that all babies be breast-fed for the first 6 to 12 months of life; iron-fortified infant formula is the only acceptable substitute. Solids are typically introduced at 4 to 6 months and progress from strained cereal, fruits, meat, vegetables, and/or vegetable-meat dinners. Infants with diabetes do well following the same schedule. Eventually when the infant begins eating 2 to 3 tablespoons of baby foods and/or table food (other than low-calorie vegetables), basic carbohydrate counting can be introduced as a guideline. It is recommended to establish a feeding schedule despite somewhat erratic eating behaviors in the infant.

One to 4 Years of Age

A 1992 report in the *New England Journal of Medicine* proposed a possible link between drinking cow's milk as an infant and the development of type 1 diabetes. Upon further inspection the association of exposure to cow's milk and type 1 diabetes is unlikely.[32,33] Although whole cow's milk should not be given during the child's first year, after the first year cow's milk should not be removed from the diets of infants who have a family history of type 1 diabetes.

Between 12 and 15 months of age, the milk intake may begin to decrease and the intake of solid food increases. A total revision of the meal plan is needed at this time. During this time, a child may begin to be more accepting of meat and cheese, which can be added to the meal plan. Although fruits are included in the meal plan, fruit juice should be limited or avoided due to its effect on appetite, weight, and blood glucose.

As the toddler develops more mobility, interest in the environment also increases, and interest in food may wane. In some instances, getting the toddler to eat anything at a meal is an accomplishment. Erratic eating behaviors in toddlers require careful insulin therapy monitoring. In some cases, insulin is given after the meal, when the toddler has consumed the food and the dose of insulin can be titrated based on the amount of food consumed. Food-behavior guidelines for this young group, with or without diabetes, should be firmly established by caregivers at the time the child begins solid foods.

School-Age Children

Adjusting diabetes around the school schedule rather than changing PE classes or lunch periods to accommodate an insulin regimen communicates to the child that the child is more important than the diabetes. It is possible to arrange snacks and injections around most school schedules. Parents should be encouraged to address food and diabetes-treatment issues with school personnel; however, some parents may require assistance from their health care team. School-age children will ordinarily need three meals and two to three snacks a day, scheduled according to their insulin regimen. However, some children can omit the morning snack without creating a problem as long as lunch is not delayed. Children should be instructed to carry a fast-acting carbohydrate with them at all times in case of emergency. The use of chocolate candy bars or other high-fat items is discouraged as a treatment for hypoglycemia because fat ingestion slows the absorption of the carbohydrate needed to raise the blood glucose to a safe level. Most schools will offer lunch items appropriate to meet the needs of children following a meal plan, such as low-fat milk and fresh fruit. If school personnel are unwilling to cooperate, reference can be made to Section 504 of the Rehabilitation Act of 1973, Individuals with Disabilities Education Act of 1991 (originally the Education for All Handicapped Children Act of 1975), commonly referred to as Public Law No. 94-142, which mandates that handicapped students, including children with diabetes, have access to all services necessary to assist in full participation in school.[34]

Adolescents

The advent of adolescence may bring a great deal of conflict into the lives of family members. Adolescents strive for independence and expect parents to trust them to manage their own diabetes. Children may for the first time vent their anger about having diabetes during the adolescent period. The key to working successfully with adolescents is for the parents and the health care team to make every effort to provide positive reinforcement and negotiated support. Parents should continue their involvement and supervision of monitoring blood glucose and insulin administration at home. It is often more effective for team members to see teenagers and their parents individually, while at the same time respecting the teenagers' confidentiality. More flexibility in food choices and an increase in calories during this period of growth is usually necessary. Food choices may improve in a nonjudgmental atmosphere and with assistance for the teen to work favorite foods into the meal plan. On clinic visits, the teen should be routinely asked if a change in the meal plan is desired. Even if no change is made, the teen will enjoy having some control over the meal plan.

GROWTH MAINTENANCE

Routine charting of a child's height, weight, and BMI is an excellent way to monitor the growth pattern. Deviation from the child's normal growth curve (except for increased height or decreasing weight in a child who has reached full height potential) needs close monitoring. In a child whose diabetes is poorly controlled, weight percentile will often remain stationary or decrease. After about 6 months of little or no weight gain, height velocity may also begin to slow. Achieving optimal height potential can be used to motivate boys and girls to strive for better blood glucose control. Adolescents are more likely to be interested in improved self-care when they understand the relationship between good control, appropriate weight gain, consistent height increase, and/or normal menses.

WEIGHT CONTROL AND DISORDERED EATING

Weight control can become an important issue to children prior to and when entering adolescence. Parents and the health care team must take concerns about body image seriously. Some weight gain is usually seen prior to growth spurts. If a child's weight is disproportionate to height, the weight should be kept stable until the height fits the weight. Calorie reduction and food restriction are not recommended for children at any time during growth and development. Rather, the child should be encouraged to become involved in active play and physical exercise and to incorporate more fresh fruits and vegetables into his/her daily intake.

Children who are overly concerned about weight gain but who find it hard to reduce their intake may choose to skip insulin injections to promote quick weight loss. When significant weight loss is noted, the etiology should be explored. Signs of insulin omission or misuse may include:

- Weight fluctuations of 10 pounds or more
- Uncontrolled diabetes based on glycosylated hemoglobin measures
- Controlled diabetes only when hospitalized
- Multiple hospital admissions with unexplained diabetic ketoacidosis
- Reluctance or refusal to take more insulin
- Blaming insulin for weight problems
- Preoccupation with body weight or shape
- Engaging in excessive exercise
- Depression with low self-esteem

Referral to a registered dietitian or certified diabetes educator is the first line of defense when a child or adolescent exhibits weight dissatisfaction but does not exhibit clinical eating pathology. Strict guidelines regarding food and blood glucose should not be implemented because this may actually promote binge eating or weight gain. Adolescents should be advised that glucose fluctuations could create increased hunger and result in weight gain. Education should also be provided about serious short and long-term consequences of destructive food behaviors. Referral to a mental health professional who is knowledgeable about diabetes and disordered eating, or hospitalization, is often necessary to break the disordered eating cycle.

TYPE 2 DIABETES

In the last 10 years, the number of children being diagnosed with type 2 diabetes has been labeled an epidemic.[35] By 1999, depending on geographic location, between 8 and 45% of all new cases of diabetes in children were type 2.[36] The increase of type 2 diabetes in children is proportional with the increase of childhood obesity. Many of the cases occur in children of ethnic minorities including African-American, Mexican-American, Native-American, and Asian-American.[37] Type 2 diabetes in children, as in adults, is due to the combination of insulin resistance and beta-cell failure. At present time, there have been few studies done to determine the most effective way to manage these children. Incorporating physical activity and nutrition counseling to help the child or adolescent to maintain or lose weight is often prescribed, coupled with either Metformin or insulin. Metformin is presently the only oral diabetes medication that is approved by the FDA for pediatric use.

The increased rate of children being diagnosed with type 2 diabetes is a public health problem. In a position statement of the American Diabetes Association and the National Institute of Diabetes, Digestive and Kidney Diseases,[38] the following recommendations were made:

- Children of families at risk should be aware of the benefits of weight maintenance or moderate weight loss, and the health benefits of regular physical activity.
- Intervention strategies should involve counseling on weight loss and physical activity, with follow-up, which appears to be important for success.
- Drug therapy should not be routinely used to prevent diabetes until more information is known.

In 2002, the Diabetes Prevention Program published the results of a study comparing lifestyle intervention to administering Metformin in the prevention or delay of developing type 2 diabetes in adults. There was a 58% reduction of diabetes progression in the lifestyle group as compared to a 31% reduction in the Metformin group.[39] These results are particularly important to those who are interested in preventing type 2 diabetes in U.S. youth. Providing education for a healthy and active lifestyle might be the best defense against this ever-growing public health epidemic.

PREGNANCY

To help ensure a healthy pregnancy and a positive outcome to the woman with diabetes, optimal medical care must begin *before* conception. However, many unplanned pregnancies occur shortly after puberty among young people with and without diabetes, putting those with pregestational diabetes mellitus (PGDM) at a higher risk for early pregnancy loss or very costly congenital malformations in infants. The deterioration of metabolic control in combination with other obstetric and medical complications during an unplanned pregnancy can lead to serious complications of diabetes such as retinopathy, nephropathy, hypertension, and neuropathy. It is the responsibility of the health care team to provide prepregnancy counseling, including information on the risk of congenital malformations, to those of child-bearing age who have diabetes.

Unplanned pregnancies should be addressed immediately by a multidisciplinary team approach including a diabetologist, obstetrician, and diabetes educators, including a nurse, a registered dietitian, a social worker, and possibly an exercise physiologist. The team approach can guide the mother toward a goal of a healthy pregnancy and offspring.[40] Members of the adolescent or young adult's immediate family are encouraged to attend and participate in all learning sessions.

A preconception, interactive care plan outlined by the ADA to facilitate reimbursement for all elements of the program by health insurance organizations includes the following[40]:

- Patient education related to interaction of diabetes, pregnancy, and family planning
- Education in diabetes self-management skills
- Physician-directed medical care and laboratory testing
- Counseling by a mental health professional to reduce stress and improve adherence to the diabetes treatment plan

Nutrition management during pregnancy should begin at the earliest possible time. Caloric intake should be evaluated as soon as possible in the first trimester and at the start of each trimester thereafter to ensure adequate intake. Guidelines for medical nutrition therapy for pregnancy for preexisting diabetes are listed in Exhibit 20–2.

Breastfeeding

Breastfeeding is encouraged for mothers with diabetes and provides to the mother and infant the same benefits as it does for any woman (insulin is not ingested by the baby through breast milk). Not only does breast milk contain immunoglobulins and antibodies, which protect the infants from diseases, intestinal distress, and allergic reactions,

Exhibit 20–2 Medical Nutrition Therapy (MNT)

Recommendations are the same for pre-existing diabetes and gestational diabetes (GDM) except where noted.

Counseling and education

- All pregnant women should receive MNT counseling by a registered dietitian (RD)/certified diabetes educator (CDE).
- All pregnant women should receive self monitoring blood glucose (SMBG) training by a CDE.
- Daily food records and SMBG record are required to assess effectiveness of MNT.
- Carbohydrate (carb)-counting skills are taught for either consistent carb intake or a personalized insulin-to-carbohydrate ratio so the patient can adjust insulin based on carb intake.
- At least three encounters with a RD are recommended:
  1. Visit 1 (60–90 min) for assessment and meal planning. This could be SMBG instruction if the RD has received training.
  2. Visit 2 (30–45 min) in 1 week to assess and modify meal plan
  3. Visit 3 (15–45 min) 1–3 weeks to assess and modify plan as needed
  4. Additional visits every 2–3 weeks p.r.n. until delivery and one visit 6–8 weeks after delivery.

Calories

BMI Range		Kcal/kg prepreg wt*	Recommended wt gain (lbs)
Normal weight	(19.8–26)	30	25–35
Underweight	(<19.8)	36–40	28–40
Overweight	(26–29)	24	15–25
Obese	(>29)	not < 1800 kcal	15
Twins**			35–45
Triplets**			45–55

*an additional 150 –300 kcals/day in the 2nd and 3rd trimesters

**150 kcals/day above singleton pregnancy or amount that is consistent with target weight gain

Distribution of calories

- Individualize based on usual intake, preferences and medical regimen.
- 6–8 small meals/snacks. More frequent meals decrease postprandial hyperglycemia.

Carbohydrate	**Gestational Diabetes**	**Preexisting Diabetes**
Breakfast	40–45% total calories	45–55% total calories
HS Snack	15–30 grams*	Individualize as per usual intake and blood glucose levels
Fiber		
	15–30 grams carbs	15–30 grams carbohydrate
	20–35 grams	20–35 grams

*may be increased if insulin added

Protein

- 0.8 grams protein per kg dry body weight plus an additional 10 grams/day.
- 20–25% of total calories is usual.

Fat

- Preexisting diabetes: 30–35% total calories, with <10% total calories from saturated fat.
- GDM: <40% total calories with 10% total calories from saturated fat.
- Encourage use of polyunsaturated and monounsaturated fats instead of saturated fats.

continues

Exhibit 20–2 continued

Artificial sweeteners	• Nonnutritive sweeteners considered safe during pregnancy: aspartame, acesulfame potassium (ace-K), and sucralose. • Because saccharin remains on the "anticipated" carcinogen list, it is not recommended during pregnancy.
Vitamin/mineral supplements	Prenatal multivitamin and mineral supplement including: • Iron (30 mg/day for 12 weeks) • Folic Acid (1 mg) daily to decrease risk of neural tube defects • Additional calcium supplementation may be needed to meet daily requirements of 1200 mg per day (begin prior to conception)
Physical activity	• Regular physical activity is recommended after clearance by provider. • Benefits include reducing insulin resistance, postprandial hyperglycemia, and excessive weight gain. • Hypoglycemia is more likely with prolonged exercise (over 60 minutes). • Encourage activity after meals to reduce postprandial hyperglycemia.

Source: Reprinted with permission from Joslin Diabetes Center and Joslin Clinic Guideline for Detection and Management of Diabetes and Pregnancy (Rev. 02/22/02). Joslin's Clinical Guidelines are reviewed periodically and modified as needed to reflect changes in clinical practice and available pharmacological information. Check Joslin's Web site for the latest version (www.joslin.org).

but the process of breastfeeding also encourages mother-infant bonding. Breastfeeding, however, increases the need for fluids, and mothers should be encouraged to drink 2 to 3 liters (8 to 12 cups) of caffeine-free liquids per day to cover the fluid needs of the mother and replace what is used in breast milk.

Meal planning during breastfeeding requires assistance from a dietitian and physician. Insulin requirements are usually reduced during breastfeeding; however, caloric intake requires an additional 500 calories per day above what was consumed before the pregnancy. Extra calories may be added in the form of protein and calcium-rich foods such as milk, yogurt, tofu, and cheese. The calcium requirement for lactating women is 1200 mg per day. Calcium intake should be routinely assessed by a dietitian to prevent calcium loss from the mother during breastfeeding. If the mother is not able to consume adequate sources of calcium-rich foods, a calcium supplement may be required. It is important to keep a carbohydrate food source (15 to 20 gms) available while nursing because hypoglycemia may occur while breastfeeding. To prevent possible nocturnal hypoglycemia, an extra snack including 20 to 30 gms of carbohydrate and a source of protein may be added to the meal plan in the middle of the night.

CONTROLLING BLOOD GLUCOSE

The glycosylated hemoglobin measures the weighted average amount of glucose in the blood over a 2- to 3-month period. Used in conjunction with regularly monitored blood glucose results, glycosylated hemoglobin levels can help evaluate the level of control. However, the glycosylated hemoglobin level reflects an average amount of glucose in the blood and can be the result of very high and low blood glucose levels, which is not indicative of good control. Although "excellent control" for an adult with diabetes is 6 percent or less, the activity levels and eating habits of children and adolescents vary, so a level even under 7 percent can be unsafe and difficult to achieve in children. Glycosylated hemoglobin goals should be set by the child's diabetes team and tailored to each individual case.

Home blood glucose monitoring devices provide the child and family with immediate feedback on the effects of food, exercise, insulin, and stress on blood glucose levels, allowing for more flexibility in lifestyle and food intake.

A child with diabetes has many self-care responsibilities. Checking and recording the blood glucose level may be one of the most bothersome responsibilities for a child because it must be done so often and because others may inappropriately evaluate and judge the results. Blood glucose results are not totally reliable as a monitor of compliance with meal plans. If, by reporting a high blood glucose reading, a child risks accusations of sneaking food or overeating, the child may choose to record more acceptable but false levels. This practice may result in poor diabetes management. Establishing a nonjudgmental and honest atmosphere for the exchange of information is imperative for the parent, the dietitian, and other health care providers. When monitoring blood glucose, use the word "check" rather than "test" and use positive words to describe the results, such as *"high"* or *"low"* rather than *"good"* or *"bad."* Any information received from monitoring provides positive feedback, regardless of the number.[41]

High or low blood glucose levels will occur in most children even when insulin and exercise schedules and the meal plan are followed closely. When a high or low level occurs, it is useful to review the day's activities to see if there is an obvious explanation. The extent to which children should monitor blood glucose levels is variable, depending on many factors such as the type of insulin therapy, increased activity or exercise, sickness or infection, new food choices, change in lifestyle, increased stress, change in insulin type or dose, episodes of hypoglycemia, or overall poor control. A general guideline for blood glucose checking for infants and children on traditional insulin therapy is before each meal and before the bedtime snack.

Exercise/Activity

Regular exercise or activity is an important element in controlling blood glucose, lowering lipid levels, and maintaining appropriate body weight. Aerobic exercise is necessary to maintain a healthy cardiovascular system as well as to improve glucose control. To prevent obesity in children, emphasis should be placed on the importance of routinely scheduled activity. A minimum of 30 minutes to 1 hour of daily activity is a reasonable goal. However, exercising when ketones are present, which may occur when the blood glucose level is above 240mg/dL, or if the blood glucose is 400 mg/dl or higher without ketones, is not recommended.

To prevent hypoglycemia during activity, food intake may need to be increased or the dose of insulin decreased. Generally, children choose to increase food intake unless the activity occurs routinely, then the insulin can be adjusted accordingly. If the child's overall activity increases and the child is experiencing increased number of hypoglycemic events, the diabetes team should be consulted for insulin adjustment. Older children may be instructed on how to reduce their own insulin dose when participating in sports. It is wise to avoid exercise when insulin is peaking; however, sports events and practices are usually scheduled when the insulin is working hardest. In this instance, a larger snack, which includes carbohydrate as well as protein, may be needed prior to the activity. Some children may find it difficult to eat a large volume of food prior to prolonged activity and plan ahead to reduce their insulin dose.

The amount of insulin reduction depends on the results of blood sugar tests done before and after the activity. Food adjustments will depend on the duration and intensity of the exercise and on the blood glucose level prior to exercise (Exhibit 20–3). A general rule is to add 10 to 15 g of carbohydrate for every hour of extra activity. Prolonged activity may utilize a majority of the glucose stores in the muscle. The body replaces these stores when blood glucose becomes available. It is important for the child and adolescent to realize that an adequate snack, probably containing protein as well as carbohydrate, may need to be eaten after prolonged exercise to avoid drops in blood glucose level, which may occur after the activity has stopped.

Exhibit 20–3 Snack Guidelines for Exercise

Types of Exercise and Examples	*If Blood Glucose is (mg/dl)*	*Suggestions of Food to Use*
Exercise of short duration (30 min or less) and of moderate intensity Examples: walking a mile or bicycling for less than 30 min	Less than 100 100–180 180 or more	30 g carbohydrate + 1 protein 30 carbohydrate choices Snack may not be necessary
Exercise of intermediate duration (1 hr) and moderate intensity Examples: Tennis, swimming, jogging, leisurely bicycling, gardening, golfing, or vacuuming for 1 hour	Less than 100 100–180 180–240 240 or more	30 grams carbohydrate + 1 protein 15 grams carbohydrate + 1 protein 15 grams carbohydrate Snack may not be necessary
Exercise of long duration (2 hr or more) and/or high intensity Examples: football, hockey, racquetball, or basketball games; strenuous bicycling or swimming: shoveling heavy snow; skiing; hiking	Consult with your physician or exercise physiologist. Insulin may need to be decreased by 30–75%. Begin with a snack of 30 grams Carbohydrate + 2 oz protein, then eat at least 15 grams carbohydrate per hour of exercise. Test hourly. If blood glucose is 180 or more, an extra snack may not be needed for that hour.	

Sources: Adapted from Joslin Diabetes Center. *The Snack Guidelines for Exercise Handout*. and Beaser RS, Hill JVC. *The Joslin Guide to Diabetes*. 1995, Simon & Schuster (Fireside), p. 79.

HYPOGLYCEMIA

The most common emergency in insulin-dependent diabetes is hypoglycemia. The exact blood glucose level that produces symptoms of hypoglycemia is an individual response and differs with level of glucose control. Symptoms may occur below a certain level (i.e., 60, 70, 80 mg/dl) or when blood glucose levels are dropping rapidly even when the level is still in normal range. Exhibit 20–4 lists suggestions for treating hypoglycemia. Children with diabetes should be instructed to wear medical alert identification at all times to ensure proper treatment of hypoglycemic reactions, which may render the child unable to communicate.

SICK DAYS

Illness in the child with diabetes always presents a challenge. Insulin must always be given and may need to be increased during these periods. The blood glucose should be monitored every 3 to 4 hours during illness. Parents need to know when to call the doctor for assistance in managing illness because certain symptoms, such as prolonged vomiting and fever, can lead to rapid de-

Exhibit 20–4 Treatment for Hypoglycemia

Item	5 yrs of age and younger (5–10 grams carb)	6–10 yrs of age (10–15 grams carb)	Over 10 yrs of age (15–20 gram carb)
Glucose tablets			
(4–5 gram carb/ea)	1–2 tablets	2–3 tablets	3–4 tablets
Insta-glucose			
(24 gram carb tube)	1/3–1/2 tube	1/2–2/3 tube	2/3–1 tube
Glutose 45			
(45 gram per tube)	1/6–1/4 tube	1/4–1/3 tube	1/3–1/2 tube
Orange juice			
(1/2 cup = 13–15 grams carb)	1/4–1/2 cup	1/2–3/4 cup	3/4–1 cup
Apple juice			
(1/2 cup = 15 grams carb)	1/6–1/3 cup	1/3–1/2 cup	1/2–2/3 cup
Sugar			
(1 tsp = 4 grams)	2 teaspoons	3 teaspoons	4–5 teaspoons
Cake icing			
(1 tsp = 4 grams)	2 teaspoons	3 teaspoons	4–5 teaspoons
Honey, maple, or Karo Syrup			
1 teaspoon = 4–5 grams carb)	2 teaspoons	3 teaspoons	4–5 teaspoons
Regular soda or tonic			
(1 fl oz = 3–4 grams carb)	2–3 fl oz	4–5 fl oz	5–6 fl oz
Life Savers			
(1 ea = 3 grams)	2–3 each	4–5 each	5–6 each
Marshmallows			
Mini (2 = 5 grams)	2–4	4–6	6–8
Large (1 = 5 grams)	1–2	2–3	3–4
Raisins			
(1 Tbs = 7 1/2 grams)	1 Tbs	1 1/2–2 Tbs	2 1/2 Tbs

Source: Joslin Diabetes Center.

Carb = carbohydrate.

hydration and diabetic ketoacidosis. During brief illness, the meal plan should be maintained as much as possible, using foods that can be tolerated. If the child cannot tolerate food, it is important to replace the usual amount of carbohydrate consumed with sugar-containing liquids that can be easily used by the body for energy. Liquids also help to prevent dehydration. Some examples of easily tolerated liquids that contain 15 g of carbohydrate include 8 ounces of a regular carbonated beverage (with sugar), 4 ounces of fruit juice or a frozen fruit bar, or 1/2 cup of regular gelatin. It is recommended to sip on room temperature liquids at a rate of about 15 g of carbohydrate per hour. Exhibit 20–5 provides guidelines for diabetes management during illness.

CONCLUSION

Nutrition management of the child with diabetes is one of the most important factors in attaining and maintaining good metabolic control. Devising meal plans that provide flexibility while conforming to guidelines based on current research is a challenge to the dietitian. A thorough understanding of all the components of diabetes

Exhibit 20–5 Sick Day Guidelines

1. NEVER OMIT INSULIN. Continue to give insulin, although the dose may need to be changed.
2. Check the child's blood glucose and urine ketones every 3–4 hours.
3. Prevent dehydration; know the signs and symptoms, such as dry mouth, cracked lips, dry skin, sunken eyes, not making tears, and weight loss.
   - Sip on 8 ounces of room temperature fluid every 1/2–1 hour to prevent dehydration.
   - Use sugar-free drinks if blood sugar remains above 120–150 mg/dl.
   - Fluids with sodium and potassium, such as broth, Pedialyte, Ricelyte, may be alternated with other fluids.
   - Use sugar-containing fluids if blood sugar is below 80 mg/dl or below 120–150 mg/dl and your child is not able to eat the usual meal.
   - Keep a scale in your house. A child should be weighed once to twice a day during illness. If the child is losing weight (2 or 3 pounds), CALL YOUR DOCTOR!
4. A sick day nutrition cupboard should be maintained at the home in case your child becomes suddenly ill.
   - A copy of "Sick Day Guidelines"
   - Aspirin-free products (liquid, chewable) and/or suppositories
   - Broth, bouillon, or noncreamy soups
   - Cans of soda—sugared and sugar-free
   - Cans, bottles, or boxes of juice (do not need refrigeration)
   - Gelatin—sugared and sugar-free
   - Punch drinks—sugared and sugar-free
   - Rehydration products for the very young child (Pedialyte or Ricelyte)
5. When able to eat the usual amount of carbohydrate-containing foods, use food appropriate for a sick day:

milk	oatmeal	saltines	Popsicles
custard	cold cereal	toast	sherbet
yogurt	cream soup	applesauce	eggnog

Source: Adapted from Lawlor MT, Laffel L, Anderson B, Bertorelli A. *Caring for Young Children Living with Diabetes—Parent Manual*, pp. 68–77. Adapted with permission.

management will help the family adapt diabetes into their lifestyle instead of fitting their lifestyle into the diabetes. It is the role of the diabetes team members to empower the family and child with the knowledge to make the healthy decisions for long-term maintenance of good control.

REFERENCES

1. Lockwood D, Frey ML, Gladish NA, Hiss RG. The biggest problem in diabetes. *Diabetes Educ.* 1986;12:30–33.
2. American Diabetes Association. Nutrition principles and recommendations in diabetes. *Diabetes Care.* 2004;27: S36–S46.
3. The Diabetes Control and Complications Trial Research Group. The effect of intensive treatment of diabetes on the development and progression of long-term complications in insulin-dependent diabetes mellitus. *N Engl J Med.* 1993;329:977–986.
4. Drash AL. The child, the adolescent, and the Diabetes Control and Complications Trial. *Diabetes Care.* 1993; 16:1515–1516.
5. Franz MJ, Horton ES Sr, Bantle JP, Beebe CA, Brunzell JD, Coulston AM, Henry RR, Hoogwerf BJ, Stacpoole PW. Nutrition principles for the management of diabetes and related complications. *Diabetes Care.* 1994;17:490–518.
6. Butler DA, Lawlor MT. It takes a village: Helping families live with diabetes. *Diabetes Spectrum.* 2004;17:26–31.
7. Laffel LM, Brackett J, Ho J, Anderson BJ. Changing the process of diabetes care improves metabolic outcomes and reduces hospitalizations. *Qual Manag Health Care.* 1998;6:53–62.
8. U.S. Department of Agriculture and U.S. Department of Health and Health Services. *Report of the Dietary*

Guidelines Advisory Committee on the Dietary Guidelines for Americans, 2000. 2000.

9. U.S. Food and Nutrition Board. *Recommended Dietary Allowances.* Washington, DC: National Academy of Sciences; 1989.
10. Jenkins DJ, Wolever TM, Taylor RH, Barker H, Fielden H, Baldwin JM, Bowling AC, Newman HC, Jenkins AL, Goff DV. Glycemic index of foods: A physiological basis for carbohydrate exchange. *Am J Clin Nutr.* 1981;34: 362–366.
11. Gillespie S. Implementing liberized carbohydrate guidelines: Nutrition free-for-all or a more rational approach to carbohydrate consumption? *Diabetes Spectrum.* 1996; 9:165–167.
12. Bantle JP, Swanson JE, Thomas W, Laine DC. Metabolic effects of dietary fructose in diabetic subjects. *Diabetes Care.* 1992;15:1468–1476.
13. Duffy VB, Anderson GH. Position of the American Dietetic Association: Use of nutritive and nonnutritive sweeteners. *J Am Diet Assoc.* 1998; 98:580–587.
14. Payne ML, Craig WJ, Williams AC. Sorbitol is a possible risk factor for diarrhea in young children. *J Am Diet Assoc.* 1997;97:532–534.
15. Butchko HH, Stargel WW, Comer CP, Mayhew DA, Benninger C, Blackburn GL, de Sonneville LM, Geha RS, Hertelendy Z, Koestner A, Leon AS, Liepa GU, McMartin KE, Mendenhall CL, Munro IC, Novotny EJ, Renwick AG, Schiffman SS, Schomer DL, Shaywitz BA, Spiers PA, Tephly TR, Thomas JA, Trefz FK. Aspartame: Review of safety. *Regul Toxicol Pharmacol.* 2002;35:S1–S93.
16. Morrison AS, Buring JE. Artificial sweeteners and cancer of the lower urinary tract. *N Engl J Med.* 1980;302: 537–541.
17. Marlett JA, McBurney MI, Slavin JL. Position of the American Dietetic Association: Health implications of dietary fiber. *J Am Diet Assoc.* 2002;102:993–1000.
18. Randecker GA, Smiciklas-Wright H, McKenzie JM, Shannon BM, Mitchell DC, Becker DJ, Kieselhorst K. The dietary intake of children with IDDM. *Diabetes Care.* 1996;19:1370–1374.
19. American Diabetes Association. Nephropathy in diabetes. *Diabetes Care.* 2004;S79–S89.
20. National Cholesterol Education Program. *Report of the Expert Panel on Blood Cholesterol Levels in Children and Adolescents.* National Heart, Lung, and Blood Institute pub. no. 91-2732. Bethesda, MD, U.S. Department of Health and Human Services; 1991.
21. Virtanen SM, Ylonen K, Rasanen L, Ala-Venna E, Maenpaa J, Akerblom HK. Two year prospective dietary survey of newly diagnosed children with diabetes aged less than 6 years. *Arch Dis Child.* 2000;82:21–26.
22. American Diabetes Association. Management of dyslipidemia in children and adolescents with diabetes. *Diabetes Care.* 2004;26:2194–2197.
23. Alaimo K, McDowell MA, Briefel RR, Bischof AM, Caughman CR, Loria CM, Johnson CL. *Dietary Intake of Vitamins, Minerals, and Fiber of Persons Ages 2 Months and Over in the United States: Third National Health and Nutrition Examination Survey, Phase 1, 1988–1991.* Adv Data 1994;258:1–28.
24. Nakamura T, Higashi A, Nishiyama S, Fujimoto S, Matsuda I. Kinetics of zinc status in children with IDDM. *Diabetes Care.* 1991;14:553–557.
25. Madison LL, Lochner A, Wulff J. Ethanol-induced hypoglycemia. II. Mechanism of suppression of hepatic gluconeogenesis. *Diabetes.* 1967;16:252–258.
26. Arky RA. Current principles of dietary therapy of diabetes mellitus. *Med Clin North Am.* 1978;62:655-662.
27. Grinvalsky M, Nathan DM. Diets for insulin pump and multiple daily injection therapy. *Diabetes Care.* 1983;6: 241–244.
28. Tamborlane WV, Sherwin RS, Genel M, Felig P. Outpatient treatment of juvenile-onset diabetes with a preprogrammed portable subcutaneous insulin infusion system. *Am J Med.* 1980;68:190–196.
29. Tamborlane WV, Sherwin RS, Koivisto V, Hendler R, Genel M, Felig P. Normalization of the growth hormone and catecholamine response to exercise in juvenile-onset diabetic subjects treated with a portable insulin infusion pump. *Diabetes.* 1979;28:785–788.
30. Steindel BS, Roe TR, Costin G, Carlson M, Kaufman FR. Continuous subcutaneous insulin infusion (CSII) in children and adolescents with chronic poorly controlled type 1 diabetes mellitus. *Diabetes Res Clin Pract.* 1995;27:199–204.
31. Anderson BJ. Diabetes and adptations in family systems. In: Holmes C, ed., *Neuropsychology and Behavioral Aspects of Diabetes.* New York: Springer-Verlag; 1990: 85–101.
32. Couper JJ, Steele C, Beresford S, Powell T, McCaul K, Pollard A, Gellert S, Tait B, Harrison LC, Colman PG. Lack of association between duration of breastfeeding or introduction of cow's milk and development of islet autoimmunity. *Diabetes.* 1999;48:2145–2149.
33. Kimpimaki T, Erkkola M, Korhonen S, Kupila A, Virtanen SM, Ilonen J, Simell O, Knip M. Short-term exclusive breastfeeding predisposes young children with increased genetic risk of type I diabetes to progressive beta-cell autoimmunity. *Diabetologia.* 2001;44:63–69.
34. American Diabetes Association. Diabetes care in the school and day care setting. *Diabetes Care.* 2004;27: S122–S128.
35. American Diabetes Association. Type 2 diabetes in children and adolescents. *Diabetes Care.* 2000;23:381–389.
36. Rosenbloom AL, Joe JR, Young RS, Winter WE. Emerging epidemic of type 2 diabetes in youth. *Diabetes Care.* 1999;22:345–354.

37. Fagot-Campagna A, Pettitt DJ, Engelgau MM, Burrows NR, Geiss LS, Valdez R, Beckles GL, Saaddine J, Gregg EW, Williamson DF, Narayan KM. Type 2 diabetes among North American children and adolescents: An epidemiologic review and a public health perspective. *J Pediatr.* 2000;136:664–672.

38. American Diabetes Association. The prevention or delay of type 2 diabetes. *Diabetes Care.* 2002;25:742–749.

39. Knowler WC, Barrett-Connor E, Fowler SE, Hamman RF, Lachin JM, Walker EA, Nathan DM. Reduction in the incidence of type 2 diabetes with lifestyle intervention or metformin. *N Engl J Med.* 2002;346:393–403.

40. American Diabetes Association. Gestational diabetes mellitus. *Diabetes Care.* 2004;27 Suppl 1:S88–S90.

41. Lawlor MT, Anderson B, Laffel L. *Blood Sugar Monitoring Owner's Manual Booklet.* Boston, MA: Joslin Diabetes Center; 1997.

CHAPTER 21

Pediatric Human Immunodeficiency Virus

Lauren R. Furuta and Lynne Lewis

HIV AND AIDS OVERVIEW

The first cases of acquired immunodeficiency syndrome (AIDS) were reported in a small cohort of gay men in 1981.[1] Since that time, it is estimated that 56 million people worldwide have been infected with the human immunodeficiency virus (HIV, the virus that causes AIDS) and nearly 20 million people have died. AIDS has become a leading cause of death, and in some African countries it is actually lowering the life expectancy by as much as 15 years.[2–4]

HIV is a sexually transmitted and blood-borne disease. Modes of transmission include exposure to blood and body fluids such as sexual contact, breastfeeding, sharing of contaminated needles, and transmission from mother to child during the perinatal period or during labor and delivery. The greatest impact of the AIDS epidemic is among men who have sex with men (MSM), racial and ethnic minorities with a growing number of infected minority women, and cases attributed to heterosexual transmission.[2] Nearly all transfusion-associated cases occurred prior to screening of the blood supply in 1985.[2]

The first pediatric cases of HIV were described in 1982.[5] The majority of pediatric cases were associated with perinatal transmission, which peaked in 1992 (901 cases) and sharply declined after 1994 with the advent of zidovudine therapy protocols to prevent/reduce perinatal transmission. From 1985 to 1999, AIDS cases among children declined 81%. In 2000, children less than 19 years accounted for approximately 3800 cases or 1.4% of the cases of AIDS in the United States.[2]

The prognosis of children with HIV and AIDS has improved tremendously in much of the developed world. Once a fatal disease, HIV can now be described as a chronic, manageable disease. Where treatment is available and affordable, most children are maintaining healthy states and thriving. Many children are reaching adulthood in a state of health, allowing them to attend college and gain employment.

The medical, nutritional, and social implications of pediatric HIV and AIDS are numerous and complex. Effective management of the disease requires a coordinated and comprehensive approach that involves early diagnosis and aggressive medical, nutritional, and psychosocial intervention. This chapter gives a brief overview of pediatric HIV infection and AIDS and an in-depth description of the goals and strategies of nutritional management of the pediatric patient with HIV infection and AIDS.

IMMUNE FUNCTION AND HIV/AIDS

HIV is a retrovirus that primarily infects cells of the immune system, a system comprised of lymphocytes and other white blood cells. The lymphocytes are divided into two types known as T-cells and B-cells. T-cells are responsible for cellular immunity or fighting off invading antigens and B-cells are responsible for humoral immunity or antibody (immunoglobulin) production. T-cells express different antigens and HIV targets T-cells expressing the CD4 antigen (referred to as CD4 cells). HIV integrates itself into the host CD4 cell's DNA and then replicates itself, creating additional virus that ultimately cause the immune cell's destruction and death. The cell's destruction and death leads to a weakened immune system without enough immune cells to fight infections.[6]

AIDS is an advanced disease caused by acquisition of the human immunodeficiency virus (HIV-1 or HIV-2) and subsequent destruction of the immune system. This decrease in cellular immunity impairs the host's ability to fight off infection and results in the host acquiring opportunistic infections and malignancies. Untreated HIV infection allows for the continued destruction of CD4 cells, resulting in a progression of HIV disease. When the immune system deteriorates to specified and measurable levels (described later), the disease is termed acquired immune deficiency syndrome or AIDS.

DEFINITIONS OF AIDS SURVEILLANCE OF CHILDREN

The term HIV disease covers the spectrum of individuals from healthy to seriously ill. The term AIDS is employed by the Centers for Disease Control (CDC) to refer to those individuals who typically display specific "indicator" diseases as a result of HIV infection.[7]

As shown in Table 21–1, the current CDC definition criteria for children less than 13 years of age are based on clinical disease conditions/diagnoses and laboratory criteria. Only those children who meet the strict diagnostic criteria are classified as having AIDS. The classification categories include a letter designation (i.e., N, A, B, C) indicative of the presence of clinical conditions and a number designation indicative of immune status, which is based on CD4 T-cell counts and the CD4 percentage of total lymphocytes. The immune categories (see Table 21–2) are further delineated by age groups, because CD4 T-cell norms differ according to age, usually being higher in younger children at baseline.[7]

As the immune system declines, the likelihood of symptomatic HIV infection increases. The AIDS diagnosis is reserved for those patients in category C: severely symptomatic. Today, the child carrying a diagnosis of AIDS may be in significantly better health than in the days when treatment was unavailable. An undiagnosed infant may present to the medical system with pneumocystis *carinii* pneumonia (PCP), an AIDS-defining illness. With the advent of medical therapies, that same child may have immune reconstitution (recovery of the CD4 T-cell number and percentage), which places the child in category 1 (no immune suppression), and remain quite healthy. The clinical category provides a snapshot for categorizing the historical "sickest" that the child has been. The immune category is a reflection of the child's current immune status.

DIAGNOSIS

Ideally, pregnant women are screened for HIV infection as part of routine prenatal care. This screening provides for antenatal, peripartal, and neonatal HIV treatment that significantly decreases the rate of perinatal transmission to infants (approximately 1–4% versus 15–30% transmission without treatment).[8]

Infants are screened and diagnosed with laboratory testing that can usually confirm or exclude infection by 6 months of age. The DNA and RNA PCR tests are used to determine an infant's HIV infection status. Children older than 18 months can be tested using the ELISA and Western Immunoblotting methods that screen for the presence of antibodies to HIV. This is the same test utilized for adult HIV testing. The Elisa and Western Blot cannot be used on children younger than 18 months because they give false positive readings by detecting maternal antibody that is passed to the infant in utero.[9] There should be a high index of suspicion when the mother's HIV status is unknown. Infants born to high-risk mothers or with symptoms as described in the clinical categories for children with HIV should be tested for HIV infection.

CLINICAL MANIFESTATIONS OF HIV INFECTION AND AIDS

Children with HIV infection display a wide array of clinical features. Some untreated children have rapid disease progression while other

Table 21–1 Clinical Categories for Children with HIV Infection

CATEGORY N: NOT SYMPTOMATIC

Children who have no signs or symptoms considered to be the result of HIV infection or who have only one of the conditions listed in Category A.

CATEGORY A: MILDLY SYMPTOMATIC

Children with two or more of the conditions listed below but none of the conditions listed in Categories B and C.

—Lymphadenopathy (≥0.5 cm at more than two sites; bilateral = one site)
—Hepatomegaly
—Splenomegaly
—Dermatitis
—Parotitis
—Recurrent or persistent upper respiratory infection, sinusitis, or otitis media

CATEGORY B: MODERATELY SYMPTOMATIC

Children who have symptomatic conditions other than those listed for Category A or C that are attributed to HIV infection. Examples of conditions in clinical Category B include but are not limited to:

—Anemia (<8 gm/dL), neutropenia (<1,000/mm3), or thrombocytopenia (<100,000/mm3) persisting ≥30 days
—Bacterial meningitis, pneumonia, or sepsis (single episode)
—Candidiasis, oropharyngeal (thrush), persisting (>2 months) in children over 6 months of age
—Cardiomyopathy
—Cytomegalovirus infection, with onset before 1 month of age
—Diarrhea, recurrent or chronic
—Hepatitis
—Herpes simplex virus (HSV) stomatitis, recurrent (more than two episodes within 1 year)
—HSV bronchitis, pneumonitis, or esophagitis with onset before 1 month of age
—Herpes zoster (shingles) involving at least two distinct episodes or more than one dermatome
—Leiomyosarcoma
—Lymphoid interstitial pneumonia (LIP) or pulmonary lymphoid hyperplasia complex
—Nephropathy
—Nocardiosis
—Persistent fever (lasting >1 month)
—Toxoplasmosis, onset before 1 month of age
—Varicella, disseminated (complicated chickenpox)

CATEGORY C: SEVERELY SYMPTOMATIC

Children who have any condition listed in the 1987 surveillance case definition for acquired immunodeficiency syndrome, with the exception of LIP.

Source: Data from endnote reference 7.

children appear quite healthy and present after many years of immune decline. Presenting symptoms include lymphadenopathy, hepatosplenomegaly, failure to thrive, diarrhea, and multiple bacterial infections. As the clinical course progresses, the child may have severe cases of common childhood infections such as varicella (chicken pox), herpes simplex, and cytomegalovirus. With profound immunosuppression, severe infections such as disseminated mycobacterium *avium* complex (MAC/MAI), cryptococcal meningitis, and esophageal candidiasis may occur. Many

Table 21–2 Immunologic Categories Based on Age-Specific CD4+ T-lymphocyte Counts and Percent of Total Lymphocytes

	Age of child					
	<12 mos		*1–5 yrs*		*6–12 yrs*	
Immunologic category	*μL*	*(%)*	*μL*	*(%)*	*μL*	*(%)*
1: No evidence of suppression	≥1,500	(≥25)	≥1,000	(≥25)	≥500	(≥25)
2: Evidence of moderate suppression	750–1,499	(15–24)	500–999	(15–24)	200–499	(15–24)
3: Severe suppression	<750	(<15)	<500	(<15)	<200	(<15)

Source: Data from endnote reference 7.

of these infections and/or conditions are found in the description of the clinical categories cited previously.[7,9]

In untreated children or children with advanced HIV disease or AIDS, conditions such as oral or esophageal candidiasis, diarrhea, severe bacterial infections, MAI, tuberculosis (both pulmonary and extrapulmonary), and encephalopathy can severely affect enteral intake and/or absorption of nutrients. Failure to thrive is a common issue in the untreated child, compounding the disease effects on the immune system.[7,9]

HIV treatment can also negatively impact the child's nutritional intake. Frequent doctor visits, blood draws, tests, and hospitalizations may result in emotional upset and decreased appetite. Medication regimens used to treat HIV infection and prophylactic medications used to prevent opportunistic infections may consist of several pills taken two to three times per day and may have gastrointestinal side effects such as nausea, vomiting, indigestion, and diarrhea. Some of the more severe medication side effects that can severely compromise intake include anemia, pancreatitis, and liver steatosis.[9]

MEDICATIONS

Highly active antiretroviral therapy (HAART) is the hallmark of current treatment for HIV infection. HAART consists minimally of a three-drug regimen utilizing drugs from two different HIV drug classes. As of January 2004, there were 20 drugs available for treatment of HIV infection, although only 12 had approved pediatric indications. Antiretroviral drug classes include four major categories:[9]

1. nucleoside analogue or nucleotide reverse transcriptase inhibitors (NRTIs/NtRTIs)
2. nonnucleoside reverse transcriptase inhibitors (NNRTIs)
3. protease inhibitors (PIs)
4. fusion inhibitors

These drugs work on specific areas of the cell targeted by HIV and must be taken consistently and in combination to be effective. Efficacy of drug therapies is measured by clinical assessment, rebound, and/or maintenance of the CD4+ lymphocyte counts, and on the amount of HIV virus in the blood, commonly referred to as viral load. Effective medication therapy decreases the patient's viral load, allowing the CD4 cell counts to increase and be maintained. Common drug combinations include a protease inhibitor and two drugs from the NRTI class or an NNRTI and two drugs from the NRTI class. All of the drugs have significant side effects (see Table 21–3). Many are available in liquid and tablet/capsule

Table 21–3 Antiretrovirals and Common Side Effects*

Class	*Drug/Formulation*	*Side Effects*
NRTI	**zidovudine** (ZDV/AZT) capsule/liquid	Anemia, granulocytopenia
	didanosine (ddI) tablet/liquid	Peripheral neuropathy
	lamivudine (3TC) tablet/liquid	Pancreatitis, peripheral neuropathy
	stavudine (d4T) capsule/liquid	Pancreatitis, peripheral neuropathy
	zalcitabine (ddC) tablet	Pancreatitis, peripheral neuropathy
	abacavir (ABC) tablet/liquid	Potentially lethal hypersensitivity reaction
	emtricitabine (FTC) capsule	Pancreatitis, lactic acidosis, hepatic steatosis
NtRTI	**tenofovir disoproxil fumerate** tablet	Pancreatitis, lactic acidosis, hepatic steatosis
NNRTI	**nevirapine** tablet/liquid	Skin rash
	efavirenz capsule/liquid	Skin rash, central nervous system effects
	delavirdine tablet	Skin rash
PI	**nelfinavir** tablet/powder	Diarrhea
	ritonavir soft gel capsule/liquid	Severe GI upset, lipid abnormalities
	amprenavir soft gel capsule/liquid	Parasthesias, lipid abnormalities, rash
	lopinavir/ritonavir soft gel capsule/liquid	Fat redistribution, lipid abnormalities
	indinavir soft gel capsule	Nephrolithiasis, fat redistribution
	saquinavir soft gel capsule	Fat redistribution, lipid abnormalities
	atazanavir soft gel capsule	Elevation of indirect bili, prolongation of PR interval (EKG changes)
	fosamprenavir soft gel capsule/liquid	Parasthesias, rash
Fusion Inhibitor	**enfuvirtide** (T-20) injection	Local injection site reaction

Source: Data adapted from endnote reference 9.

*This list highlights the most common side effects of specific drugs and is not exhaustive. Please review drug side effects with a pharmacist and seek written documentation from the drug manufacturer.

formulation. The fusion inhibitors are injectable only. Rarely, patients may be on suboptimal therapy such as one or two drugs from the same class. This can be seen with patients with medication-related side effects or with poor adherence while medical, behavioral, psychiatric, and/or psychosocial interventions can be instituted. Monotherapy (the use of one drug) is utilized with neonates. Zidovudine (AZT/ZDV) is administered to a mother during labor and delivery and then to the neonate for 6 weeks to decrease the risk of perinatal transmission.

In addition to HAART, the pediatric patient may be taking medications regularly for prophylaxis or prevention of opportunistic infections. Many of the drugs used to treat HIV and prevent opportunistic infection have significant side effects and interactions. Foods, herbal treatments, and home remedies can significantly affect drug levels, leading to suboptimal drug levels or severe side effects. Although little research exists regarding pediatric HIV and the use of herbal treatments, thorough assessment of nutritional adjuncts is essential to optimize medical therapy.

NUTRITIONAL IMPLICATIONS

The growth and cellular immune function of HIV-infected children is impacted by their nutritional state. The majority of children infected with HIV will experience nutritional deficits during the course of their illness.[10] Pre-HAART nutritional issues affecting growth deficits and malnutrition include impaired absorption,[11] decreased dietary intake,[12] increased nutrient requirements, and the disease itself (see Table 21–4). Malnutrition has a deleterious effect on immune function, compromising the ability to produce effective antibodies; thus, it increases risks of life-threatening infections.[13]

In the current era of HIV and HAART, children in developed countries are living longer with fewer opportunistic infections. When seen, malnutrition is more likely associated with drug-resistant virus, noncompliance with therapy, and/or end-stage viral disease. Nutritional issues have become further complicated by potent drug therapies and possibly by the consequences of living longer with the disease itself. Some of the clinical and metabolic complications seen in adult HIV populations are now being seen in children. These include body fat redistribution, altered serum lipid levels, insulin resistance, and decreased bone mineral density.

GROWTH AND BODY COMPOSITION

Research results have demonstrated a variety of growth patterns in HIV-infected children, reflecting a broad spectrum of clinical course and disease activity. A large study in the United States reported that both HIV-positive and -negative children born to HIV-infected mothers are small at birth.[13] No significant differences in birth weights and lengths between HIV-infected and noninfected children born to these infected mothers were identified.[14] However, in this and a similar European study infancy[14] and childhood[15] weights and heights were significantly lower in the HIV-infected group and these differences persisted and increased with age. Several other studies of HIV-positive children reflect disturbed growth patterns including acute wasting, slow weight gain, and chronic slow linear growth.[12,16]

Table 21–4 Causes of Malnutrition

1. Decreased Intake
   (etiology: nausea, anorexia, oral ulceration, esophagitis, chewing difficulties, pain, dementia, depression)
2. Increased Losses
   (etiology: lactose intolerance, pancreatic insufficiency, malabsorption)
3. Increased Requirements
   (etiology: fever, opportunistic infections, metabolic abnormalities)
4. Psychosocial Barriers
   (etiology: inadequate access to food, unsafe food practices, caretaker substance abuse)

Growth is defined as an important possible prognostic indicator for children with HIV.[17–19] In particular, height velocity is an independent predictor of survival when controlling for age, viral load, and CD4+ count.[19] With this in mind, maintenance of normal growth is taking on increased importance. Because children with HIV are living longer, studies have looked at antiretroviral therapy and its effects on growth. This data requires careful consideration. Each study examines different patient populations with different drug treatment experience and various stages of the disease. For example, children receiving PI-containing regimens experienced a wide spectrum of effect on growth ranging from weight gain,[20] improved height,[21] significantly improved height,[22] and small improvement in weight and height[23,24] to decline in weight and height.[25] Despite this wide range of findings, collectively these studies show a trend toward improved growth on PI-containing regimens. Virologic response to HAART may be a key factor to positive effect on weight and height.[26]

Lipodystrophy syndrome in HIV-positive adults is characterized by several changes in body composition. Classifications of lipodystrophy include lipoatrophy or arm, leg, buttock, and/or facial wasting; lipohypertrophy or truncal obesity; or mixed lipodystrophy including a combination of peripheral wasting and truncal obesity. In addition, affected individuals may exhibit metabolic complications including hypercholesterolemia, hyperlipidemia, and/or insulin resistance. Many, but not all, of these features have recently been described in children[27–32] using various methods of diagnosis including XA (dual X-ray absorptometry), MRI,[28] and clinical assessment.[27] Although the causes of these abnormalities are not entirely clear, they seem to be at least in part due to drug therapies, particularly those containing PIs. Development of symptoms may be related to duration of HAART therapy[28] and increasing doses of medications.[27] Chemical abnormalities including high cholesterol and triglycerides have been described in children with or without clinical features of lipodystrophy[31] and thus serial anthropometry, clinical assessment, and laboratory values can provide valuable information about a child trending toward lipodystrophy.

BONE DENSITY

HIV-infected adults have increased rates of osteoporosis and osteopenia that may also be a side effect of HAART therapy. Lower bone mineral densities have also been found in HIV-positive children compared to healthy age matched controls;[33–35] however, the relationship to drug therapy is still unclear. One study showed significantly lower bone mineral density among children on HAART with lipodystrophy compared to untreated HIV-positive children. A third group of HAART-treated children without lipodystrophy fell somewhere in between these two groups.[33] In contrast, others found that length of time on antiretroviral therapy and PI use were not significant factors in differences in BMD between HIV-positive children and healthy controls.[34] Bone mineral density is best measured by DXA; however, it is too expensive and not widely available for routine use. Given the existing data just highlighted and the crucial time during childhood of laying down the majority of bone mass, thoughtful consideration should be given to dietary prevention of osteopenia and osteoporosis.

CALORIC REQUIREMENTS

Caloric requirements of HIV-infected children are not completely known. Although children with HIV were once thought to have an increased resting metabolic rate caused by viral infection, subsequent research suggests that clinically stable children have normal caloric needs.[36] Despite this fact, the benefit of caloric intake beyond the RDA has been demonstrated. In a group of HIV-positive children consuming at least the RDA for calories,[12] children with normal growth patterns were shown to take in significantly more calories than those with poor growth. The resting energy expenditure (REE) and total energy expenditure (TEE) of both of these groups was similar.[12] Supplemental gastrostomy tube feeding restores weight gain but not subsequent height and lean body mass gains.[37,38] Therefore, lower caloric intake among growth failure/HIV-positive children is suggested as only one piece of the puzzle.[12] Weight loss in HIV-positive children can be linked to inadequate intake, increased requirements imposed by opportunistic infections, or malabsorptive losses.[39] Caloric requirements should be calculated according to additional needs subsequent to stress, fever, increased respiratory needs, and careful monitoring of serial growth measures.

NUTRITIONAL INTERVENTION

The most appropriate nutrition plan for HIV-infected children is tailored to their clinical manifestations, growth, dietary history, gastrointestinal function, and social situation (Table 21–5). The child's caretakers should receive ongoing education to optimize growth, ensure access to food, promote safe food handling, and accommodate any necessary dietary modifications. Because of the risk of micronutrient deficiency in the HIV-infected child, it is prudent to consider a complete multivitamin/mineral supplement that provides one to two times the dietary reference intakes (DRI).[40,41] Emerging data on risk of low bone mineral density suggests that attention should be given to ensure adequacy of calcium and vitamin D in the diet.

In the HIV-infected child with slow growth, prescribing a high-calorie, high-protein, nutrient-dense diet early on is indicated. If enhancement of the typical diet is not sufficient to promote

Table 21–5 Nutritional Evaluation and Management of the HIV-Infected Child

Nutritional Assessment

Dietary intake and nutrient analysis
- 24-hour diet recall or 3-day food diary
- Access to food
- Stability of home environment/caretakers

Anthropometry and body composition measurements
- Four-site skinfolds (if possible)
- Serial height (length), weight, and head circumference (until 36 mo)
  - z-scores (particularly with measurements <3 percentile)
  - BMI and BMI percentage

Biochemical evaluation
- Albumin, lipid profile (fasting, if possible), fasting glucose/insulin, iron, other vitamin/mineral levels as indicated by degree of malnutrition and malabsorption

Drug/Nutrient Interactions
- Amprenavir: Avoid excess vitamin E supplementation because it contains ~100 IU/pill

Nutritional Intervention

Diet modifications and education (based on growth, gastrointestinal function, lipid abnormalities)
- Nutrient dense with supplements as needed to optimize growth
- Lactose free (if evidence of diarrhea/malabsorption)
- High fiber or low fiber
- Heart healthy, balanced with adequate calories for growth

Food safety assessment and counseling

Vitamin and mineral supplementation
- Multivitamin:1 to 2 times RDA/DRI depending on diet
- Calcium and vitamin D supplement to achieve at least DRI

Tube feedings/total parenteral nutrition (when enteral diet alone fails)

---

desired growth, oral nutritional supplementation, including shakes and commercial formulas, should be considered. When oral measures alone cannot achieve the nutritional goals, enteral tube supplementation should be administered. Gastrostomy tubes are beneficial in providing both complete or supplemental feedings, as well as medication administration. Children with anorexia, neurological impairment, swallowing difficulty, or those taking a significant number of pills may benefit from a gastrostomy tube.

Nocturnal tube feedings are often preferred because they can allow the child to eat normally during the day without interrupting daily activities. Formula selection should be determined based on the child's need for any modification from a polymeric formula. This may include fiber-containing, lactose-free, or more elemental formulas for those patients with enteropathy. Studies show improvements in weight gain (primarily as increased fat mass) in response to the increased caloric provisions and suggest improvements in morbidity and mortality as a result of such nutritional rehabilitation.[38]

Total parenteral nutrition, despite its associated infection risks, may be warranted if hydration, electrolyte balance, or weight gain cannot be achieved through enteral means. Candidates for parenteral nutrition include children with intractable diarrhea with accompanying weight loss or severe recurrent or chronic pancreatic or biliary tract dysfunction.[10,38] For children experiencing oroesophageal ulcers, soreness, or inflammation, care should be given to selecting foods that are soft and nutrient dense, and not highly spiced or acidic. Drug side effects (see Table 21–3) may lead to anorexia, nausea/vomiting, epigastric distress, diarrhea, and/or glossitis and could result in a child's refusal to eat. Appetite stimulants such as megestrol acetate (Megace) increase oral intake in some anorectic children. Although Megace was associated with improvements in weight gain and increased fat mass, concurrent improvements in linear growth were not appreciated. In addition, weight-gain effects may not be sustained once the medication is discontinued.[42,43]

Dysphagia, developmental delay, and poor gross motor control secondary to neurologic complications associated with HIV may also contribute to poor intake. Neurologically impaired children should be closely monitored to ensure adequate intake and to prevent aspiration.

CONCLUSION

Optimal nutritional status has been associated with improvements in immune function and morbidity in the HIV-infected child. Close nutrition surveillance and intervention results in improved clinical outcome and quality of life. Malnutrition in HIV-infected children is a serious complication. Early and aggressive nutritional support is indicated in all children infected with HIV and should include nutrient-dense oral feedings and enteral and parenteral supplementation when necessary. Anthropometric and body composition changes should be serially monitored, and biochemical parameters should be assessed so that necessary nutrition intervention can occur. These measures can provide crucial information regarding tendency towards some of the complications seen with HIV and HAART therapy such as fat redistribution, hyperlipidemias, and poor bone health. Ongoing research continues to augment the understanding of interrelationships between nutrition and HIV and will elucidate more definitive nutrition intervention strategies.

REFERENCES

1. Centers for Disease Control. Pneumocystis pneumonia—Los Angeles. *MMWR.* 1981;30:250–252.
2. Centers for Disease Control. HIV/AIDS—United States, 1981–2000. *MMWR.* 2001;50:430–433.
3. Centers for Disease Control. The global HIV/AIDS epidemic, 2001. *MMWR.* 2001;50.
4. Piot P, Bartos M, Ghys PD, Walker N, Schwartlander B. The global impact of HIV/AIDS. *Nature.* 2001;410:968–973.
5. Centers for Disease Control. Unexplained immunodeficiency and opportunistic infections in infants—New York, New Jersey, California. *MMWR.* 1982;31(49):665–667.
6. Weiss RA. Gulliver's travels in HIV land. *Nature.* 2001;410:963–967.
7. Centers for Disease Control. Revised classification system for human immunodeficiency virus infection in children less than 13 years of age. *MMWR.* 1994;43.
8. Centers for Disease Control. U.S. public health service task force recommendations for use of antiretroviral drugs in pregnant HIV-1 infected women for maternal health and interventions to reduce perinatal HIV-1 transmission in the United States. *MMWR.* 2002;51:1–38.
9. Working Group on Antiretroviral Therapy and Medical Management of HIV-Infected Children. Guidelines for the use of antiretroviral agents in pediatric HIV infection. *AIDSinfo.nih.gov.* 2004:1–79.
10. Miller TL. Nutritional aspects of pediatric HIV infection. In: Walker, Watkins, ed., *Nutrition in Pediatrics,* 2nd ed. Hamilton, Ontario Canada: B. Dekker; 1996:534–550.
11. Miller TL, Orav EJ, Martin SR, Cooper ER, McIntosh K, Winter HS. Malnutrition and carbohydrate malabsorption in children with vertically transmitted human immunodeficiency virus 1 infection. *Gastroenterology.* 1991;100:1296–1302.
12. Arpadi SM. Growth failure in children with HIV infection. *J Acquir Immune Defic Syndr.* 2000;25 Suppl 1:S37–42.
13. Chandra RK. Mucosal immune responses in malnutrition. *Ann NY Acad Sci.* 1983;409:345–352.
14. Miller TL, Easley KA, Zhang W, Orav EJ, Bier DM, Luder E, Ting A, Shearer WT, Vargas JH, Lipshultz SE. Maternal and infant factors associated with failure to thrive in children with vertically transmitted human immunodeficiency virus-1 infection: The prospective, P2C2 human immunodeficiency virus multicenter study. *Pediatrics.* 2001;108:1287–1296.
15. Newell ML, Borja MC, Peckham C. Height, weight, and growth in children born to mothers with HIV-1 infection in Europe. *Pediatrics.* 2003;111:E52–60.
16. Hilgartner MW, Donfield SM, Lynn HS, Hoots WK, Gomperts ED, Daar ES, Chernoff D, Pearson SK. The effect of plasma human immunodeficiency virus RNA and CD4(+) T lymphocytes on growth measurements of hemophilic boys and adolescents. *Pediatrics.* 2001;107:E56.
17. Benjamin DK Jr, Miller WC, Benjamin DK, Ryder RW, Weber DJ, Walter E, McKinney RE. A comparison of height and weight velocity as a part of the composite endpoint in pediatric HIV. *AIDS.* 2003;17:2331–2336.

18. Carey VJ, Yong FH, Frenkel LM, McKinney RE Jr. Pediatric AIDS prognosis using somatic growth velocity. *AIDS.* 1998;12:1361–1369.

19. Chantry CJ, Byrd RS, Englund JA, Baker CJ, McKinney RE Jr. Growth, survival and viral load in symptomatic childhood human immunodeficiency virus infection. *Pediatr Infect Dis J.* 2003;22:1033–1039.

20. Wintergerst U, Hoffmann F, Solder B, Notheis G, Petropoulou T, Eberle J, Gurtler L, Belohradsky BH. Comparison of two antiretroviral triple combinations including the protease inhibitor indinavir in children infected with human immunodeficiency virus. *Pediatr Infect Dis J.* 1998;17:495–499.

21. Fiore P, Donelli E, Boni S, Pontali E, Tramalloni R, Bassetti D. Nutritional status changes in HIV-infected children receiving combined antiretroviral therapy including protease inhibitors. *Int J Antimicrob Agents.* 2000;16:365–369.

22. Dreimane D, Nielsen K, Deveikis A, Bryson YJ, Geffner ME. Effect of protease inhibitors combined with standard antiretroviral therapy on linear growth and weight gain in human immunodeficiency virus type 1-infected children. *Pediatr Infect Dis J.* 2001;20:315–316.

23. Buchacz K, Cervia JS, Lindsey JC, Hughes MD, Seage GR III, Dankner WM, Oleske JM, Moye J. Impact of protease inhibitor-containing combination antiretroviral therapies on height and weight growth in HIV-infected children. *Pediatrics.* 2001;108:E72.

24. Miller TL, Mawn BE, Orav EJ, Wilk D, Weinberg GA, Nicchitta J, Furuta L, Cutroni R, McIntosh K, Burchett SK, Gorbach SL. The effect of protease inhibitor therapy on growth and body composition in human immunodeficiency virus type 1-infected children. *Pediatrics.* 2001; 107:E77.

25. Nachman SA, Lindsey JC, Pelton S, Mofenson L, McIntosh K, Wiznia A, Stanley K, Yogev R. Growth in human immunodeficiency virus-infected children receiving ritonavir-containing antiretroviral therapy. *Arch Pediatr Adolesc Med.* 2002;156:497–503.

26. Verweel G, van Rossum AM, Hartwig NG, Wolfs TF, Scherpbier HJ, de Groot R. Treatment with highly active antiretroviral therapy in human immunodeficiency virus type 1-infected children is associated with a sustained effect on growth. *Pediatrics.* 2002;109:E25.

27. Amaya RA, Kozinetz CA, McMeans A, Schwarzwald H, Kline MW. Lipodystrophy syndrome in human immunodeficiency virus-infected children. *Pediatr Infect Dis J.* 2002;21:405–410.

28. Vigano A, Mora S, Testolin C, Beccio S, Schneider L, Bricalli D, Vanzulli A, Manzoni P, Brambilla P. Increased lipodystrophy is associated with increased exposure to highly active antiretroviral therapy in HIV-infected children. *J Acquir Immune Defic Syndr.* 2003;32:482–489.

29. Arpadi SM, Cuff PA, Horlick M, Wang J, Kotler DP. Lipodystrophy in HIV-infected children is associated with high viral load and low CD4+-lymphocyte count and CD4+-lymphocyte percentage at baseline and use of protease inhibitors and stavudine. *J Acquir Immune Defic Syndr.* 2001;27:30–34.

30. Lainka E, Oezbek S, Falck M, Ndagijimana J, Niehues T. Marked dyslipidemia in human immunodeficiency virus-infected children on protease inhibitor-containing antiretroviral therapy. *Pediatrics.* 2002;110:E56.

31. Jaquet D, Levine M, Ortega-Rodriguez E, Faye A, Polak M, Vilmer E, Levy-Marchal C. Clinical and metabolic presentation of the lipodystrophic syndrome in HIV-infected children. *AIDS.* 2000;14:2123–2128.

32. Beregszaszi M, Jaquet D, Levine M, Ortega-Rodriguez E, Baltakse V, Polak M, Levy-Marchal C. Severe insulin resistance contrasting with mild anthropometric changes in the adipose tissue of HIV-infected children with lipohypertrophy. *Int J Obes Relat Metab Disord.* 2003;27:25–30.

33. Mora S, Sala N, Bricalli D, Zuin G, Chiumello G, Vigano A. Bone mineral loss through increased bone turnover in HIV-infected children treated with highly active antiretroviral therapy. *AIDS.* 2001;15:1823–1829.

34. Arpadi SM, Horlick M, Thornton J, Cuff PA, Wang J, Kotler DP. Bone mineral content is lower in prepubertal HIV-infected children. *J Acquir Immune Defic Syndr.* 2002;29:450–454.

35. O'Brien KO, Razavi M, Henderson RA, Caballero B, Ellis KJ. Bone mineral content in girls perinatally infected with HIV. *Am J Clin Nutr.* 2001;73:821–826.

36. Alfaro MP, Siegel RM, Baker RC, Heubi JE. Resting energy expenditure and body composition in pediatric HIV infection. *Pediatr AIDS HIV Infect.* 1995;6:276–280.

37. Henderson RA. Effect of enteral tube feeding on growth of children with symptomatic human immunodeficiency virus infection. *J Pediatr Gastroenterol Nutr.* 1994; 18:429–434.

38. Miller TL, Awnetwant EL, Evans S, Morris VM, Vazquez IM, McIntosh K. Gastrostomy tube supplementation for HIV-infected children. *Pediatrics.* 1995;96:696–702.

39. Coodley GO, Loveless MO, Merrill TM. The HIV wasting syndrome: A review. *J Acquir Immune Defic Syndr.* 1994;7:681–694.

40. Heller LS, Shattuck D. Nutrition support for children with HIV/AIDS. *J Am Diet Assoc.* 1997;97:473–474.

41. Galvin T. Micronutrients: Implications in human immunodeficiency virus disease. *Top Clin Nutr.* 1992;7:63–73.

42. Clarick RH, Hanekom WA, Yogev R, Chadwick EG. Megestrol acetate treatment of growth failure in children infected with human immunodeficiency virus. *Pediatrics.* 1997;99:354–357.

43. Antiretroviral therapy and medical management of pediatric HIV infection and 1997 USPHS/IDSA report on the prevention of opportunistic infrections in persons infected with human immunodeficiency virus. *Pediatrics.* 1998;99:354–357.

CHAPTER 22

Oncology and Hematopoietic Cell Transplantation

Karen V. Barale and Paula M. Charuhas

Childhood cancer is the most common cause of death from disease in children between the ages of 1 and 14 years of age.[1] The incidence of malignancies in children under the age of 15 is 14.1 per 100,000 among whites and 11.8 per 100,000 among blacks.[2–4] Table 22–1 lists common childhood tumors with their standard treatment. Leukemias and cancer of the brain and other nervous systems account for more than half of the cancers among children. Prognosis depends upon tumor histology and stage, age of patient, and certain laboratory indexes.[5] Treatment may include chemotherapy, surgery, radiation therapy, and hematopoietic cell transplantation (HCT). In many instances, initial treatment is curative because of excellent response to multimodal therapy. The overall cure rate now exceeds 70% and is projected to reach 85% by the year 2010.[6] Advances in nutrition support have paralleled improvements in treatment, making optimum care of these patients possible. Pediatric nutrition support goals in oncology are to prevent or reverse nutritional deficits, promote normal growth and development, minimize morbidity and mortality, and maximize quality of life.[7,8] The disease, its therapy, and any complications will affect the nutritional status of the child.

NUTRITIONAL EFFECTS OF CANCER

Protein-Energy Malnutrition

Protein-energy malnutrition (PEM) is a common secondary diagnosis in pediatric patients with cancer.[7] At diagnosis, the incidence ranges from 6% in children with newly diagnosed leukemia to as high as 50% in children with stage IV neuroblastoma.[9] Patients with advanced disease during initial intense treatment and those who relapse or do not respond to treatment are most likely to develop PEM.[10,11] Additionally, certain types of treatment promote the development of PEM: major abdominal surgery; radiation of the head, neck, esophagus, abdomen, or pelvis; or intense, frequent courses of chemotherapy (3-week intervals or less).[12] Complications such as pain, fever, and frequent or severe infections decrease appetite and may increase energy requirements.

PEM ultimately results from decreased energy intake, increased energy requirements, and malabsorption.[9] Organ systems most readily affected by PEM (hematopoietic, gastrointestinal [GI], and immunological) are also the most sensitive to oncologic treatment. Malnutrition in these children leads to intolerance of chemotherapy and radiotherapy as well as increased local and systemic infections.[13] Thus, the prevention or reversal of PEM to maximize the function of these organ systems seems prudent in childhood cancer.[9]

Cachexia

Cancer cachexia is a poorly understood syndrome that includes tissue wasting, anorexia, weakness, anemia, hypoalbuminemia, hypoglycemia, lactic acidosis, hyperlipidemia, impaired liver function, glucose intolerance, accelerated

Table 22–1 Cancers in Childhood

Malignancy	*% of Cases*	*Standard Treatment*	*Comment*
Hematologic			
Leukemia	42.8		
Acute lymphoblastic leukemia (ALL)		Induction chemo Consolidation chemo CNS prophylaxis (RT or IT chemo) Oral maintenance chemo with intermittent IV Rx lasts about 3 years HCT for persistent relapse or second remission	65–70% 5-year disease-free survival
Acute nonlymphoblastic leukemia (ANL)		Remission induction with intensive chemo Continuation therapy up to 18 mo CNS prophylaxis HCT for persistent relapse or first remission	30–50% 3-year continuous complete remission
Chronic myelocytic leukemia (CML)		Chronic phase: oral chemo for symptomatic relief, HCT Length of Rx based on symptoms & phase Blast crisis: aggressive chemo, HCT Oral chemo	<5% incidence in children Blast crisis <20% survival Usually diagnosed before 2 years of age
Juvenile chronic myelocytic leukemia (JCML)		HCT	Median survival <9 mo
Hodgkin's disease and lymphoma	11.3		
Hodgkin's disease			
Stages I–IV, with involvement ranging from single node region to diffuse or disseminated involvement to extralymphatic organs		Chemo vs. RT controversial for all stages; multimodal therapy often used HCT for failure to achieve remission or relapse	In children <10 years, male incidence higher Chemo has the advantage of avoiding high-dose radiation to the growing spine 70–96% survival

Nonlymphoblastic lymphoma		Chemo with/without RT for 6–18 mo	Therapy depends on extent of disease Cure rate 10—40% with bone marrow involvement; to 90% with limited disease
Lymphoblastic lymphoma		Aggressive chemo, autologous or allogeneic HCT during early remission, plus whole-brain RT, IT chemo	Adverse prognostic factors: extensive marrow or CNS involvement
Brain tumors Astrocytoma (most prevalent) Medulloblastoma Brain stem glioma Ependymomas	20.7	Surgical removal/debulking Chemo and RT	Survival based on tumor type & location 5-year survival 15–70% Brain stem gliomas lead to CNS dysfunction and swallowing problems Can have cranial nerve palsies or paresis
Neuroblastoma Stages I–IV, wth involvement ranging from localized disease to metastatic disease	7.3	Surgical resection of local disease Palliative RT to shrink tumor size Chemo HCT, allogeneic or autologous, for advanced disease	2 years = median age at diagnosis 50–90% survival, depending on stage & location Most common primary site is adrenal gland, which produces an abdominal mass, metastatic disease Most common extracranial solid tumor in childhood; comprises up to 50% of malignancies in infants
Wilms' tumor Stages I–IV, with involvement ranging from well-encapsulated tumor to bilateral disease and metastases	6.1	All stages: Surgery for staging and tumor removal Chemo—preferred therapy Metastatic disease to bone, liver, or lung: RT	Usually seen between ages 1 and 5 years 59–90% survival, stages I–III Survival dependent on stage at presentation

continues

Table 22–1 continued

Malignancy	*% of Cases*	*Standard Treatment*	*Comment*
Bone tumors Rhabdomyosarcoma Stages I–IV, with involvement ranging from localized disease to distant metastasis	6.0	Surgery—total excision if possible Chemo RT 5000—6000 cGy to primary tumor with wide ports	Most common soft tissue sarcoma in children 28–71% survival, depending on stage
Osteogenic sarcoma		Surgery: Amputation or limb salvage Chemo to prevent metastasis	Resistant to RT Common sites: Around knee joint and below shoulder Primary malignant tumor of bone Peak incidence during adolescent growing spurt 60% survival
Ewing's sarcoma	2.1	RT, based on site and leg length growth: If length discrepancy won't be excessive, 6000–7000 cGy; if it will be excessive, amputation and chemo or salvage procedures	Males predominate 2:1 Peak age of incidence: 11–12 years, female; 15–16 years, male Small-cell bone tumor 2-year disease-free survival 70%
Retinoblastoma Stages I–V, based on number and size of lesions	2.9	Surgery RT Chemo for advanced disease	90% <5 years of age; average age is 18 mo Increased risk for other sarcoma, secondary to therapy 90% survival

Note: HCT, Hematopoietic cell transplant; chemo, chemotherapy, CNS, central nervous system; IV, intravenous; IT, intrathecal; RT, radiation therapy; Rx, treatment.

Source: Data from endnote references 1–5.

gluconeogenesis, skeletal muscle atrophy, visceral organ atrophy, and anergy.[10,13] It produces a metabolic environment that prevents the appropriate use of nutrients.[14] Some studies are looking at the possibility of anti-inflammatory agents such as fish oil in combination with nutritional supplementation to reverse aspects of cachexia.[15] This syndrome is a major source of morbidity for young cancer patients.[16] Children with progressive and metastatic disease have an incidence of cachexia as high as 40%.[17]

NUTRITIONAL EFFECTS OF CANCER THERAPY

Multimodal treatments can have an additional adverse effect on nutritional status.[8] Antitumor therapies may produce only mild, transient nutritional disturbances or may lead to severe, permanent problems.

Chemotherapy

The nutritional consequences of chemotherapeutic agents are shown in Table 22–2. These drugs affect normal as well as malignant cells, targeting rapidly dividing cells such as the epithelial cells of the GI tract. The degree to which GI function is altered depends on the particular drug, dosage, duration of the treatment, rate of metabolism, and the child's susceptibility.

Nausea and vomiting are the most common problems interfering with adequate oral intake.[18] These symptoms occur as a result of a direct central nervous system effect as drugs are administered. Complications of chemotherapy-induced emesis include weight loss, dehydration, fluid and electrolyte imbalances, and metabolic alkalosis.[19] Management of chemotherapy-induced nausea and vomiting includes the judicious use of antiemetics. Single agent or combination antiemetics are frequently used and can decrease the child's discomfort. Antiemetics such as ondansetron and diphenhydramine assist in controlling symptoms of nausea and vomiting. Nonpharmacologic interventions such as music therapy, hypnosis, and muscle relaxation have also been described as effective techniques of treating nausea and vomiting.[20]

Alterations in taste and smell as a result of chemotherapy may persist well beyond periods of nausea and vomiting and result in prolonged anorexia.[21] In addition, children may develop food aversions that can limit intake.

Mucositis is a major GI complication and is usually intensified by concurrent radiation therapy.[22] Mucositis may affect any part of the GI tract and lead to ulceration, bleeding, and malabsorption. Chemotherapy-induced neutropenia accentuates these complications. Rigorous mouth care prevents additional oral breakdown.[9] Fortunately, the renewal rate of the GI tract mucosa is rapid, so that mucositis from chemotherapy is usually short-lived.

Certain chemotherapy and antibiotic agents cause malabsorption and alterations in the gut flora, with associated weight loss and intractable diarrhea.[9,23] Constipation related to use of vincristine or narcotics or inactivity may result in significant abdominal discomfort and loss of appetite.

Surgery

Surgical removal of a tumor may lead to insufficient oral intake over several days during a time of increased requirements. Depending on the surgical site, nutrient intake and absorption may be significant. Radical surgery of the head and neck can result in chewing and swallowing problems. Massive intestinal resection may cause malabsorption of vitamins and fat, as well as fluid and electrolyte imbalance.[23]

Radiation

Complications of radiation (see Table 22–3) may develop acutely or become chronic and progress after completion of therapy.[24] Side effects and their intensity vary according to[24]

1. the region of the body irradiated
2. dose, fractionation, length of time, and field size of the radiation administered

Table 22–2 Chemotherapeutic Agents and Toxicities Affecting Nutritional Status

Drug	*Synonyms*	*Antitumor Spectrum*	*Toxicities*
Alkylating agents			
Cyclophosphamide	Cytoxan, CTX	Lymphomas, leukemias, sarcomas, neuroblastoma	N&V, cystitis, water retention; cardiac (HD)
Ifosfamide	IFOS, IFEX	Sarcomas, germ cell	N&V, cystitis, NT, renal
Cisplatin	Platinol, CDDP	Testicular and other germ cell, osteosarcoma, brain tumors, neuroblastoma	N&V, renal, NT
Busulfan	Myleran	Leukemia (CML) Used in conditioning regimens for HCT	N&V, mucositis, NT, hepatic (HD); do not eat for 1 hr before or after taking medication
Dacarbazine	DTIC	Neuroblastoma, sarcomas	N&V, flulike syndrome, hepatic
Melphalan	Akeran, L-PAM	Rhabdomyosarcoma, sarcomas, neuroblastoma, and leukemias	N&V, mucositis and diarrhea (HD)
Mechlorethamine	Mustargen, HN_2, nitrogen mustard	Hodgkin's	N&V, mucositis; NT (HD)
Procarbazine	Matulan, PCZ	Hodgkin's, brain tumors	N&V, NT, rash, mucositis; low tyramine diet indicated
Lomustine	CCNU	Brain tumors, lymphomas, Hodgkin's	N&V, renal & pulmonary toxicity
Antimetabolites			
Methotrexate	MTX	Leukemia, lymphoma, osteosarcoma	Mucositis, rash, hepatic; renal NT (HD)
6-Mercaptopurine	Purinethal, 6-MP	Leukemia (ALL, CML)	Hepatic, mucositis
6-Thioguanine	6-TG	Leukemia (ANL)	N&V, mucositis, hepatic
Cytarabine	Cytosine arabinoside, Cytosar, Ara-C	Leukemia, lymphoma	N&V, mucositis, GI; NT, ocular, skin (HD)
Antibiotics			
Doxorubicin	Adriamycin, ADR	Leukemia (ALL, ANL), lymphoma, most solid tumors	Mucositis, N&V, cardiac (acute and chronic)
Daunomycin	Daunorubicin, DNR	Leukemia (ALL, ANL), lymphoma	Same as doxorubicin
Bleomycin	Blenoxane, BLEO	Lymphoma, testicular cancer	N&V, lung, skin, hypersensitivity; Raynaud's

Dactinomycin	Cosmegen, ACT-D, actinomycin D	Wilms' tumor, sarcomas	N&V, mucositis, hepatic
Plant alkaloids			
Vincristine	Oncovin, VCR	Leukemia (ALL), lymphomas, most solid tumors	NT, SIADH, hypotension
Vinblastine	Velban, VLB	Histiocytosis, Hodgkin's, testicular	Mucositis, mild NT
Etoposide	VePesid, VP-16, VP-16-213	Leukemias (ALL, ANL), lymphomas, neuroblastoma, sarcomas, brain tumors	N&V, mucositis, mild NT, hypotension
Miscellaneous			
Prednisone (po)	Deltasone, PRED	Leukemia, lymphoma	Increased appetite, centripetal obesity, myopathy, osteoporosis, aseptic necrosis of hip, peptic ulceration, pancreatitis, hyperactivity, hypertension, diabetes, growth failure, amenorrhea, impaired wound healing, atrophy of subcutaneous tissue
Prednisolone (IV)		Leukemia, lymphoma	
Dexamethasone	Decadron, DEX	Leukemia, lymphoma, brain tumors	
L-Asparaginase	Elspar, L-ASP	Leukemia (ALL), lymphoma	N&V, acute pancreatitis, decreased serum albumin, insulin, and lipoproteins

Note: ALL, acute lymphoblastic leukemia; ANL, acute nonlymphoblastic leukemia; CML, chronic myelogenous leukemia; GI, gastrointestinal toxicity; HD, high-dose; IV, intravenous; N&V, nausea and vomiting; NT, neurotoxicity.

Source: Adapted with permission from Balls FM, Holcenberg S, Poplack, DG. General principles of chemotherapy. In: Pizzo DH, Poplack DG, eds., *Principles and Practice of Pediatric Oncology,* © 1989, Lippincott Williams & Wilkins.

Table 22–3 Radiation Effects in Pediatric Patients

Head and neck
- Nausea, anorexia
- Mucositis, esophagitis
- Decreased taste and smell
- Damage to developing teeth
- Decreased salivation ⟶ thick, viscous mucus
- Decreased jaw mobility

Thoracic
- Pharyngeal and esophageal inflammation and cell damage
- Sore throat, dysphagia

Abdominal or pelvic
- Nausea, vomiting, diarrhea
- Ulceration
- Colitis
- Malabsorption
- Fluid, electrolyte imbalance

Total body
- Nausea, vomiting, diarrhea
- Mucositis, esophagitis
- Decreased taste and salivation
- Anorexia
- Delayed growth and development

Source: Data from endnote references 9, 10, and 24.

3. concurrent use of other antitumor therapy such as surgery or chemotherapy
4. the child's initial nutritional status

Hematopoietic Cell Transplantation

HCT has become an established treatment modality for certain pediatric disorders[25] (see Table 22–4). Children receiving an HCT are prepared with a conditioning regimen consisting of high doses of chemotherapy, with or without total body irradiation (TBI). The intense conditioning regimen is designed to eliminate active and residual malignant cells or a defective hematopoietic system to restore normal hematopoiesis and immunologic function.[26] An intravenous infusion of autologous (patient's own), syngeneic (identical twin), or allogeneic (from a histocompatible related or unrelated donor) stem cells follows conditioning. The source of the stem cells may be marrow, peripheral blood, or umbilical cord blood.

Posttransplant Course

Severe pancytopenia lasts from 2 to 6 weeks posttransplant. Children are at the greatest risk for bacterial and fungal infections until the stem cells engraft. During this period, supportive care including frequent red blood cell and platelet transfusions, systemic antibiotic therapy, and parenteral nutrition (PN) support are instituted.

Nutrition effects of HCT are due to conditioning therapy, infections, graft-versus-host disease (GVHD), and medications, including anti-infectious and immunosuppressive agents.[26] Complications interfering with nutrient intake include mucositis, esophagitis, altered taste, xerostomia, viscous saliva, nausea, vomiting, anorexia, diarrhea, steatorrhea, and multiple-organ dysfunction.[26] The duration and intensity of symptoms, as well as the stress of treatment, preclude oral intake for a minimum of 3 to 4 weeks posttransplant and necessitate the use of PN support.

Oral intake is encouraged as soon as tolerated. Calorie, protein, and fluid goals should be defined for each child. Some facilities restrict certain foods or require a modified diet during neutropenia.[27] Educating caregivers on safe food handling during immunosuppression is also important.

At hospital discharge, some children are still unable to eat an adequate amount of nutrients and partial PN and/or enteral tube feeding may be prescribed. Although enteral feedings are not commonly used in the immediate posttransplant period, they may be an option for children with chronic food aversions and long-term anorexia posttransplant. Supplemental intravenous hydration may also be necessary. Follow-up nutrition counseling and assessment are imperative throughout the child's posttransplant course to ensure provision of adequate nutrition support.

Table 22–4 Conditions for Application of Hematopoietic Cell Transplantation in the Pediatric Population

Hematologic Malignancies
Acute leukemia
Chronic leukemia
Recurrent lymphomas
Myelodysplastic syndrome
Malignant Solid Tumors
Advanced-stage neuroblastoma
Refractory Ewing's sarcoma
Immunodeficiency Disorders
Severe combined immunodeficiency disease
Wiskott-Aldrich syndrome
Other cellular immunodeficiencies
Nonneoplastic Disorders
Severe aplastic anemia
Thalassemia major
Fanconi's anemia
Diamond-Blackfan syndrome
Sickle cell disease
Paroxysmal nocturnal hemoglobinuria
Shwachman-Diamond syndrome
Lysosomal storage diseases (i.e., Gaucher's disease; Niemann-Pick syndrome; metachromatic leukodystrophy)
Mucopolysaccharidoses (i.e., Hurler's disease; Hunter's disease)
Infantile osteopetrosis

Source: Data from endnote reference 25.

Graft-Versus-Host Disease

Children who receive allogeneic transplants are at risk for the development of graft-versus-host disease (GVHD) following engraftment. GVHD is an immunologic reaction in which the newly engrafted stem cells react against the host's tissue antigens. The ensuing immunologic response can cause multiple-organ damage.[28] GVHD may occur as an acute reaction early posttransplant or progress to a chronic condition. Because of its potentially devastating effects, efforts are directed at prevention of GVHD. Medications and therapy used for prophylaxis and treatment of GVHD[29] are shown in Table 22–5.

Acute GVHD can affect the skin, liver, or GI tract. Clinical symptoms include a maculopapular rash, cholestatic liver dysfunction, or nausea, vomiting, diarrhea. Intestinal GVHD can involve either the upper or lower GI tract.[28] Upper intestinal GVHD symptoms include early satiety, anorexia, nausea, and vomiting. In lower intestinal GVHD, diarrhea may be severe and, at its worst, associated with crampy abdominal pain and bleeding. Children with severe disease often require a period of bowel rest with PN support. Refeeding guidelines[30] include slow diet progression and feeding one new food at a time, as illustrated in Table 22–6.

NUTRITION ASSESSMENT

Nutritional status at diagnosis has been associated with treatment outcome in children with cancer.[31–34] Nutrition assessment should begin at diagnosis and continue through and following treatment.[7,35] Techniques for the newly diagnosed patient do not differ from normal assessment recommendations as presented in Chapter 2. Table 22–7 provides guidelines for ongoing assessment in the pediatric cancer patient.

Anthropometry

Initial measurements should include age, height (recumbent length in children less than 2 years of age), weight, and, in children younger than 3 years of age, head circumference (see growth charts, Appendix A). Any measurement below the 10th percentile should be investigated as a sign of growth impairment due to inadequate nutrition. Weight-height percentile is believed to be the most reliable anthropometric indicator of nutritional status in the child with cancer.[7,10,12] It can be used to reliably predict nutritional status because of its high direct correlation with triceps skinfold and mid-arm muscle circumference measurements. In the pediatric cancer patient, current or previous chemoradiotherapy may depress growth. Catch-up growth has been observed in these patients.[36] However, patients who receive cranial irradiation may develop long-

Table 22-5 Therapies Used for Prophylaxis and Treatment of GVHD

Therapy	*Nutritional Implications*
Antithymocyte Globulin	Nausea and vomiting; diarrhea; stomatitis
Azathioprine	Nausea and vomiting; anorexia, diarrhea; mucosal ulceration; esophagitis; steatorrhea
Beclomethasone Dipropionate	Xerostomia; dysgeusia; nausea
Budesonide	None known
Corticosteroids	Sodium and fluid retention resulting in weight gain or hypertension; hyperphagia; weight gain; hypokalemia; skeletal muscle catabolism and atrophy; gastric irritation and peptic ulceration; osteoporosis; growth retardation in children; decreased insulin sensitivity and impaired glucose tolerance hyperglycemia or steroid-induced diabetes; hypertriglyceridemia
Cyclosporine	Nausea and vomiting; renal insufficiency; magnesium wasting; potassium wasting
Extra Corporeal Photopheresis	IV fluid may be necessary to maintain adequate hydration status; monitor calcium status if citrate anticoagulant is used as it may bind calcium and induce hypocalcemia
Methotrexate	Nausea and vomiting (mild to moderate); anorexia; mucositis and esophagitis; diarrhea; renal and hepatic changes; decreased absorption of vitamin B12, fat, and D-xylose; hepatic fibrosis; change in taste acuity
Methoxsalen (in conjunction with Psoralen + Ultraviolet A Light)	Nausea; hepatotoxicity
Monoclonal Antibodies	Nausea and vomiting
Mycophenolate Mofetil	Nausea and vomiting; diarrhea
Sirolimus	Hypertriglyceridemia
Tacrolimus	Nephrotoxicity; hyperglycemia; hyperkalemia; hypomagnesemia
Thalidomide	Constipation; nausea; xerostomia
Ursodeoxycholic acid	Nausea and vomiting; diarrhea; dyspepsia

Source: Data from endnote reference 29. Used with permission.

Table 22–6 Gastrointestinal GVHD Diet Progression

Phase	*Clinical Symptoms*	*Diet*	*Nutrition Support*
1. Bowel rest	GI cramping Large volume watery diarrhea or active GI bleeding Depressed serum albumin Severely reduced transit time Small bowel obstruction or diminished bowel sounds Nausea and vomiting	Oral: NPO	TPN with supplemental zinc and possibly copper
2. Introduction of oral feeding	Minimal GI cramping Diarrhea less than 500 mL/day Guaiac-negative stools Improved transit time (minimum 1.5 hours) Infrequent nausea and vomiting	Oral: isosmotic, low-residue, low-lactose beverages, initially 60 mL every 2 to 3 hours, for several days	TPN Trophic enteral feeds of semielemental formula if patient unable to eat
3. Introduction of solids	Minimal or no GI cramping Formed stool	Oral: allow introduction of solid food, once every 3 to 4 hours: minimal lactose, low fiber, low fat (20 to 40 g/day), low total acidity, no gastric irritants	Begin to cycle and decrease TPN Advance feeds slowly (small boluses or continuous infusion) if patient unable to eat
4. Expansion of diet	Minimal or no GI cramping Formed stool	Oral: minimal lactose, low fiber, low total acidity, no gastric irritants; if stools indicate fat malabsorption: low fat	Nighttime supplemental TPN if oral intake less than needs or unable to maintain weight owing to malabsorption Enteral feed schedule and formula dependent on any residual GI symptoms

continues

Table 22–6 continued

Phase	*Clinical Symptoms*	*Diet*	*Nutrition Support*
5. Resumption of regular diet	No GI cramping Normal stool Normal transit time Normal albumin	Oral: progress to regular diet by introducing one restricted food per day: acid foods with meals, fiber-containing foods, lactose-containing foods; Order of addition will vary, depending on individual tolerances and preferences Patients no longer exhibiting steatorrhea should have the fat restriction liberalized slowly	Discontinue TPN Supplemental enteral feeds if patient unable to eat adequate nutrients

Source: Data from endnote reference 30.

term growth disturbances.[37] Growth velocity should be plotted yearly to detect deviations from normal growth patterns in children receiving long-term therapy or post-HCT.[29]

Evaluation of Nutrient Intake

For a thorough evaluation of intake, daily food intake records provide a basis for decisions regarding supplemental or nonvolitional feeding. Parenteral or enteral nutrient solutions, other intravenous fluids, and oral intake must all be included when evaluating intake. Patients and family members may assist with record keeping and provide valuable intake information.

Determination of feeding skills in the young child will facilitate choices for self-feeding. Many children's feeding skills will regress during acute illness.[38]

Biochemistry

The disease or treatment may affect laboratory data used for nutrition assessment. Hemoglobin and hematocrit values in children with leukemia, lymphoma, and Hodgkin's disease reflect the disease state rather than nutritional status.[7] Many chemotherapeutic agents cause bone marrow suppression and decreased total lymphocyte count. The complete blood count must also be interpreted cautiously in patients with solid tumors, because once therapy begins, complete blood counts primarily reflect treatment effects.

A concentration of serum albumin of less than 3 g/dl may reflect PEM; however, infection, excessive GI or renal losses, impaired liver function, certain chemotherapy agents, and overhydration can all depress serum albumin level. Furthermore, serum albumin level does not clearly reflect weight-height percentiles, calorie intake, or dietary protein intake in pediatric cancer patients.[39] Serial prealbumin may be a more effective measure; however, it is also altered by infection and fever.[12] Biochemical indices on visceral protein status, as well as renal and hepatic function, serum lipids, glucose, and electrolytes should be reviewed for detection of nutrient deficiencies.

Table 22–7 Ongoing Nutrition Assessment Measurements that Identify Real or Impending Nutritional Depletion in Children with Cancer

Measurements	*Risk Criteria and Interpretation*	*Comments*
Nutrient intakes		
Energy (kcal/kg)		
% of healthy children	<80% of median intake: low intake	Energy intakes calculated from records kept by trained parents or personnel and reviewed by a dietitian for completeness, explicitness, and use of acceptable measures. Adjust for emesis: emesis within half hour—do not include in calculations; emesis 1–2 hours after eating—calculate as half intake; emesis 3–4 hours later—calculate as all intake. Energy intakes >80% of medium intake may be low when diarrhea occurs.
Anthropometric		
Height		
Height for age	<5th percentile: growth stunting—may be due to chronic PEM*	
Weight		
% change	>5% loss: acute PEM (with adequate hydration state)	Percentage weight loss derived from highest previous weight. Weight is inaccurate when child has edema, large tumor masses and organs extensively infiltrated with tumor, effusions or organ congestion, solid mass, or excess fluid administration (twice maintenance) for chemotherapy.
Weight for age	<5th percentile: acute or chronic PEM	Weight losses of >2% a day suggest dehydration.
Weight for height	<5th percentile: acute PEM when height for age is <10th percentile	
Skinfold thickness measurements		Steroid therapy may increase fat deposition. Measurements are inaccurate when child has edema.
Triceps	<10th percentile: depleted body fat stores	
Subscapular	>0.3 mm decrease: subclinical PEM†	

continues

Table 22–7 continued

Measurements	*Risk Criteria and Interpretation*	*Comments*
Biochemical		
Albumin % change	<3.2 gm/dL;‡ acute or chronic PEM >10% decrease;§ subclinical PEM	Biological half-life of 14 days. May be decreased in presence of overhydration, severe liver dysfunction, or zinc deficiency.
Transferrin % change	<200 mg/dL: subclinical PEM > 20% decrease;§ subclinical PEM	Biological half-life of 8 days. May be decreased in the presence of liver dysfunction; may be elevated in the presence of infection or iron deficiency.
Prealbumin % change	<20 mg/dL; subclinical PEM > 20% decrease;§ subclinical PEM	Biological half-life of 2 days. May be decreased in the presence of severe liver dysfunction, vitamin A deficiency, or zinc deficiency; can be useful in assessing adequacy of nutrition support regimens.
Retinol-binding protein %change	<4 mg/dL: subclinical PEM >20% decease;§ subclinical PEM	Biological half-life of 12 hours. May be elevated in the presence of renal failure; can be useful in assessing adequacy of nutrition support regimens.

*PEM, protein-energy malnutrition.

†More than twice coefficient of variation (method error) determined from 265 data sets of measurements obtained by two trained examiners.

‡Lowest percentile of healthy children.

§More than twice coefficient of variation.

Source: From Rickard KA, Grosfeld JL, Coates TD, Weetman R, Baehner RL. Advances in nutrition care of children with neoplastic disease: A review of treatment, research and application. Copyright The American Dietetic Association. Reprinted by permission from *Journal of The American Dietetic Association* (1986;86:1666).

NUTRIENT REQUIREMENTS

Energy and Protein

Energy requirements should be based on age, weight, gender, therapy, and growth needs.[40] Although the dietary reference intakes (DRI) for energy and protein are categorized by age and gender, they may not be appropriate in this population. Factors affecting nutrient needs include inactivity, bacterial sepsis, fever secondary to neutropenia, or secondary complications such as neutropenic enterocolitis. Basal metabolic rate[41,42] with additions for growth, infection, and stress can be used to determine energy needs. Multiplying basal metabolic rate by a factor of 1.6 to 1.8 for very young or malnourished children will allow for growth, stress, and light activity.[29] Nitrogen balance and actual energy balance can be measured to ensure that desired results have been achieved. The best long-term indicator of adequate nutrient intake is growth (refer to Chapter 1 for additional information).

The Harris-Benedict formula and other equations have been used to estimate calorie needs in adults and may be appropriate for children who have completed their growth.[40]

Vitamin and Mineral Requirements

Vitamin and mineral requirements have not been determined for children with cancer. Recommendations are based on the DRI (Appendix I). Marginal nutrient deficiencies can occur in the pediatric patient with cancer. Patients are especially susceptible to nutrient deficiencies due to malabsorption or inadequate supplementation when they are receiving PN secondary to limited GI function for an extended period; have sustained radiation or surgical damage to an area of the intestine; or are receiving antibiotics for chronic infections.[10] Specific nutrient deficiencies can be masked by therapy effects and are difficult to identify. For example, thiamin deficiency has been noted in children maintained on long-term PN.[43] The peripheral neuropathy that can accompany this deficiency mimics chemotherapy toxicity.

NUTRITION SUPPORT

Oral Supplementation

Suboptimal oral intake of short duration during treatment is of less concern if the child is initially well-nourished and can compensate when feeling well. These children may benefit from high-density foods that increase energy and other nutrient levels of the diet. Suggestions for boosting the nutrient density of foods consumed are shown in Table 22–8. Dietary guidelines for common problems[44] seen during and following therapy are presented in Table 22–9.

Refeeding a child following intensive cancer therapy may be a slow process because the child's appetite and tolerance for food fluctuate widely. Individualizing the child's diet by including frequent servings of foods enjoyed (in the absence of oral and GI symptoms) may enhance oral intake. Although many commercial liquid nutritional supplements designed for pediatric patients are currently available, taste acceptance may be a limiting factor. Shakes made with familiar products and supplemented by glucose polymers or other nondetectable modular components are usually best tolerated. Supplements are often acceptable if offered in an unobtrusive manner as part of the regular meal or snack pattern. For the lactose-intolerant child, lactose-free or soy-based products can be useful. Oral and esophageal lesions may limit tolerance for oral supplements. Hyperosmolar or lactose-containing products may aggravate diarrhea. Encouragement from staff, patient education, and nutrition classes can help improve acceptance of supplements.

Tube Feeding

Children who cannot or will not eat may benefit from enteral tube feeding. Enteral nutrition has several practical advantages over PN. These include lower risk of infection or other catheter-related complications, maintenance of gut integrity, more normal play activities, and decreased cost.

The utility and safety of enteral tube feedings in pediatric cancer patients have been demonstrated.[45–47] Pietsch and colleagues[46] reported adequate provision of nutrition support via nasogastric feeds in 17 children with high-risk cancer. Another study by Barron and colleagues[47] showed that gastrostomy tube feedings provided to nutritionally compromised pediatric cancer patients were effective in reversing malnutrition.

Nasogastric feeds may not be appropriate in the older infant, toddler, and preschool-age groups because of psychologic trauma associated with insertion and maintenance of tubes. In addition, nausea and vomiting, as well as decreased intestinal motility and absorption secondary to oncologic therapy, make tube feedings less favorable and less effective.

Enteral feedings for children undergoing HCT have been used infrequently in the immediate posttransplant period due to severe regimen-related toxicities, thrombocytopenia, and neutropenia. Complications such as dislodgement of nasoenteral tubes and inadequate energy support have been reported.[48,49] The combined use of enteral feedings with PN during HCT is an acceptable and cost-effective alternative.[50] Enteral nutrition should be considered in children with mild or controlled intestinal GVHD, low-risk HCT (autologous or matched sibling) with long-term eating problems, adequate platelet recovery

Table 22–8 Suggestions for Increasing Nutrient Density

- Add butter or margarine to soup, mashed and baked potatoes, hot cereal, grits, rice, noodles, and cooked vegetables. Stir butter or margarine into sauces and gravies.
- Add cream to soups, egg dishes, batters, puddings, custards, and dry or hot cereal. Substitute cream for milk in recipes. Make cocoa with cream and add marshmallows.
- Add nondairy whipped topping to pudding, pies, hot cocoa, fruit, and gelatin.
- Add sour cream to soups, baked potatoes, vegetables, sauces, salad dressings, stews, baked meat and fish dishes, gelatin desserts, and bread and muffin batter. Use sour cream as a dip for raw fruits and vegetables.
- Spread mayonnaise on sandwiches and crackers. Combine mayonnaise with meat, fish, or boiled eggs.
- Add honey to cereal, milk drinks, fruit desserts, or smoothies; add to yogurt as a dessert.
- Sprinkle granola on yogurt, ice cream, pudding, custard, and fruit. Mix granola with dried fruits and nuts for a snack.
- Stir roasted nuts or sunflower seeds into cereals, pancakes, or waffles. Sprinkle them on salads.
- Add dried fruits and nuts to muffins, cookies, breads, cakes, rice and grain dishes, cereals, pudding, and stuffing.
- Spread peanut butter or cream cheese on crackers, toast, bread, or apple slices.
- Instead of drinking water, select beverages that contain calories, such as fruit juice.
- Combine yogurt or milk with fresh or frozen fruit and whip in a blender.
- Eat small, frequently scheduled meals throughout the day. Six feedings a day may help to meet caloric requirements without too much effort.
- Notice the time of day when the appetite is best and plan for higher-calorie foods then. Eat a good snack before bedtime.
- Add powdered milk to hot or cold cereals, scrambled eggs, soups, gravies, casserole dishes, desserts, and in baking.

Source: Adapted from Gallagher LM, et al. Pediatric Acquired Immunodeficiency Syndrome. In: Queen PM, Langs CE, eds., *Handbook of Pediatric Nutrition.* pp. 384–399. © 1993; Aspen Publishers, Inc.

or support, need for long-term nutrition support, adequate family support, and social problems that preclude the use of PN.[51] Enteral feedings may also be appropriate for children with long-term eating problems who receive a non-myeloablative HCT, in which lower doses of chemotherapy and radiation are delivered. Further research exploring optimal time for initiation of feedings, types of tubes, methods of delivery, and appropriate formulas is vital.

Parenteral Nutrition

PN provides nutrients for children who cannot ingest, digest, or absorb food via the GI tract. Nutrition support has been demonstrated to improve treatment tolerance in children with advanced neoplastic disease.[32,52] Fewer treatment delays and accelerated recovery of bone marrow function have also been reported in pediatric oncology patients maintained on PN.[53,54]

Due to intensive treatment regimens, PN has been the standard nutrition support therapy for children undergoing HCT.[55] Improved visceral protein status,[56] maintenance of body weight,[57] and earlier engraftment following cytoreductive therapy[58] have been observed in pediatric transplant patients. Improved disease-free survival has been reported in allogeneic transplant patients who received prophylactic PN.[59]

Table 22–9 Dietary Guidelines for Managing Common Nutrition Problems of Pediatric Oncology Patients

Oral and esophageal mucositis
- Try soft, puree-textured or blenderized liquid diet.
- Try smooth, bland, or moist foods (custard, cream soups, mashed potatoes).
- Offer soft, nonirritating, cold foods (popsicles, ice cream, frozen yogurt, slushes).
- Encourage frequent mouth rinsing to remove food and bacteria and to promote healing.

Xerostomia (oral dryness)
- Offer moist foods (stews, casseroles, canned fruit) and liquids.
- Add extra sauces, gravies, margarine, butter, and broth to foods.
- Encourage liquids with meals.
- Add vinegar and pickles to foods to help lessen xerostomia.
- Offer lemon-flavored, sugarless candy to help stimulate saliva.
- Encourage good oral hygiene.
- Try commercial saliva substitutes.

Thick, viscous saliva and mucous
- Encourage adequate fluid intake.
- Offer clear liquids (tea, popsicles, slushes, warm broth).
- Encourage good oral hygiene.

Dysgeusia (impaired taste)
- Flavor poultry, fish, eggs, or dairy products.
- Enhance the taste of foods with herbs, spices, flavor extracts, and marinades.
- Offer cold, nonodorous foods.
- Offer fruit-flavored beverages.
- Try highly aromatic foods.
- Try tart foods like oranges or lemonade that may have more taste.
- Encourage good oral hygiene.
- Offer fluids with meals to help take away a bad taste in the mouth.

Anorexia
- Offer small, frequent meals of nutrient-dense foods.
- Use carbohydrate supplements and protein powders.
- Create a pleasant mealtime atmosphere with enhancing food aromas, colorful place settings, and varied color and textures of foods.

Nausea and vomiting
- Try high carbohydrate foods and fluids (crackers, toast, gelatin); nonacidic juices.
- Try small, frequent feedings.
- Offer cold, clear liquids and solids.
- Avoid overly sweet or high fat foods.
- Avoid feeding the patient in a stuffy, too-warm room or one filled with cooking odors or other odors that might be disagreeable.
- Encourage drinking or sipping liquids frequently throughout the day; using a straw may help.
- Encourage rest periods after meals.
- Avoid offering favorite foods when nauseated; it may cause a permanent dislike of the food.
- Observe if there is a pattern or regularity to when nausea occurs or what causes it (specific foods, events, surroundings); suggest appropriate changes in diet or schedule.

continues

Table 22–9 continued

Diarrhea
- Try a low-fat, low-fiber diet.
- Avoid caffeine.
- Offer cold or room-temperature foods and beverages that may be better tolerated.
- Offer low-lactose intake.
- Encourage adequate fluids to prevent dehydration.
- Avoid excessive fruit juice ingestion.

Constipation
- Encourage fluids.
- Offer a hot beverage in the morning or evening that may stimulate a bowel movement.
- Offer high-fiber foods.

Source: Data from endnote reference 44.

The decision to use central or peripheral PN is based on the child's nutrition status, expected duration of nutrition therapy, and availability of peripheral veins. Central venous catheters are often placed for delivery of chemotherapy and make central PN the appropriate choice. Multiple-lumen catheters help to simplify the delivery of medications, blood products, and nutrient solutions. Cyclic/home PN can be used to provide nutrition support while allowing the child time out of the hospital. A home health agency can work with caregivers to provide PN solutions, education, and monitoring. See also Chapter 25, Parenteral Nutrition.

SPECIAL CONSIDERATIONS

Long-Term Nutritional Sequelae

The growing child receiving antineoplastic therapy is susceptible to adverse effects of the treatment modalities, which may not become apparent until the child matures. Endocrine complications such as gonadal dysfunction, hypothyroidism, and impaired growth and development have been described.[60,61]

Growth hormone deficiency with decreased growth velocity and delayed onset of puberty have been observed in children following HCT.[61,62] Children who have received cranial irradiation prior to HCT show growth hormone deficiency with deceleration of normal growth rates.[62,63] Regular evaluations to determine occurrence of endocrine gland dysfunction are recommended.

Neuropsychologic complications, cardiac complications, and dental abnormalities are other consequences of cancer therapy.[61,64]

Integrative Medicine

Parents may use integrative medicine/alternative treatments out of desperation to cure their child's condition. The use of herbals and megavitamin therapy in the treatment of childhood cancer raises several concerns, including:

1. Unexpected or undesirable interactions between preparations and prescribed medications may affect the action of drugs routinely used during the course of chemotherapy and HCT.
2. Potential contamination of preparations derived from plants poses the risk of bacterial, fungal, or parasitic infections. A few specific preparations have been associated with serious toxic side effects or infections.[29]
3. Alternative nutrition therapy may be chosen as the sole source of treatment.

Herbals and botanicals are frequently explored as alternative therapies. These preparations are derived directly from plants and may be sold as tablets, capsules, liquids, extracts, teas, or powered and topical preparations. A common herbal taken by cancer patients to boost the immune system is echinacea. This herb is claimed to boost the body's immune system by stimulating macrophage activity to attack cancer cells.[65] It is available in tincture, capsule, or liquid form; however, the dose is dependent on the potency of the preparation. Recommendations regarding the effectiveness of echinacea as an adjunct to traditional childhood cancer therapy cannot be made at this time because no studies in the pediatric population have been reported.

Some herbals are contraindicated in children with cancer because of their association with serious side effects. Garlic and gingko biloba may reduce blood-clotting factors.[65,66] Other botanicals containing pyrrolizidine alkaloids, such as comfrey and maté tea, may induce hepatotoxicity.[67] Herbal preparations should be discontinued during HCT. Dietetic professionals must be sensitive to the family's views and biases and educate the family and health care team appropriately.

Guidelines for Oral Intake

Diet for the Immunosuppresed Patient

The goal of the diet for the immunosuppressed patient is to maximize healthy food options while minimizing GI exposure to pathogenic organisms.[68,69] Although no empirical research exists on the relative benefits of restricting specific food groups, most facilities place restrictions ranging from no raw fresh fruits or vegetables to a specific low microbial diet.[70,71]

Table 22–10 shows an example of diet restrictions for HCT patients undergoing treatment in the hospital and at home. High-risk foods, iden-

Table 22–10 Recommended Foods to Restrict for Immunosuppressed Patients

- Raw and undercooked meat (including game), fish, shellfish, poultry, eggs, sausage, bacon
- Raw tofu, unless pasteurized or aseptically packaged
- Luncheon meats (including salami, bologna, hot dogs, and ham) unless heated until steaming
- Refrigerated smoked seafood typically labeled as lox; kippered, nova-style, smoked or fish jerky (unless contained in a cooked dish)
- Pickled fish
- Nonpasteurized milk and raw milk products, nonpasteurized cheese and non-pasteurized yogurt
- Soft and blue-veined cheeses, including Brie, Camembert, feta, farmer's, blue, Gorgonzola, Roquefort, Stilton
- Mexican-style soft cheese, including queso blanco and quesco fresco
- Cheese containing chili peppers or other uncooked vegetables
- Fresh salad dressings (stored in the grocer's refrigerated case) containing raw eggs or contraindicated cheeses
- Unwashed raw vegetables and fruits and those with visible mold
- All raw vegetable sprouts (alfalfa, mung bean, all others)
- Unpasteurized commercial fruit and vegetable juices
- Raw honey
- All miso products (miso soup); tempe (tempeh); maté tea
- All moldy and outdated food products
- Raw, uncooked brewer's yeast
- Well water, unless boiled for 1 minute

Source: Reprinted with permission from Diet for immunosupressed patients 2004, Seattle Cancer Care Alliance, Washington.

tified as potential sources of organisms known to cause infection in immunosuppressed patients, are restricted. Recommendations on the duration of the diet are based on treatment.

Food Safety

Educating patient and caregiver on food safety may be more important in reducing food-borne illness than extensive diet restrictions.[72–74] A food-handling observational study has shown that healthy people repeatedly make food-handling errors in their home, increasing risk.[75] Improper holding temperatures and/or personal hygiene of food handlers contribute most to disease incidence.[76] Education should emphasize hand washing, high-risk foods, proper temperatures for storage, defrosting, and cooking, cross-contamination issues, correct cooling and reheating procedures, and sanitation.

Several infections are of particular concern with this population, including *Salmonella enteritidis, Campylobacter jejuni, E. coli 0157:H7,* and *Listeria monocytogenes*. The Centers for Disease Control publishes food-borne illness diagnosis and management recommendations for health care professionals.[77]

Special Food Service Needs

The food service for oncology patients should be designed to provide a variety of foods served at frequent intervals to meet patient tolerance. Traditional hospital food services with set menus, trayline service, rigid meal hours, and 24-hour advance menu selection often do not meet the needs of many oncology and transplant patients. A more flexible food service, such as unit nourishment centers or satellite kitchens, will provide opportunities for oral intake.[71,72]

Some facilities have implemented hotel-style room service with extended hours (up to 24 hour/day), telephone ordering systems, short delivery times, and elimination of wasted trays.[74,78] At one facility, patients' caloric intake improved significantly and protein intake increased by 18% after the introduction of room service. Patient satisfaction with hospital food service improved with excellent ratings increasing 35%.[79]

Promoting Oral Intake during Hospitalization

Encouraging oral intake in the pediatric cancer patient can be a challenge.[80] Anxious, scared, or depressed children do not feel like eating. Chronic pain may also decrease the child's interest in eating. Providing a calm, relaxed hospital atmosphere for eating, with uninterrupted time for feeding (door closed, sign posted), may improve intake. Small children require a secure feeding position (high chair or toddler feeding table), a bib, towel, and covered floor area to limit anxiety over spills.

Children should not be forced to eat. A maximum mealtime of 20 to 30 minutes should be adequate with food texture and portion size provided that is age appropriate. Older children may benefit from group eating situations (such as a playroom area) or participatory food preparation times, as well as by knowing their oral intake goals for hospital discharge. Many facilities implement an outside food policy, allowing the patient's family or caregivers to bring food into the hospital. Outside food items should conform to the medical diet order. These items are usually not stored on the unit; perishable foods must be consumed immediately. Family education in food safety is important.

For patients refusing to eat, behavior modification techniques may be necessary.[81] Children transitioning from tube feeding may exhibit oral, motor, sensory, and developmental feeding problems that make weaning difficult. A weaning process based on developmental stages is recommended.[82]

CONCLUSION

The nutritional needs of the child with cancer are an important consideration in the treatment plan. The goal is to ensure a nutritional intake adequate for growth and development. Dietetics professionals serving this population have a challenging task of promoting appropriate intake while encouraging a well-balanced diet. Additional dietary modifications may also be necessary due to therapy-induced adverse nutritional effects.

Ongoing patient and family education provides an opportunity to teach age-appropriate nutrition and food safety concepts to support cancer therapies.

REFERENCES

1. Ross JA, Severson RK, Pollock HB, Robison LL. Childhood cancer in the United States. A geographical analysis of cases from the Pediatric Cooperative Clinical Trials Group. *Cancer.* 1996;77:201–207.
2. Guerney JG, Davis, S, Severson RK, et al. Trends in cancer incidence among children in the US. *Cancer.* 1996;78:532–541.
3. Gloeckler Ries LA. Cancer rates and risks. Retrieved March 12, 2004, from http://seer.cancer.gov/publications/raterisk.
4. Gurney JG, Severson RD, Davis S, Robison LL. Incidence of cancer in children in the United States. Sex-, race-, and 1-year age-specific rates by histologic type. *Cancer.* 1995;75:2186–2195.
5. Smith MA, Gloeckler Ries LA. Childhood cancer: Incidence, survival and mortality. In: Pizzo PA, Poplack DG, eds., *Principles and Practice of Pediatric Oncology.* Philadelphia: Lippincott Williams & Wilkins; 2002; 1–34.
6. Harras A. *Cancer Rates and Risks,* 4th ed. NIH publication no. 96-691. Bethesda, MD: National Cancer Institute; 1996.
7. Novy MA, Saavedra JM. Nutrition therapy for the pediatric cancer patient. *Top Clin Nutr.* 1997;12:16–25.
8. Mauer AM, Burgess JB, Donaldson SS, et al. Special nutritional needs of children with malignancies: A review. *J Parenter Enter Nutr.* 1990;14:315–324.
9. Coates TD, Rickard KA, Grosfeld JL, et al. Nutritional support of children with neoplastic diseases. *Surg Clin North Am.* 1986;66:1197–1212.
10. Bechard LJ, Adiv OE, Jaksic T, Duggan C. Nutritional supportive care. In: Pizzo PA, Poplack DG, eds., *Principles and Practice of Pediatric Oncology*. Philadelphia: Lippincott Williams & Wilkins; 2002: 1285–1300.
11. Reilly JJ, Weir J, Mcool JH, Bison BE. Prevalence of protein-energy malnutrition at diagnosis in children with acute lymphoblastic leukemia. *J Pediatr Gastroenterol Nutr.* 1999;29:194–197.
12. Sala A, Pencharz P, Barr RD. Children, cancer and nutrition–A dynamic triangle. *Cancer.* 2004;100:677–687.
13. Andrassy RJ, Chwals WJ. Nutritional support of the pediatric oncology patient. *Nutrition.* 1998;14:124–129.
14. Strasser F, Bruera ED. Update on anorexia and cachexia. *Hem Onc Clin N Amer.* 2002;16(3):589–617.
15. Barber MD. Cancer cachexia and its treatment with fish-oil–enriched nutritional supplementation. *Nutrition.* 2001; 17:751–755.
16. Kern KA, Norton JA. Cancer cachexia. *J Parenter Enter Nutr.* 1988;12:286–298.
17. Van Eys J. Nutrition and cancer: Physiological interrelationships. *Ann Rev Nutr.* 1985;5:435–461.
18. Berde CD, Bilett AL, Collins JJ. Symptom management in supportive cancer care. In: Pizzo PA, Poplack DG, eds., *Principles and Practice of Pediatric Oncology.* Philadelphia: Lippincott Williams & Wilkins; 2002; 1301–1332.
19. Eldridge B. Chemotherapy and nutritional implications. In: McCallum PD, Polisen CG, eds., *The Clinical Guide to Oncology Nutrition.* Chicago: American Dietetic Association; 2000;61–69.
20. Keller VE. Management of nausea and vomiting in children. *J Pediatr Nurs.* 1995;10:280–286.
21. Sherry VW. Taste alterations among patients with cancer. *Clin J Oncol Nurs.* 2002;6:73–76.
22. Kennedy L, Diamond J. Assessment and management of chemotherapy-induced mucositis in children. *J Ped Onc Nurs.* 1997;14(3):164–174.
23. Eldridge B, Hamilton KK. *Management of Nutrition Impact Symptoms in Cancer and Educational Handouts,* 2nd ed. Chicago: American Dietetic Association; 2004; 27–28.
24. Polisena CG. Nutrition concerns with the radiation therapy patient. In: McCallum PD, Polisena CG, eds., *The Clinical Guide to Oncology Nutrition.* Chicago, IL: American Dietetic Association; 2000;70–77.
25. Horowitz MM. Uses and growth of hematopoietic cell transplantation. In: Blume KG, Forman SJ, Appelbaum FR, eds., *Thomas' Hematopoietic Cell Transplantation,* 3rd ed. Malden, MA: Blackwell Publishing; 2004;9–15.
26. Charuhas PM. Pediatric hematopoietic stem cell transplantation. In Hasse JM, Blue LS, eds., *Comprehensive Guide to Transplant Nutrition.* Chicago: American Dietetic Association; 2002;226–247.
27. French MR, Levy-Milne R, Zibrik D. A survey of the use of low microbial diets in pediatric bone marrow transplant programs. *J Am Diet Assoc.* 2001;101:1194–1198.
28. Vogelsang GB, Lee L, Bensen-Kennedy DM. Pathogenesis and treatment of graft-versus-host disease after bone marrow transplant. *Ann Rev Med.* 2003;54:29–52.
29. Seattle Cancer Care Alliance. *Hematopoietic Stem Cell Transplantation Nutrition Care Criteria,* 2nd ed. Seattle, WA: Seattle Cancer Care Alliance; 2002.
30. Gauvreau JM, Lenssen P, Cheney CL, et al. Nutritional management of patients with intestinal graft-versus-host disease. *J Am Diet Assoc.* 981;79:673–677.
31. Donaldson SS, Wesley MN, DeWys WD, et al. A study of the nutritional status of pediatric cancer patients. *Am J Dis Child.* 1981;135:1107–1112.

32. Rickard KA, Detamore CM, Coates TD, et al. Effect of nutrition staging on treatment delays and outcome in stage IV neuroblastoma. *Cancer.* 1983;52:587–598.
33. Deeg HJ, Sediel K, Bruemmer B, et al. Impact of patient weight on non-relapse mortality after marrow transplantation. *Bone Marrow Transplant.* 1995;15:461–468.
34. Murry DJ, Riva L, Poplack DG. Impact of nutrition on pharmacokinetics of anti-neoplastic agents. *Internat J Cancer-Supp.* 1998;11:48–51.
35. Motil KJ. Sensitive measures of nutrition status in children in hospital and in the field. *Internat J Cancer-Supp.* 1998;11:2–9.
36. Katz JA, Chambers B, Everhart C, et al. Linear growth in children with acute lymphoblastic leukemia treated without cranial irradiation. *J Pediatr.* 1991;118:575–578.
37. Moshang T Jr, Grimberg A. The effects of irradiation and chemotherapy on growth. *Endocr Metab Clinics of North Am.* 1996;25:731–741.
38. O'Neil SM, Pipes PL. Managing mealtime behaviors. In: Trahms CM, Pipes PL, eds., *Nutrition in Infancy and Childhood,* 6th ed. Dubuque, IA: WCB/McGraw-Hill; 1997.
39. Merritt RJ, Kalsch M, Roux, LD, et al. Significance of hypoalbuminemia in pediatric oncology patients: Malnutrition or infections? *J Parenter Enter Nutr.* 1983;9: 303–306.
40. Nevin-Folino NL, ed. *Pediatric Manual of Clinical Dietetics,* 2nd ed. Chicago: American Dietetic Association; 2003.
41. Altman PL, Dittmer DS. *Metabolism.* Bethesda, MD: Federation of American Societies for Experimental Biology; 1968:344.
42. Nelson JK, Moxness KE, Gastineau CF, Jenson MD. *Mayo Clinic Diet Manual: A Handbook of Nutrition,* 7th ed. St. Louis, MO: Mosby; 1994.
43. Alexander HR, Rickard KA, Godshall B. Nutritional supportive care. In: Pizzo PA, Poplack DG, eds. *Principles and Practice of Pediatric Oncology.* Philadelphia: Lippincott-Raven; 1997:1167–1181.
44. Charuhas PM. Introduction to marrow transplantation. *Oncol Nutr Diet Pract Group Newsletter.* Chicago: American Dietetic Association; 1994:2:2–9.
45. Deswarte-Wallace J, Firouzbakhsk S, Finklestein JZ. Using research to change practice: Enteral feedings for pediatric oncology patients. *J Pediatr Oncol Nurs.* 2001; 18:217–223.
46. Pietsch JB, Ford C, Whitlock JA. Nasogastric tube feedings in children with high-risk cancer: A pilot study. *J Pediatr Hematol Oncol.* 1999;21:111–114.
47. Barron MA, Duncan DS, Green GJ, et al. Efficacy and safety of radiologically placed gastrostomy tubes in paediatric haematology/oncology patients. *Med Pediatr Onc.* 2000;34:177–182.
48. Sefcick A, Anderton D, Byrne JL, et al. Naso-jejunal feeding in allogeneic bone marrow transplant recipients: Results of a pilot study. *Bone Marrow Transplant.* 2001 28:1135–1139.
49. Langdana A, Tully N, Molloy E, et al. Intensive enteral nutrition support in paediatric bone marrow transplantation. *Bone Marrow Transplant.* 2001;27:741–746.
50. Hopman GD, Pena EG, le Cessie S, et al. Tube feeding and bone marrow transplantation. *Med Pediatr Oncol.* 2003;40:375–379.
51. Ringwald-Smith K, Krance R, Strickin L. Enteral nutrition support in a child after bone marrow transplantation. *Nutr Clin Pract.* 1995;10:140–143.
52. Rickard KA, Coates TD, Grosfel JL, et al. The value of nutrition support in children with cancer. *Cancer.* 1986; 58:1904–1910.
53. Rickard KA, Detamore CM, Coates TD, et al. Effect of nutrition staging on treatment delays and outcome in stage IV neuroblastoma. *Cancer.* 1983;52:587–598.
54. Hays DM, Merritt RJ, White L, et al. Effect of total parenteral nutrition on marrow recovery during induction therapy for acute nonlymphocytic leukemia in childhood. *Med Pediatr Oncol.* 1983;11:134–140.
55. American Society for Parenteral and Enteral Nutrition. Guidelines for the use of parenteral and enteral nutrition in adult and pediatric patients. *J Paren Enter Nutr.* 2002; 1S:124SA–126SA.
56. Uderzo C, Rovelli A, Bonomi M, et al. Total parenteral nutrition and nutritional assessment in leukemia children undergoing bone marrow transplantation. *Eur J Cancer.* 1991;27:758–762.
57. Yokoyama S, Fujimoto T, Mitomi T, et al. Use of total parenteral nutrition in pediatric bone marrow transplantation. *Nutrition.* 1989;5:27–30.
58. Weisdorf S, Hofland C, Sharp HL, et al. Total parenteral nutrition in bone marrow transplantation: A clinical evaluation. *J Pediatr Gastroenterol Nutr.* 1984;3:95–100.
59. Weisdorf SA, Lynse J, Wind D. Positive effect of prophylactic total parenteral nutrition on long-term outcome of bone marrow transplantation. *Transplantation.* 1987; 43:833–838.
60. DeLaat CA, Lampkin BC. Long-term survivors of childhood cancer: Evaluation and identification of sequelae of treatment. *Ca-A-Cancer Journal for Clinicians.* 1992; 42:263–282.
61. Sanders JE. Growth and development after hematopoietic cell transplantation. In: Blume KG, Forman SJ, Appelbaum FR, eds., *Thomas' Hematopoietic Cell Transplantation,* 3rd ed. Malden, MA: Blackwell Publishing; 2004:929–943.
62. Sanders JE, Pritchard S, Mahoney P, et al. Growth and development following marrow transplantation for leukemia. *Blood.* 1986;68:1129–1135.

63. Copeland DR. Neuropsychological and psychosocial effects of childhood leukemia and its treatment. *Ca-A Cancer Journal for Clinicians.* 1992;42:283–295.

64. Uderzo C, Fraschini D, Balduzzi A, et al. Long-term effects of bone marrow transplantation on dental status in children with leukemia. *Bone Marrow Transplant.* 1997; 20:865–869.

65. American Cancer Society. *American Cancer Society's Guide to Complementary and Alternative Cancer Methods.* Atlanta, GA: American Cancer Society; 2000; 204–205.

66. Gardiner P, Kemper KJ. Herbs in pediatric and adolescent medicine. *Pediatrics in Review.* 2002;21:44–57.

67. McGee J, Patrick RS, Wood CB, Blumgart LH. A case of veno-occlusive disease of the liver in Britain associated with herbal tea consumption. *J Clin Path.* 1976; 29: 788–794.

68. Henry L. Immunocompromised patients and nutrition. *Prof Nurse.* 1997;12:655–659.

69. Moe G. Enteral feeding and infection in the immunocompromised patient. *Nutr Clin Pract.* 1991;6(2):55–64.

70. Moody K, Charlson ME, Finlay J. The neutropenic diet: What's the evidence? *J Pediatr Hematol Oncol.* 2002;24:717–721.

71. Stern JM, Lenssen P. Food and nutrition services for the BMT patient. In Buschsel PC, Whedon MB, eds., *Bone Marrow Transplantation: Clinical and Administrative Strategies.* Boston, MA: Jones and Bartlett; 1995: 113–136.

72. Altekruse SF, Swerdlow DL. The changing epidemiology of foodborne disease. *Am J Med Sci.* 1996;311(1): 23–29.

73. Newman KA, Schimpff SC. Hospital hotel services as risk factor for infection among immunocompromised patients. *Rev Infect Dis.* 1987;9:206–213.

74. Lenssen P. Hematopoietic Cell Transplantation. In: Matarese LE, Gottschlich MM, eds., *Contemporary Nutrition Support Practice: A Clinical Guideline,* 2nd ed. Philadelphia: WB Saunders; 2003;574–594.

75. Anderson JB, Shuster TA, Hanson KE, et al. A camera's view of consumer food-handling behaviors. *J Am Diet Assoc.* 2004;104:186–191.

76. Collins JE. Impact of changing consumer lifestyles on the emergence/reemergence of foodborne pathogens. *Emerging Infect Dis.* 1997;3:471–479.

77. Diagnosis and management of foodborne illnesses: A primer for physicians and other heath care professionals. *MMWR.* 2004;53:1–33.

78. Lowe M, Mortensen S. "Room service"—Feeding on demand succeeds for cancer patients. *J Amer Diet Assoc.* 1995;95(suppl):A82.

79. Williams R, Virtue K, Adkins A. Room service improves patient food intake and satisfaction with hospital food. *J Ped Onc Nurs.* 1998;15(3):183–189.

80. Sherry ME, Aker SN, Cheney CL. Nutrition assessment and management of the pediatric cancer patient. *Top Clin Nutr.* 1987;2:38–48.

81. Handen BL, Mandell F, Russo DC. Feeding induction in children who refuse to eat. *Am J Dis Child.* 1986;140: 52–54.

82. Schauster H, Dwyer J. Transition from tube feedings to feeding by mouth in children: Preventing eating dysfunction. *J Amer Diet Assoc.* 1996;96:277–281.

EDUCATION RESOURCES

National Cancer Institute Education Materials:
www.cancer.gov or 1-800-4CANCER

- *National Cancer Institute Research on Childhood Cancers*
- *Questions and Answers About Care for Children and Adolescents with Cancer*
- *When Someone in Your Family Has Cancer*
- *Young People With Cancer. A Handbook for Parents.*

Leukemia and Lymphoma Society Education Material: www.leukemia.org or 1-800-955-4572

- *Emotional Aspects of Childhood Leukemia.*

INTERNET RESOURCES AND NEWSLETTERS

BMT Infonet: www.bmtnews.org

Nutrition for Kids: www.nutritionforkids.com

Kids Cancer Network: www.kidscancernetwork.org

Tiny Tummies: www.TinyTummies.com

CHAPTER 23

Nutrition for the Burned Pediatric Patient

Michele Morath Gottschlich and Theresa Mayes

Trauma is a major cause of mortality in children, and a significant number of these deaths are from burns. Burn injury poses a complex metabolic challenge that is directly related to subsequent morbidity and mortality. As such, an important determinant of outcome is adequacy of energy and nutrient provision. If nutriture becomes impaired, wound healing and organ function will suffer. In addition, malnutrition will induce deterioration of immune defenses and profound catabolism of lean body mass and bone tissue.

The purpose of this chapter is to point out metabolic changes, physiologic deficiencies, and nutritional requirements of burned infants and children. Because the common denominator to which all nutrients are related is adequacy of energy intake, methods for evaluating caloric requirements will be emphasized. The basis for selecting the safest and most efficacious route of support and ratio of nutrients will be addressed. This section will also review enteral and parenteral feeding techniques, as well as present options available for assessing and monitoring the nutrition rehabilitation program.

ANATOMIC AND PHYSIOLOGIC CONSIDERATIONS

Pediatric burn injury has a high mortality rate, compared with that of adults with equivalent burns,[1,2] although outcome has clearly improved with advancements in burn care.[3] The higher incidence of complications in pediatric burn patients is partially attributable to the fact that the unique physical and metabolic features of infants and children are frequently overlooked. It is important to recognize that the burned youngster in need of medical and nutritional therapy presents a separate and often much more complex therapeutic problem than does his or her adult counterpart.

Although the older child rapidly approaches the physical and metabolic makeup of the adult and responds to injury and treatment in a corresponding fashion, specialized nutritional care is required by younger age groups due to their anatomic and physiologic immaturity (Table 23–1). All burned children, however, pose a special challenge to meet obligatory growth needs. Burn injuries represent a particular threat to growth through imposition of a catabolic state. Bone growth is slowed during the acute phase postburn.[4] Furthermore, height and weight gain velocities have been documented during the first 3 years following the burn injury without significant catch-up growth.[5]

A burned child, with more limited endogenous reserves and greater caloric and protein requirements than an adult, quickly reaches negative nitrogen balance with a smaller area of burn. Furthermore, the functional immaturity of the infant's gastrointestinal tract and renal system[6–8] poses a unique challenge to his or her ability to tolerate nonvolitional feeding regimens and nutrient-dense products. They are extremely susceptible to diarrhea, dehydration, and malnutrition, which only worsen the degree of catabolism.

Table 23–1 Anatomic and Physiologic Immaturities of Children of Various Ages

System	*Deficit*	*Clinical Implications*	*Age Maturation*
Temperature regulation	Labile system Surface area/body weight ratio greatly increased	Increased radiant and evaporative heat loss Increased metabolic rate in an attempt to maintain core temperature	10–12 years
Integument	Thin skin	Heat penetrates more rapidly, with resultant deeper burn	16–18 years
Gastrointestinal	Immature tract Limited surface area of the small intestinal mucosa Decreased gastric volume capacity	Limited capacity to digest or assimilate some nutrients Prone to antigen absorption High incidence of diarrhea	1–2 years
Renal	Glomerular immaturity Young kidneys inefficient in excretion of sodium chloride and other ions, as well as in water resorption	Renal concentrating ability low; therefore, more water required to excrete the renal solute load produced by the metabolism of protein and electrolytes	1–2 years

METABOLIC MANIFESTATIONS OF THERMAL INJURY

In addition to developmental immaturities, the burned child must respond to the metabolic challenges associated with thermal injury. Extensive burn injury initiates the most marked alterations in body metabolism that can be associated with any illness. The pattern of physiologic events following thermal injury falls into two phases: the ebb and the flow responses.[9,10] The initial, or ebb, response of the burn syndrome is short, lasting 3 to 5 days postinjury. This phase is characterized by general hypometabolism and is manifested by reductions in oxygen consumption, cardiac output, blood pressure, and body temperature (Table 23–2). Fluid resuscitation is conducted during this time in response to the tremendous fluid losses that occur during the early postburn period.

With the resuscitative restoration of circulatory blood volume, the body advances to a prolonged state of hypermetabolism and increased nutrient turnover, termed the flow phase. This second phase is influenced by elevations in circulating levels of catecholamines,[11,12] glucocorticoids,[13–15] and glucagon.[16–19] Insulin levels are usually in the normal range or even elevated. However, the rise in the glucagon/insulin ratio,[19,20] in combination with other hormonal derangements, initiates gluconeogenesis, lipolysis, and protein degradation. Hypermetabolism and hypercatabolism also vary with the time postburn. The classic studies of Wilmore and colleagues[12,21] show that, following the ebb phase, catabolic hormone production and oxygen consumption increase dramatically, peaking between the 6th and 10th day following burns.[12,21] Thereafter, metabolic rate slowly begins to decrease, and a gradual recession of catabolism occurs. These metabolic and hormonal sequelae

Table 23–2 Metabolic Alterations Following Burns

		Flow Response	
	Ebb Response	*Acute Phase*	*Adaptive Phase*
Dominant factors	Loss of plasma volume Shock Low plasma insulin	Elevated catecholamines Elevated glucagon Elevated glucocorticoids Normal or elevated insulin High glucagon to insulin ratio	Stress hormone subsiding response
Symptoms	Hyperglycemia Decreased oxygen consumption Depressed resting energy expenditure Decreased blood pressure Reduced cardiac output Decreased body temperature	Catabolism Hyperglycemia Increased respiratory rate Increased oxygen consumption Hypermetabolism Increased body temperature Increased cardiac output Redistribution of polyvalent cations, such as zinc and iron Mobilization of metabolic reserves Increased urinary excretion of nitrogen, sulphur, magnesium, phosphorus, and potassium Accelerated gluconeogenesis	Anabolism Normoglycemia Energy turnover diminished Convalescence

Source: Adapted from Gottschlich MM, Alexander JW, Bower RH. Enteral nutrition in patients with burns or trauma. In: Rombeau JL, Caldwell MD, eds., *Enteral and Tube Feeding.* With permission of WB Saunders Co, 1990.

have important implications from a nutritional perspective.

FLUID REQUIREMENTS

Water is the most critical of all nutrients. It is an essential component of all cellular structures and is the medium in which all chemical reactions of the host take place. The body composition of the infant is 70–75% water, in contrast to that of an adult, which is 60–65% water. The extracellular fluids of the infant constitute approximately 50% of the total body weight, compared with 20–25% in the adult. Excesses or deficits in water of more than 5% of the optimal value produce measurable effects, and large deviations may lead to death.

Immediately after burns, altered capillary permeability results in the escape of fluid, electrolytes, and protein from the vascular compartment to the interstitial area surrounding the burn wound. The injured area also loses its ability to act as a barrier to water evaporation. In children, with their relatively larger surface area per weight, the insensible water loss is of critical magnitude. Infants and young children are particularly susceptible to a lack of sufficient water intake because of their considerably higher obligatory urinary and insensible water losses, compared with those of adults. Hemodynamic dysfunction as a consequence of fluid shifts necessitates prompt provision of intravenous fluid resuscitation to restore tissue blood flow and to prevent shock following burns. Children require more fluid per square meter of body surface area than do adults with burns.[22]

The most popular pediatric fluid replacement formula is the Parkland formula,[23] modified for children (Table 23–3). The modified Parkland formula includes a factor for basal fluid needs, in addition to compensation for losses from the burn wound. The application of this formula should not replace assessment of the patient's vital signs, blood pressure, and urinary output, because these are the ultimate determinants of the adequacy of replacement.

CALORIC NEEDS

Increases in energy expenditure accompany burn injury. The degree of hypermetabolism is generally related to the size of the burn,[21] with burns of approximately 50% body surface area encountering a peak in energy expenditure. It was once thought that the increase in metabolic rate was a response to the tremendous evaporative heat loss from the wound,[24,25] supported by the finding that raising ambient temperature partially reduced the hypermetabolic response. However, even in very warm environments, burn patients remained hypermetabolic, and their core and skin temperatures persisted. Other causes of hypermetabolism were sought after Zawacki and associates[26] demonstrated that blocking evaporation by application of impermeable dressings to the burn wound produced only a modest reduction in metabolic rate.

The root cause of hypermetabolism continues to be an active area of investigation. A number of studies support the role of cytokines in postburn metabolism.[27–31] Following injury, cytokines appear to produce neuromediators that activate endocrine organs to produce higher concentrations of catecholamines, glucagon, and cortisol. Sleep pattern disturbance has also been suggested as a factor contributing to increased metabolism following burn injury.[32] Prevention of infection and reducing wound size are the primary means of decreasing metabolic rate. However, sufficient pain and anxiety control are crucial means of reducing metabolism in the pediatric population as well. Application of a reliable pain scale index is vital in preverbal children, so that severity of pain is understood and therefore treated appropriately. Age-appropriate explanations of procedures prior to performance may appear trivial, but offer huge rewards toward the reduction of anxiety. Finally, promotion of routine, scheduled breaks, and uninterrupted sleep with attention to duration and quality should be viewed as intricate components of the care plan.

The provision of sufficient calories to meet the increased metabolic expenditure is a critical factor in the management of the burned child. Energy needs may be estimated or measured. A number of pediatric energy equations have been applied

Table 23–3 Pediatric Fluid Calculations for Resuscitation and Maintenance

	Modified Parkland Formula
Total resuscitation fluids = (mL/24 hr)	[4 mL × % burn × weight (kg)] + [basal fluid requirements (1500 × m²)]
	1/2 of calculated fluid volume given in the first 8 hours 1/2 of calculated fluid volume given in the next 6 hours
	Maintenance Fluid Calculation
Total maintenance fluids = (mL/hr)	basal fluids + evaporative losses
	$\frac{1500 \text{ mL} \times \text{m}^2 + (35 + \% \text{ burn}) \times \text{m}^2}{24 \text{ hr}}$

Source: Courtesy of the Shriners Hospitals for Children, Cincinnati, OH.

Table 23–4 Formulas for Calculating Energy Requirements of Burned Children

Reference	*Age*	*% BSAB*	*Calories/Day*
Curreri[33]	0–1 yr	<50	Basal + (15 × % BSAB)
	1–3 yr	<50	Basal + (25 × % BSAB)
	4–15 yr	<50	Basal + (40 × % BSAB)
Davies and Liljedal[34]	Child	Any	60W + (35 × % BSAB)
Hildreth[35–37]	<15 yr	>30	(1800/m^2 BSA) + (2200/m^2 burn)
Hildreth[38]	<12 yr		(1800/m^2 BSA) + (1300/m^2 burn)
Mayes[39]	0–3 yr	10–50	108 + 68W + (3.9 × % BSAB)
			818 + 37.4W + (9.3 × % BSAB)

W, weight in kg, BSA, body surface area, BSAB, body surface area burn

successfully in burns (Table 23–4). Studies support reduced energy demands in this population.[38,39] It has been suggested that during stress, there is a shift in energy expenditure necessary for growth to that needed for acute illness. Energy needs for activity are also greatly reduced in the acute postburn phase.

The wide range of formulas for calculating energy needs is an indication of the uncertainties of this approach. Most mathematic derivations utilize body weight, age, and burn size as the only determinants of caloric requirements. Although these three factors represent significant effectors of metabolic rate, energy expenditure is also influenced by surgery, pain, anxiety, sepsis, body composition, gender, thermal effect of food, sleep deprivation, and physical activity. Therefore, mathematic formulas could derive fairly inaccurate caloric goals, considering the variability among individuals. If caloric needs are underestimated, some tissues, as well as exogenous substrates, will be consumed for energy. Although it is important to provide pediatric burn patients with the energy needed to compensate for hypermetabolism, as well as for growth and development, reports also caution against the delivery of an overabundance of calories.[40] Administering a surfeit of calories has been associated with increased metabolic rate, hyperglycemia, and liver abnormalities and can cause an increase in carbon dioxide production.[41,42]

Indirect calorimetry remains a viable option in the assessment of energy expenditure in pediatric burn patients. The use of indirect calorimetry in burn care has been extensively reviewed elsewhere.[43,44] In general, the patient's caloric goal should be calculated at 120–130% of the measured resting energy expenditure (REE).[45–47] Although there is some degree of error possible with this extrapolation, it is more accurate than estimates based solely on weight, age, and burn size. To ensure the clinical validity of this goal, tests must be repeated regularly. Because hypermetabolism undergoes transient variation during the recovery phase, it is recommended that indirect calorimetry be conducted twice weekly, at minimum, for proper adjustment of the nutritional support regimen.

CARBOHYDRATE NEEDS

Metabolic changes that occur following thermal injury include deranged carbohydrate metabolism. Early in the response to burns, glycosuria and hyperglycemia frequently occur. A similar response is observed in patients with supervening sepsis. Predisposition to glucose intolerance is correlated with the severity of the burn injury.

Elevated blood glucose is also modulated by the phase of injury. During the shock phase, hyperglycemia is primarily caused by decreased peripheral tissue utilization in lieu of impaired tissue perfusion and low insulin levels.[48–50] Glucose intolerance typically persists during the flow phase, but it appears to be the result of enhanced hepatic glucose production and gluconeogenesis.[50,51]

Carbohydrate plays an important role in the nutritional support of the burned child. It appears to be the most important nonprotein calorie source in terms of nitrogen retention in burned patients,[52,53] although a limit exists to its effectiveness as an energy source.[41] Excessive glucose loads, which can increase carbon dioxide production, heighten glucose intolerance, and induce hepatic fat deposition, should be avoided.[42,54–56] Therefore, all burn patients should be monitored for hypercapnia and hyperglycemia. When these symptoms are present, the intake of total calories or carbohydrate may need to be reduced. Exogenous insulin administration is often necessary to improve blood glucose levels and to achieve maximal glucose utilization.

PROTEIN REQUIREMENTS

Thermal injury also brings about momentous changes in protein metabolism. There is increased proteolysis as energy needs are met by deamination of amino acids in the generation of carbon skeletons for glucose.[47,50] Transamination of amino acids likewise occurs as an intermediary step in the formation of nonessential amino acids and priority proteins associated with host defense, wound healing, and survival. Reservoirs of amino acids that are mobilized to the liver include skeletal muscle, connective tissue, and gastrointestinal mucosa. The degree of amino acid mobilization is related to the size of the burn and adequacy of protein intake.[57]

The protein requirements of the burned infant and child are elevated because of accelerated tissue breakdown and exudative losses during a period of rapid repair and growth. Failure to meet heightened protein needs can be expected to yield suboptimal clinical results in terms of wound healing and resistance to infection. The infant and child further adapt to inadequate protein intake by curtailing growth of cells, conceivably sacrificing genetic potential.

Studies have shown that enteral fortification using large quantities of protein can accelerate the synthesis of visceral proteins and promote positive nitrogen balance and host defense factors.[45,58–64] For example, Alexander and colleagues[58] demonstrated that severely burned children on enteral diets containing approximately 22% of calories as protein had higher levels of total serum protein, retinol-binding protein, prealbumin, transferrin, C3, and immunoglobulin G (IgG), and better nitrogen balance than patients receiving 15% of calories as protein. In addition, the high-protein group had improved survival and fewer episodes of bacteremia. Therefore, in planning a nutritional intervention strategy for a burned youngster, an important goal is the provision of a sufficient quantity of protein. Patients greater than 6 months of age with burns in excess of 30% TBSA, should receive 20–23% of calories as protein.[9,58,64] This translates to 2.5–4.0 g/kg, for a nonprotein calorie/nitrogen ratio of 80:1. An ongoing study at the Shriners Hospital for Children in Cincinnati, Ohio supports the safe provision of this approximate high level of protein in the less-than-3-year-old population. Preliminary evidence further suggests improved clinical outcomes with higher protein provision in this age group. Other factors that influence protein repletion, assuming an adequate intake of energy, include the quality of dietary protein and the source of nonprotein energy that the patient receives.

Close monitoring of protein intake is necessary because excessive protein loads or amino acid imbalances may result in azotemia, hyperammonemia, or acidosis. Particular care must be taken when administering high-protein feedings to children younger than 12 months of age because excessive amounts can have adverse effects on immature or compromised kidneys. Ongoing assessment of fluid status, blood urea nitrogen (BUN), plasma proteins, and nitrogen balance is recommended for individual evaluation of tolerance and adequacy. However, when fluid intake is not restricted, renal or hepatic dysfunction does not exist, and pathways of intermediary metabolism are relatively mature, a high-protein diet is usually tolerated well.

FAT NEEDS

During the flow phase, burn-mediated increases in catecholamine and glucagon levels stimulate an accelerated rate of fat mobilization and oxidation. It is recognized, however, that lipid is important to the diet of the burned child because of its high caloric density, its role in myelination of nerve cells and brain development, the palatability it imparts to food, and its role as a carrier for the fat-soluble vitamins. In addition, fat in the form of the essential fatty acid linoleate provides vital components for cellular membranes and is a precursor for dienoic prostaglandin synthesis.

The minimum requirement for linoleic acid needed to prevent omega-6 fatty acid deficiency is considered to be approximately 2–3% of the calories consumed. This requirement is usually not difficult to accomplish because most enteral feeding supplements and intravenous fat emulsions contain high levels of fat and linoleic acid.[45,64,65] An overabundance of dietary lipid, however, can be detrimental to recovery from burns.[66] Complications ascribed to excessive fat intake have been reported. These include lipemia, fatty liver, diarrhea, and decreased resistance to infection.[65–67] Furthermore, lipid appears to represent an inefficient source of calories for the maintenance of nitrogen equilibrium and lean body mass following major injury.[68–70]

Therefore, conservative administration of fat, particularly linoleic acid, given its immunosuppressive metabolites, is recommended.[5,45] Given its competitive effects on the down-regulation of linoleic acid, provision of omega-3 fatty acid, a proven anti-inflammatory and immune-enhancing agent, is recommended.[45,67]

MICRONUTRIENT NEEDS

The functions of vitamins and trace elements pertinent to burn injury have been summarized elsewhere.[64,71–74] Optimal vitamin and mineral intake of the burned child remains to be determined, because few satisfactory data are available in this area of nutrition. Nevertheless, several facts are indisputable and bring to mind the importance of micronutrient supplementation. First, vitamin and mineral requirements increase with severity of thermal injury, related to heightened protein synthesis, enhanced caloric expenditure, and increased micronutrient losses. Second, individual vitamin and mineral needs are also dependent on preburn status.

Undoubtedly, a deficiency of vitamins and minerals would compromise reparative processes. However, oral, tube feeding, and intravenous hyperalimentation regimens frequently do not meet the heightened needs for certain micronutrients. Thus, it is recommended that additional supplementation be provided,[64,65,71–78] especially of those vitamins and trace elements associated with energy expenditure, wound healing, immune function, bone mineral density, coagulation, and those likely to have enhanced urinary and wound losses. Thiamine, riboflavin, niacin, folate, biotin, vitamin K, magnesium, phosphorus, chromium, and manganese are all cofactors for energy-dependent processes. The requirement for pyridoxine is closely related to dietary protein intake and protein metabolism. Vitamin B12, folate, and zinc are cofactors necessary for collagen synthesis. Furthermore, inadequacy of many micronutrients, particularly vitamins A, C, E, and pyridoxine, as well as zinc, copper, and iron inadequacies, can adversely affect immune function. Iron supplementation, however, remains controversial,[45] because excessive iron also appears to enhance susceptibility to infection.[79]

Recently, a high incidence of hypovitaminosis D was demonstrated in pediatric burn patients.[74] Recent evidence also suggests a high rate of bone demineralization and increased risk of fractures in the acute post burn phase.[80–82] Burn patients are at risk for bone disease from a variety of sources. Vitamin D depletion appears to be one such causative factor, which may require therapeutic intervention; however, the most effective means to treat this deficiency remains elusive at this time.

Daily intakes of a multivitamin and supplemental vitamin A, vitamin C, and zinc (Table 23–5) are usually suggested. Many centers administer folate and vitamin D as well, although there is much less information on which to base levels of intake at this time. Although select vitamin and mineral replacement in excess of RDAs appears to be justified in burned children, some micronutrients, particularly fat-soluble vitamins, are toxic in large amounts. Thus, all micronutrients should be administered judiciously.

NUTRITIONAL INTERVENTION STRATEGIES

Specialized nutrition support is extremely important in the rehabilitation of the infant or child who has sustained a burn injury. Many children with thermal injuries previously died from malnutrition and sepsis because nutritional support was not possible or was inadequate. There have been exceptional clinical advances in applied nutrition support in the past 25 years. The marketing of oral supplements and improvements in enteral and parenteral hyperalimentation techniques has improved nutrition supplementation options. This technological progress has had a significant positive impact on the survival of extensively burned victims.

The goal of nutritional support for the pediatric burn patient is to provide adequate calories and nutrients to offset the increased metabolic demands induced by injury and growth. Ideally, nutrition intervention should be aimed at facilitating wound healing, maximizing immunocompetence, maintaining or improving organ function, and preventing loss of lean body mass. Specific objectives vary, however, according to the underlying metabolic and nutritional status of each patient. Special consideration is indicated whenever fluid restriction, organ failure, septicemia, mechanical ventilation, or any other presenting condition limits the ability to obtain vital nutrients.

Small burns (less than 20% surface area) not complicated by facial injury, psychologic problems, inhalation injury, or preburn malnutrition can usually be supported by an oral high-protein, high-calorie diet. Between-meal snacks should be encouraged. Commercial meal-replacement beverages or the addition of nutrient modules to

Table 23–5 Vitamin and Trace Mineral Recommendations

Children and adolescents (3 years or older)

1. Major burn
   - One multivitamin daily
   - 500 mg ascorbic acid twice daily*
   - 10,000 IU vitamin A daily
   - 220 mg zinc sulfate daily*
2. Minor burn (<20%) or reconstructive patient
   - One multivitamin daily

Children (less than 3 years of age)

1. Major burn
   - One children's multivitamin daily
   - 250 mg ascorbic acid twice daily*
   - 5000 IU vitamin A daily
   - 100 mg zinc sulfate daily*
2. Minor burn (<20%) or reconstructive patient
   - One multivitamin daily

*Recommended delivery in suspension for tube feeding because oral vitamin C and zinc in large doses may precipitate nausea or vomiting.

menu selections may be helpful in boosting a marginal intake of calories or protein.

Children with burns covering a larger surface area (20% or more) generally cannot meet their nutrient requirements by oral intake alone. In these cases, alternative forms of feeding must be implemented. Nutrients should be provided enterally to the burned youngster whenever possible. The enteral route is preferred over intravenous because it is safer, gastrointestinal function is preserved, and the integrity of the small intestinal mucosal surface is better maintained,[65,83,84] thus possibly minimizing bacterial translocation from the gastrointestinal tract.[83,85,86] In general, gastric feedings are not supported for a number of reasons. These include the fact that postburn gastric ileus often inhibits the initial advancement and full-volume delivery of enteral feedings. In addition, the multiple position changes that patients undergo for dressing changes, physical therapy, and operative procedures increase the aspiration risk when fed nasogastrically. Gastric feedings also potentiate limited oral intake because the patient minimally experiences hunger.

Owing to the grave concern for possible aspiration, enteral alimentation that bypasses the stomach and uses the functional small intestine is desirable. Fluoroscopically or endoscopically placing feeding tubes into the third portion of the duodenum can be a safe means of enteral nutritional support, even during critical periods such as resuscitation, surgery, anesthesia for major dressing changes, or septic ileus.[86,87] Small bowel feedings permit minimal interruption of the nutrition regimen, thereby maximizing nutrient intake.

Determining the correct time for initiating a tube feeding program requires consideration. In general, enteral nutrition support should commence as soon as possible postburn. The obvious reasons include the fact that a significant nutrient deficit can develop when alimentation is delayed following thermal injury, which has a direct bearing on morbidity and mortality. In addition, aggressive enteral support has been associated with improved tube feeding tolerance and sustained bowel mucosal integrity.[65,84,88] Furthermore, when tube feeding is initiated within the first few hours postburn, the hypermetabolic response can be partially suppressed, as evidenced by decreased energy expenditure and improvements in measurements of nitrogen balance, visceral proteins, and catabolic hormones.[59,84,89,90]

A recent study conducted by Gottschlich and colleagues evaluated the effects of early versus delayed enteral feeding on various outcomes postburn.[91] Patients were randomized to receive enteral feedings within 24 hours (study group) or 48 hours (control) of burn injury. Results indicate that early feeding reduces cumulative caloric deficits and potentially stimulates insulin secretion while conserving lean body mass. Feeding within 24 hours of injury did not limit postburn hypermetabolism, nor did it improve nutritional status, reduce infection, or decrease hospital stay. Some question the definition of early feeding (initiated within 24 hours) applied in this study. Perhaps benefit would have been increasingly apparent if nutrition support was initiated within a few hours of insult or if the control group delayed feeds for a greater period of time. Nevertheless, this is the only prospective clinical feeding trial of its nature in pediatric burns. Additional studies are recommended to establish feeding times that maximize clinical benefit and minimize morbid outcomes.

Riegel and associates recently examined the effects of fluid resuscitation, inotrope use, and early feeding on the development of bowel necrosis.[92] Results indicated that patients with bowel necrosis had similar characteristics that divided them from those who did not infarct. Patients who sustained bowel necrosis required more fluid resuscitation during burn shock and tended to have prolonged (greater than 24 to 48 hours) burn shock. This subgroup of patients required higher doses of dopamine during burn shock and tended to receive dopamine more frequently during burn shock. Initiation of enteral feeds within 24 hours of insult did not increase the incidence of bowel necrosis in this study. As a result of this study, patients who are underresuscitated and require inotropic support greater than renal dose dopamine should be monitored for bowel necrosis during the postresuscitation phase. In addition, some recommend that trophic enteral feeds be employed for this subpopulation until fluid resuscitation is complete.

Because burn patients usually have unscathed digestive and absorptive capabilities, products containing intact nutrients should be used. Elemental or dipeptide formulations are unnecessary, unless dictated by concomitant disease or anatomic anomalies,[93] and appear to yield less-favorable results in burns.[94] Most tube feedings can be started at full strength. The initial hourly infusion rate should begin at approximately half of the final desired volume and be increased by 5 mL/hour in the infant and toddler, 10 mL/hour in the school-age child, and 20 mL/hour in the teenager, as tolerated, until the final hourly rate is achieved.

As oral intake improves and nutrient needs decrease, the child can be gradually weaned from the tube feeding regimen. Initially, tube feedings can be held at mealtime to stimulate appetite. Once the patient demonstrates the ability to consume 25–50% of caloric needs by mouth, the tube feeding program may be necessary only at night. Eventually, when the patient is able to meet approximately 75% or greater of his or her caloric needs orally, tube feedings can be discontinued.

The composition of the enteral infusate should take into account the unique metabolic and age-related alterations in nutrient utilization that accompany an extensive burn injury. Suggested tube feeding regimens for pediatric burn patients can be divided into two major categories: (1) those appropriate for children younger than 6 months of age and (2) those for patients 6 months of age or older.

Enteral protocols for infants less than 6 months of age are generally conservative, relying on commercial infant formulas. The normal dilution of infant formula is 20 kcal/oz (0.66 kcal/mL). Gradually advancing the concentration to 24 kcal/oz is routinely safe. Further progression to 27–30 kcal/oz to meet the infant's energy needs must be monitored carefully, due to the resulting increased renal solute load.

The protein content of infant formulas ranges from 9% to 12% of total calories. This level is sometimes insufficient in those with large surface area burns. The addition of a protein module to the infant formula may be indicated in such cases if, once again, the patient is carefully monitored. Infant formulas derived from soy protein should not be used unless casein or whey intolerances have been confirmed, because the biologic value of soy protein is less than that of animal protein. Nutritional support regimens containing significantly reduced-fat content are likewise not routinely recommended during infancy because fat is an extremely important nutrient during the period of central nervous system maturation.

Tube feeding products for children over 6 months of age can generally be selected from formularies established for adults. The coincident fluid needs and energy requirements normally result in utilizing a tube feeding concentration of 30 kcal/oz or 1 kcal/mL. If the tube feeding product selected is low in protein, according to the guidelines established for burn patients,[8,58,64,95] products should be enriched with protein modules to yield 20–23% of their energy content as protein.

To date, there are no commercially manufactured tube feeding formulas specifically designed for the burn patient. However, it is clear from recent studies that this patient population has atypical nutritional needs that transcend traditional recommendations for a high-calorie, high-protein solution. Modular tube feeding recipes have evolved that not only take into consideration energy and quantitative protein guidelines but also currently offer the only means of incorporating findings regarding unique fat, amino acid, vitamin, and mineral requirements.[45,65,90,96,97] Employment of modular tube feeding prescriptions has been correlated with statistically significant reductions in infection rates and length of hospital stay.[14] However, because complex recipes are not feasible at many institutions, due to the laborious, complicated preparation procedures involved, protein enrichment of commercial substrates or careful scrutiny of the formulary for a high-protein, low-fat, low linoleic acid, omega-3 fatty acid–enriched product is recommended as a practical alternative.

PARENTERAL HYPERALIMENTATION

During the late 1960s, when intravenous feeding was shown to permit growth and development, it became possible to provide nutritional support to virtually any child.[98] Although the gastrointestinal tract is the preferred route of nutritional support, under certain circumstances intravenous feeding can become a necessary, and even lifesaving, part of burn management.

Appropriate indications for intravenous feeding in burns are listed in Table 23–6. There are two general categories of pediatric patients for whom parenteral nutrition is indicated. The first major category includes youngsters with protracted diarrhea or serious tube feeding intolerance, resulting in caloric insufficiency. If at all possible, however, at least some nutrients should be administered enterally via trophic feeds during episodes of diarrhea. Children with gastrointestinal disease or injury form a second group that frequently requires total parenteral nutrition (TPN).

In general, peripheral parenteral support does not provide adequate calories and nitrogen, and the delivery of intravenous nutrients via a central line is necessary to promote anabolism in the presence of burns.[99] Standard central venous regimens for the thermally injured patient usually consist of a final concentration of 25% dextrose and 5% crystalline amino acids, although individualized balancing is often warranted.

Table 23–6 Indications for Total Parenteral Nutrition in Burns

- Gastrointestinal trauma
- Curling's ulcer
- Severe pancreatitis
- Superior mesenteric artery syndrome
- Obstructions of the gastrointestinal tract
- Severe vomiting or abdominal distention
- Intractable diarrhea
- Adjunct to insufficient enteral support
- Necrotic bowel

If essential fatty acid requirements are being met in the trophic enteral feeds, then additional intravenous fat is not necessarily warranted. Patients receiving 100% of their energy needs via the parenteral route require the administration of modest amounts of intravenous fat. Five hundred milliliters of 10% lipid emulsion (or 250 mL of 20% lipid emulsion) infused two to three times weekly will suffice in meeting essential fatty acid requirements.

The application of parenteral nutrition has undoubtedly contributed to improved outcome in pediatric burn victims unable to be supported enterally. No longer does the thermally injured patient need to deteriorate when enteral feeding is insufficient or contraindicated. However, the metabolic and mechanical complications of parenteral hyperalimentation and the high incidence of septic morbidity in burns speak for reserving TPN for those whose nutritional needs cannot be met by the enteral route. Adherence to strict protocols of infection control, along with continuous monitoring of tolerance, will most often promote a successful intravenous feeding program. Every attempt to advance the enteral feeding rate with subsequent decrease in parenteral feeds should be made to minimize the immunosuppression concomitant with the intravenous route.

NUTRITIONAL ASSESSMENT

Nutritional assessment is the process of identifying an individual's energy and nutrient requirements and evaluating the adequacy of enteral or parenteral nutrition support programs in meeting these needs. Clinical nutrition protocols for the care of burned children have been published; however, there is little specific information regarding their precise nutritional requirements.[100] Therefore, assessment and monitoring of patient response to diet therapy are especially important, so that the clinician can react to alterations in metabolism that occur over time and reduce the opportunity for complications. Tables 23–7 and 23–8 summarize the nutrition assessment program successfully employed at the Cincinnati Shriners Hospital for Children.

CONCLUSION

Burn injury in pediatrics has important ramifications for nutrition. Decisions regarding what and how to feed patients continue to pose perplexing problems. Prompt provision of individually tailored diet therapy is of paramount importance in preventing malnutrition in burned children. This nutritional challenge is complicated by the fact that the knowledge of these patients' precise nutrient requirements remains incomplete. Burned infants and children represent separate and much more complex diet therapy problems, compared with their adult counterparts, because requirements for growth and development must be considered, as well as the increased nutrient needs imposed by burns. It is obvious that there is much to learn regarding optimal feeding practices in pediatric burn patients. Further research is needed to establish more definitive guidelines for nutritional intervention in burned children.

Table 23–7 Acute Burns—Guidelines for Initial Nutrition Assessment

Collect Objective Data	*Obtain Appropriate Histories*	*Determine Preburn Nutritional Status*	*Calculate*	*Determine Appropriate Route of Feeding*	*Initiate Assessment Tools*
Age Percent total body surface area burn Percent third degree burn Body areas burned Inhalation injury Ventilatory status Gastric decompression initiated Anthropometrics: • Weight • Height/length • Head circumference (<3 years)	Past medical history Social history Concomitant injuries Routine medications Referring hospital course as applicable	Diet history Food restrictions/ allergies Dentition Appetite Vitamin/ mineral supplementation	Calorie and protein needs Vitamin/ mineral supplementation recommendations Weight percentage: Percent ideal body weight (>18 years) *NCHS growth chart percentile (≤18 years)	Oral Nasoenteral Parenteral	Obtain indirect calorimetry within 24 hours of admission Begin 24–hour urinary urea collection for nitrogen balance determination Obtain serum prealbumin Begin monitoring calorie and protein intake

*National Center for Health Statistics

Source: Reprinted from Mayes T, Gottschlich M. Burns and wound healing. *In*: The Science and Practice of Nutrition Support. A Case-Based Core Curriculum. Gottschlich MM, ed. Kendall/Hunt Publishing Co. 2001:401.

Table 23–8 Acute Burns—Recommendations for Nutrition Reassessment

Daily	*Weekly*	*Upon Discharge*
Calorie and protein intake Labs: • BUN/creatinine • Glucose • Electrolytes • Nitrogen balance Tolerance (nausea, vomiting, distention, diarrhea, constipation) Clinical course (sepsis, infection, surgeries, fluid status, medications, respiratory status) Appropriateness of diet/enteral or parenteral nutrition order	Weight (once edema resolved) Prealbumin Nitrogen balance trend Wound healing (% open wound) Indirect calorimetry: • REE • RQ	Percent preburn weight of discharge Adequacy of oral intake Nutrition supplementation requirements Need for nutrition follow-up in the outpatient setting

Source: Reprinted from Mayes T, Gottschlich MM. Burns and wound healing. *In:* The Science and Practice of Nutrition Support. A Case-Based Core Curriculum. Gottschlich MM, ed. Kendall/Hunt Publishing Co. 2002:402.

REFERENCES

1. Curreri PW, Luterman A, Braun DW, et al. Burn injury: Analysis of survival and hospitalization time for 937 patients. *Ann Surg.* 1980;192:472–478.
2. Erickson EJ, Merrell SW, Saffle JR, Sullivan JJ. Differences in mortality from thermal injury between pediatric and adult patients. *J Pediatr Surg.* 1991;26: 821–825.
3. Sheridan RL, Remensnyder JP, Schnitzer JJ, et al. Current expectations for survival in pediatric burns. *Arch Pediatr Adolesc Med.* 2000;154:245–249.
4. Klein GL, Herndon DN, Rutan TC, et al. Bone diseases in burn patients. *J Bone Miner Res.* 1993;8(3):337–345.
5. Rutan RL, Herndon DN. Growth delay in postburn pediatric patients. *Arch Surg.* 1990;125:392–395.
6. Grybowski JD. Gastrointestinal function in the infant and young child. *Clin Gastroenterol.* 1977;6:253–265.
7. Lebenthal E, Lee PC. Development of functional response in human exocrine pancreas. *Pediatrics.* 1980; 66:556–560.
8. Spitzer A. The role of the kidney in sodium homeostasis during maturation. *Kidney Int.* 1982;21:539–545.
9. Gottschlich M, Alexander JW, Bower RH. Enteral nutrition in patients with burns or trauma. In: Rombeau JL, Caldwell MD, eds., *Enteral and Tube Feeding,* 2nd ed. Philadelphia: WB Saunders Co.; 1990:306–324.
10. Cuthbertson DP, Zagreb H. The metabolic response to injury and its nutritional implications: Retrospect and prospect. *J Parenter Enter Nutr.* 1979;3:108–130.
11. Aikawa N, Caulfield JB, Thomas RJS, et al. Post burn hypermetabolism: Relation to evaporative heat loss and catecholamine level. *Surg Forum.* 1975;26:74–76.
12. Wilmore DW, Long JM, Mason AD, et al. Catecholamines: Mediators of the hypermetabolic response to thermal injury. *Ann Surg.* 1974;180:653–669.
13. Bane JW, McCaa RE, McCaa CS. The pattern of aldosterone and cortisone blood levels in thermal burn patients. *J Trauma.* 1974;14:605–611.
14. Dolocek R, Adamkova M, Sotornikova T. Endocrine response after burn. *Scand J Plast Reconstr Surg.* 1979; 13:9–16.
15. Vaughn GM, Becker RA, Allen JP, et al. Cortisol and corticotrophin in burned patients. *J Trauma.* 1982;22: 263–273.
16. Wilmore DW, Lindsey CA, Moylan JA, et al. Hyperglucagonemia after burns. *Lancet.* 1974;1:73–75.
17. Johoor F, Herndon DH, and Wolfe RR. Role of insulin and glucagon in the response of glucose and alanine kinetics in burn-injured patients. *J Clin Invest.* 1986;78: 807–814.
18. Orton CI, Segal AW, Bloom SR, et al. Hypersecretion of glucagon and gastrin in severely burned patients. *Br Med J.* 1975;2:170–172.

19. Shuck JM, Eaton RP, Shuck LW, et al. Dynamics of insulin and glucagon secretions in severely burned patients. *J Trauma.* 1977;17:706–713.
20. Shuck JM. Insulin-glucagon ratios and catabolic state. *J Trauma.* 1979;19:909–910.
21. Wilmore DW. Nutrition and metabolism following thermal injury. *Clin Plast Surg.* 1974;1:603–619.
22. Merrell SW, Saffle JR, Sullivan JJ, et al. Fluid resuscitation in thermally injured children. *Am J Surg.* 1986; 152:664–669.
23. Baxter CR, Shires T. Physiological response to crystalloid resuscitation of severe burns. *Ann NY Acad Sci.* 1968;150:874–894.
24. Caldwell FT. Energy metabolism following thermal burns. *Arch Surg.* 1976;111:181–185.
25. Caldwell FT, Bowser BH, Crabtree JH. The effect of occlusive dressings on the energy metabolism of severely burned children. *Ann Surg.* 1981;193:579–591.
26. Zawacki BE, Spitzer KW, Mason AD, et al. Does increased evaporative water loss cause hypermetabolism in burn patients? *Ann Surg.* 1970;171:236–240.
27. Cerami A. Inflammatory cytokines. *Clin Immunopathol.* 1992;62:S3–S10.
28. Tracey KJ. TNF and other cytokines in the metabolism of septic shock and cachexia. *Clin Nutr.* 1992;11:1–11.
29. Tredgett EE, Yu YM, Zhong S, et al. Role of interleukin-1 and tumor necrosis factor on energy metabolism in rabbits. *Am J Physiol.* 1988;255:E760–E768.
30. Dinarello CA. Overview: Interleukin-1 and tumor necrosis factor in inflammatory disease and the effect of dietary fatty acids on their production. In: Kinney JM, Tucker HN, eds., *Organ Metabolism and Nutritional Ideas for Future Critical Care.* New York: Raven Press; 1994:181–195.
31. Warren RS, Starnes HF, Gabrilove JL. The acute metabolic effects of tumor necrosis factor administration. *Arch Surg.* 1987;122:1396–1400.
32. Gottschlich MM, Jenkins ME, Mayes T, et al. A prospective clinical study of the polysomnographic stages of sleep following burn injury. *J Burn Care Rehabil.* 1994;15:486–492.
33. Day T, Dean P, Adams MC, et al. Nutritional requirements of the burned child: The Curreri Junior Formula. *Proc Am Burn Assoc.* 1986;18:86.
34. Davies JWL, Liljedahl SL. Metabolic consequences of an extensive burn. In: Polk HC, Stone HH, eds., *Contemporary Burn Management.* Boston: Little Brown; 1971:151–169.
35. Hildreth M, Caravajal HF. Caloric requirements in burned children: A simple formula to estimate daily caloric requirements. *J Burn Care Rehabil.* 1982;3: 78–80.
36. Hildreth MA, Herndon DN, Desai MH, Duke MA. Calorie needs of adolescent patients with burns. *J Burn Care Rehabil.* 1989;10:523–526.
37. Hildreth MA, Herndon DN, Parks DH, et al. Evaluation of a caloric requirement formula in burned children treated with early excision. *J Trauma.* 1987;27:188–189.
38. Hildreth MA, Herndon DN, Desai MH, Broemeling LD. Current treatment reduces calories required to maintain weight in pediatric patients with burns. *J Burn Care Rehabil.* 1990;11:405–409.
39. Mayes TM, Gottschlich MM, Khoury J, Waden GD. An evaluation of predicted and measured energy requirements in burned children. *J Am Diet Assoc.* 1996;96: 24–29.
40. Wolfe RR. Burn injury and increased glucose production. *J Trauma.* 1979;19:898–899.
41. Burke JF, Wolfe RR, Mullany CJ, et al. Glucose requirements following the burn injury: Parameters of optimal glucose infusion and possible hepatic and respiratory abnormalities following excessive glucose intake. *Ann Surg.* 1979;190:274–283.
42. Askanazi J, Elwyn DH, Silverberg PA, et al. Respiratory distress secondary to high carbohydrate load. *Surgery.* 1980;87:596–598.
43. Saffle JR, Medina E, Raymond J, et al. Use of indirect calorimetry in the nutritional management of burned patients. *J Trauma.* 1985;25:32–39.
44. Ireton-Jones CS. Use of indirect calorimetry in burn care. *J Burn Care Rehabil.* 1988;9:526–529.
45. Gottschlich MM, Jenkins M, Warden GD, et al. Differential effects of three enteral regimens on selected outcome parameters. *J Parenter Enter Nutr.* 1990;14: 225–236.
46. Kagan RJ, Gottschlilch MM, Mayes T, Warden GD. Estimation of calorie needs in the thermally injured child. *Proc Am Burn Assoc.* 1995;27:283.
47. Wilmore DW, Goodwin CW, Aulick LH, et al. Effect of injury and infection on visceral metabolism and circulation. *Ann Surg.* 1980;192:491–500.
48. Wilmore DW, Mason AD, Pruitt BA. Insulin response to glucose in hypermetabolic burn patients. *Ann Surg.* 1976;183:314–320.
49. Wolfe RR, Burke JF. Effect of burn trauma on glucose turnover, oxidation and recycling in guinea pigs. *Am J Physiol.* 1977;223:80–85.
50. Wolfe RR, Durkot MJ, Allsop JR, et al. Glucose metabolism in severely burned patients. *Metabolism.* 1979;28:1031–1039.
51. Wilmore DW, Orcutt TW, Mason AD, et al. Alterations in hypothalamic function following thermal injury. *J Trauma.* 1975;15:697–703.
52. McDougal WS, Wilmore DW, Pruitt BA. Effect of intravenous near isosmotic nutrient infusions on nitrogen

balance in critically ill injured patients. *Surg Gynecol Obstet.* 1977;145:408–414.

53. Hart DW, Wolf SE, Zhang X-J, et al. Efficacy of a high-carbohydrate diet in catabolic illness. *Crit Care Med.* 2001;29:1318–1324.

54. Barrocas A, Tretola R, Alonso A. Nutrition and the critically ill pulmonary patient. *Respir Care.* 1983;28: 50–61.

55. Askanazi J, Rosenbaum SH, Hyman AI, et al. Respiratory changes induced by large glucose loads of total parenteral nutrition. *JAMA.* 1980;243:1444–1447.

56. Young VR, Motil KJ, Burke JF. Energy and protein metabolism in relation to requirements of the burned pediatric patient. In: Suskind RM, ed., *Textbook of Pediatric Nutrition.* New York: Raven Press; 1981:309–340.

57. Hart DW, Wolf SE, Chinkes DL, et al. Determinants of skeletal muscle catabolism after severe burn. *Ann Surg.* 2000;232:455–465.

58. Alexander JW, MacMillan BG, Stinnett JD, et al. Beneficial effects of aggressive protein feeding in severely burned children. *Ann Surg.* 1980;192:505–517.

59. Dominioni L, Trocki O, Mochizuki H, et al. Prevention of severe postburn hypermetabolism and catabolism by immediate intragastric feeding. *J Burn Care Rehabil.* 1984;5:106–112.

60. Serog P, Baigts F, Apfelbaum M, et al. Energy and nitrogen balances in 24 severely burned patients receiving 4 isocaloric diets of about 10 MJ/m2/day (2392 kcal/m2/day). *Burns.* 1983;9:422–427.

61. Saito H, Trocki O, Wang S, et al. Metabolic and immune effects of dietary arginine supplementation after burn. *Arch Surg.* 1987;122:784–789.

62. Dominioni L, Trocki O, Fang CH, et al. Nitrogen balance and liver changes in burned guinea pigs undergoing prolonged high-protein enteral feeding. *Surg Forum.* 1983;34:99–101.

63. Dominioni L, Trocki O, Fang CH, et al. Enteral feeding in burn hypermetabolism: Nutritional and metabolic effects of different levels of calorie and protein intake. *J Parenter Enter Nutr.* 1985;9:269–279.

64. Gottschlich MM. Acute thermal injury. In: Lang CE, ed., *Nutritional Support in Critical Care.* Gaithersburg, MD: Aspen Publishers; 1987;159–181.

65. Gottschlich MM, Warden GD, Michel MA, et al. Diarrhea in tube-fed burn patients: Incidence, etiology, nutritional impact and prevention. *J Parenter Enter Nutr.* 1988;12:338–345.

66. Mochizuki H, Trocki O, Dominioni L, et al. Optimal lipid content for enteral diets following thermal injury. *J Parenter Enter Nutr.* 1984;8:638–646.

67. Gottschlich MM, Alexander JW. Fat kinetics and recommended dietary intake in burns. J *Parenter Enter Nutr.* 1987;11:85–89.

68. Long JM, Wilmore DW, Mason AD, et al. Effect of carbohydrate and fat intake on nitrogen excretion during total intravenous feeding. *Ann Surg.* 1977;185: 417–422.

69. Souba WW, Long JM, Dudrick SJ. Energy intake and stress as determinants of nitrogen excretion in rats. *Surg Forum.* 1978;29:76–77.

70. Freund H, Yoshimura N, Fischer JE. Does intravenous fat spare nitrogen in the injured rat? *Am J Surg.* 1980; 140:377–383.

71. Gottschlich MM, Warden GD. Vitamin supplementation in the burn patient. *J Burn Care Rehabil.* 1990; 11:275–279.

72. Gamliel Z, DeBiasse MA, Demling RH. Essential microminerals and their response to burn injury. *J Burn Care Rehabil.* 1996;17:264–272.

73. Jenkins ME, Gottschlich MM, Kopcha R, et al. A prospective analysis of serum vitamin K and dietary intake in severely burned pediatric patients. *J Burn Care Rehabil.* 1998;19:75–81.

74. Gottschlich MM, Mayes T, Khoury J, Warden GD. Hypovitaminosis D in acutely injured pediatric burn patients. *J Am Diet Assoc.* 2004;104:931–941.

75. Pochon JP. Zinc and copper replacement therapy: A must in burns and scalds in children? *Prog Pediatr Surg.* 1981;14:151–172.

76. King N, Goodwin CW. Use of vitamin supplements for burned patients: A national survey. *J Am Diet Assoc.* 1984;84:923–925.

77. Council on Scientific Affairs. Vitamin preparations as dietary supplements and as therapeutic agents. *JAMA.* 1987;257:1929–1936.

78. Shippee RL, Wilson SW, King N. Trace mineral supplementation of burn patients: A national survey. *J Am Diet Assoc.* 1987;87:300–303.

79. Weinberg ED. Iron and susceptibility to infectious disease. *Science.* 1974;184:952–956.

80. Klein GL, Herndon DN, Langman CB, et al. Long term reduction in bone mass after severe burn injury in children. *J Pediatr.* 1995;126:252–256.

81. Klein GL, Herndon DN, Rutan TC, et al. Bone disease in burn patients. *J Bone Miner Res.* 1993;8:337–345.

82. Mayes T, Gottschlich MM, Scanlon J, Warden GD. Four year review of burns as an etiologic factor in the development of long bone fractures in pediatric patients. *J Burn Care Rehabil.* 2003;24:279–284.

83. Saito H, Trocki O, Alexander JW, et al. The effect of route of nutrient administration on the nutritional state, catabolic hormone secretion, and gut mucosal integrity after burn injury. *J Parenter Enter Nutr.* 1987;11:1–7.

84. Saito H, Trocki O, Alexander JW. Comparison of immediate postburn enteral versus parenteral nutrition. *J Parenter Enter Nutr.* 1985;9:115.

85. Herek O, Kara IG, Kaleli I. Effects of antibiotics and Saccharomyces boulardii on bacterial translocation in burn injury. *Surg Today.* 2004;34:256–260.

86. Gottschlich MM. Early and perioperative nutrition support. In: Matarese L, Gottschlich MM, eds., *Contemporary Nutrition Support Practice.* Philadelphia: WB Saunders Co.; 1998:265–278.

87. Jenkins M, Gottschlich M, Baumer T, et al. Enteral feeding during operative procedures. *J Burn Care Rehabil.* 1994;15:199–205.

88. Mochizuki H, Trocki O, Dominioni L, et al. Mechanism of prevention of postburn hypermetabolism and catabolism by early enteral feeding. *Ann Surg.* 1984;200: 297–310.

89. Jenkins M, Gottschlich M, Waymack JP, et al. An evaluation of the effect of immediate enteral feeding on the hypermetabolic response following severe burn injury. *Proc Am Burn Assoc.* 1988;20.

90. Jenkins M, Gottschlich MM, Alexander JW, et al. Enteral alimentation in the early postburn phase. In: Blackburn GL, Bell SJ, Mullen JL, eds., *Nutritional Medicine: A Case Management Approach.* Philadelphia: WB Saunders Co.; 1989:1–5.

91. Gottschlich MM, Jenkins MJ, Mayes T. An evaluation of the safety of early versus delayed enteral support and effects on clinical, nutritional and endocrine outcomes after severe burns. *J Burn Care Rehabil.* 2002;23: 401–415.

92. Riegel T, Allgeier C, Gottschlich M, et al. Fluid resuscitation, inotropic agents and early feeding: Is there a relationship to bowel necrosis? *J Burn Care Rehabil.* 2003;24:S61.

93. Gottschlich MM. Managing chylothorax in a pediatric burn patient. *RD.* 1987;7:10–12.

94. Trocki O, Mochizuki H, Dominioni L, et al. Intact protein versus free amino acids in the nutritional support of thermally injured animals. *J Parenter Enter Nutr.* 1986;10:139–145.

95. Gottschlich MM, Alexander JW, Jenkins M, et al. Burns. In: Blackburn GL, Bell SJ, Mullen JL, eds., *Nutritional Medicine: A Case Management Approach.* Philadelphia: WB Saunders Co.; 1989:6–9.

96. Bell SJ, Molnar JA, Carey M, et al. Adequacy of a modular tube feeding diet for burned patients. *J Am Diet Assoc.* 1986;86:1386–1391.

97. Gottschlich MM, Stone M, Havens P, et al. Therapeutic effects of a modular tube feeding recipe in pediatric burn patients. *Proc Am Burn Assoc.* 1986;18:84.

98. Dudrick SJ, Wilmore DW, Vars HM, et al. Can intravenous feeding as the sole means of nutrition support growth in the child and restore weight loss in an adult? *Ann Surg.* 1969;169:974–984.

99. Gottschlich MM, Warden GD. Parenteral nutrition in the burned patient. In: Fischer JE, ed., *Total Parenteral Nutrition.* Boston: Little Brown & Co.; 1991:270–298.

100. Mayes T, Gottschlich MM, Warden GD. Clinical nutrition protocols for continuous quality improvements in the outcomes of patients with burns. *J Burn Care Rehabil.* 1997;18:365–368.

CHAPTER 24

Enteral Nutrition

Nancy Nevin-Folino and Myrna Miller

[Note that enteral feeding of the premature infant is addressed in Chapter 3 of this text.]

INTRODUCTION

Infants and children who are unwilling or unable to ingest, digest, or absorb an adequate amount of nutrients orally are candidates for supplemental feedings and/or an alternate route of nutritional support. If the patient's gastrointestinal tract is functioning, enteral nutrition is indicated.

Enteral nutritional support (ENS) refers to the nonvolitional delivery of nutrients by a tube to the gastrointestinal tract. Enteral nutrition is preferred over parenteral feeding because it is more physiologic, is associated with fewer technical and infectious complications, and is also less expensive.[1–3] Additionally, enteral feedings may be nutritionally superior to parenteral feedings because more is known about enteral nutrient requirements and utilization.[4] Advances in commercial formulas and equipment for their delivery have made enteral feeding safe and efficacious to administer to pediatric patients in either the hospital or home setting.

This chapter provides practical guidelines for:

1. selecting appropriate candidates for enteral nutrition, ranging in age from birth to 18 years
2. selecting specific products
3. administering and monitoring enteral feedings
4. considering specific factors of the pediatric population

PATIENT SELECTION

The health care team should establish criteria for consideration of ENS. Nutrition screening should identify patients who are failing to thrive or progress by self-initiated hunger or consumption of oral feeds. Factors to evaluate would include:[1,5]

1. usual calorie intake of less than 80% of needs
2. weight maintenance or loss
3. weight/length or weight/height ratio under the 5th percentile
4. excessive feeding time or physical inability to keep liquids from dribbling out of the mouth
5. oral aversion
6. mechanical problems with mastication, swallowing, or peristalsis

Pediatric patients with a variety of diseases are at nutritional risk and have been shown to benefit from ENS (Exhibit 24–1). Specific screens can be developed for a particular disease state or condition, as the need arises.[6–9]

However, when enteral nutrition is contraindicated, due to severe intestinal dysfunction (Exhibit 24–2), parenteral nutrition constitutes the appropriate route for specific nutritional support (see Chapter 25).

Exhibit 24–1 Indications for Enteral Nutrition in the Pediatric Patient

Functional
1. Neurologic disorders
2. Neuromuscular disorders
3. Prematurity
4. Inability to take in adequate nutrition
5. Genetic/metabolic disorders

Structural
1. Congenital anomalies
   a. Tracheoesophageal fistula
   b. Esophageal atresia
   c. Cleft palate
   d. Pierre Robin syndrome
2. Obstruction
   a. Cancer of head/neck
   b. Intubation
3. Injury
   a. Ingestions
   b. Trauma
   c. Sepsis
4. Surgery

Exhibit 24–2 Potential Complications for Enteral Nutrition in Pediatric Patients

Acute pancreatitis
Gastrointestinal obstruction
Inflammatory bowel disease
Intestinal atresia
Limited or impaired absorptive surface
Necrotizing enterocolitis
Overwhelming sepsis
Side effects of cancer therapy

PRODUCT SELECTION

A wide variety of commercial infant, pediatric, and adult enteral formulas can be utilized for pediatric patients. However, proper product selection is contingent on a number of factors related to the specific medical and nutritional status of the patient. Patient-specific factors include age, gastrointestinal function, history of feeding tolerance, nutrient requirements, and feeding route. Other important factors to take into consideration are formula specific. These factors include osmolality, renal solute load, nutrient complexity, product availability, cost, and caloric density.

Infants Less than 1 Year of Age

Human milk and/or commercial infant formulas constitute the most appropriate feedings for infants who are less than 1 year of age.

The available formula choices contain macronutrients in either complex or semi-elemental forms, which are suited for a variety of medical problems found in pediatrics and are listed in Table 24–1. Most manufacturers' product guides have detailed information about the indicated use of formulas and absorption/utilization routes.[10–15] The use of highly specialized formulas for infants and children with inborn errors of metabolism is addressed in Chapter 13.

The standard dilution for infant formulas is 20 kcal/oz. However, infants who have increased metabolic needs and/or a decreased fluid tolerance may not be able to consume an adequate volume of standard formulas to promote growth. In this instance, a more concentrated formula may be needed. Formulas with a caloric density greater than 20 kcal/oz are most commonly provided to infants with chronic lung disease and congenital heart disease or to those infants with chronic renal failure who require continuous ambulatory peritoneal dialysis. Concentrated infant formulas may also be useful for infants with nonorganic failure to thrive during periods of catch-up growth.

Infant formulas can be concentrated cautiously to a maximum of 30 kcal/oz (without modular additives) by adding less water to a concentrated liquid or powdered formula base.[16] If human milk is used in lieu of infant formulas, it can be "concentrated" with the addition of powdered infant formula. When this formula base (or human milk) is concentrated, the infant's water balance in relation to renal solute load should also be

Table 24–1 Characteristics of Selected Enteral Formulas

Formula Classification	*Product Characteristics*	*Possible Indications for Use*	*Infant Formula (Manufacturer)*	*Pediatric Formula (Manufacturer)*	*Adult Formula (Manufacturer)*
Standard milk based (SMB)	Intact protein Contains lactose Long-chain triglycerides Moderate residue Low to moderate osmolality	Normally functioning gastrointestinal tract Lactose tolerant	Human milk Similac Advance (Ross Products) Enfamil Lipil (Mead Johnson) Good Start (Nestles)		Compleat (Novartis)
Standard milk based, altered	Intact protein Electrolyte manipulation (low iron)	Renal, endocrine conditions	PM 60:40[†] (Ross Products)	Pediasure[‡§] (Ross Products)	Ensure (Ross Products) Osmolite[‡] (Ross Products) Isocal[‡] (Mead Johnson)
	SMB Lactose free	Lactose intolerant	Lactofree (Mead Johnson)	Resource Just for Kids[§] (Novartis)	
	Added rice starch	Mild reflux	Enfamil AR (Mead Johnson)		
Standard soy, lactose free	Intact protein Low to moderate residue Low to moderate osmolality	Primary lactase deficiency Secondary lactase deficiency (intestinal injury or PEM) Galactosemia	Isomil Advance (Ross Products) Prosobee (Mead Johnson) Alsoy (Nestles)		

continues

Table 24–1 continued

Formula Classification	*Product Characteristics*	*Possible Indications for Use*	*Infant Formula (Manufacturer)*	*Pediatric Formula (Manufacturer)*	*Adult Formula (Manufacturer)*
Standard fiber containing[¶]	Intact protein Lactose free 4.3–14 g fiber per 1,000 mL Low to moderate osmolality	Constipation Diarrhea Normal digestive and absorptive capacity		Pediasure with fiber[§] (Ross Products) Kindercal[§] (Mead Johnson) Compleat Pediatric (Novartis) Resource Just for Kids (Novartis)	Ensure with fiber (Ross Products) Jevity[‡] (Ross Products) Boost with fiber (Mead Johnson) Compleat (Novartis)
Lactose free/ modified fat	Intact protein Fat content is 88% medium-chain triglycerides and 12% long-chain triglycerides	Chylothorax Intestinal lymphangiecatasia Severe steatorrhea Cholestasis Liver disease		Portagen[‡‖] (Mead Johnson)	Portagen[‡‖] (Mead Johnson)
Semi-elemental	Hydrolyzed protein (peptides and amino acids) Lactose free Low to moderate osmolality Partial medium-chain triglyceride content	Steatorrhea Intestinal resection Cystic fibrosis Chronic liver disease Inflammatory bowel disease Diarrhea associated with hypoalbuminemia Allergy to cow's milk and soy proteins Not needed for jejunal feedings in patients with normal gastro-intestinal function	Pregestimil Lipil[‡] (Mead Johnson) Alimentum Advance[‡] (Ross Products) Nutramigen Lipil[¶] (Mead Johnson)		Vital HN[‡] (Ross Products) Reabilan[‡] (O'Brien) Subdue (Mead Johnson)

continues

Elemental	Protein in form of free amino acids Lactose free High osmolality Low fat Carbohydrate in form of glucose oligo-saccharides	Intestinal fistula Glycogen storage disease Chylothorax or intestinal lymphangiectasia not responsive to Portagen Short gut syndrome HIV+ Inflammatory bowel disease	Neocate (SHS) Ele-Care (Ross Products)	Neocate One[+§] (SHS) Ele-Care (Ross Products) Vivonex Pediatric[§] (Novartis) Peptamen Junior[§] (Nestles)	Vivonex (Novartis) Peptamen (Nestles) Perative (Nestles)
Calorically dense	Intact protein Lactose free High renal solute load High osmolality 1.5–2.0 kcal/mL	Fluid restriction Increased metabolic needs Not recommended for transpyloric feedings			Boost Plus (Mead Johnson) Ensure Plus (Ross Products) Magnacal (Sherwood Medical)
Follow-up	Increased nutrients Increased calories	Ex-premature babies for first year of life	Neocare Advance[‡] (Ross Products) Enfacare Lipil[‡] (Mead Johnson)		
	Over 1 year of age Iron fortified Balanced formulation with vitamins and minerals			Similac Advance-2 (Ross Products) Isomil Advance-2 (Ross Products) Enfamil Next Step and Next Step Soy (Mead Johnson)	

*Blenderized feedings, contain 6 g dietary fiber per liter
†Altered calcium and phosphorus, low iron
‡Contains medium-chain triglycerides as part of its total fat
§Designed for children from ages 1 to 10
‖30 kcal/oz dilution for children and adults.
¶Does not contain medium-chain triglycerides

Sources: Data from endnote references 10–13.

monitored. Patients on formulas concentrated to more than 120% (24 kcal/oz)[17,18] should be monitored frequently for signs of:

- dehydration
- irregular output (urine, stool, or emesis)
- urine specific gravity
- renal solute load
- serum electrolytes
- intolerance or nutrient toxicity

For initial fluid prescription, it is general practice to use 100 mL/kg for the first 10 kg of body weight; for weight between 10–20 kg, use 1000 mL plus 50 mL/kg for each kg over 10 kg; and for weight over 20 kg, use 1500 mL plus 20 mL/kg for each kg over 20 kg.[23,24] Adjust fluid delivery frequently based on weight gain changes. Insensible water loss should be factored, as well as additional needs caused by any medical condition.

If insensible water losses are high, it would be advisable to concentrate the base formula (or human milk) only to 24 kcal/oz. The caloric density can be then increased by utilizing modular additives of carbohydrate (glucose polymers) or fat (vegetable oil or medium-chain triglycerides). Carbohydrate and fat additives do not increase the renal solute load. However, carbohydrate additives can cause a moderate increase in osmolality. With the addition of a long-chain triglyceride, the gastric emptying time may also be decreased. This effect may be clinically significant for those patients who are at risk for aspiration and already have delayed gastric emptying.

Increases in caloric density are best tolerated by the patient when advanced gradually in increments of 2–4 kcal/oz/day.[16] Formulas that consist of a base concentration of 24–26 kcal/oz and also contain modular additives of fat (e.g., 0.25–0.50 g corn oil/oz, 2.5–5.0 kcal/oz, respectively) and/or carbohydrates (e.g., 0.5–1.0 g glucose polymer/oz, 2–4 kcal/oz, respectively) are generally tolerated by infants. Adding modulars to increase calories will change the percentage of calories from carbohydrate and fat and the ratio of protein/100 calories.

In Table 24–2, there are three comparisons of nutrient percentages and the percentage change with modulars. Patients on nutrient-skewed formula recipes should be monitored closely and changed to a more appropriate distribution of macronutrients, as tolerated.

The distribution of calories in breast milk is approximately 6–7% calories from protein, 50–52% calories from fat, and 40–43% from carbohydrate. Infant formula's distribution of macronutrients is 8–9% calories from protein, 48% calories from fat and 42–44% calories from carbohydrate.[10,11]

Protein intakes accounting for more than 16% of calories could contribute to azotemia and negative water balance if associated fluid intakes are low. Established protein needs are 2.5 to 3.3 grams

Table 24–2 Nutrients in Different Concentrations and Formula Recipes

Formula	*20 kcal/oz Standard Dilution*	*24 kcal/oz from Formula Powder or Liquid Concentrates*	*24 kcal/oz from 20 kcal/oz + 4 kcal/oz Corn Oil*
Oz per 100 calories	5	4.16	3.57
CHO (g/oz)	2.4	2.5	2.5
% calories	43	43	36
Pro g/oz	0.43	0.51	0.51
% calories	9	9	7
Fat (g/oz)	1.08	1.3	1.82
% calories	48	48	57
Protein (g per 100 kcal)	2.14	2.14	1.82

per 100 calories.[17] A minimum of 2.2 g/kg is recommended for infants younger than 3 months and a minimum of 1.8 g/kg for infants older than 3 months.[17] Additionally, high carbohydrate intakes may contribute to osmotic diarrhea, and fat intakes that exceed 60% of the formula calories could lead to ketosis.

Diluting formula to less than 20 kcal/oz should be done only with careful consideration and monitoring because of the risk of hyponatremia, diluted or insufficient nutrients, and/or excess fluid.[1,18] It is important to explain the exact amount of water to use without variance when giving formula recipe instructions to caregivers.

Children Older than 1 Year

Feedings for children who are older than 1 year of age include a choice of concentrated infant formulas, pediatric follow-up formulas, pediatric enteral formulas, various homemade blenderized feedings, and/or a number of commercial adult formulas. The caloric density of feedings utilized for children in this age group is approximately 30 kcal/oz. Once again, the caloric density may need to be increased further if the patients have increased metabolic needs and/or decreased fluid tolerance.

Formulas designed for pediatric enteral feedings meet the daily recommended dietary allowances (RDAs) for children who are younger than 11 years of age in approximately 1,000 to 1,100 mL per day (see Appendix I). These enteral products are isotonic and lactose free, with a partial medium-chain triglyceride content to facilitate absorption.

Under specific conditions, infant formulas can be continued through 4 years of age. These formulas can be concentrated to provide higher levels of nutrients, but also have a higher osmolality. Additional vitamin or mineral supplementation may also be needed, depending on the specific volume provided. Altered formulas have not been tested in vitro or processed by the manufacturer to be absorbed or used by the body as the original product. Adding nutrient supplementation, such as calcium or phosphorus, to a formula does not guarantee that the patient will be able to utilize the extra nutrients. Infant formulas have a lower renal solute load than do products designed for patients who are older than 1 year of age. These formulas may be more appropriate for malnourished toddlers who may actually be infant size.

Adolescents

For children between 10 and 18 years, many factors require consideration, such as maturation level, physical ability or limitations, calorie requirements, and volume tolerance. Adolescent nutrient needs increase with the last growth phase. Their calorie and protein needs may be met in a pediatric formula but not other nutrients, such as calcium and iron. Micronutrient analysis is helpful in matching a formula or combination of pediatric and adult formulas to meet the unique needs of the teen. There are a variety of computer nutrition assessment programs available, and when selecting one, pediatric parameters and pediatric formulas within the database should be considered in the selection criteria.

Blenderized Feedings

Blenderized feedings consist of a mixture of various meats, fruits, vegetables, milk (or formula), carbohydrates, fats, water, vitamins, and minerals. These blenderized feeding recipes can be made for use in an institution or in the home setting. Blenderized feedings are moderate in residue and moderate to high in osmolality and viscosity. Because their high viscosity hinders flow through small feeding tubes, these feedings are most often administered as gastrostomy tube feedings. Other disadvantages of blenderized feedings include a potentially high bacteria count[19–22] and the additional labor required for preparation. Homemade blenderized feedings:

1. provide a more variable nutrient content than do commercially manufactured products
2. are not emulsified

3. can be used only when enteral feeding is delivered into the stomach
4. do not necessarily contain all essential nutrients in the level that a pediatric patient requires

Blenderized feedings are considered for use today in the health care arena when third-party reimbursement or support is not provided. Although homemade formulas seem to be more economic in the home setting using food products, nutrient adequacy or variety is not taken into account. Economics becomes particularly important to families of children with chronic diseases, and blenderized concoctions will continue to represent a viable feeding alternative when a pediatric specific product is not covered.

Because inappropriate homemade tube feedings can result in hypernatremic dehydration[23] and a number of nutrient deficiencies, it is important to perform a periodic analysis of the recipe, including verification of how the family is making the formula at home, the adequacy of the nutrients, and the associated fluids. It is equally important to monitor the intake of protein and electrolytes because excess may lead to a negative water balance in the patient.[23]

Commercial Adult Formulas

A large variety of adult enteral products is commercially available. These products contain macronutrients in various forms and percentages. They can be divided into several general categories: standard milk based, lactose free, elemental, fiber containing, and calorically dense. General characteristics of selected adult enteral products with possible indications for use are covered in Table 24–1. This list is not inclusive of all products that are commercially available but is intended to provide examples of products that are available in each general category. Information regarding the complete nutrient composition of commercial adult formulas is readily available from various manufacturers.

It should be noted that adult enteral products have not been designed for use in children nor have they been extensively tested in the pediatric population. Specific concerns regarding the use of these products in children are addressed in the upcoming discussions of renal solute load and nutrient requirements.

Renal Solute Load and Fluid Balance

The renal solute load of a formula consists primarily of electrolytes and metabolic end products of protein metabolism that must be excreted in the urine.[18] These solutes require water for urinary excretion. Infants have an immature renal system with limited concentrating ability, and they require more free water to excrete solutes than do older children and adults. Therefore, infants are at particular risk for negative water balance and subsequent dehydration. Potential renal solute load (PRSL) does not need to be calculated routinely, but is important with patients who have medical problems or formula prescriptions that would influence renal metabolism. Equations for PRSL vary in the units of measurement for solute load.[1] An example equation is as follows:

$$\text{PRSL (mOsm/L)} = \text{mEq sodium/L} + \text{mEq potassium/L} + \text{mEq chloride/L} + [4 \times \text{protein(g)/L}]$$

The renal solute load and fluid balance should be closely monitored when infants have a low fluid intake, are receiving calorically dense feedings, or have increased extrarenal fluid losses (i.e., fever, diarrhea, sweating) and/or impaired renal concentrating ability.[18] Neurologically impaired infants and children who are unable to indicate thirst may also be at risk for dehydration.

Infant formulas at standard dilution contain approximately 95% water[10] (preformed water plus water of oxidation). In contrast, standard adult enteral formulas contain approximately 85% water. Because adult formulas are also higher in protein and electrolytes, this contributes to a higher renal solute load. Therefore, when administering adult products to infants and toddlers, proper precautions should be taken. For example, additional water may be required and can usually be given while flushing the feeding tube.

Osmolality

Osmolality refers to the number of particles in a kilogram of solution. The osmolality of a formula may affect the tolerance. Feeding intolerances associated with delivering a hyperosmolar formula may include delayed gastric emptying, abdominal distention, vomiting, or diarrhea.

Carbohydrates, electrolytes, and amino acids are the major factors that determine the gastrointestinal osmotic load of a formula. Smaller particles, such as glucose and free amino acids, contribute more to a higher osmolality than do larger particles, such as polysaccharides or intact protein molecules. Thus, formulas that contain hydrolyzed protein and monosaccharides will tend to have a higher osmolality than will formulas with intact protein and glucose polymers.

Recommendations for infant formulas are an osmolality less than 460 mOsm/kg.[18] Therefore, the osmolality in formulas for infants and children younger than 4 years should be less than 400 mOsm/kg and for older children under 600 mOsm/kg.[1,18] The osmolality of infant formulas at a caloric density of 20 kcal/oz generally falls below this suggested limit (range of 150–380 mOsm/kg). However, several adult enteral products exceed this limit at a caloric density of 30 kcal/oz and may require a dilution to two thirds strength prior to use in infants. Medications can increase osmolality significantly and should be evaluated.[24] The osmolality of Pregestimil concentrated to 27 kcal/ oz is approximately 496 mOsm/kg, whereas a multivitamin with iron (Poly-Vi-Sol with Iron) at 10 mg/1mL Fe is 10,683 mOsm/kg.[24]

Nutrient Requirements

The DRIs published by the National Academy of Sciences (Food and Nutrition Board) are the standards most frequently used for the assessment of enteral intakes of children.[25] It should be noted that the RDAs were intended to be recommendations for a healthy population and may not reflect the needs imposed by specific disease states or treatment modalities. In addition, the RDAs (with the exception of energy) include a safety factor that exceeds the requirements of most people to ensure that the specific needs of the majority of the population will be met.

DRIs (RDAs) used as a standard for comparison with nonambulatory, ill, or physically delayed children must be done with consideration. Values for specific conditions such as spina bifida, Down syndrome, and bronchopulmonary dysplasia have been established.[26–28] Calorie levels are based on cm/height or percentage of RDAs.

The DRI and the RDA may both be lower than potential therapeutic needs dictated by specific disease or deficiency states. In specific circumstances, both infant and adult formulas may require vitamin and/or mineral supplementation.

Again, supplements may not be absorbed or utilized in the body as desired and should be evaluated frequently. Infant formulas that contain iron generally provide adequate amounts of vitamins and minerals with a volume of 1 quart. However, infants who have restricted fluid intakes (e.g., infants with congenital heart disease) may require vitamin and mineral supplementation.

Adult enteral formulas are designed to provide the adult RDAs for vitamins and minerals when a volume of 1,500–2,000 mL/day is administered. However, when these adult enteral products are administered to children at lower volumes, some nutrients may not be adequate. A micronutrient analysis may be warranted.

PRODUCT AVAILABILITY AND COST

The cost of commercial enteral formulas may exceed the financial resources of some families. Therefore, whenever medically possible, the least specialized enteral product should be considered. The more specialized the feedings are (i.e., hydrolyzed protein and medium-chain triglyceride oil), the higher will be the cost.

Formula costs do not necessarily constitute a socioeconomic barrier. Infants and children who range in age from birth to 5 years may be enrolled in the Women, Infant, and Children (WIC) nutrition program if their family income falls below a certain level. A variety of infant formulas is available through this program. The Medicaid program and private insurance companies may cover enteral formulas and needed supplies, such as tubes, bags, or pumps. Coverage varies and the health care team should work closely with home care companies and insurers to ensure that the patient obtains the best coverage possible.

Selection of Specific Feeding Routes

Common routes for enteral nutrition in pediatric patients include nasogastric, nasoduodenal, nasojejunal, gastrostomy, and jejunostomy feedings. The risk of aspiration becomes a major consideration when determining whether the tube should be placed in the stomach or small intestine. Evaluation process for gastroesophageal reflux (GER) may include UGI, modified barium swallow, pH probe, and occasional esophageal motility. See Figure 24–1 for a decision tree as to the use of nasogastric or enterostomy feeding routes. If the patient is determined to have a high risk of aspiration due to GER, surgical placement of a gastrostomy is done, along with a fundoplication (surgical repair for GER). Figure 24-1 gives criteria for making a decision to use a nasogastric or enterostomy feeding route.[29]

Gastric Feeding

A direct gastric feeding is preferable to an intestinal feeding because it allows for a more normal digestive process. This is generally true because the stomach serves as a reservoir and

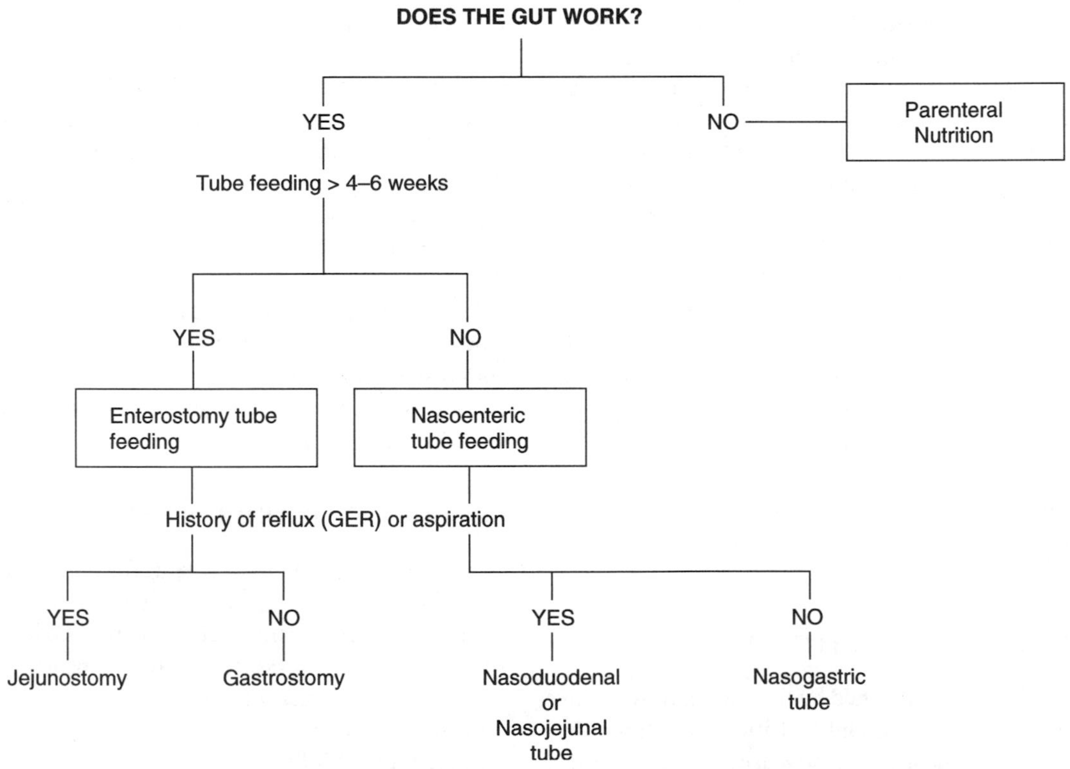

Figure 24–1 Decision Making for Selecting the Feeding Site. *Source:* Adapted with permission from Enteral and tube feedings. In: Rombeau JL, Caldwell MD, eds., *Clinical Nutrition*, vol. 1. © 1984, WB Saunders Co.

provides for a gradual release of nutrients into the small bowel. Gastric feedings are associated with a larger osmotic and volume tolerance, a more flexible feeding schedule, easier tube insertions, and a lower frequency of diarrhea and dumping syndrome. In addition, gastric acid has a bactericidal effect that may be an important factor in decreasing the patient's susceptibility to various infections. See Table 24–3 for enteral feeding sites and routes.

Nasogastric feeding tubes are used for the short term (4 to 6 weeks). Patients requiring long-term enteral nutrition are then evaluated to determine the best enteral device to meet their needs.

Nasogastric feeding is contraindicated in patients with severe esophagitis or who have an obstruction between the nose and stomach. In addition, nasogastric tubes may not be tolerated in neonates, who are obligate nose breathers. To prevent airway occlusion in this instance, orogastric tubes are often used when tube feeding is indicated.

Transpyloric Feedings

Nasoduodenal, nasojejunal, or gastrojejunal feeding is desirable for patients who are at risk of aspiration. Typically, this includes patients who have a diminished gag reflex, delayed gastric emptying, frequent vomiting, or severe gastroesophageal reflux. Nasoenteric tube placement is the most common route of enteral access. These tubes may fail secondary to tube occlusion or tube dislodgement and interrupt tube feeding and medication schedule.[30]

Nasojejunal feeding may be more efficacious than nasoduodenal feeding in preventing aspiration. Gastric reflux of duodenally administered solutions can be a problem. Additionally, nasoduodenal tubes may fail to enter or stay in the duodenum, resulting in aspiration.[30] Nasojejunal tubes may also be less likely than nasoduodenal tubes to become dislodged in children with cystic fibrosis, who may experience severe coughing episodes. This is also true for children with cancer, who may have vomiting associated with chemotherapy. Specific procedures for nasoduodenal or nasojejunal intubation have been outlined by Wesley.[31] The enteric position of the tube requires radiographic verification before feeding is initiated. A potential complication of transpyloric feeding is intestinal perforation with use of stiff, large-bore tubes.[31] Use of small-bore tubes made of polyurethane or silicone might decrease the incidence of this complication; however, there may be an increase in tube clogging.

Jejunostomy Feeding

Many enteral feeding devices are currently available. Endoscopically placed gastrostomies or jejunostomies (PEG/PEJ) are becoming very popular because they are less invasive and require less anesthesia time or even conscious sedation.[32]

Low-profile gastrostomy devices are frequently used as replacement devices after the stoma tract is well healed (usually 6 to 8 weeks). There are also low-profile devices that can be placed initially as a one-step procedure.[32] Enteral feedings, although safer than parenteral nutrition, are not without complications (see Table 24–4).

ADMINISTRATION OF FEEDING

Methods of Delivery

The specific method utilized for feeding delivery is contingent on the clinical condition of the patient and the anatomic location of the tube (gastric or transpyloric). Continuous drip and intermittent bolus administration are the two methods most often used for delivery of enteral feedings to infants and children. Intermittent bolus feedings are generally delivered to the stomach by gravity over 15 to 30 minutes on a schedule of every 2 to 4 hours. In contrast, the continuous drip method provides an infusion of nutrients at a constant rate over several hours. Continuous drip feedings are beneficial for patients with altered gastrointestinal function and essential for those receiving enteral transpyloric or nocturnal feedings. Each method of delivery provides a number of specific advantages and

Table 24–3 Enteral Feeding Sites and Routes

Site	*Route*	*Advantage*	*Disadvantages*	*Indications*	*Contraindication*
Stomach		Anti-infective mechanism Allows for normal processes and hormonal responses Tolerances of larger osmotic loads Decreased incidence of dumping syndrome Greater mobility between feedings Greater flexibility in feeding schedule and formula choice		As the first consideration for enteral nutrition	Delayed gastric emptying Pulmonary aspiration GER Intractable vomiting Impaired or absent gag reflex
	Orogastric	Does not obstruct nasal passage	May increase salivary flow and make clearance more difficult	< 34-wk gestation with gag; doesn't obstruct nasal passage	> 34-wk gestation or when patient acquires a gag
	Nasogastric	Easy intubation Surgery not required	Nasal, esophageal, or tracheal irritation Local skin care required Easily dislodged by a toddler Easily dislodged by a forceful cough May stimulate gag Caretaker must be well-trained Limited long-term compliance in the home care setting	For short- term use	Same as for the stomach
	Gastrostomy	Allows patient greater mobility Feedings are generally well-tolerated	Requires a surgical procedure for placement May result in increased GER	Prolonged enteral nutrition support	Same as for the stomach

		Larger diameter feeding tube lessens chances of obstruction/clogged feeding tube Doesn't obstruct the airway	Occasional leakage around the insertion site Skin irritation and infection Difficulty hiding the external portion of the tube under clothing Risk of intra-abdominal leak with peritonitis		
Small Bowel		Can feed enterally despite poor gastric motility and persistent high gastric residuals Lessens the chances of gastric distention	Less mixing of formula with pancreatic enzymes Tube easily malpositioned Greater exposure to radiation when checking placement Greater risk of bacterial overgrowth Changes small bowel intestinal flora May limit choices of feeding schedule and formula selection	Congenital upper GI anomalies Inadequate gastric motility After upper GI surgery Patients with increased risk of aspiration	Nonfunctioning GI tract
	Nasojejunal		Requires radiographic proof of adequate placement Takes a long time to pass without radiographic placement Tube easily displaced during peristalsis	For short-term nutrition support	
	Jejunostomy		Technically difficult to place	Jejunal feedings for >6 mo For postop nutritional management of abdominal surgery while an ileus exists	Patient at operative risk

Source: Copyright © 1990, K. Hendricks and W. Walker.

disadvantages (see Exhibit 24–3). In practice, the individual patient's tolerance ultimately dictates the method of delivery.

Pumps

Enteral feeding pumps are typically utilized to control the rate of delivery of continuous drip feedings. A number of enteral feeding pumps are available for use in pediatric patients.[33] Portable enteral pumps allow for greater patient mobility.

Important features of enteral pumps for use in the pediatric population include the ability to provide low delivery rates (less than 5 mL/hour) and to advance in small increments (1 to 5 mL/hour). Other desirable features of pediatric pumps include tamper-proof controls, an occlusion alarm, and a low-battery indicator.[34] These features all contribute to the safe and efficient delivery of continuous tube feedings for the pediatric population.

Initiation and Advancement of Feedings

There are published recommendations for advancing enteral nutrition in pediatric patients.[35] Many of these recommendations are based on institutional practices and modification of adult regimens. Generally, the rate of advancement of a feeding regimen (Exhibit 24–4) is contingent on the structure and function of the patient's gastrointestinal tract. Plan for a 2 to 5 day time frame to meet the nutritional goal. Use isotonic feedings initially and avoid making changes in volume and concentration simultaneously. Dilute feedings can be considered for patients with altered gastrointestinal function or when transitioning to enteral feeding from parenteral nutrition. For gut sensitive patients, advancing every 2 to 3 days may be warranted. Increase volume before concentration when administering transpyloric feedings. Advance concentration before volume when delivering gastric feedings. If feeding intolerance develops, return to the pre-

Exhibit 24–3 Methods of Delivering Enteral Feedings

Continuous Drip Feedings

Advantages	*Disadvantages*
1. Ability to increase volume of formula more rapidly	1. More expensive feeding method because a pump is required for delivery
2. Improved absorption of major nutrients in infants with intestinal diseases	2. Restricts patient ambulation
3. Reduced stool output in hypermetabolic patients	3. Less physiologic
4. Associated with a reduced incidence of vomiting in infants with gastroesophageal reflux	
5. Greater caloric intake when volume tolerance may be a problem	

Intermittent Feedings

Advantages	*Disadvantages*
1. More physiologic because a normal feeding schedule is mimicked	1. Associated with a longer time to reach nutritional goals
2. Less expensive because an enteral pump is not required	2. Reduced weight gain and nutrient absorption in infants with malabsorption
3. Greater flexibility in feeding schedule	3. Larger-bore tube may be required for gravity administration
4. Freedom from infusion equipment	4. More time required for administration than for pump-delivered feedings
5. Improved nitrogen retention with less fat and fluid accumulation	

Exhibit 24–4 Initiation and Advancement of Feedings

Continuous Drip Feeding*

Age	Weight Range (kg)	Volume Range (ml/kg/d)	Initial Rate (ml/h)	Advancement Rate (ml/h)	Maximum Rate (ml/h)
Infant	3–10	125–160	1 ml	1.5–3	25–50
Toddler/preschool	10–20	110–130	1 ml	5–10	60–70
School age	20–40	70–110	2 ml	5–10	80–100
Teenage	>40	60–80	2 ml	20–100	100–150

Intermittent Feedings**

Age	Weight (kg)	Kcal/kg	Suggested Advancement*** 1st day (ml)	advance to and evaluate for tolerance (ml)
Infant	3–10	98–108	250	1000
Toddler/preschool	10–20	70–100	450	1800
School age	20–40	60–90	675	2700
Teenage	>40	40–55	700	2800

*Adjust per needs, tolerance, and medical condition
**Adjust to needs and intake by mouth
***Divided over number of feeds

viously tolerated concentration and volume, and advance with caution.

For intermittent feeding, determine the total volume of formula needed to provide the nutritional goal. Advance to total desired volume (4 to 8 feedings) over a 4-day period. Administer by gravity over 15 to 30 minutes.[34]

Long-term parenteral nutrition support or malnutrition can cause a number of physiologic alterations of the gastrointestinal tract that may affect a child's ability to digest and absorb nutrients. The various functional and histologic changes generally associated with malnutrition include:[35,36]

1. shortened microvilli
2. decreased production of a number of pancreatic enzymes, including lipase, trypsin, and amylase
3. decreased brush border enzyme activities of maltase, sucrase, and lactase

Parenteral nutrition support without concomitant enteral feeding also has been shown to lead to a decrease in enteric mucosal mass and associated brush border enzymes.[2] Therefore, children who are being weaned from parenteral nutrition and/or who are malnourished generally require a more conservative feeding progression than what is typically administered to children who have normal gastrointestinal function.

Breast Milk Tube Feedings

Human milk provides the optimal feeding for infants and offers many immunologic and nutritional benefits. Infants who are unable to nurse at the breast can receive pumped breast milk through a feeding tube. However, the delivery of breast milk by tube requires some unique considerations. First of all, the mother must be taught safe methods for the collection and storage of her milk.[34] Breast milk administration techniques also should be devised and implemented.

Continuous drip feedings of human milk have been associated with appreciable fat losses, which result in a significant reduction of energy delivered to the infant.[37] These losses occur because the fat in human milk separates and collects in the infusion system. A caloric loss of approximately 20% is typical. The delivery of essential fatty acids, phospholipids, cholesterol, and associated fat-soluble vitamins may also be diminished. It should be noted that when residual milk is flushed from the tubing, a large fat bolus may be delivered to the patient. Patients with impaired gastrointestinal function may not tolerate a fat bolus.

Short-term refrigeration of human milk has been shown to increase the delivery of fat during continuous feedings.[38] Unfortunately, significant fat losses still occur. Therefore, when delivering a continuous feeding of breast milk, the use of refrigerated milk may be advantageous. If continuous feedings of expressed breast milk are required, combining the expressed breast milk with a liquid fortifier or other liquid formulas can promote more efficient delivery of breast milk nutrients via tube.[34]

Intermittent bolus feeding of human milk, in contrast, does not result in a significant loss of fat in the tubing or the terminal delivery of a large fat bolus.[37] Therefore, intermittent bolus feeding is the preferred method of delivery for the tube feeding of human milk, whenever possible.

PREVENTION AND TREATMENT OF COMPLICATIONS

Potential complications are generally classified into gastrointestinal, mechanical (tube-related), metabolic, and psychologic categories. Some pediatric studies have reported complications that include various mechanical problems related to gastrostomy[39,40] and to nasogastric tubes,[41,42] metabolic disturbances, and feeding disorders that are related to the delayed introduction of oral feedings.[43] Additionally, gastrointestinal complications have been associated with low serum albumin levels in pediatric surgical patients,[44] delayed enteral support in pediatric burn patients,[45] and with contaminated feedings. A summary of the most common complications and associated management suggestions is presented in Table 24–4.

Formulas that require reconstitution or manipulation (dilution or additives) are at the greatest risk for bacterial contamination.[46] In contrast, the use of sterile, undiluted "ready-to-feed" products minimizes the risk of contamination (see Exhibit 24-5).

Precautions that should be taken to guard against the contamination of enteral feedings include the frequent changing of the feeding bag tubing, careful attention to clean technique during handling of the feedings, and limiting of the hang time of the formulas. Specific recommendations for preparation, administration, and monitoring of enteral feedings to maximize bacteriologic safety have been published.[47,48] Of note, disposable enteral feeding bags should not be reused.

WEANING

When the patient's medical condition allows for normal oral feedings, weaning from tube feedings can be initiated. The management of the transition back to oral feedings is multifaceted and involves the medical team, the patient, and the caregivers.[49] A complete weaning from ENS should not be considered until the patient has achieved a satisfactory nutritional status, because the patient may stop gaining weight for a time during the transition.

The weaning time may vary from a few days to several months. Records of the patient's oral intake should be kept during this time because it is important to maintain an adequate intake. Tube feedings should be continued until the patient can demonstrate that nutrient requirements can be met consistently by the oral intake. Some patients use enteral nutrition in combination with parenteral nutrition and/or oral intake.[50] The combination of enteral and cycled parenteral nutrition is controlled on the basis of patient tolerance. Monitoring for intolerance or complications would be completed similarly to any nutrition

Table 24–4 Complications of Enteral Feeding

Complication	*Possible Cause*	*Management/Prevention*
	Gastrointestinal	
Aspiration Pneumonia	Aspiration of feedings Emesis Displacement or migration Supine position during feeds Gastroesophageal reflux	Confirm tube placement prior to administration of feedings Elevate head 30 to 45 degrees
	Presence of nasogastric tube preventing complete closure of esophagus	Tube placement into the duodenum
	Delayed gastric emptying	Use of prokinetics
Bloating/Cramps/Gas	Air in tubing	Remove as much air as possible when setting up feeding
Diarrhea	Bacterial contamination of formula	Proper storage, preparation, and administration of feedings Change feeding bag daily Limit hang time of formulas to 8–12 hrs for commercially manufactured products Undiluted "ready-to-feed" products minimize risk
	Food allergies	Consider changing to formula that is lactose free
	Hyperosmolar formulas	Consider changing formula to an isotonic product
	Too rapid infusion	Slow down rate of infusion to previously tolerated rate
	Low fiber intake	Consider using a fiber-containing product
	Fat malabsorption	Consider changing formula to a product with partial medium-chain triglyceride content
	Medications (antibiotics), antacids, sorbitol, magnesium, antineoplastic agents	
Dumping Syndrom	Cold formula	Administer formula at room temperature
	Rapid feeding	Slow down rate of feeding
Vomiting	Hyperosmolar formulas Delayed gastric emptying	Consider changing formula to an isotonic product Consider transpyloric route for feeding

continues

Table 24–4 continued

Complication	*Possible Cause*	*Management/Prevention*
	Gastrointestinal	
		Consider continuous infusion Elevate head of bed 45 degrees during feeding administration Check residuals prior to feedings Consider utilizing prokinetics
	Obstruction	Discontinue feedings
	Too rapid advancement of volume and/or concentration	Return to previously tolerated strength and volume, and advance more slowly
	Mechanical	
Clogged Tube	Inadequate flushing	Flush tube before and after aspirating residuals, after bolus feedings, and every 4–8 hours during continuous feedings
	Inadequate crushing of medications	Dissolve crushed tablets in warm water Use liquid form of medication instead of crushed tablet whenever possible
	Formula and medication residue	Flush tube before and after medication administration Avoid mixing formula with medication
	Kinking of the feeding tube	Replace feeding tube
	Highly viscous fiber-rich formulas	
Tube Displacement	Coughing Vomiting Inadvertent dislodgment Removal of tube by patient	Replace the tube
	Metabolic	
Dehydration	Inadequate free water	Monitor intake and output Monitor hydration status of patient routinely
	Hyperosmolar formulas	Assess renal solute load of formula
Overhydration	Excessive fluid administration	Advance feedings slowly
	Too rapid refeeding or patients with moderate to severe PEM	Allow a 5- to 7-day period to meet nutritional goals
Electrolyte imbalance	Formula components	Evaluate electrolyte adequacy of specific formula and appropriateness of formula dilution

Table 24–4 continued

Complication	*Possible Cause*	*Management/Prevention*
	Metabolic	
	Medical condition/diagnosis	Monitor electrolytes, phosphorus, BUN, creatinine, glucose
Failure to achieve appropriate weight gain	Inadequate nutrient intake	Evaluate adequacy of nutrient intake Perform routine nutritional assessments
	Psychologic	
Fear of tube insertion	Psychologic trauma associated with insertion of nasogastric tube/ gastrostomy	Utilize relaxation techniques Medical play—child to handle tube tube and insert tube in doll Comfort child after tube insertion Consider sedation prior to replacement of gastrostomy tube
Altered body image	Visible presence of nasogastric tube or gastrostomy tube	Consider nocturnal feedings and removal of tube during the day Consider use of low-profile gastrostomy device
Food refusal	Deprivation of normal oral feeding experiences	Initiate oral feedings when medically possible Provide positive oral experiences during tube feedings Referral to speech therapist

Source: Data from endnote reference 27.

delivery that is provided and not patient initiated. A combination of enteral and oral feedings is more difficult to project. Total daily requirements in fluid and calories are calculated, then enteral feedings are used to complete what the oral feedings lack. To stimulate hunger, the enteral feeds will need to be decreased. A guideline is to begin with a 25% decrease in the caloric intake by tube, then start to offer oral feeds. This transition will require evaluation frequently because of the risk of decrease in growth with a lower caloric intake or if the child has trouble or delay in progressing. If the oral intake varies from day to day, a sliding scale for supplemental enteral feeds should be created. To summarize the recommendations at the time of transition, Glass and Lucas[51] suggest normalizing the tube feeding schedule to approximate the timing of meals and snacks, altering the feeding schedule to promote hunger, reducing the calories from tube feedings, providing adequate fluids, and, as oral intake increases, adjusting the tube feedings accordingly.

Feeding Disorders

Infant and toddler feeding disorders constitute a tube-feeding complication that is unique to the pediatric population. Many times, when a chronically ill infant is medically ready to begin oral feedings, the infant or toddler may display no

Exhibit 24–5 Guidelines for Storage and Administration of Enteral Feedings (in hours)

(See references for neonates and immune–compromised patients)

Manufacturer's guidelines and/or hospital policy should be followed for any manipulation of enteral nutrition products. Equipment with ice packs may be used in overnight delivery, but temperatures must be checked routinely to ensure safety.
All enteral nutrition products should be placed in food-grade containers.

	Storage Time		*Hang Time*[1]	*Bag Change*	*Tubing Change*
Product	*Room Temp*	*Refrigerator*			
EBM/EBM with fortifiers[2]	2	24	2 / 2–4[5]	4	4
Sterile formula[3], nonsterile with additives, or powdered formula[4]	≤4	24	4	4	4
Infant, pediatric, and adult sterile, canned-bottled liquid products	8	48	8	8	Infants 8 Pediatric 24

1. Hang time includes all periods of time that the product is not refrigerated below 45°F, i.e., transport time; tubing or equipment set-up.
2. For hospitalized infants.
3. Sterile feeds include industrially produced, prepacked-liquid formulas that are "commercially sterile."
4. Nonsterile feedings are those that may contain live bacteria and include hospital- or home-prepared formulas, reconstituted powered feedings, and commercial liquid formulas to which nutrients and/or other supplements have been added in the hospital kitchen, pharmacy, unit, school, or home. Powdered formula is not recommended for neonates or immune compromised patients, unless there is no alternative available.
5. One manufacturer recommends 2 hours and other companies recommend 4 hours.

Source: Data from endnote references 19, 47, and 48.

interest in eating or may respond with actual hysteria when food, liquid, or utensils are near the face. In this situation, the child typically refuses, cries, gags, or vomits when offered feedings. This oral aversion can occur in children with or without mechanical eating problems.

Due to the emotional component of eating/feeding, a dysfunctional or uninformed family may further the trauma of eating by force feeding. Children who have been given ENS often do not have normal hunger cycles, normal eating experiences at a table, or a mealtime routine. All of these points should be addressed when the transition to oral feeding occurs. Severe cases of oral aversion require intervention and behavior modification from pediatric psychologists, as well as other health professionals such as speech pathologists, dietitians, and occupational therapists.[52]

Illingsworth and Lister[53] suggest that resistant feeding behavior may be due to missing a "critical period" in the development of the child's feeding skills. They indicate that the critical period for the development of chewing skills is 6 to 7 months of age; if solids are not introduced during this time, the child typically will have difficulty accepting them later.

Other important oral experiences during the first year of life include the development of the rooting and sucking reflexes, the oral exploration of objects, and the association of hunger with feeding.[53] When a child is deprived of these normal oral feeding experiences during the first year of life, he or she may subsequently experience feeding difficulties that last throughout the toddler and preschool years. These children may also demonstrate significant delays in gross motor and personality development.[43] Daily oral therapy or "mouth play" can help to eliminate or reduce the problems that typically occur in the patient with nonoral nutrition support. Most feeding problems can be resolved or improved through medical, oral motor, and behavioral therapy.[54,55]

Initiating oral feedings as soon as medically possible can minimize feeding disorders. Concomitant speech or feeding therapy with ENS can help to alleviate oral aversion.[56] Nonnutritive sucking during tube feedings in infancy can help to stimulate oral sucking and swallowing behavior. Pediatric occupational therapists or speech pathologists are the health professionals most qualified to assess an infant's feeding potential and to design an appropriate, ongoing oral motor stimulation program. Intervention should be considered during enteral feeding rather than at the termination of enteral feeding. Lastly, textured foods ideally should be offered, if medically feasible, when the infant is at a developmental age of 6 to 7 months. Positive caregiver-child mealtime interactions are critical for achieving feeding success.[57]

Swallowing Disorders

Eating/swallowing disorder therapy often includes recommendations to thicken liquids for therapy in the management of an infant or child who has been diagnosed with misswallowing by modified barium swallow studies using videofluoroscopy. This diagnosis means that, on regular fluid consistency, the patient is at risk for aspiration or actually aspirates. Several disease states or conditions contribute to misswallowing.[58]

Swallowing dysfunction is compounded in infants or young children who have not learned the act of swallowing. A behavioral eating plan is a complicated process because the family and/or medical team are often trying to avoid an alternative feeding delivery. Developmental progress, therapy, and nutrition all must be considered as the patient's plan is developed.[59]

Adding a thickening agent or food to the formula or liquid thickens the fluid so that the patient can swallow liquid with decreased risk of aspiration. If at all possible, a gel thickener should be considered. They are made from gum substances and contribute no calorie or carbohydrate value.[60] Powdered thickeners have nutritional consequences. The more thickener that is required, the more effect this will have on the nutrition content of the intake. Available powdered commercial thickening agents are carbohydrate based, with few or no other nutrients. Adding a carbohydrate product will skew the nutrients, add calories, and increase free water needs in a medically unstable patient or one who is at risk for dehydration. The recipe for thickened consistency is included with the package label, and the categories for thickening generally are nectar, honey, and pudding consistencies.

An example is a baby who is 3 months old, taking 22 oz of 20 kcal/oz formula, growing well, and is diagnosed with misswallowing. The recommended therapy is liquid thickened to honey consistency. The thickener is 15 calories per tablespoon. The recipe for this consistency is 1 tablespoon plus 1 teaspoon (4 teaspoons or 1 teaspoon/oz) of thickener per 4 oz of fluid. The baby previously was receiving 440 calories and 660 mL of fluid. With the addition of thickener (7 tablespoons plus 1 teaspoon), 553 calories (126% of the original) and 660 mL of fluid are provided. In addition, free water needs vary by status of patient. For patients who are at fluid risk, it has been suggested to use 1 mL of water for every kilocalorie consumed.[61] Added calories will increase the gain per day for this infant if the formula amount continues at 22 oz per day. It is a dilemma whether to add calories and risk rapid weight gain or to decrease the formula intake to match the previous caloric intake.

There is an option of using baby rice cereal as a thickener, which will provide some nutrients other than carbohydrate. Dehydrated baby cereal flakes are difficult to blend with the formula in a liquid form, do not thicken evenly, are not an exact measured substitute for thickener, and vary in the amount of time they take to thicken. In older children, a variety of other food products may be used as a thickening agent.[61]

In all situations, there may be an increased need for fluid or free water with no method of delivery unless ENS is considered as a means of alternative delivery. Because of these factors, judicious prescription and follow-up must be made. Time frames for trial therapy should be established. A well-developed behavioral and skill progression feeding plan is helpful and should include a multidisciplinary team familiar with pediatric dysphagia. Oral intake is important to encourage—as much as is medically safe. At the conclusion of the trial therapy, the patient should be evaluated for progress and/or level of rehabilitation. If there has been no change in ability, a different modality for fluid delivery should be established, with swallowing therapy to work with oral skills. Lefton-Grief has published a detailed skill list matched with nutrition modality recommendations that is helpful to use as an evaluation tool.[59]

For a growing infant, 3 to 4 weeks on an altered regime would be the maximum for a trial period, as would 2 to 3 months for a toddler or older child.

In summary, the management plan for dysphagia should focus on the reduction or elimination of factors that potentially contribute to airway compromise, provide adequate nutrition and hydration, and facilitate a workable interaction between the caregiver and the child.[59]

PLANNING FOR HOME ENTERAL SUPPORT

Whenever possible, ENS should be provided in the home rather than in the hospital. Advantages of home enteral support include a number of psychosocial benefits for the child and the family, and an economic benefit is also provided because the costly hospital stay is minimized. Often, third-party payers are making the decision of home enteral support because of the much-reduced cost of home management. A patient who is a candidate for home enteral feedings should be evaluated on the following criteria:[62]

1. The patient must be medically stable and have demonstrated a tolerance to the feeding regimen in the hospital.
2. A safe home environment is required, with available running water, electricity, refrigeration, and adequate storage space.
3. The family (or patient) must be willing and capable of administering the feedings at home.
4. A payment source is needed for the formula and associated tube-feeding equipment.
5. A home care agency should be available to service the patient in his or her home locale. If an agency is not available, a hospital team that takes responsibility for home monitoring must be identified (pediatric nurse, dietitian, and pharmacist).
6. A physician must be willing to assume responsibility for following the patient after discharge from the hospital.
7. Supplies and equipment must be available.
8. Patient/caregiver education must be arranged.
9. A nutrition plan is established.
10. A social support system is identified.
11. Outpatient follow-up is established.

Monitoring forms should be used for these patients to document data collected between medical evaluations (see Exhibit 24–6). Any forms used or developed should allow for quality improvement monitoring or the collection of data to measure outcomes.[63] Lastly, arrangements should be made for outpatient follow-up.

Successful ENS can be delivered in the medical or home environment to provide for a patient's

Exhibit 24–6 Pediatric Home Care Monitoring Form

Date ______________

Patient DOB	Primary Care Physician
Caregiver	Hospital RD
Address	Monitoring Comments ______________
	______________
Phone no.	Nutrition Support Contact Person ______________

Age:	Last measurements, date: ______________	Last nutrition Rx: Date ______________
Wt:	Wt:	Formula:
Ht:	Ht:	Total Volume
OFC	OFC	Delivery Schedule

Procurement Enteral ☐ Parenteral ☐ **Supporting Medical Equipment**

Formula ______________	Provider ______________	Monitor	☐ provider ______________
Equipment ______________	Provider ______________	Oxygen	☐ provider ______________
Supplies ______________	Provider ______________	Other	☐ provider ______________
Problems ______________		Problems ______________	

Formula and Delivery ☐ Same ☐ Change to ______________

Formula Concentration

Vol/day Substitute Formula

Infusion and Schedule

☐ By mouth (po)—attach diet history

☐ PO in combination with—attach diet history

☐ Intermittent Infuse ________ ml over ________ minutes ________ times per day

☐ Continuous Infuse ________ ml/hr for ________ hours from ______ to ______

☐ Parenteral Infuse ________ ml/hr for ________ hours from ______ to ______

(See formula that follows)

Feeding Tube Type: ______________ Size: ______________

☐ Nasogastric ☐ PEG ☐ Gastrostomy ☐ Jejunostomy ☐ Other

Water Flushes: Vol/day ________ ml ________ ml water per flush ______ flushes/day

Medications and methods of delivery: ______________

____

____

continues

Exhibit 24–6 continued

Monitoring Instructions (labs, anthropometrics, nutrition, specialists, etc.)

____

____

____

Referral Recommendations ______________________________

____

____

Care Giver Issues ______________________________

____

____

Home Nutrition Support Information given to

____

Signature ______________________________

Home Care Staff ______________________________
Telephone: ______________________________
Comments: ______________________________

____

____

____

Problems: ☐ Vomiting ☐ Reflux ☐ Aspiration ☐ Gagging ☐ Diarrhea ☐ Illness ☐ Constipation ☐ Weight loss ☐ Behavioral ☐ Sepsis ☐ Equip. Malfunction ☐ Other ________

Parenteral Rx	Date ________
Dextrose	________
Amino Acid	________
NaCl	________
KCl	________
Kphos	________
CaGlu	________
Mg	________
Na Acetate	________
Other	________
	________
	________
	________
Calories provided	________
Amt. Protein	________

PLAN OF CARE

____

____

____

____

____

____

____

____

____

____

____

____

____

signature

nutritional needs. The improvement in products and supplies and the reduction in complications of ENS have enabled many ill children to improve nutrition and health outcomes in a more naturalized setting.

REFERENCES

1. Klawitter BM. Pediatric enteral nutrition support. In: Nevin-Folino NL, ed., *Pediatric Manual of Clinical Dietetics,* 2nd ed. Chicago: The American Dietetic Association; 2003.
2. ASPEN Board of Directors. Guidelines for the use of parenteral and enteral nutrition in adult and pediatric patients. *J Parenter Enter Nutr.* 2002;26 (supp.).
3. Schwart, DB. Enhanced enteral and parenteral nutrition practice and outcomes in an intensive care unit with a hospital-wide performance improvement process. *J Am Diet Assoc.* 1996;96:484–489.
4. Parrish CR. Enteral feeding: The art and science. *Nutr in Cl Prac.* 2003;18:76–85.
5. Lucas B, ed. *Children with Special Health Care Needs: A Community Nutrition Pocket Guide,* 2nd ed. Chicago: The American Dietetic Association; 2004.
6. Cox JH, ed. *Nutrition Manual for At-Risk Infants and Toddlers.* Appendix B. 1997;183–186.
7. Theriot L. Routine nutrition care during follow-up. In: Groh-Wargo S, Thompson M, Cox JH, eds., *Nutritional Care for the High Risk Newborn,* 3rd ed. Chicago: Pre cept Press; 2000.
8. Campbell MK, Kelsey KS. The PEACH survey: A nutrition screening tool for use in early intervention programs. *J Am Diet Assoc.* 1994;94(10):1156–1158.
9. Feldhausen J, Thomson C, Duncan B, Taren D. *Referral Criteria in Pediatric Nutrition Handbook.* New York: Chapman & Hall; 1996:65.
10. Ross Products Division, Abbott Laboratories. Retrieved April 10, 2004, from www.rosspediatrics.com.
11. Mead Johnson & Company. Retrieved April 10, 2004, from www.meadjohnson.com.
12. Nestles Clinical Nutrition. Retrieved April 10, 2004, from www.nestlesclinicalnutrition.com.
13. Novartis Nutrition Corporation. Retrieved April 10, 2004, from www.novartisnutrition.com.
14. Scientific Hospital Supplies, Inc. Retrieved April 12, 2004, from www.shsna.com.
15. Wyeth-Ayerst Labs. Retrieved April 12, 2004, from www.parentschoiceformula.com.
16. Sapsford AB. Human milk and enteral nutrition products. In: Groh-Wargo S, Thompson M, Cox JH, eds., *Nutritional Care for the High Risk Newborn,* 3rd ed. Chicago: Precept Press; 2000:286–287.
17. Denne, SC. Protein requirements. In: Polin RA, Fox WW, eds., *Fetal and Neonatal Physiology,* 2nd ed. Philadelphia, PA: Sanders; 1998:315–325.
18. Fomon SJ. *Nutrition of Normal Infants.* St. Louis, MO: Mosby-Year Book; 1993:100.
19. Campbell S. *Preventing Microbial Contamination of Enteral Formulas and Delivery.* Ross Product Division, Abbott Laboratories, Inc; 2002. Retrieved April 14, 2004, from http://www.rossce.com.
20. Bar-Oz B, Preminger A, Peleg O, Block C, Arad I. *Enterobacter sakazakii* infection in the newborn. *Acta Pediatr.* 2001;90:356–358.
21. Vanek VW. Closed versus open enteral delivery systems: A quality improvement study. *Nutr in Clin Prac.* 2000; 15:234–243.
22. Fink MJ. Ban the blender. In: *ONN News, The Newsletter of the Ohio Neonatal Nutritionists.* Spring 1998.
23. Cowen SL. Feeding gastrostomy: Nutritional management of the infant or young child. *J Pediatr Perinat Nutr.* 1987;1:51.
24. Jew RK, Owen D, Kaufman D, Balmer D. Osmolality of commonly used medications and formulas in the neonatal intensive care unit. *Nutr Clin Pract.* 1997;12:158–163.
25. Food and Nutrition Board. The Institute of Medicine, National Academy of Sciences. *Dietary Reference Intakes.* Retrieved February 23, 2004, from www.nap.edu.
26. Cloud HH. Nutrition management of developmental disabilities. In: Nevin-Folino NL, ed., *Pediatric Manual of Clinical Dietetics,* 2nd ed. Chicago: The American Dietetic Association; 2003:193–206.
27. Cox JH, ed. *Nutrition Manual for At-Risk Infants and Toddlers.* Chicago: Precept Press; 1997.
28. Lucas B, ed. *Children with Special Health Care Needs: A Community Nutrition Pocket Guide,* 2nd ed. Chicago: The American Dietetic Association; 2004.
29. Walker WA, Hendricks KM, eds. Enteral nutrition: Support of the pediatric patient. In: *Manual of Pediatric Nutrition.* Philadelphia, PA: WB Saunders Co; 1990.
30. Delegge, MH. Enteral access: The foundation of feeding. *J Parenter Enter Nutr.* 2000:25:S8–S13.
31. Wesley JR. Special access to the intestinal tract. In: Balistreri WF, Farrell MK, eds., *Enteral Feeding: Scientific Basis and Clinical Applications.* Report of the 94th Ross Conference on Pediatric Research. Columbus, OH: Ross Products; 1988:57–62.
32. Lord LM. Enteral access devices. *Nurs Clin North Am.* 1997;32(4):685–702.
33. Walker WA, Hendricks KM, eds. Enteral nutrition support of the pediatric patient. In: *Manual of Pediatric Nutrition.* Philadelphia, PA: WB Saunders Co; 1985.
34. Wessel JJ. Feeding methodologies. In: Groh-Wargo S, Thompson M, Cox JH, eds., *Nutritional Care for the High Risk Newborn.* 3rd ed. Chicago: Precept Press; 2000:321–339.

35. Cooning SW. Unique aspects in pediatric care. In: Lang C, ed., *Nutrition Support in Critical Care.* Gaithersburg, MD: Aspen Publishers; 1987:395–404.
36. Braunschweig CL, Wesley JR, Clark SF, et al. Rationale and guidelines for parenteral and enteral transition feeding of the 3- to 30-kg child. *J Am Diet Assoc.* 1988;88: 479.
37. Greer FR, McCormick A, Loker J. Changes in fat concentration of human milk during delivery by intermittent bolus and continuous mechanical pump infusion. *J Pediatr.* 1984;105:745–749.
38. Lavine M, Clark RM. The effect of short-term refrigeration of milk and addition of breast milk fortifier on the delivery of lipids during tube feeding. *J Pediatr Gastroenterol Nutr.* 1989;8:496–499.
39. Grumow JE, Al-Hafidh AS, Tunell WP. Gastroesophageal reflux following percutaneous endoscopic gastrostomy in children. *J Pediatr Surg.* 1989;24:44–45.
40. Canal DF, Vane DW, Goto S, et al. Reduction of lower esophageal sphincter pressure with Stamm gastrostomy. *J Pediatr Surg.* 1987;22:54–57.
41. Kellie SJ, Fitch SJ, Kovnar EH, et al. A hazard of using adult-sized weighted-tip enteral feeding catheters in infants. *Am J Dis Child.* 1988;142:916–917.
42. Allen DB. Postprandial hypoglycemia resulting from nasogastric tube malposition. *Pediatrics.* 1988;81:582–584.
43. Rommel N, DeMeyer A, Feenstra L, Veereman-Wauters G. The complexity of feeding problems in 700 infants and young children presenting to a tertiary care institution. *J of Ped Gastro Nutr.* 2000;37:75–84.
44. Ford EG, Jennings M, Andrassy RJ. Serum albumin (oncotic pressure) correlates with enteral feeding tolerance in the pediatric surgical patient. *J Pediatr Surg.* 1987;22: 597–599.
45. Gottschlich MM, Warden GD, Michel M, et al. Diarrhea in tube-fed burn patients: Incidence, etiology, nutritional impact, and prevention. *J Parenter Enter Nutr.* 1988;12: 388–445.
46. Patchell CJ, Anderton A, MacDonald A, George RH, Booth JW. Bacterial contamination of enteral feeds. *Arch Dis Child.* 1994;70:327–330.
47. Hutsler D. Delivery and bedside management of infant feedings. In: Robbins S, Beker L, eds., *Infant Feedings: Guidelines for Preparation of Formula and Breast Milk in Health Care Facilities.* Chicago: The American Dietetic Association; 2003.
48. Arnold LDW. *Recommendations for Collection, Storage, and Handling of a Mother's Milk for Her Own Infant in the Hospital Setting.* Denver, CO: Human Milk Banking Association of North America, Inc.; 1999.
49. Lucas B, ed. *Children with Special Health Care Needs: A Community Nutrition Pocket Guide,* 2nd ed. Chicago: The American Dietetic Association; 2004.
50. Issacs JS. Nutritional care for the gastrostomy-fed child with neurological impairments. *Top Clin Nutr.* 1993;8(4): 58–65.
51. Glass RP, Lucas B. *Making the Transition from Tube Feeding to Oral Feeding. Nutrition Focus for Children with Special Health Care Needs.* Seattle, WA: Children's Development and Mental Retardation Center, University of Washington; 5:1–4.
52. Stein, K. Children with feeding disorders: An emerging issue. *J Am Diet Assoc.* 2000;100(9):1000–1001.
53. Illingsworth RS, Lister J. The critical or sensitive period, with special reference to certain feeding problems in infants and children. *J Pediatr.* 1964;65:8.
54. Rudolph, CD, Link D. Feeding disorders in infants and children. *Ped Gastro Nutr.* 2002;49:97–112.
55. Burklow KA, McGrath AM, Allred KE. Parent perceptions of mealtime behaviors in children fed enterally. *Nutr Cl Prac.* 2002;17:291–295.
56. Camp KM, Kalscheur MC. Nutritional approach to diagnosis and management of pediatric feeding and swallowing disorders. In: Tuchman DN, Walter RS, eds. *Disorders of Feeding and Swallowing in Infants and Children: Pathophysiology, Diagnosis, and Treatment.* San Diego, CA: Singular Publishing Group; 1994:153–185.
57. Manikam R, Perman JA. Pediatric feeding disorders. *J Cl Gastro.* 2000;30:34–46.
58. American Academy of Pediatrics. *Pediatric Nutrition Handbook,* 4th ed. Elk Grove, IL: 1998;108.
59. Lefton-Grief MA. Diagnosis and management of pediatric feeding and swallowing disorders: Role of the speech-language pathologist. In: Tuchman DN, Walter RS, eds., *Disorders of Feeding and Swallowing in Infants and Children: Pathophysiology, Diagnosis, and Treatment.* San Diego, CA: Singular Publishing Group; 1994: 97–113.
60. Phagia-Gel Technologies, LLC. Retrieved May 29, 2004, from www.simplythick.com.
61. Feucht S. Guidelines for the use of thickeners in foods and liquids. In: *Nutrition Focus for Children with Special Health Care Needs.* Seattle, WA: Children's Developmental and Mental Retardation Center, University of Washington; 10(6):1–6.
62. Vanderhoff JA, Young RJ. Overview of considerations for the pediatric patient receiving home parenteral and enteral nutrition. *Nutrition in Clinical Practice.* 2003:18: 221–226.
63. Gallagher AL, Onda RM. Using quality assurance procedures to improve compliance with standards to nutrition care for patients receiving isotonic tube feeding. *J Am Diet Assoc.* 1993;93:678–679.

CHAPTER 25

Parenteral Nutrition

Janice Hovasi Cox and Ingrida Mara Melbardis

INTRODUCTION

The use of parenteral nutrition (PN) in pediatrics has greatly evolved over the past years. It has been viewed as an almost routine aspect of care in the treatment of a wide variety of conditions. Technological advances and refinements in delivery systems that have made PN so commonplace in the hospital setting have propelled this complex form of nutritional support into the home setting. In more recent years, enteral feedings have been found to be beneficial and cost effective in a variety of settings. These advances require medical professionals to rethink the circumstances under which PN is currently utilized.[1–4] This chapter summarizes the complexities of pediatric PN as it is utilized in the hospital and in the home.

PN is the intravenous delivery of nutrients, including water, carbohydrates, fat, protein, electrolytes, vitamins, minerals, and trace elements. The proportions of these nutrients are individualized, based on an assessment of the child's clinical and nutritional needs. The goal of PN is to support normal growth and development as well as to promote tissue repair and maintenance while oral/enteral feedings are precluded.

CLINICAL INDICATIONS

Parenteral nutrition is needed when an infant or child is unable to meet ongoing nutrition needs with an oral diet and/or enteral feedings. In extremely premature infants, gastrointestinal tract immaturity may prevent sufficient enteral feedings for several weeks. Because premature infants have low nutritional stores, PN should be started within 24 hours of birth. Undernourished infants and children require nutrition support within 1 to 2 days if they will not be able to consume adequate feedings. Initially, well-nourished infants and children are better able to tolerate longer periods without nutrition intervention, up to 3 to 5 and 5 to 7 days, respectively.[5,6] Intravenous solutions (dextrose/sodium chloride/potassium chloride) are usually provided during this time to meet fluid needs and prevent hypoglycemia.

It is important to ensure that PN is used appropriately and that the infants and children who receive PN are managed effectively to support the best outcome at the lowest cost. Policies and decision trees can help practitioners choose the most suitable form of nutrition support (see Figure 25–1).[6] Conditions that may require PN are listed in Exhibit 25–1. Some hospitals utilize interdisciplinary nutrition support teams (physicians, dietitians, nurses, and pharmacists)[7] and clinical pathways[8,9] to help evaluate and manage patients requiring enteral or parenteral nutrition.[10]

Gastrointestinal (GI) tract dysfunction can occur at any age due to disease, injury, or radiation/chemotherapy.[5,11] In GI conditions requiring surgical resection, the extent of macronutrient and micronutrient malabsorption depends on the amount of bowel resected, the presence or absence of the ileocecal valve, and the function of the remaining bowel. Often children with short gut syndrome are able to tolerate at least partial enteral feedings. When the ileocecal valve is not

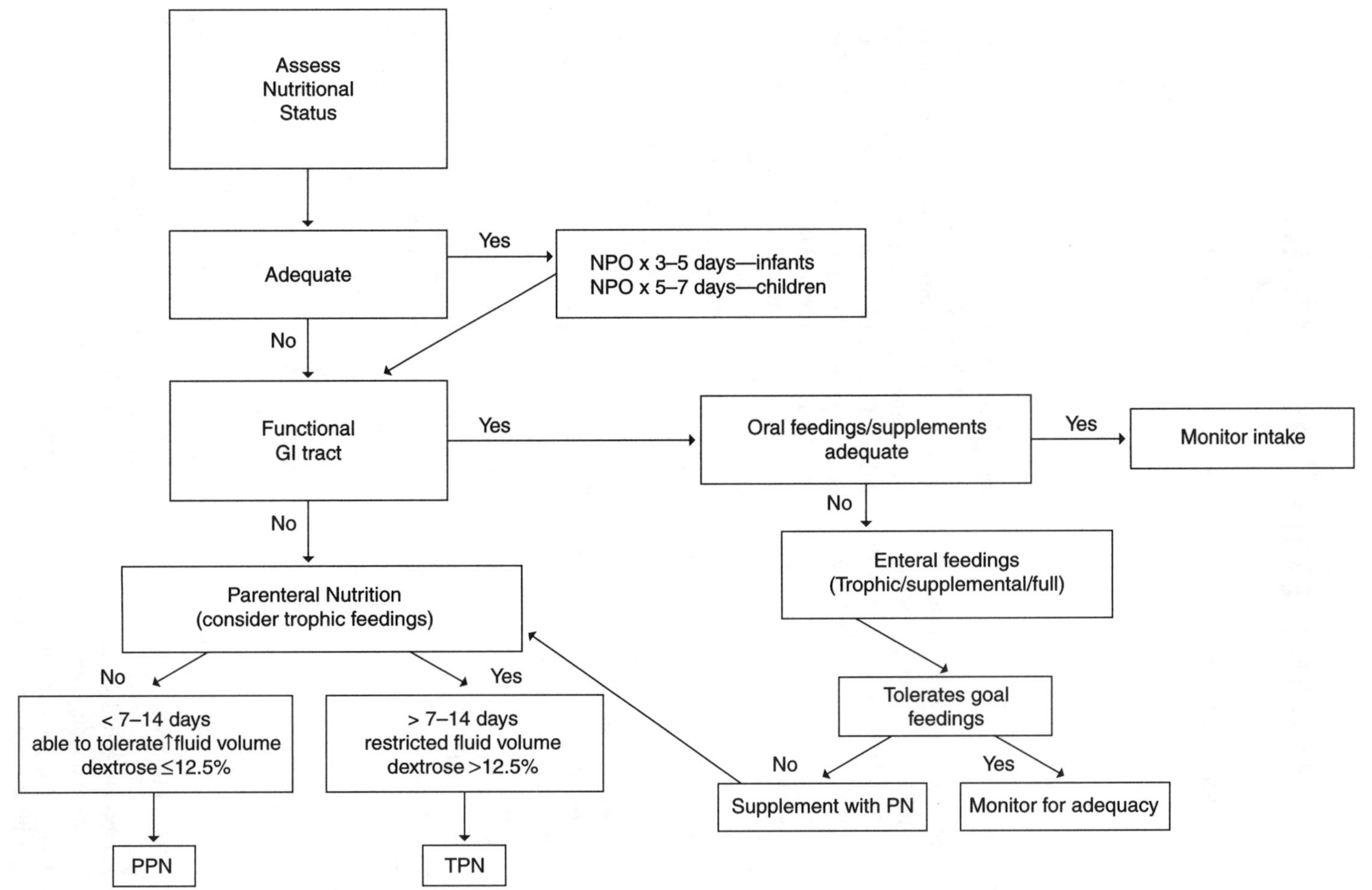

Figure 25–1 Pediatric Nutrition Support Algorithm

Exhibit 25–1 Conditions that May Require Parenteral Nutrition

GI Conditions		*Other Circumstances*
bowel obstruction	meconium ileus	anorexia nervosa
Crohn's disease	necrotizing enterocolitis	bronchopulmonary dysplasia
diaphragmatic hernia	neuromuscular intestinal disorders	cancer cachexia
gastroschisis	omphalocele	chylothorax
high-output fistulas	radiation enteritis	low-birth-weight neonate (<1,500 g)
intestinal atresia	severe Hirschsprung's disease	
intractable diarrhea	short bowel syndrome	
intussusception	ulcerative colitis	
malrotation/volvulus		

intact, the rapid transit time of enteral formulas through the bowel may require a greater dependence upon PN.[12] The extent of the resection, paired with the tolerance of enteral feedings, can help predict the duration of a neonate's dependence on PN.[13,14]

Although PN may help bring about disease remission in children with irritable bowel disease (IBD), ulcerative colitis, or Crohn's disease, relapse occurs soon after a normal diet is resumed.[15] Elemental enteral feedings may be more beneficial for inducing remission of IBD, improving nutrition status, and reversing growth failure.[16] Parenteral nutrition should be reserved only for those children who are unable to tolerate enteral feedings. Gastrointestinal disorders requiring nutritional support are discussed in detail in Chapter 16.

Children with cancer are at increased risk for malnutrition. The causes for cancer cachexia seem to be multifaceted and include anorexia, anxiety, and increased metabolic needs.[11] Whether enteral feeding has been impeded by the side effects of radiation and chemotherapy or by surgical procedures, the child with cancer may have an improved quality of life with PN.[17–20] Helping children maintain optimal nutrition during therapy may promote improved growth and better tolerance of therapies.[21] Some children may be able to tolerate small gastric feedings along with PN to meet nutrition needs. Most practitioners agree that children receiving aggressive cancer therapy should also receive supportive nutrition therapy, but the benefits of PN should be weighed against the potential risks of PN, which include increased infection rates and metabolic abnormalities.[22,23]

Parenteral nutrition may be used in the refeeding process for children with anorexia nervosa simply because it has less resemblance to food than the enteral feeding. The use of PN in these patients depends on the severity of malnutrition and on the patient's tendency to interfere with the infusion apparatus.[24,25]

VASCULAR ACCESS

Peripheral Venous Access

Parenteral nutrition needs may be met through a peripheral or central venous route, depending on the anticipated length of therapy, nutrition needs, and the volume of the solution to be given. A final concentration of no more than 12.5% dextrose with a maximum solution osmolarity of under 900 mOsm/L with lipids or less than 600 mOsm/L without lipids[4] is recommended in the administration of peripheral parenteral nutrition (PPN). A simple equation can be used to estimate osmolarity.[26] It is difficult to provide sufficient nutrients to meet the long-term needs of most children using this route. Because PPN solutions are not as calorie dense as total PN (TPN) solutions, greater fluid volumes are required to provide comparable nutrition. Peripheral parenteral nutrition is typically feasible when the anticipated length of therapy will be less than 2 weeks. The major complications associated with PPN are soft tissue sloughs and phlebitis (this is more common with solutions with an osmolarity of more than 900 mOsm/L). Limiting calcium to a maximum of 8 mEq/liter may also help decrease the risk of phlebitis.[4] The peripheral delivery route may also be more restrictive to normal activity, depending on the site and stability of venous access.

Central Venous Access

Providing TPN through a central vein is indicated when the child requires fluid restriction or long-term nutrition therapy or when the child is a candidate for home PN. The tip of these central venous catheters (CVCs) should be at the top of the right atrium. Infusion of TPN is safer into the central vein because the high blood flow rapidly dilutes the hypertonic solution. Location of the catheter tip should be verified every 6 to 12 months for children undergoing significant linear growth.[27] The major complications associated with central venous catheter (CVC) insertion and use include infection and thrombosis.[28,29]

Central venous catheters are used to provide PN, chemotherapy, prolonged antibiotic therapy, and blood components. Blood sampling can also be done from a CVC site. Central venous access can be temporary or permanent. Permanent catheters are indicated when long-term access (over 3 weeks) is needed.[29] The surgically placed right atrial catheter (e.g., Broviac, Hickman) is the most suitable CVC for pediatric patients who require long-term or home TPN. The catheter is placed in the external jugular or the facial vein and threaded through the internal jugular vein and down into the superior vena cava. The distal end of the catheter is tunneled subcutaneously and exits midchest. The Dacron cuff affixed to the tunneled portion of the catheter helps secure the catheter because subcutaneous fibrous tissue adheres to the cuff.

The peripherally inserted central catheter (PICC line) provides reliable central venous access and may be inserted at the bedside using strict sterile techniques.[30–33] Many of the insertion-related complications inherent in the surgically placed CVC, such as pneumothorax and hemothorax, are virtually eliminated with the PICC line. Some studies have also found that sepsis rates tend to be lower in neonates and children with PICC lines versus surgically placed central catheters.[34,35] PICC lines are being used in increasing numbers both in neonates and older children because they provide central venous access less invasively, with lower risks, and at lower cost than surgically placed CVCs or multiple insertions of peripheral lines.[29,36–38]

Although a single-lumen CVC is the venous access device most often used for the pediatric PN patient, two- and three-lumen CVCs have also been used for the pediatric population. Double and triple lumen catheters are particularly useful in patients who require frequent infusions of blood products and medications in addition to the nutrition solution. Any lumens not in use must be heparinized and capped. Multiple-lumen catheters may be more suitable for the larger child rather that the neonate because of total catheter size. Strict aseptic technique is critical when a multilumen CVC is in place.[39,40]

In order to avoid some of the problems associated with the externalized CVC, a totally implantable vascular device consisting of a catheter connected to a chamber or port was developed.[41] The advantages of the implantable port are that it eliminates the daily dressing change when not in use and it is not as disruptive to body image.

For the child on home PN, the implanted CVC requires daily access. Daily percutaneous puncture or leaving a Huber needle in place with a dressing for days at a time may negate the overall benefits of the implanted device. Skin irritation and breakdown have been associated with frequent port access, and other CVC-related complications such as occlusion and infection remain risks with the implanted CVC.[29]

The P.A.S. Port and CathLink are recently developed central access devices. They are peripherally inserted implanted devices. Use in pediatric patients has not been widely reported.

SOLUTION ADMINISTRATION

Parenteral nutrition can be ordered in various ways. Nutrients can be ordered based on the infant's or child's weight (per kg), per liter, or in combinations of both. Standard ranges for the various nutrients can be included on order forms to help ensure the design of an appropriate, nutritionally complete solution[42] (see Exhibit 25–2). Computerized and Web-based programs are also available to simplify order entry for PN.[43–45]

Parenteral nutrition solutions should be initiated slowly and advanced gradually as the child's fluid and glucose tolerance permits. Infusion pumps are used to maintain a constant flow rate, thereby maintaining steady glucose delivery. If the PN infusion is interrupted or discontinued abruptly, a 10% dextrose solution may be infused to maintain euglycemia (or to prevent hypoglycemia) until the PN solution can be replaced.

There are two ways of preparing PN solutions. In 2-in-1 solutions, dextrose and amino acids are combined, and this solution is infused through one arm of a Y-connector while lipids are infused in the other. A 2-in-1 solution allows for the visualization of potential calcium phosphate precipitates. Running lipids separately can also permit infusion of the lipids over a shorter time span, but this may lead to hypertriglyceridemia in the preterm infant.[46]

A 3-in-1 or total nutrient admixture (TNA) combines the lipid emulsion, amino acid, and dextrose solutions in the same container. Although the TNA is more convenient to use, there has been concern about the stability and safety of these solutions. TNAs, unlike 2-in-1 solutions, are emulsions and, therefore, are more significantly influenced by pH and temperature.[47,48] Of concern also is the potential peroxidation of lipid emulsions by phototherapy lights.[49]

Exhibit 25–2 Recommendations for Writing Parenteral Nutrition Prescriptions

1. Use standard order forms specifically developed for infants and for children.
2. Identify prescription with patient name and date of birth.
3. Provide patient's current weight; provide dosing weight if different than current weight due to malnutrition, edema, or obesity.
4. Identify whether intravenous access route is peripheral or central because this determines dextrose concentration limitations.
5. Include fluid prescription, accommodating other fluids needed for administration of flushes, medications, other intravenous fluids, and/or enteral feedings.
6. Specify total daily volume, hourly rate of delivery, and number of hours of delivery.
7. Each nutrient should be clearly identified, including chloride and acetate.
8. Include guidelines for nutrient requirements for various ages and/or acceptable ranges of nutrient concentration in admixture, including mineral content compatibility.
9. List of nutrients in prescription should be in the same order and units as in guidelines and on label. For example, do not use "mEq" for calcium in the prescription list, but "mg" of calcium in the guidelines or "mL" of calcium gluconate on the label.
10. Avoid using percent concentration. Use amount per volume, amount per kg, or amount per day.
11. Use one zero before the decimal to hold a place, but do not use trailing zeros. For example, use "0.5" but do not use ".5"; use "5" but do not use "5.0".
12. Complete form for all subsequent orders, even if only one nutrient is changed.
13. If standard solutions are used, provide options for decreasing lipid, copper, and manganese and other modifications that may be clinically indicated.
14. Establish standard guidelines for laboratory monitoring.

Shielding the bag and the tubing from phototherapy lights with aluminum foil can prevent this from happening. Opaque tubing is also available.[50] Infusion of an MVI preparation along with shielding the tubing may fully protect the solution from peroxidation.[51]

In TNAs, three main variables affect the overall stability of the final product:[52,53] (1) the final concentration of the macronutrients, (2) the amount of added cations (especially polyvalent cations such as iron, magnesium, calcium, and zinc), and (3) the compounding order. If parenteral medications are to be infused simultaneously via a Y-site, compatibility with the TNA solution should be verified.[54] Care must be taken to identify any precipitates or emulsion breakdown in the TNA before infusion occurs. The most commonly found precipitate is calcium phosphate. Emulsion breakdown or "creaming" (liberation of free oil) can result when higher amounts of cations are used in the mixture. The presence of yellow-brown oil droplets at or near the TNA surface is an indicator that the solution is unsafe for administration.[53] Various methods of in-process end-product testing are described in the American Society for Parenteral and Enteral Nutrition (ASPEN) guidelines to ensure and document the safety of the end TNAs.[53]

Of greatest concern with neonatal and pediatric PN solutions is the solubility of calcium and phosphorus.[52] Although the addition of lipids to the PN solution does not directly affect the solubility of calcium and phosphorus, the opacity of the admixture makes visual detection of precipitates difficult. Computer and Web-based programs are available to help maximize the amount of calcium and phosphorus that can be provided safely in PN solutions.[44,53]

For neonates and children receiving home PN, the stability of the PN needs to be assured for longer periods of time. Using dual-chamber bags to separate the lipid from the rest of the solution and adding vitamins and trace minerals just before infusion helps improve the shelf-life of TNAs used in this setting.[52,55] Use of a MCT/LCT-based TNA may also improve stability.[56,57] Caretakers administering PN in the home need to be trained on how to visually assess the stability of the emulsion.

The use of filters with PN provides additional safety.[53,58] Filters can prevent the infusion of particulate matter, air, and microorganisms. Different types of filters are used for 2-in-1 and 3-in-1 solutions. Positively charged filters and 0.2 mm filters can be used with 2-in-1 solutions. These filters remove microorganisms and pyrogens (gram-negative endotoxins) and reduce the risk of air embolism. For TNAs, larger 1.2 mm filters are used to allow administration of lipid droplets. These filter out particulate matter and larger organisms, such as *Candida albicans,* but are unable to filter out common smaller bacterial contaminants.

CYCLING

Administration of PN in cycles provides for planned interruption of the nutrient infusion. Cycling more closely simulates normal patterns of food ingestion and fasting and may help prevent PN-associated hepatic complications.[59] Whether at home or in the hospital, cyclic PN allows a more normal daytime routine, enhancing mobility and activity patterns and also leaving a "window" of time for lipid clearance.

The nutrition needs of the child, compared with the ability to tolerate oral/enteral feedings, should be taken into consideration when deciding on cyclic PN. Infants younger than 4 to 6 months of age who are receiving all of their nutrition parenterally may be able to tolerate breaks from PN up to only 4 hours in duration. Older infants and children may tolerate interruptions of up to 6 to 8 hours. Infants and children who are receiving enteral feedings or are eating in addition to their PN may receive adequate PN in shorter spans of time. Supplemental PN can usually be provided over 8 to 12 hours. Children who are more tolerant of the necessary fluid load can receive their total required nutrition and fluid loads condensed into 10- to 16-hour cycles.

Gradually increasing the rate when starting the infusion and slowly weaning the rate at the end of the infusion may lessen the likelihood of hyper/hypoglycemia. The rate should be adjusted over a period of 1 to 2 hours (i.e., run at half rate for the first and last hour) to maintain euglycemia. Infusion pumps that can be programmed to accomplish the gradual introduction and weaning of PN are available.

As an infant or child is able to make a transition to enteral/oral feedings, the volume of PN should be gradually decreased (by means of decreased hourly rate and/or decreased infusion time). Total energy intake needs to be adjusted as the percentage of nutrition provided by an enteral route is increased. (PN energy needs are usually lower than enteral needs because energy is not required for digestion and there are no absorptive losses.) Providing PN at night provides supplemental nutrition with limited suppression of appetite during the day, which may better support a transition to oral feedings.[46]

FLUID AND ELECTROLYTES

Guidelines for the administration of parenteral fluids to infants and children are based on normal maintenance estimates with adjustments for increased or decreased losses due to disease or environmental conditions (see Table 25–1). During the first week of life, infants experience three phases of fluid and electrolyte homeostasis.[63] Renal excretion of fluid, sodium, and potassium is minimal and insensible water loss (IWL) may be high during the first 12 to 36 hours of life or prediuretic phase. The onset of the diuretic phase usually occurs within the first 2 days and accounts for most of the weight, sodium, and potassium loss that occurs during the first week of life. The postdiuretic phase usually begins between 3 and 5 days of age and is characterized by improved homeostasis of fluid, sodium, and potassium.[63] This adjustment to extrauterine life usually results in up to 10% weight loss in term infants. Prematurely born infants may lose 10% to 20% of their body weight during the first week of life. This is primarily due to their greater percentage of total body water as extracellular water and increased IWL associated with their relatively large body surface area to body mass ratio and their more permeable epidermis.[60] Weight loss greater than 15% to 20% of birth weight may represent some loss of lean tissue due to energy deficit.[64]

Fluid losses through urine and the gastrointestinal tract may be relatively easy to measure, although IWL through the respiratory tract and skin is more elusive and may be affected by environmental conditions. Radiant heat warmers and ultraviolet light therapy may increase IWL by 20% to 25%.[65] Use of double-walled isolettes may prevent this increase in water loss.[66] Use of mist tents and humidified air may decrease IWL. In older infants and children, hyperventilation and visible sweating often associated with fever may increase IWL by 20% to 25%.[67]

Low-birth-weight infants may require up to 200 ml/kg/d due to their renal immaturity and

Table 25–1 Daily Maintenance Fluid Requirements

Clinical Condition	*Fluids Required per Day*
Sick newborn, day 1	40–80 mL/kg
Sick newborn, week 1	80–150 mL/kg
Anuria, extreme oliguria	45 mL/kg
Diabetes insipidus	up to 400 mL/100 kcal
1–10 kg body weight	100 mL/kg
11–20 kg body weight	1000 mL + 50 mL/kg above 10 kg
Body weight above 20 kg	1500 mL + 20 mL/kg above 20 kg
Body surface area	1500–1800 mL/m^2

Source: Data from endnote references 60–62.

increased IWL. They may also be intolerant of excessive fluid intake. Patent ductus arteriosus, bronchopulmonary dysplasia, intraventricular hemorrhage, and necrotizing enterocolitis have each been linked with excessive fluid administration.[62,68–71] Frequent monitoring of fluid and electrolyte intake, serum and urine electrolyte levels, weight changes, and urine output may be needed to appropriately manage fluid and electrolyte balance during the neonatal period.

Beyond the first week of life and throughout childhood, maintenance fluid and electrolyte requirements are directly related to metabolic rate.[72] Infants and children generally require at least 115 mL of fluid for every 100 kcal of energy provided[73] (see Table 25–1). The amount of fluid needed to maintain adequate hydration often does not provide adequate nutrition when using peripheral venous access, though administration of fluids 30–50% above maintenance levels are usually well tolerated. Changes in metabolic rate, respiratory rate, IWL, and water production from the oxidation of protein, carbohydrate, and fat also affect fluid needs. Older infants and children may initially require fluids and electrolytes in excess of maintenance requirements to establish normal hydration if they have had prolonged or excessive vomiting or diarrhea.

Losses of fluid and electrolytes through the GI tract in disease states may be measured directly for replacement or estimated by monitoring changes in body weight every 8 or 24 hours. Gastrointestinal losses may be due to vomiting, nasogastric suctioning, diarrhea, or ostomy drainage.[74] Due to the wide range in electrolyte composition of various GI fluids, direct measurement may be required to provide adequate replacement.

Urinary losses of fluid and electrolytes depend largely on intake and renal maturity. Infants less than 1 year of age can dilute urine to 50 mOsm/kg of water. Concentrating ability at birth is about 600 mOsm/kg of water and gradually increases to 1000 to 1200 mOsm/kg of water during the first year. During periods of growth, the renal solute load is lower, as nitrogen, phosphorus, sodium, potassium, and chloride are retained as constituents of body tissues. During periods of stress and tissue catabolism, the renal solute load is higher.

Various conditions may alter urinary losses of fluid and electrolytes. Preterm infants have an immature capacity to either excrete or retain electrolytes and maintain acid-base balance.[75,76] Excessive sodium losses are common and may require up to 12 mmol/kg/day of sodium. Inappropriate or excessive antidiuretic hormone (ADH) secretion, often associated with hypoxia, hemorrhage, central nervous system insult, hypotension, anesthesia, pneumothorax, or pain requires fluid restriction and sodium supplementation to maintain normal extracellular fluid volumes and prevent hyponatremia.[75] However, hyperchloremic acidosis in preterm infants is associated with excessive chloride intake when sodium is provided solely as sodium chloride. Using sodium acetate (up to 14.2 mmol/kg/d) has been shown to reduce the incidence of metabolic acidosis and hyperchloremia.[76] If IWL (which is all free water) is high in prematurely born infants, particularly during the diuretic phase of initial fluid and electrolyte homeostasis, hypernatremia may develop.[63,77]

Fluid and electrolyte restriction may be necessary in some disease states such as congestive heart failure, head trauma, and renal insufficiency. Medications may be a significant source of fluid and/or electrolytes. Saline flushes used in routine care of intravenous lines may be a significant source of sodium and chloride.[78] Some medications may cause increased excretion or retention of some electrolytes. Direct measurement of urine volume and electrolytes may be necessary to provide appropriate replacement.

ENERGY

Parenteral energy needs are probably about 10% to 15% lower than estimated enteral needs for most infants and children due to reduced fecal losses and reduced energy required for digestion and absorption (see Table 25–2). While meeting basal energy needs prevents catabolism and weight loss, energy needs to support catch-up growth, or even normal growth and activity levels, may be nearly double basal energy needs.[87] Energy requirements for postoperative infants and children may be closer to basal needs possibly due to administration of sedative medications and temporary interruption of growth, although energy needs generally return to normal within 1 to 3 days of surgery and may even exceed normal levels.[5,88] Energy needs during the acute phase of critical illness, sedation, or paralysis may be lower than normal.

Several elaborate equations have been developed to include length, specific age, body temperature, and heart rate to estimate individual energy needs.[46] When considering fluctuations in clinical condition, activity levels, growth spurts, and so forth, these methods may be cumbersome and perhaps no more accurate than simpler methods based on estimated lean weight and general age category (see Table 25–2). Energy intakes that are below needs may result in poor growth and nutritional status. Energy intakes that exceed needs may result in hepatic steatosis, increased risk of infection, and obesity. As indirect calorimetry has become more readily available for infants and children, individual energy needs can be measured specific to carbohydrate and fat utilization.[1,5,89,90] Whatever method is used to estimate energy needs, frequent monitoring of anthropometric, clinical, and laboratory parameters allows adjustment of energy delivery to meet individual energy needs.

The percentage contribution of protein, carbohydrate, and fat to total energy intake varies with individual tolerance to fluid, carbohydrate, lipid infusion, clinical condition, and the route of delivery. General guidelines for energy distribution are 8% to 15% protein, 45% to 60% carbohydrate, and 25% to 40% fat.[60] Positive nitrogen balance is best achieved when the nonprotein calorie to nitrogen ratio is 150 to 300 to 1.[84,91]

CARBOHYDRATE

Nearly all centers use glucose (dextrose monohydrate, 3.4 kcal/g) as the primary source of parenterally administered carbohydrate. Glycerol, found in parenterally administered fat emulsions, is also a source of carbohydrate. Dose recommendations for infants and children are found in Table 25–2. Glucose infusions of less than 2 mg/kg/min (3 gm/kg/d) may be insufficient to prevent ketosis caused by mobilization of fat stores as a source of energy. Glucose utilization by infants (6–8 mg/kg/min or 8.6–9.5 g/kg/day) is significantly different from adults (2 mg/kg/min or 3 g/kg/day) primarily due to brain metabolism. The brain requires glucose as the primary source of energy, and the brain to body weight ratio in infants is 12% compared to 2% in adults.[85,92] Brain utilization of glucose may account for as much as 90% of basal glucose needs. In addition, infants and children require glucose to support normal growth. Prematurely born infants may require as much as 16 mg/kg/min (24 g/kg/day) of glucose if fat is poorly tolerated as a source of energy.[85,91] Net fat synthesis is shown to occur in infants when glucose intake exceeds 12.5 mg/kg/min (18 g/kg/day) or 6 mg/kg/min (8.6 g/kg/day) in older children. Prematurely born infants often require lipogenesis because they may lack adequate fat stores that normally accumulate during the last trimester of fetal growth. Glucose given in excess of need is not recommended because this may be associated with hyperglycemia, hepatic steatosis, and/or excess carbon dioxide production.[1,84,87] Maximum glucose tolerance varies with age, total energy expenditure, and clinical condition.[46,85,92]

Insulin is not generally added to parenteral nutrient admixtures because dose response varies widely, particularly in the low-birth-weight infant. Insulin, when needed, may be given in a separate infusion starting at 0.1 U/kg/h and increased or decreased as needed to maintain euglycemia.[93,94] Small glycogen stores in low-birth-weight infants and undernourished infants and children place them at a greater risk of developing hypoglycemia following abrupt cessation of parenteral glucose. Gradual weaning from parenteral glucose and adequate enteral feeding help prevent the development of hypoglycemia.

The recommended dose of carbohydrate may be delivered while meeting normal fluid requirements by using a 10% to 12.5% dextrose solu-

Table 25–2 Recommendations for Daily Parenteral Administration of Macronutrients, Electrolytes, and Minerals

	Dose Unit	*Premature Infants*	*Term Infants*	*1–3 Years*	*4–6 Years*	*7–10 Years*	*11–18 Years*	*Maximum Dose*
Basal Energy[1]	kcal/kg	46–55	55	40–55	38–40	25–38	23–25	
Total Energy[2]	kcal/kg	85–105	90–108	75–90	65–80	55–70	30–55	
Dextrose[3]	mg/kg/min	5–15	5–15	5–12	5–11	6–10	4–7	see text
Carbohydrate	g/kg	8–21	8–21	8–18	8–16	8–14	6–10	see text
Protein[4]	g/kg	2.5–4	2.5–3.5	1.5–2.5	1.5–2.5	1.5–2.5	0.8–2	4
Fat[5]	g/kg	0.6–3	0.6–3	0.6–2.5	0.5–2.5	0.5–2.5	0.4–1.8	4
Sodium	mEq/kg	2–4	2–4	2–4	2–4	2–4	60–150 mEq/d	150 mEq/d
Potassium	mEq/kg	2–4	2–4	2–4	2–4	2–4	70–180 mEq/d	180 mEq/d
Chloride	mEq/kg	2–4	2–4	2–4	2–4	2–4	60–150 mEq/d	150 mEq/d
Calcium[6]	mEq/kg	2.5–3	1–2	0.5–1	0.5–1	0.5–1	10–40 mEq/d	see text
Phosphorus[7]	mmol/kg	1–1.5	1–1.5	0.5–1.3	0.5–1.3	0.5–1.3	9–30 mEq/d	see text
Magnesium[8]	mEq/kg	0.5–1	0.25–1	0.25–0.5	0.25–0.5	0.25–0.5	8–24 mEq/d	see text
Zinc[9]	mcg/kg	325–400	100–250	100	100	50	2–5 mg/d	5000 mcg/d
Copper[9]	mcg/kg	20	20	20	20	5–20	200–300 mcg/d	300 mcg/d
Chromium[9]	mcg/kg	0.14–0.2	0.14–0.2	0.14–0.2	0.14–0.2	0.14–0.2	5–15 mcg/d	15 mcg/d
Manganese[9]	mcg/kg	1	1	1	1	1	40–50 mcg/d	50 mcg/d
Selenium[9]	mcg/kg	2	2	2	2	1–2 mcg/d	40–60 mcg/d	60 mcg/d
Molybdenum[9]	mcg/kg	0.25	0.25	0.25	0.25	0.25	5 mcg/d	5 mcg/d
Iron[10]	mg/kg	see text	0.1/see text	see text	see text	see text	see text	see text

Table 25–2 continued

[1]Basal energy needs increase: 12% for every degree of fever, 15–25% in cardiac failure, 20–30% in traumatic injury or major surgery, 25–30% in severe respiratory distress or bronchopulmonary dysplasia, 40–50% in severe sepsis, 6 kcal/g weight gain for catch-up growth.

[2]Total parenteral energy needs include basal energy needs but do not include energy required for digestion or energy losses in stool that occur with enteral feeding.

[3]Peripheral venous access limits dextrose concentration to 12% solutions due to high osmolality and increased risk of tissue damage. Central venous access allows up to 25% dextrose solutions.

[4]Protein needs may vary with diagnoses: 0.8–2 g/kg/d for renal failure; 3 g/kg/d for necrotizing enterocolitis, major surgery, traumatic injury, sepsis; 4–8 g/kg/d for thermal injury. Most efficient protein utilization occurs when nonprotein/calorie ratio is 150–250:1 (100–150:1 in burns and multiple trauma).

[5]Minimum fat dose to meet essential fatty acid requirements varies depending upon fat source and total energy needs. See text.

[6]Calcium conversions: 1 mEq = 0.5 mMol = 20 mg elemental calcium; 1 mL calcium gluconate 10% contains 100 mg calcium gluconate = 9.3 mg elemental calcium = 0.47 mEq = 0.25 mMol calcium.

[7]Phosphorus conversions: 1 mMol = 31 mg elemental phosphorus; 1 mL sodium phosphate contains 3 mMol or 93 mg elemental phosphorus (and 4 mEq sodium); 1 mL potassium phosphate contains 3 mMol or 93 mg elemental phosphorus (and 4.4 mEq potassium).

[8]Magnesium conversions: 1 mEq = 0.5 mMol = 12.5 mg elemental magnesium; magnesium sulfate 50% contains 500 mg magnesium sulfate heptahydrate or 4.1 mEq (or 51.3 mg) elemental magnesium.

[9]Trace mineral additives are currently available individually and in various combinations/concentrations for various ages. Doses vary. Copper and manganese needs may be lower with cholestasis. See Table 25–6..

[10]Many institutions do not routinely include iron in parenteral admixtures due to incompatibility with other nutrients, contraindication during sepsis, and risks associated with overdose with multiple blood transfusions.

Source: Data from endnote references 5, 11, 60, 64, 79–86, and 203.

tion. This concentration is compatible with peripheral intravenous infusion. Greater concentrations of carbohydrate are given by central venous infusion, generally up to a maximum concentration of 25%.[95] These may be needed when caloric needs are greater than normal, when parenterally administered fat is poorly tolerated, or when fluid restriction is necessary.

PROTEIN

Studies attempting to define parenteral protein needs are more abundant for preterm infants than for older infants and children. Parenteral administration of 1.1 to 2.5 g/kg/day along with 30 to 60 kcal/kg/day supports neutral or positive nitrogen balance in very-low-birth-weight (VLBW) infants during the first 24 hours of life. Subsequently, 3.0 to 3.5 g/kg/day (3.5 to 4.0 g/kg/day in infants less than 1000 g) is needed to support normal tissue accretion.[96–102] Early amino acid delivery may improve glucose tolerance by enhancing endogenous insulin secretion.[87,101] Insulin-like growth factor I (IGR-I) is lower in prematurely born infants and may be further reduced by inadequate protein intake. Low levels of IGR-I are associated with increased risk of retinopathy of prematurity, bronchopulmonary dysplasia, intraventricular hemorrhage, and necrotizing enterocolitis.[103] Recommendations beyond infancy are more empirical or disease related.[84,102,104] General recommendations for protein administration for infants and children are given in Table 25–2. Protein usually comprises about 10 to 15% of total energy intake. Individual protein needs can be determined from nitrogen balance studies.

Unlike energy needs, protein needs do not decrease during periods of acute stress.[104] The administration of amino acids during periods of acute stress does not completely prevent endogenous protein catabolism, but, in conjunction with enough energy to meet basal requirements, helps maintain normal plasma amino acid concentrations, increases nitrogen retention, and may stimulate endogenous insulin secretion to improve glucose tolerance.[5,87,101] Protein status is generally evaluated by monitoring serum total protein and albumin levels, although changes in serum prealbumin, transferrin, retinol binding protein, or blood urea nitrogen (BUN) levels may identify changes in protein status more quickly. Monitoring acid-base balance and BUN or ammonia levels helps identify excess protein intake. Recommendations concerning monitoring and complications of protein administration are found in Tables 25–3 and 25–4.

Crystalline amino acid (CAA) products have been developed for infants reflecting the amino acid composition of human milk or plasma aminograms of healthy term infants fed mature human milk. Metabolic immaturity has also been considered, as cystine, taurine, tyrosine, and histidine may be essential amino acids for the neonate and young children.[105–109] Methionine, phenylalanine, and glycine concentrations have been decreased in these solutions, while histidine, tyrosine, taurine, arginine, glutamic acid, and aspartic acid may be added or their concentrations increased.[109] Although cystine may be a conditionally essential amino, it is not included in CAA solutions because it is unstable in solution for prolonged periods of time.[110] It is available as L-cystine hydrochloride to be added separately at the time of administration. Cystathionase activity matures to 70% of adult activity by 9 days of age in preterm infants and by 3 days of age in term infants. Cystine supplementation does not increase overall nitrogen retention or improve growth in neonates when 120 mg methionine per kilogram per day is provided, suggesting that cystine may not be needed beyond the neonatal period.[111,112] However, children 1 to 7 years of age receiving home parenteral nutrition with short bowel syndrome demonstrate low serum taurine levels that are increased to within normal reference range by the addition of cystine to their pediatric amino acid preparation, even though the preparation itself contains taurine.[113] The most commonly recommended dose for cystine is 30 to 40 mg/g of protein for pediatric CAA products, although cystine may not be needed for standard solutions due to higher methionine content.[112–115] Adding L-cystine hydrochloride

Table 25–3 Suggested Laboratory Monitoring During Pediatric Parenteral Nutrition

Laboratory Index	*Initial*	*Stable*	*Home Monitoring*
Blood glucose	Daily	Daily to 3x/week	Daily to 3x/week
Acid-base status	Daily to weekly	Every other week	Monthly < 6 months Every 3 months < 1 year Every 6 months > 1 year
Electrolytes Na, K, Cl, CO_2	Daily	Weekly or every other week	
Chemistry profile: total protein albumin BUN, creatinine Ca, P, Mg triglyceride	Weekly	Weekly or every other week	Monthly < 6 months Every 3 months < 1 year Every 6 months > 1 year
Liver profile: total bilirubin alk phos LDH, ALT, AST PTT	Weekly	Monthly	Monthly < 6 months Every 3 months < 1 year Every 6 months > 1 year
Hematology profile: HBG/HCT platelet count	Baseline	Weekly	Monthly < 6 months Every 3 months < 1 year Every 6 months > 1 year
CBC w/diff	Weekly	Monthly or as indicated*	As above or as indicated*
iron/TIBC/ferritin	As indicated*	As indicated*	As indicated*
Other: trace minerals vitamins carnitine	As indicated*	As indicated*	As indicated*
Urine glucose specific gravity pH	2–4 times a day	Daily to weekly	As indicated*

*as indicated = clinical condition or symptoms indicating deficiency, imbalance, or abnormality

Note: BUN = blood urea nitrogen; LDH = lactic dehydrogenase; ALT = alanine amino transferase; AST = aspartate amino transferase; PTT = prothrombin time; HGB = hemoglobin; HCT = hematocrit; CBC = complete blood count; TIBC = total iron binding capacity.

Table 25–4 Metabolic Complications of Pediatric Parenteral Nutrition

Complication	*Cause*	*Treatment*
Hyperglycemia, glycosuria, osmotic diuresis, hyperosmolar nonketotic dehydration, coma	Excessive dose or rate of glucose infusion	Decrease rate, concentration of glucose; use insulin with caution, results are often erratic in the very low birth weight infant
Hypoglycemia	Abrupt discontinuation of glucose infusion; excess insulin	Maintain constant glucose infusion; decrease glucose infusion rates slowly; decrease insulin
Metabolic acidosis, hyperammonemia, prerenal azotemia	Excessive amino acid infusion, inappropriate protein/calorie ratio	Decrease amino acids, increase nonprotein calories
Hyperchloremic metabolic acidosis	Excessive chloride administration causing cation gap	Provide equal amount of sodium and chloride in infusate; neutralize cation gap with lactate or acetate if respiratory status allows
Hypokalemia	Inadequate potassium infusion relative to increased requirements for protein anabolism	If potassium needs are greater than the potassium provided by potassium phosphate, potassium acetate is generally recommended
Hyperkalemia	Excessive potassium administration, especially in metabolic acidosis	Decrease potassium in infusate
Volume overload, congestive heart failure	Excessive rate of fluid administration	Monitor weight daily; monitor intake and output daily to prevent volume overload; do not attempt to "catch up" by increasing rate of infusion; to treat, decrease rate of infusion
Hypocalcemia	Inadequate calcium administration or phosphorus administration without simultaneous calcium infusion; hypomagnesemia or hypoalbuminemia	Increase calcium infusion, maintaining appropriate phosphorus and magnesium infusion
Hypophosphatemia	Inadequate phosphorus administration especially relative to increased needs of protein anabolism	Increase phosphorus infusion, maintaining appropriate calcium/phosphorus precipitation

continues

Table 25–4 continued

HypeHypomagnesemia	Inadequate magnesium infusion relative to increased gastrointestinal losses in chronic diarrhea or increased needs for protein anabolism	Increase magnesium infusion
Essential fatty acid deficiency	Inadequate linoleic acid infusion	Provide at least 4–8% of total calories as intravenous fat emulsion to provide 1–4% of total calories as linoleic acid
Hypertriglyceridemia, hypercholesterolemia	Lipids infused at a rate greater than the capacity to metabolize	Decrease or interrupt lipid infusion; add heparin to infusate*
Anemia	Deficiency of iron, folic acid, vitamin B12, or copper	Administer appropriate nutrient
Cholestatic jaundice	Sepsis, prematurity, starvation, essential fatty acid deficiency, lipid infusion, amino acid deficiency, amino acid excess, carbohydrate excess, decreased bile flow, bowel obstruction, lack of enteral feedings	Begin enteral feedings as soon as possible, maintain adequate but not excessive intake; liver function generally returns to normal within 6–9 months after cessation of therapy, but may progress to chronic liver disease

* Data from reference 43, Chapter 7.

Source: Adapted with permission from Groh-Wargo S, et al., *Nutritional Care for High-Risk Newborns,* pp. 56–58, © 1994, Precept Press, Inc.

decreases the solution's pH, which increases calcium and phosphorus solubility, thus increasing mineral delivery.[116,117]

Although glutamine is not routinely added to parenteral nutrition solutions due to solubility problems, this amino acid may be conditionally essential during periods of sepsis, trauma, surgery, or shock when circulating levels decrease and needs, particularly in maintaining GI mucosal cell integrity, are increased.[118,119] For extremely low-birth-weight infants, glutamine added to parenteral nutrition in amounts of 0.3 to 0.5 gm/kg/day (or 20% of amino acid intake) appears safe and may support lower occurrence rates of GI dysfunction and severe neurological sequellae and earlier achievement of full enteral feedings.[120,121]

Most of the studies comparing or evaluating the efficacy of pediatric and standard CAA products have been done in small numbers of patients over relatively short duration (5 to 21 days).[93,105–107,117] While greater weight gain and nitrogen balance with pediatric products may be statistically significant, these differences may not be clinically significant. The greatest advantage seems to be that plasma amino acid patterns are similar to those of healthy breastfed neonates. Implications for use with older infants or children have not been clearly identified. Although the data are inconclusive, there may be a decreased incidence of cholestatic liver disease during specific pediatric CAA product administration.[115,122–125]

In practice, based on current literature, pediatric CAA products may be of benefit to the prematurely born infant or the infant who requires long-term parenteral nutrition. Pediatric CAA products may require cystine supplementation with 55 to 77 mg/kg/day for infants less than 4 months of age due to inadequate cystathionase activity. All other infants and children may need 3 to 22 mg cystine per gram of total amino acid content due to reduced methionine content.[93,110,112–115]

Special solutions of L-isomer CAA formulated for adults with severe hepatic or renal failure appear to also be efficacious in children with severe hepatic or chronic renal failure, though standard CAA solutions may better meet the amino acid needs of children with acute renal failure.[126–130] Older children with sepsis or traumatic injury may benefit from using formulations with increased amounts of branched-chain amino acids.[131]

FAT

Fat is included in parenteral nutrition regimens for infants and children as a source of essential fatty acids (EFA) and energy. Linoleic acid (LA) deficiency is clinically manifested as dry, flaky skin; dry hair; poor growth; decreased platelets; and impaired wound healing. Biochemical deficiency of LA precedes these clinical manifestations. Plasma levels of LA and arachidonic acid (AA) decline, and the ratio of plasma eicosatrienoic acid to AA (triene:tetraene) becomes elevated. Numbness, paresthesia, weakness, inability to walk, and blurring of vision may occur if linolenic acid (LNA) deficiency is present, and docosapentaenoic acid (DPA) levels increase while docosahexaenoic acid (DHA) levels decrease.[5,132,133] Long-chain polyunsaturated acids AA and DHA are involved in the structure and function of cell membranes, specifically retinal and central nervous system structures, and dietary manipulation of these fatty acids is the subject of current research.[134] Very-low-birth-weight infants or infants and children with depleted body stores of fat or with a chronic history of fat malabsorption are at greatest risk of developing EFA deficiencies.[135]

Providing as little as 1% to 2.7% of the total daily caloric intake as LA and 0.54% to 1.0% of the total daily caloric intake as LNA can prevent deficiency in most infants and children.[11,60,136] Parenteral lipids available contain linoleic acid as 50%, 54.5%, or 65.8% of total fat and LNA as 4.2%, 8.3%, or 9% of total fat, depending upon the product used.[109] Usual recommendations for prevention of EFA deficiency are 0.5 g/kg/day or 2.5 mL of 20% lipid emulsion/kg/day, but this may not provide adequate amounts of LNA for infants or young children. Doses of parenteral lipid that meet estimated LNA needs for infants and young children are 0.6 g/kg/day (or 6.5% of total calories as fat) if the lipid emulsion contains at least 50% of total fatty acids as LA and 8% of total fatty acids as LNA. Children over 4 years of age require only 0.5 g/kg/day and adolescents require only 0.4 g/kg/d to meet estimated essential fatty acid needs. Somewhat larger doses may be necessary for lipid emulsions containing lesser amounts of LNA. Products made with medium-chain triglyceride (MCT) oil are not available in the United States, but are available in Europe. Products containing MCT oil may provide advantages of more rapid hydrolyzation and oxidation with improved tolerance and better energy delivery, but they also contain lower amounts of essential fatty acids.[87,137,138]

Limitations of glucose or fluid tolerance and high energy needs usually dictate a greater intake of lipid than that which prevents deficiency. Fifty percent of energy intake is derived from fat in the breastfed infant. Parenteral lipid doses of 2.5 to 3.0 g/kg/d provide infants with only 25–35% of total energy intake as fat, but higher doses may be poorly tolerated, especially in prematurely born or small for gestational age infants.[60,84,139,140] In children over 2 years of age, it may be advisable to limit fat to 30% of total calories (generally 1.0 to 2.5 g/kg/d), as recommended by the American Academy of Pediatrics.[141] Fat should not provide more than 60% of total calories in any patient, because ketotic acidosis may occur.[142]

The rate of administration may be just as significant a factor in lipid tolerance as daily dose. Adverse effects of intravenous fat when given in boluses or in doses exceeding 0.15 g/kg/hr or 3.6 g/kg/d have been reported, including altered pulmonary function, impaired neutrophil function, and an increased risk of kernicterus in infants with elevated serum bilirubin level.[143–145] Preterm or malnourished infants and children may be at greater risk for impaired fat tolerance due to decreased adipose tissue mass, reduced lipoprotein lipase activity, hepatic immaturity, or carnitine deficiency. While heparin stimulates the release of lipoprotein lipase, it may not significantly affect lipid clearance over time and is not routinely recommended for that purpose.

Parenteral lipid is available in 10% or 20% emulsions of soybean oil or a combination of safflower and soybean oils. These emulsions also contain egg phospholipid as an emulsifying agent. Because phospholipids interfere with enzymes that help metabolize and clear plasma lipids, 20% emulsions are recommended over 10% emulsions due to lower phospholipid to lipid ratio.

Parenteral lipid emulsions also contain glycerol and are relatively isotonic and pH neutral, providing a favorable environment for the proliferation of several common pathogens. When infused separately, lipid emulsions are associated with an increased incidence of coagulase negative staphylococcal bacteremia, particularly when hang times exceed 12 hours. When administered as a component of a TNA, this association is no longer apparent, likely due to the hypertonic and relatively acidic environment provided by the presence of other nutrients.[145] However, both of these factors may decrease the stability of the lipid emulsion, causing separation, particularly when higher amounts of amino acids and minerals are used, as for low-birth-weight infants. The opacity of TNAs may also mask the presence of incompatibilities and precipitates, resulting in adverse outcomes, although use of a 1.2 micron filter can remove larger organisms, particles, precipitates, and fat globules.[147]

Intravenous fat may be safely given if:

1. The initial dose is 0.5 g/kg/d and it is gradually increased by 0.25 to 0.5 g/kg/d.
2. The highest dose is under 0.12 to 0.15 g/kg/hr (3 to 3.6 g/kg/d) or less than 0.08 gm/kg/h (2 g/kg/d) during periods of acute sepsis.
3. Serum triglycerides are monitored and kept within the normal range, although there are various recommendations given in the literature for the acceptable upper limit of normal, ranging from 100 to 200 mg/dL.[136,143,144]
4. Whenever possible, lipids are administered as a component of a TNA over 24 hours using a 1.2 micron filter to best maintain physiochemical stability and minimize infectious risk.[146,147]

When lipids must be infused separately due to higher protein and mineral needs, as for low-birth-weight infants, recommendations for reducing risk of nosocomial bacteremia include: (1) aseptic transferal of lipid emulsion from the original container directly to infusion devices by pharmacy personnel under a class "A" laminar air flow hood, and (2) hang times limited to 12 hours whenever possible.[148] Limiting hang times to 12 hours ultimately limits total lipid dose to 1.8 g/kg/day or 17–20% of total energy intake. When energy needs exceed 95 kcal/kg/day and fluid tolerance is limited to 120–150 mL/kg/day, dextrose solutions of 15–18% given through centrally placed catheters may be required. Because this may exceed glucose tolerance particularly in extremely low-birth-weight infants, using administration sets up to 24 hours to accommodate a second lipid infusion has been suggested.[146]

If serum bilirubin levels are greater than 8–10 mg/dl (while the serum albumin level is 2.5 to 3 g/dl), lipids should be given only in amounts adequate to prevent essential fatty acid deficiency.[145] If intravenous fat is given in greater amounts or given in bolus doses, the free fatty acid to serum albumin molar ratio should be maintained at less than 6 while bilirubin levels remain elevated.[60] (See Chapter 3 for further discussion on this issue.)

Carnitine facilitates transport of long- and medium-chain fatty acids across mitochondrial membranes. Carnitine is normally synthesized by the liver from methionine and lysine. Pediatric amino acid solutions are lower in methionine than standard solutions, and patients at risk for carnitine deficiency demonstrate lower plasma concentrations of carnitine when receiving carnitine-free parenteral products as their single source of nutrition.[149] Patients at highest risk for carnitine depletion include those who are less than 30 weeks' gestation, have a birth weight under 1500 g or a history of fetal malnutrition, or have hepatic or renal dysfunction, infection, or medium-chain acetyl-dehydrogenase deficiency.[150]

Studies are somewhat conflicting as to whether or not routine carnitine supplementation is needed, even in high-risk individuals, or if carnitine supplementation significantly affects parenteral lipid utilization.[151–156] Carnitine supplementation may be considered in patients identified at high risk if parenteral nutrition is expected to be the single source of nutrition longer than 2 weeks, or if hypertriglyceridemia, hypoglycemia, and low serum carnitine are present.[150,152] Dose recommendations for oral or intravenous supplementation of carnitine vary from 50 to 100 mmol/kg/day (approximately 10–20 mg/kg/day).[151–155] Doses of 300 mmol/kg/day (50 mg/kg/day) or greater are not recommended, because these doses are associated with increased metabolic rate, decreased protein deposition, and impaired growth.[150,155] Although carnitine is not routinely added to parenteral nutrition solutions in all institutions at this time, it is available for parenteral use.

VITAMINS

Recommendations for term infants and children up to 11 years of age were established by the Nutrition Advisory Group of the American Medical Association in 1975.[157] They are based on the 1974 recommended dietary allowances (RDAs), which are guidelines for enteral nutrient intake. Recommendations for adolescents are based on guidelines for adults. Vitamin requirements of prematurely born infants may vary from those of term infants due to the immaturity of vitamin absorption, excretion, enterohepatic recirculation, and renal tubular reabsorption mechanisms. Current estimates of need are based on numerous studies and extrapolations from term infant data.[82] Two different vitamin dose regimens for infants who weigh less than 2500 g have been suggested. Doses based on broad weight categories are more likely to underdose larger infants and/or overdose smaller infants, particularly with vitamins E and K and B-complex vitamins.[158–160] Either dose regimen is likely to underdose vitamin A, particularly for smaller infants, though vitamin A is often dosed separately for these infants and given intramuscularly.[158,161]

Studies have shown the Food and Drug Administration's current dose recommendations to produce serum levels at or above the reference range for α-tocopherol, 25-hydroxycholecalciferol, thiamin, riboflavin, niacin, pyridoxine, folate, pantothenic acid, cyanocobalamin, and biotin.[162,163] There are no reports of toxic vitamin levels using these recommended doses. Thiamin deficiency has been reported in infants and children during shortages of parenteral multivitamin (MVI) products. Oral or enteral administration of thiamin, and perhaps other vitamins, may not be sufficient in patients who require total or partial delivery of nutrition parenterally. Thiamin should be given as a separate intravenous additive during MVI shortages.[164] The vitamin content of MVI Pediatric for Infusion and MVI-12 Multivitamin Infusion (Astra USA, Inc.) are compared to the current vitamin dose recommendations in Table 25–5.

Levels of several vitamins may decrease over time in parenteral nutrient admixtures due to light degradation, decomposition in the presence of bisulfite (an antioxidant additive) or varying pH, and adsorbance to plastic or glass. For these reasons, it is recommended that multivitamins be added to parenteral nutrient solutions immediately prior to administration, excessive light exposure (direct sunlight or phototherapy light) should be avoided, and administration of these admixtures completed within 24 hours.

MINERALS

Magnesium

Magnesium deficiency is identified by decreased serum levels. Hypomagnesemia may be seen in protein-calorie malnutrition, chronic malabsorption, proximal jejunal resection, ileostomy, cystic fibrosis, neonatal hepatitis, congenital biliary atresia, DiGeorge's syndrome, hypokalemia; in infants born to diabetic mothers; or during chronic diuretic therapy, aminoglycoside therapy, or during chemotherapy.[13] If serum levels are below 1.4 mg/dL or if seizures occur, repletion dose is 0.2 mEq/kg given intramuscularly or intravenously every 6 hours until symptoms subside. Older children may require 0.8–1 mEq/kg/day for repletion or during critical illness.[86] Blood pressure should be monitored with intravenous magnesium repletion, because hypotension may occur.[60]

Parenteral doses of 0.5–1 mEq/kg/d may be needed to allow adequate retention for prematurely born infants, though general dose recommendations for all other infants and children are 0.25 to 0.5 mEq/kg/d of magnesium with a maximum allowable dose of 24 mEq/d.[60,91,140] Upper-range doses may be needed during rapid growth phases, diuretic therapy, or chronic malabsorption. Lower range doses may be indicated if renal function is impaired. Magnesium is added to parenteral admixtures as magnesium sulfate (50% $MgSO_4$), which contains 4.1 mEq (49.3 mg) of magnesium per milliliter. Excessive doses may cause central nervous system depression and hypotonia.[82]

Calcium

Calcium deficiency is not usually identified by low serum levels. If calcium intake is insufficient, serum calcium is maintained at the expense of bone stores in most infants and children.[82] Hypocalcemia is most common during the neonatal period, particularly in infants born prematurely due to their relatively low calcium stores and inappropriately low parathyroid hormone levels. This initial hypocalcemia usually resolves within the first few days of life when treated with intravenous administration of calcium 1 to 2 mEq/kg/d.[105]

Nutrition recommendations for parenteral calcium administration to prematurely born infants range from 50 to 80 mg/kg/d (which is 1.3–2 mmol/kg/d or 2.5–3 mEq/kg/d).[82,144,166,167] Most published sources empirically recommend 10–50 mg/kg/d (which is 0.25 to 1.3 mmol/kg/d or 0.5 to 2 mEq/kg/d) for all other ages[49] (see Table 25–2). Calcium should be administered over 24 hours because parenteral calcium administered chronically as bolus doses over 20 minutes to 1 hour has been associated with hypercalcemia and hypercalciuria.[168,169] Nephrolithiasis and hypercalciuria have been associated with furosemide therapy and inadequate phosphorus intake.[166,170] Older children receiving cyclic parenteral nutrition may have greater urinary losses of calcium due to higher rates of infusion.[171]

Table 25–5 Recommendations for Pediatric Parenteral Daily Vitamin Dosage

	A *IU*	*D* *IU*	*E* *mg*	*K* *mcg*	*C* *mg*	*B1* *mg*	*B2* *mg*	*B3* *mg*	*B6* *mg*	*B12* *mcg*	*FA* *mcg*	*PA* *mg*	*Biotin* *mcg*
Recommended amount/kg/day													
Preterm infant (≤ 2.5 kg)	1700	160	2.8	80	25	0.35	0.15	6.8	0.18	0.3	56	2	6
MVI Pediatric** doses													
30% dose/day (0.5–1 kg)	700–1400	120–240	2.1–4.2	60–120	24–48	0.4–0.7	0.3–0.6	5–10	0.3–0.6	0.3–0.6	42–84	1.5–3	6–12
65% dose/day (1–2.5 kg)	600–1500	100–260	1.8–4.5	50–130	21–52	0.3–0.8	0.4–0.9	4–11	0.3–0.6	0.3–0.6	36–90	1.5–3	5–13
40% dose/kg/day (≤2.5 kg)*	920	160	2.8	80	32	0.48	0.56	6.8	0.4	0.4	56	2	8
Recommended amount/day													
Preterm infant (> 2.5 kg)	700–1500	40–160	2–4	6–10	35–50	0.3–0.8	0.4–0.9	5–12	0.3–0.7	0.3–0.7	40–90	2–5	6–13
Term infant/child (age 1–11 yrs)	2300	400	5–7	200	80	1.2	1.4	17	1	1	140	5	20
MVI Pediatric,** 1 dose/day	2300	400	7	200	80	1.2	1.4	17	1	1	140	5	20
Recommended amount/day													
Adolescents (11–18 yrs)	3300	200	10	150–700	100	3	3.6	40	4	5	400	15	60
MVI–12,** 1 dose/day	3300	200	10	150	100	3	3.6	40	4	5	400	15	60

Note: A = retinol, D = cholecalciferol, E = alpha-tocopherol, K = phytonadione, B1 = thiamin, B2 = riboflavin, B3 = niacin, B6 = pyridoxine, B12 = cyanocobalamin, FA = folic acid, PA = pantothenic acid

* Maximum dose not to exceed 1 full dose per day

** Pediatric MVI (Pediatric parenteral multivitamin) and MVI-12 Injection or Unit Vial, Astra USA, Inc., Westboro, MA.

Source: Data from endnote references 5, 82, 87, 144, 162, and 163.

Calcium gluconate is generally the additive of choice, though there is some concern about aluminum contamination, especially at higher doses.[172] Solutions that deliver 15 to 30 mcg aluminum/kg/d may result in tissue loading and are considered unsafe.[82,173] Calcium gluconate 10% contains 100 mg of calcium gluconate per 1 mL, providing 0.5 mEq, 0.25 mmol, or 10 mg of elemental calcium per 1 mL.

Phosphorus

Phosphorus depletion has been reported in infants and children and may be more pronounced when calcium is given without phosphorus. Phosphorus depletion is characterized by hypercalciuria (at least 4 mg of calcium per kilogram per day), hypophosphatemia (serum levels less than 4 mg/dl), and undetectable levels of urinary phosphorus excretion.[82,174,175] Parenteral repletion of phosphorus may be accomplished by an initial one to two doses of 5 to 11 mg/kg (0.15 to 0.36 mmol/kg), each given over 6 hours. When refeeding malnourished individuals, the initial 7 to 10 days of the anabolic phase is accompanied by increased needs for phosphorus, and, to a lesser extent, potassium and magnesium, because these electrolytes are incorporated into cells of lean tissue. Phosphorus needs may be twice the normal recommended allowance during this time, though consistent monitoring is recommended to prevent excessive phosphorus administration that may cause hyperphosphatemia, hypocalcemia, and secondary hyperparathyroidism.[82]

Recommendations for parenteral administration of phosphorus to infants and children are given in Table 25–2. Doses for phosphorus are often given in proportion to calcium as 1:1 to 1.3:1 molar ratio or 1.3:1 to 1.7:1 calcium/phosphorus ratio by weight.[82] Phosphorus is added to parenteral nutrient solutions as potassium or sodium phosphate salts. Potassium phosphate contains 93 mg (3 mmol) of phosphorus and 4.4 mEq of potassium per mL. Sodium phosphate contains 93 mg (3 mmol) of phosphorus and 4 mEq of sodium per mL.

The greatest difficulty in providing adequate calcium and phosphorus parenterally is their relative insolubility in the same admixture, limited further by increasing pH and temperature. Alternating calcium and phosphorus administration is not recommended due to adverse effects including alternating elevations of serum mineral levels, increased mineral losses due to urinary excretion, and altered mineral homeostasis.[176–178] Recommendations for compounding to minimize precipitation usually include adding phosphate salts early in the process and calcium salts late (but before the lipid emulsion in 3-in-1 admixtures).[118,179] Adherence to compounding protocol is particularly important when lipid is present, as precipitates are more difficult to identify due to the opacity of the admixture. The addition of L-cysteine increases mineral solubility and the use of calcium glycerophosphate or monobasic phosphate formulations may also improve solubility.[52] Solubility studies and guidelines for simultaneous administration of calcium and phosphorus have been published for various amino acid products.[176,179–181] Filters are recommended to prevent precipitate delivery: a 1.2 micron air-eliminating filter for lipid containing admixtures and a 0.22 micron air-eliminating filter for non-lipid containing admixtures.[179] The higher doses of minerals needed for young infants are given through central intravenous access to prevent vascular damage and tissue sloughs. Separate administration of lipid may be needed to allow higher concentrations of calcium and phosphorus for prematurely born infants.

Trace Minerals

Recommendations for daily parenteral doses are given in Table 25–2.[82,182] Zinc, copper, chromium, manganese, selenium, and iodine are available singly or in combination for use in parenteral nutrition admixtures. Product concentrations and dose recommendations are given in Table 25–6. Neither clinical nor biochemical deficiency of molybdenum or iodine with parenteral nutrition has been reported in the literature, and they are generally not included in parenteral

Table 25–6 Dose Concentrations and Recommendations for Combined Trace Mineral Products

Product category	*Dose mL*	*Zinc mcg*	*Copper mcg*	*Chromium mcg*	*Manganese mcg*	*Selenium[1] mcg*
Neonatal[2]	1	1500	100	0.85	25	—
	0.2/kg	300/kg[3]	20/kg	0.17/kg	5/kg[4]	—
Pediatric	1	500 or 1000	100	0.85 or 1	25	0 or 15
	0.1/kg	50 or 100/kg	10/kg	~ 0.1/kg	2.5/kg	0 or 1.5/kg
	0.2/kg	100 or 200/kg	20/kg	~ 0.2/kg	5/kg[4]	0 or 2/kg
	2[5]	2000	200	2	50	30
	5[5]	2500 or 5000	500	4.25 or 5	125	0
Adult[6,7] (standard)	1	1000	400	4	100	0 or 20
	0.05/kg	50/kg	20/kg	0.2/kg	5/kg[4]	0 or 1/kg
Adult[6] (concentrate)	1	5000	1000	10	500	0 or 60
	0.01/kg	50/kg	10/kg	0.1/kg	5/kg[4]	0 or 0.6/kg

[1]Neonatal and select pediatric and adult products do not contain selenium or molybdenum. These may be added separately when total parenteral nutrition is required longer than 4 weeks.
[2] Neonatal products are generally recommended for preterm infants until term age. Maximum dose is 3 mL/day.
[3]Additional zinc is needed to meet recommendations for preterm neonates.
[4]Manganese dose may be excessive in cholestatic jaundice.
[5]Maximum dose of pediatric product with selenium is limited by the amount of selenium. Maximum dose of pediatric product with out selenium is limited by copper content.
[6]Adult products are generally used for adolescents, or children over 10 years of age.
[7]Iodine is included in one standard and one concentrated adult product in concentrations of 25 and 75 mcg/mL respectively; molybdenum is included in one standard adult product in a concentration of 25 mcg/mL.

Source: Data from product literature and Intravenous nutritional therapy. Trace metals. *Drug Facts and Comparisons.* St. Louis, Missouri: Wolters Kluwer Health Inc. 2003; p. 125.

nutrition admixtures. Transdermal absorption of iodine from cleansing or disinfecting solutions or ointments may be an adequate source of iodine.[183] Fluorine is not added, as its role in human nutrition is limited primarily to dental health and may be of greater benefit when administered topically once teeth have erupted around 6 months of age.[83]

Very-low-birth-weight infants and infants and children with protein-calorie malnutrition, thermal injury, neoplasms, chronic diarrhea, enterocutaneous fistulas, or bile salt malabsorption are at greatest risk for developing trace element deficiency.[182–185] Zinc supplementation without copper supplementation may interfere with copper metabolism.[183] Copper doses are reduced or eliminated, and manganese is withheld for infants and children who develop cholestatic jaundice, because these minerals are excreted primarily through bile and their accumulation is potentially hepatotoxic.[60,186,187] However, copper deficiency has been reported when omitted from parenteral nutrition due to presence of cholestasis.[188] Serum manganese levels may become markedly elevated after several months of PN. A contributory role of manganese in the development of PN-related cholestasis has been considered, particularly in individuals receiving PN longer than 30 days.[189] Selenium and molybdenum are not generally used when parenteral nutrition is required only for a short period of time. Selenium is present as a contaminant in parenteral dextrose solutions, providing up to 0.9 mg/dl. Parenteral selenium toxicity has not been reported, though lower doses may be indicated when renal function is impaired.[82]

Iron deficiency is probably the most common trace mineral deficiency. It manifests as microcytic hypochromic anemia and is characterized by low serum hemoglobin and ferritin levels, low hematocrit, and low percent transferrin saturation. Infants and children at risk for iron deficiency include those who are prematurely born, chronically ill, protein-calorie malnourished; have significant unreplaced blood loss; or who receive unsupplemented parenteral nutrition for long periods of time.

There is some controversy over whether or not iron should be routinely included in parenteral nutrition therapy. Intramuscular injections of iron may not be the best choice in the small prematurely born infant or the protein-calorie malnourished patient due to small muscle mass and increased risk of sarcoma at the site of injection.[190] Anaphylaxis has been reported in some patients with administration of iron dextran.[191] Several authors report that iron may be safely given daily in parenteral nutrition admixtures or in bolus doses given intravenously over 2 to 3 hours weekly or monthly.[190–193] Often, iron is given parenterally only in treatment of iron deficiency anemia.

Although standard dose recommendations for prematurely born infants are 0.1 to 0.2 mg/kg/d,[82,194] trials of recombinant erythropoietin have used iron supplements of 1 mg/kg/d without evidence of harmful side effects, though these are short-term studies.[195,196] Iron toxicity may be difficult to ascertain because iron is quickly stored in hepatic tissue and serum iron levels may not reflect overload. Excess iron may also increase risk of gram-negative septicemia and increase antioxidant requirements. These risks do not preclude use of standard doses of parenteral iron, but higher doses must be used with caution beyond 4 weeks duration.[82] Very-low-birth-weight infants who have received blood transfusion of at least 180 mL of packed cells may not need additional iron supplementation.[197] Doses of 0.1 mg/kg/d up to 1 mg/d are recommended for all other infants and children. Iron dextran is available as the source of iron for parenteral use. Guidelines for dosage and administration of iron dextran in treatment of iron deficiency are given in the manufacturer's package insert.

PATIENT MONITORING

A comprehensive monitoring program for infants and children receiving PN includes evaluation of laboratory measurements of metabolic and electrolyte status (see Table 25–3), anthropometric measurements (see Table 25–7), intake and output measurements, and physical examination (see Table 25–8). Baseline and regularly scheduled laboratory measurements allow timely identification of metabolic complications and assessment of nutritional adequacy. Metabolic complications that may occur during pediatric nutrition support are summarized in Table 25–4. Laboratory values obtained are compared to neonatal and/or pediatric norms that are often different from adult norms. (See Chapter 2.) Laboratory monitoring protocols may vary from one setting to another, but should take into consideration smaller blood volumes in pediatric patients, using microtechniques whenever possible and avoiding unnecessary bloodwork. For patients on long-term PN, the need and frequency for some tests can be reevaluated once a stable regimen has been established.

Suggested physical monitoring is given in Table 25–8. Temperature instability, apnea and bradycardia, and increased respiration rate and pulse may be early signs of sepsis in the pediatric patient. Records of intake provide documentation that actual administration equals planned intake. Documentation of output establishes a basis for evaluation of fluid balance, as does evaluation of skin turgor and the presence of edema. Insertion sites are monitored for redness, swelling, leaking, or other signs of infection or infiltration. Changes in behavior and/or mental status may precede other signs of sepsis or fluid and electrolyte balance.

Table 25–7 Growth Parameters Monitored During Pediatric Parenteral Nutrition

Parameter	*Frequency*
Weight	Daily (neonates up to 1 month corrected age) Weekly (1–6 months corrected age) Monthly (infants > 6 months corrected age, children)
Length or Height	Weekly (infants < 6 months corrected age) Monthly (infants > 6 months corrected age) Every 3 months (ages 1–3) Every 6 months (ages 4–18)
Head Circumference	Weekly (infants < 6 months corrected age) Monthly (infants > 6 months corrected age) Every 3 months (ages 1–3)
Body Composition Triceps Skinfold Arm Muscle Area	As clinically indicated; comparison against established norms is more useful in children > 3 years than in younger children

PSYCHOSOCIAL ISSUES

Eating is basic to life. Parents feed their infants and children. When normal feeding is replaced with PN, parents may feel helpless or useless. An infant or child of any age may feel frustrated at not being able to eat. Older children may have fears or insecurities about body function or body image. The ability of an infant or child and their family to accept and adapt to PN depends on the presenting diagnosis, the acuity or chronicity of the disease or condition, the duration and complexity of the hospitalization, the duration of nutrition support therapy, and the physical and emotional development of the infant or child.[198–199] Eighty to 90% of children requiring home TPN will likely continue to receive this support 1 year after initiation.[200] When long-term or home PN is needed, the stability of the family unit and its financial, physical, and emotional resources are important factors as well.

Table 25–8 Clinical Monitoring During Pediatric Parenteral Nutrition

Clinical Parameter	*Initial*	*Stable*
Temperature Pulse/Respirations	Hourly, then every 4–8 hr	Daily or as indicated
Intake	Hourly, then every 4–8 hr	Daily
Output	Hourly, then every 4–8 hr	As indicated
Administration system	Hourly, then every 4–8 hr	Daily
Infusion site/dressing	Hourly, then every 4–8 hr	Daily
Mental status, behavioral status, edema, skin turgor	Every 4–8 hr	Daily or as indicated

Table 25-9 Resources that Support Successful Home Parenteral Nutrition

Environment	Grounded electrical outlets; backup electricity, either battery, generator, or power company priority when there is loss of power
	Lack of physical barriers to maneuvering equipment or storing supplies
	Refrigeration to store adequate supplies of solutions
	Reliable telephone service
	Convenient and safe water supply and hand-washing facilities
Medical support	Convenient and reliable home health care agency for nursing care, ongoing nutritional assessment, supplies, laboratory assessment
	Local physician experienced and amenable to home parenteral nutrition
	Responsive local community emergency care, both ambulance and local emergency room
Family characteristics	At least two responsible adults are competent to provide all care associated with home parenteral nutrition; extended family support
	All children (both the patient and siblings, particularly small children) are protected from harm associated with home parenteral nutrition, such as needle sticks; damage to catheter, tubing, or other equipment; removal of catheter; etc.
Financial	Adequate medical insurance coverage with certified medical necessity for home parenteral nutrition
Attitude	Family and patient must see home parenteral nutrition as having a positive influence on the life of the child
	Respect for risks and safety issues associated with parenteral nutrition
	Ability and willingness to comply with medical plan and techniques

Keeping the family informed; providing consistent support through a social worker, care manager, and/or primary nurse; and involving the family and child (appropriately for age and level of understanding) in the actual care activities can empower the family and child to meet some of their own needs and lessen their feelings of helplessness. Family involvement is crucial in preparing a family for successful home PN.

Members of the hospital-based multidisciplinary team, including the physician, nurse, dietitian, pharmacist, social worker, and developmental specialist, must plan a program of home PN that is feasible, given the resources of the family and the community. Resources that support success of home PN are listed in Table 25–9. Education of family members must take into account their readiness and ability to learn. Assessment of learning includes measuring the family's ability to accurately repeat instructions or demonstrate techniques. Communication with home health care providers is essential for continuity of care.

The technical nature of parenteral nutrition must not overshadow the infant or child and his or her developmental progress. Occupational and physical therapists, speech pathologists, and child life and/or developmental specialists ensure that the hospital setting is modified as much as possible to support the normal development of the child on PN.

For the neonate whose feedings are limited or who is unable to take oral feedings, pleasant oral stimulation, nonnutritive sucking, and other sensory stimulation is needed to support normal oral development. Prolonged, early oral deprivation can lead to increased oral sensitivity and abnormal tongue movements that can adversely influence the development of future speech patterns.[201] Eating is a basic, essential function and many parents, particularly mothers, may feel responsible for their infant's problems and may suffer loss of self-esteem or have feelings of inadequacy at being unable to perform the simple caregiving task of feeding. Health care professionals can enhance the parents' involvement in "feeding" the PN-dependent infant by encouraging them to hold, cuddle, and offer other forms of oral stimulation during "normal" feeding times. When possible, the infant on PN should be offered some type of oral feeding, if only in very small amounts. If totally deprived of oral sustenance, the introduction of oral feedings may be met with gagging, vomiting, swallowing difficulties, or other signs of feeding aversion.

Infants use their mouths to explore much of their environment. Sucking on fingers or toys can be encouraged to help infants experience and develop trust in their environment. Other types of tactile and visual stimulation can be provided to distract infants from manipulating or chewing on tubes and equipment. Creative ways to protect equipment and maintain safety should be used rather than physical restraint. Clothing that covers the catheter insertion site and tubing helps prevent pulling and manipulation of equipment and allows more limited exploration of the environment.

Toddlers present many challenges to the safe delivery of PN. These challenges may include temperament, mobility, and the development of other normal milestones such as toileting. Creative strategies to allow toddlers some control and independence in their environment can promote autonomy and lessen the negative impact of hospitalization or home PN on normal development. Providing clothes, toys, and photographs from home, sibling visits, and a high level of parent involvement can help the young child deal with the fear of painful procedures, the strange hospital environment, separation from loved ones, and feelings that the illness is a punishment for being naughty. A backpack that contains solution, pump, and tubing in fastened compartments can allow mobility and prevent toddlers from handling equipment, but it allows parents easy access for managing PN. Nocturnal cyclic PN may reduce interference with developmental needs.

The school-age child who is frequently hospitalized and requires PN needs to maintain involvement in school and with friends, to have some conformity with peers in appearance, and to have as much control over personal issues as possible. In-hospital teachers or private tutors may be needed to maintain educational progress. Choices for the child are offered whenever possible, including selection of the type and placement of the CVC and assisting with dressing changes. An established routine that allows the child to accomplish as many aspects of care as possible is important to avoid feelings of inferiority and prevent excessive dependency. During home PN, children are encouraged to resume as many normal school and play activities as their clinical condition allows.

Although the technical aspects of PN in the adolescent may be easier to manage, other issues may present greater challenges. With greater intellectual and social sophistication, the adolescent may have concerns, fears, and/or anxiety regarding many issues such as loss of control; altered body image or appearance; peer acceptance or isolation; dependence on technology, technical failures, or malfunctions; health and life expectancy; ability to participate in sports and other peer group activities; financial issues; and the effects on other family members. Sleep disturbances may occur due to anxiety or frequent urination that occurs with nocturnal fluid administration. Many of these issues may cause anger or depression and lead to poor compliance with the therapeutic regimen.

Backpacks or vests designed to hold PN solutions and equipment may be used to maximize mobility and minimize changes in physical appearance. Nocturnal cyclic PN circumvents changes in appearance during the day and places less limitation on activities with peers. Other strategies to improve compliance with the PN regimen include:

1. providing information using appropriate terminology for age and educational level
2. encouraging active participation in decision making and management of PN
3. providing psychological counseling when needed

REIMBURSEMENT

In response to rapidly escalating health care costs starting in the mid-1970s, reimbursement strategies have been dramatically changing. PN is a complex and expensive therapy. Costs include nutrient solutions; technical equipment such as catheters, tubing, and automated pumps; laboratory monitoring; and health care providers such as physicians, nurses, dietitians, pharmacists, and developmental therapists. Though PN administered at home may generate fewer costs, it is still expensive.

In efforts to contain health care costs, many third-party payors have developed regulations that restrict who can be reimbursed, what is reimbursed, and place a capitation on reimbursement for PN.[202] PN provided in the hospital may be considered part of "room and board," because nutrition/feeding is considered a basic need. Because PN is not a directly reimbursed service, reimbursement often depends on the assigned primary diagnosis or specific diagnosis-related group (DRG) or comorbid condition (CC). DRGs or CCs that include the presence of malnutrition or nonfunctioning gastrointestinal tract with malabsorption are often required, particularly in the home setting. Medical necessity for PN must be justified by the prescribing physician at the initiation of therapy and periodically throughout the course of therapy. Even then, reimbursement is usually less than 100%, which leaves the family (or supplemental insurance) with the remaining costs.

Health care providers who prescribe and/or monitor PN need to keep abreast of changes in regulations governing reimbursement. Documentation is needed regarding effectiveness and outcomes with PN in terms of costs and benefits from length of hospital stay and complication rates to quality of life and functional status. If PN yields no perceived benefit, it is not needed and those who provide it will not be reimbursed. Constant efforts must be employed to control costs through exploring effective but less expensive modalities of care or designing clinical pathways or standardized policies that maximize the effectiveness of PN.

REFERENCES

1. Steinhorn DM. Nutrition in the PICU: Who needs it?! Guidelines for nutritional support of critically ill children. In: Green TP, Zucher AR, eds., *Current Concepts in Pediatric Critical Care.* Chicago: Society of Critical Care Medicine; 1996:77–86.
2. Archer S, Burnett R, Fischer J. Current uses and abuses of total parenteral nutrition. In: *Advances in Surgery.* Chicago: Mosby-Year Book, Inc.; 1996;29:165–189.
3. Chellis M, Sanders S, et al. Early enteral feeding in the pediatric intensive care unit. *J Parenter Enter Nutr.* 1996;20:71–73.
4. Acra S, Rollins C. Principles and guidelines for parenteral nutrition in children. *Pediatr Ann.* 1999;28:113–120.
5. Teitelbaum DH, Coran AG. Perioperative nutritional support in pediatrics. *Nutrition.* 1998;14:130.
6. Davis A. Pediatrics. In: Matarese LE, Gottschlich MM, eds., *Contemporary Nutrition Support Practice.* Philadelphia: WB Saunders Co.; 1998:349–351.
7. Fisher G, Opper F. An interdisciplinary nutrition support team improves quality of care in a teaching hospital. *J Amer Dietet Assoc.* 1996;96:176–178.
8. Fisher A, Poole R, Machie R, et al. Clinical pathway for pediatric parenteral nutrition. *Nutr Clin Pract.* 1997; 12:76–80.
9. Phillips S. Pediatric parenteral nutrition clinical pathway. *Building Block for Life.* 2003;Winter:1.
10. Trujillo EB, Young LS. Metabolic and monetary costs of avoidable parenteral nutrition use. *J Parenter Enter Nutr.* 1999;23:109–113.
11. American Society for Parenteral and Enteral Nutrition. Guidelines for the use of parenteral and enteral nutrition in adult and pediatric patients. *J Parenter Enter Nutr.* 1993;17 (suppl):27SA–52SA.

12. Okada A. Clinical indications of parenteral and enteral nutrition support in pediatric patients. *Nutrition.* 1988; 14:116–118.
13. Sondheimer JM, Cadnapaphornchai M, et al. Predicting the duration of dependence on parenteral nutrition after neonatal intestinal resection. *J Pediatr.* 1998;132:80–84.
14. Vantini I, Benini L, et al. Survival rate and prognostic factors in patients with intestinal failure. *Dig Liver Dis.* 2004;36:46–55.
15. Sitrin MD. Nutrition support in inflammatory bowel disease. *Nutr Clin Pract.* 1992;7:53–60.
16. Polk DB, Hattner JA, Kerner JA Jr. Improved growth and disease activity after intermittent administration of a defined formula diet in children with Crohn's disease. *J Parenter Enter Nutr.* 1992;16:499–504.
17. Rickard KA, Grosfield JL, Kirksey A, et al. Reversal of protein-energy malnutrition in children during treatment of advanced neoplastic disease. *Ann Surg.* 1979; 190:771–781.
18. Filler RM, Dietz W, Suskind RM, et al. Parenteral feeding in management of children with cancer. *Cancer.* 1979;43(suppl):2117–2120.
19. Copeland EM, MacFadgen BV, Dudrick SJ. Effect of intravenous hyperalimentation on established delayed hypersensitivity in the cancer patient. *Ann Surg.* 1976; 184:60–64.
20. Copeland EM, Daly JM, Ota DM, et al. Nutrition, cancer, and intravenous hyperalimentation. *Cancer.* 1979; 43:2108–2116.
21. Andrassay RJ, Chwals WJ. Nutritional support of the pediatric oncology patient. *Nutrition.* 1998;14:124–129.
22. Christensen ML, Hancock ML, Gattuso J, et al. Parenteral nutrition associated with increased infection rate in children with cancer. *Cancer.* 1993;72: 2732–2738.
23. Copeman MC. Use of total parenteral nutrition in children with cancer: A review and some recommendations. *Pediatr Hematol Oncol.* 1994;11:463–470.
24. Perl M. TPN and the anorexia nervosa patient. *Nutr Supp Serv.* 1981;1:13.
25. Pertschuk MJ, Forster J, Buzby G, et al. The treatment of anorexia nervosa with total parenteral nutrition. *Biol Psychiatr.* 1981;16:539–550.
26. Pereira-da-Silva L, Virella D, et al. A simple equation to estimate the osmolarity of neonatal parenteral nutrition solutions. *J Parenter Enter Nutr.* 2004;28:34–37.
27. Reed T, Phillips S. Management of central venous catheter occlusions and repairs. *J Intraven Nurs.* 1996; 19:289–294.
28. Andrew M, Marzinotto V, et al. A cross-sectional study of catheter-related thrombosis in children receiving total parenteral nutrition at home. *J Pediatr.* 1995;126: 358–363.
29. Chung D, Ziegler M. Central venous catheter access. *Nutrition.* 1988;14:119–123.
30. Chathas MK. Percutaneous central venous catheters in neonates. *J Obstet Gynecol Neonatal Nurs.* 1986;15: 324–332.
31. Dolcourt JL, Bose CL. Percutaneous insertion of Silastic central venous catheters. *Pediatr.* 1982;70: 484–486.
32. Goodwin ML. The Seldinger method of PICC insertion. *J Intravenous Nurs.* 1989;12:238–243.
33. Brown JM. Peripherally inserted central catheters: Use in home care. *J Intraven Nurs.* 1989;12:144–147.
34. Yeung CY, Lee HC, Huang FY, Wang CS. Sepsis during total parenteral nutrition: Exploration of risk factors and determination of the effectiveness of peripherally inserted central venous catheters. *Pediatr Infect Dis J.* 1998;17:135–142.
35. Chathas MK, Paton JB. Sepsis outcomes in infants and children with central venous catheters: Percutaneous versus surgical insertion. *J Obstet Gynecol Neonatal Nurs.* 1996;25:500–506.
36. Dubois J, Garel L, et al. Peripherally inserted central catheters in infants and children. *Radiology.* 1997; 204:622–626.
37. Pettit J. Assessment of infants with peripherally inserted central catheters: Part 1. Detecting the most frequently occurring complications. *Adv Neonatal Care.* 2002;2: 304–315.
38. Liossis G, Bardin C, et al. Comparison of risks from percutaneous central venous catheter and peripheral lines in infants of extremely low birth weight: A cohort controlled study of infants < 1000 g. *J Matern Fetal Neonatal Med.* 2003;13:171–174.
39. Pemberton LB, Lyman B, Lander V, Covinsky J, et al. Sepsis from triple versus single lumen catheters during total parenteral nutrition in surgical or chronically ill patients. *Arch Surg.* 1986;121:591.
40. Yeung C, May J, Hughes R. Infection rate for single lumen versus triple lumen subclavian catheters. *Inf Control Hosp Epidemiol.* 1988;9:154.
41. Hughes CB. A totally implantable central venous system for chemotherapy administration. *NITA.* 1985;8:523–527.
42. Storm HM, Young SL, Sandler RH. Development of pediatric and neonatal parenteral nutrition order forms. *Nutr Clin Pract.* 1995;10:54–59.
43. Puangco M, Nguyen H, Sheridan M. Computerized PN ordering optimizes timely nutrition therapy in a neonatal intensive care unit. *J Amer Dietet Assoc.* 1997;97: 258–261.
44. Schloerb PR. Electronic parenteral and enteral nutrition. *J Parenter Enter Nutr.* 2000;24:23–29.
45. Lehmann CU, Conner KG. Preventing provider errors: Online total parenteral nutrition calculator. *Pediatr.* 2004;113:748–753.

46. Shulman R, Phillips S. Parenteral nutrition in infants and children. *J Pediatr Gastroenterol Nutr.* 2003;36:587–607.

47. Mirtallo J. Should the use of total nutrient admixtures be limited? *Am J Hosp Pharm.* 1994;51:2831–2836.

48. Lee MD, Yoon JE, et al. Stability of total nutrient admixtures in reference to ambient temperatures. *Nutrition.* 2003;19:886–890.

49. Neuzil J, Darlow BA, Inder TE, et al. Oxidation of parenteral lipid emulsion by ambient and phototherapy lights: Potential toxicity of routine parenteral feeding. *J Pediatr.* 1995;126:785–790.

50. Laborie S, Lavoie JC. Protecting solutions of parenteral nutrition from peroxidation. *J Parenter Enter Nutr.* 1999;23:104–108.

51. Silvers KM, Sluis KB. Limiting light-induced lipid peroxidation and vitamin loss in infant parenteral nutrition by adding multivitamin preparations to Intralipid. *Acta Paediatr.* 2001;90:242–249.

52. Alwood M, Driscoll D, Sizer T, Ball P. Physicochemical assessment of total nutrient admixture stability and safety: Quantifying the risk. *Nutrition.* 1998;14:166–167.

53. National Advisory Group on Standards and Practice Guidelines for Parenteral Nutrition. Safe practices for parenteral nutrition formulations. *J Parenter Enter Nutr.* 1998;22:49–66.

54. Trissel LA, Gilbert DL. Compatibility of medications with 3-in-1 parenteral nutrition admixtures. *J Parenter Enter Nutr.* 1999;23:67–74.

55. Steger PJ, Muhlebach SF. Lipid peroxidation of intravenous lipid emulsions and all-in-one admixtures in total parenteral nutrition bags: The influence of trace elements. *J Parenter Enter Nutr.* 2000;24:37–41.

56. Driscoll DF, Bacon MN. Physicochemical stability of two types of intravenous lipid emulsion as total nutrient admixtures. *J Parenter Enter Nutr.* 2000;24:15–22.

57. Driscoll DF, Nehne J, et al. Physicochemical stability of intravenous lipid emulsions as all-in-one admixtures intended for the very young. *Clin Nut.* 2003;22:489–495.

58. Driscoll D, Bacon M, Bistrian B. Effects of in-line filtration on lipid particle size distribution in total nutrient admixtures. *J Parenter Enter Nutr.* 1996;20: 296–301.

59. Muller MJ. Hepatic complications in parenteral nutrition. *Z Gastroenterol.* 1996;34:36–40.

60. Kerner JA Jr, ed. *Manual of Pediatric Parenteral Nutrition.* New York: John Wiley and Sons; 1983.

61. Nelson WE, Behrman RE, Vaughan VC, eds. *Nelson's Textbook of Pediatrics,* 12th ed. Philadelphia: WB Saunders; 1983:231.

62. Baumgart S, Costarino AT. Water and electrolyte metabolism of the micropremie. *Clin Perinatol.* 2000;27: 131–146.

63. Lorenz JM, Kleinman LI, Ahmed G, et al. Phases of fluid and electrolyte homeostasis in the extremely low birth weight infant. *Pediatrics.* 1995;96:484–489.

64. Heimler R, Doumas BT, Jendrzejcak BM, et al. Relationship between nutrition, weight change, and fluid compartments in preterm infants during the first week of life. *J Pediatr.* 1993;122:110–114.

65. Oh W, Karechi H. Phototherapy and insensible water loss in the newborn infant. *Am J Dis Child.* 1972;124: 230–232.

66. Yeh TF, Voora S, Lillien J. Oxygen consumption and insensible water loss in premature infants in single versus double walled incubators. *J Pediatr.* 1980;97: 967–971.

67. Gruskin AB. Fluid therapy in children. *Urol Clin North Am.* 1976;3:277–291.

68. Stevenson JG. Fluid administration in the association of patent ductus arteriosus complicating respiratory distress syndrome. *J Pediatr.* 1977;90:257–261.

69. Bell EF, Acarregui MJ. Restricted versus liberal water intake for preventing morbidity and mortality in preterm infants. *Cochrane Database System Rev.* 2001;3: CD000503.

70. Goldman HI. Feeding and necrotizing enterocolitis. *Am J Dis Child.* 1980;134:553.

71. Goldberg RN, Chung D, Goldman SL, et al. The association of rapid volume expansion and intraventricular hemorrhage in the preterm infant. *J Pediatr.* 1980;96: 1060–1063.

72. Rao M, Koenig E, Li S, et al. Estimation of insensible water loss in low birth weight infants by direct calorimetric measurement of metabolic heat release. *Pediatr Res.* 1989;25:295A.

73. Ford EG. Nutrition support of pediatric patients. *Nutr Clin Pract.* 1996;11:183–191.

74. Carlson S. Acid/base balance in special care nurseries. *Support Line.* 2002;24:17.

75. Aperia A, Broberger O, Elinder G, Herin P, Zetterstrom R. Postnatal development of renal function in pre-term and full-term infants. *Acta Paediatr Scand.* 1981;70: 183–187.

76. Peters O, Ryan S, Matthew L, et al. Randomised controlled trial of acetate in preterm neonates receiving parenteral nutrition. *Arch Dis Child.* 1997;77:F12–F15.

77. John E, Klavdianou M, Vidyasagar D. Electrolyte problems in neonatal surgical patients. *Clin Perinatol.* 1989;16:219–232.

78. Groh-Wargo S, Ciaccia A, Moore J. Neonatal metabolic acidosis: Effect of chloride from normal saline flushes. *J Parenter Enter Nutr.* 1988;12:159–161.

79. Tilden SJ, Watkins S, Tong TK, Jeevanandam M. Measured energy expenditure in pediatric intensive care patients. *Am J Dis Child.* 1989;143:490–492.

80. Lowery GH. *Growth and Development of Children,* 6th ed. Chicago: Year Book Medical Publishers, 1973: 331–332.

81. Heird WC, Kashyap S, Gomez MR. Parenteral alimentation of the neonate. *Semin Perinatol.* 1991;15:493–502.

82. Greene HL, Hambidge KM, Schanler R, et al. Guidelines for the use of vitamins, trace elements, calcium, magnesium, and phosphorus in infants and children receiving total parenteral nutrition: Report of the Subcommittee on Pediatric Parenteral Nutrient Requirements from the Committee on Clinical Practice Issues of The American Society for Clinical Nutrition. *Am J Clin Nutr.* 1988;48:1324. (Revised in 1990.)

83. Kleinman RE, ed. *Pediatric Nutrition Handbook.* Elk Grove Village, IL: American Academy of Pediatrics, Committee on Nutrition; 1998:285–305.

84. Khaldi N, Coran AG, Wesley JR. Guidelines for parenteral nutrition in children. *Nutr Supp Serv.* 1984;4:27.

85. Sunehag AL, Haymond MW. Glucose extremes in newborn infants. *Clin Perinatol.* 2002;29:245–260.

86. Prelack K, Sheridan RL. Micronutrient supplementation in the critically ill patient: Strategies for clinical practice. *J Trauma.* 2001;51:601–620.

87. Adamkin DH. Total parenteral nutrition. *Neonatal Intensive Care.* 1997;Sept/Oct:24.

88. Chwals WJ. Overfeeding the critically ill child: Fact or fantasy? *New Horizons.* 1994;2:147.

89. Chwals WJ, Lally KP, Woolley MM, et al. Measured energy expenditure in critically ill infants and young children. *J Surg Res.* 1988;44:467–472.

90. Coss-Bu JA, Klish WJ, Walding D, et al. Energy metabolism, nitrogen balance, and substrate utilization in critically ill children. *Amer J Clin Nutr.* 2001;74:664–669.

91. Zlotkin SH, Bryan MH, Anderson GH. Intravenous nitrogen and energy intakes required to duplicate in utero nitrogen accretion in prematurely born human infants. *J Pediatr.* 1981;99:115–120.

92. Kalhan SC, Kilic I. Carbohydrate as nutrient in the infant and child: Range of acceptable intake. *Europ J Clin Nutr.* 1999;53:S94–100.

93. Cochran EB, Phelps SJ, Helms RA. Parenteral nutrition in pediatric patients. *Clin Pharm.* 1988;7:351–366.

94. Sajbel TA, Dutro MP, Radway PR. Use of separate insulin infusions with total parenteral nutrition. *J Parenter Enter Nutr.* 1987;11:97–99.

95. Groh-Wargo S. Prematurity/low birth weight. In: Lang C, ed., *Nutritional Support in Critical Care.* Gaithersburg, MD: Aspen Publishers; 1987:287.

96. Rubecz I, Mestyan J, Varga P, Klujber L. Energy metabolism, substrate utilization, and nitrogen balance in parenterally fed postoperative neonates and infants. *J Pediatr.* 1981;98:42–46.

97. Thureen PJ, Anderson AH, Baron KA, et al. Protein balance in the first week of life in ventilated neonates receiving parenteral nutrition. *Am J Clin Nutr.* 1998;68: 1128–1135.

98. Poindexter BB, Denne SC. Protein needs of the preterm infant. *NeoReviews.* 2003;4:E52.

99. Thureen PJ, Hay WW Jr. Intravenous nutrition and postnatal growth of the micropremie. *Clin Perinatol.* 2000; 27:197–219.

100. Kalhan SC, Iben S. Protein metabolism in the extremely low-birth weight infant. *Clin Perinatol.* 2000;27:23–56.

101. Micheli J-L, Schultz Y, Junod S, et al. Early postnatal intravenous amino acid administration to extremely-low-birth-weight infants. In: Hay WW Jr, ed., *Seminars in Neonatal Nutrition and Metabolism,* vol 2. Columbus, Ross Products Division; 1994;1.

102. Zlotkin SH, Stallings VA, Pencharz PB. Total parenteral nutrition in children. *Pediatr Clin North Am.* 1985;32: 381–400.

103. Hellstrom A, Engstrom E, Hard A-L, et al. Postnatal serum insulin-like growth factor I deficiency is associated with retinopathy of prematurity and other complications of premature birth. *Pediatr.* 2003;112: 1016–1020.

104. Adan D, LaGamma EF, Browne LE. Nutritional management and the multisystem organ failure/systemic inflammatory response syndrome in critically ill preterm neonates. *Crit Care Clin.* 1995;11:751–784.

105. Coran AG, Drongowski RA. Studies on the toxicity and efficacy of new amino acid solution in pediatric parenteral nutrition. *J Parenter Enter Nutr.* 1987;11: 368–377.

106. Helms RA, Christensen ML, Mauer EC, Storm MC. Comparison of a pediatric versus standard amino acid formulation in preterm neonates requiring parenteral nutrition. *J Pediatr.* 1987;110:466–470.

107. Chessex P, Zebiche H, Pineault M, Lepage D, Dallaire L. Effect of amino acid composition of parenteral solutions on nitrogen retention and metabolic response in very-low-birth weight infants. *J Pediatr.* 1985;106:111–117.

108. Heird WC, Dell RB, Helms RA, et al. Amino acid mixture designed to maintain normal plasma amino acid patterns in infants and children requiring parenteral nutrition. *Pediatrics.* 1987;80:401–408.

109. Intravenous nutritional therapy. Crystalline amino acid infusions. *Drug Facts and Comparisons.* 2000;96–97.

110. Heird WC. Essentiality of cyst(e)ine for neonates. Clinical and biochemical effects of parenteral cysteine supplementation. In: Kinney JM, Borum PR, eds., *Perspectives in Clinical Nutrition.* Munich, Germany: Urban Schwarzenberg; 1989:275–282.

111. Gaull GE, Sturman JA, Raiha NCR, Sturman JA. Development of mammalian sulfur metabolism. Absence of cystathionase in human fetal tissues. *Pediatr Res.* 1972;6:538–547.

112. Zlotkin SH, Bryan H, Anderson H. Cysteine supplementation to cysteine-free intravenous feeding regimens in newborn infants. *Am J Clin Nutr.* 1981;34:914–923.

113. Helms RA, Storm MC, Christensen ML, et al. Cysteine supplementation results in normalization of plasma taurine concentrations in children receiving home parenteral nutrition. *J Pediatr.* 1999;134:358–361.

114. Heird WC, Hay W, Helms RA, Storm MC, Kashyap S, Dell RB. Pediatric parenteral amino acid mixture in low birth weight infants. *Pediatrics.* 1988;81:41–50.

115. Heird WC, Dell RB, Helms RA, et al. Amino acid mixture designed to maintain normal plasma amino acid patterns in infants and children requiring parenteral nutrition. *Pediatr.* 1987;80:401–408.

116. Eggert LD, Rusho WJ, MacKay MW, Chan GM. Calcium and phosphorus compatibility in parenteral nutrition solutions for neonates. *Am J Hosp Pharm.* 1982; 39:49.

117. Battista MA, Price PT, Kalhan SC. Effect of parenteral amino acids on leucine and urea kinetics in preterm infants. *J Pediatr.* 1996;128:130–134.

118. Lowe DK, Benfell K, Smith RJ, et al. Safety of glutamine-enriched parenteral nutrient solutions in humans. *Am J Clin Nutr.* 1990;52:1101–1106.

119. Wischmeyer PE. Clinical applications of L-glutamine: Past, present, and future. *Nutr Clin Pract.* 2003;18:377.

120. Lacey JM, Crouch JB, Benfell K, et al. The effects of glutamine-supplemented nutrition in premature infants. *J Parenter Enter Nutr.* 1996;20:74–80.

121. Vaughn P, Thomas P, Clark R, et al. Enteral glutamine supplementation and morbidity in low birth weight infants. *J Pediatr.* 2003;142:662–668.

122. Adamkin DH, McClead RE, Desai NS, et al. Comparison of two neonatal amino acid formulations in preterm infants in a multicenter study. *J Perinatol.* 1991;11:375–382.

123. Forchielli ML, Gura KM, Sandler R, et al. Aminosyn PF or Trophamine: Which provides more protection from cholestasis associated with total parenteral nutrition? *J Pediatr Gastroenterol Nutr.* 1995;21:374–382.

124. Wright K, Ernst KD, Gaylord MS, et al. Increased incidence of parenteral nutrition-associated cholestasis with Aminosyn PF compared to Trophamine. *J Perinatol.* 2003;23:444–450.

125. Adamkin DH. Total parenteral nutrition-associated cholestasis: Prematurity or amino acids? *J Perinatol.* 2003;23:437–438.

126. Abitbol CL, Holliday MA. Total parenteral nutrition in anuric children. *Clin Nephrol.* 1976;5:153–158.

127. Holliday MA, Wassner S, Ramirez J. Intravenous nutrition in uremic children with protein-energy malnutrition. *Am J Clin Nutr.* 1978;31:1854–1860.

128. Motil KJ, Harmon WE, Grupe WE. Complications of essential amino acid hyperalimentation in children with acute renal failure. *J Parenter Enter Nutr.* 1980;4:32–35.

129. Takala J. Total parenteral nutrition in experimental uremia: Studies of acute and chronic renal failure in the growing rat. *J Parenter Enter Nutr.* 1984;8:427–432.

130. Helms RA, Phelps SJ, Mauer EC, Christensen ML, Storm MC. Parenteral protein use in liver disease. *Pediatr Res.* 1989;25:115A.

131. Maldonato J, Gil A, Faus MJ, Periago JL, Loscertales M, Molina JA. Differences in the serum amino acid pattern of injured and infected children promoted by two parenteral nutrition solutions. *J Parenter Enter Nutr.* 1989;13:41–46.

132. Holman RT, Johnson SB, Hatch TF. A case of human linolenic acid deficiency involving neurologic abnormalities. *Am J Clin Nutr.* 1982;35:617–623.

133. Uauy R, Mena P, Rojas C. Essential fatty acid metabolism in the micropremie. *Clin Perinatol.* 2000;27:71–93.

134. Jensen CL, Heird WC. Lipids with an emphasis on long-chain polyunsaturated fatty acids. *Clin Perinatol.* 2002;29:261–281.

135. Friedman Z, Danon A, Stahlman MT, et al. Rapid onset of essential fatty acid deficiency in the newborn. *Pediatrics.* 1976;58:640–649.

136. Baugh N, Recupero MA, Kerner JA Jr. Nutritional requirements for pediatric patients. In: Merritt RJ, ed., *The ASPEN Nutrition Support Practice Manual.* American Society for Parenteral and Enteral Nutrition. Silver Spring, MD: 1998:1–13.

137. Putet G. Lipid metabolism of the micropremie. *Clin Perinatol.* 2000;27:57–69.

138. Driscoll DF, Nehne J, Peterss H, et al. Physicochemical stability of intravenous lipid emulsions as all-in-one admixtures intended for the very young. *Clin Nutr.* 2003; 22:489–495.

139. American Academy of Pediatrics, Committee on Nutrition. Commentary on parenteral nutrition. *Pediatrics.* 1983;71:547–552.

140. Levy JS, Winters RW, Heird WC. Total parenteral nutrition in pediatric patients. *Pediatr Rev.* 1980;2:99.

141. American Academy of Pediatrics, Committee on Nutrition. Prudent life-style for children: Dietary fat and cholesterol. *Pediatrics.* 1986;78:521–525.

142. Sapsford A. Energy, carbohydrate, protein, and fat. In: Groh-Wargo S, Thompson M, Cox JH, eds. *Nutritional Care for High-Risk Newborns.* Chicago: Precept Press, Inc.; 1994:83.

143. Mitton SG. Amino acids and lipid in the total parenteral nutrition for the newborn. *J Pediatr Gastroenterol Nutr.* 1994;18:25–31.

144. Pereira GR. Nutritional care of the extremely premature infant. *Clin Perinatol.* 1995;22:61–75.

145. American Academy of Pediatric Committee on Nutrition. Use of intravenous fat emulsions in pediatric patients. *Pediatrics.* 1981;68:738–743.

146. Sacks GS, Driscoll DF. Does lipid hang time make a difference? Time is of the essence. *Nutr Clin Prac.* 2002;17:284–290.

147. Driscoll DF, Bacon MN, Bistrian BR. Effects of in-line filtration on lipid particle size distribution in total nutrient admixtures. *J Parenter Enteral Nutr.* 1996;20: 296–301.

148. Pearson ML, the Hospital Infection Control Practices Advisory Committee. Guideline for prevention of intravascular-device-related infections. *Infect Control Hosp Edpidemiol.* 1996;17:438–479.

149. Magnusson G, Boberg M, Cederblad G, et al. Plasma and tissue levels of lipids, fatty acids, and plasma carnitine in neonates receiving a new fat emulsion. *Acta Paediatr.* 1997;86:638–644.

150. McDonald CM, MacKay MW, Curtis J, et al. Carnitine and cholestasis: Nutritional dilemmas for the parenterally nourished newborn. *Support Line.* 2003;25:10.

151. Helms RA, Mauer EC, Hay WW Jr, et al. Effect of intravenous L-carnitine on growth parameters and fat metabolism during parenteral nutrition in neonates. *J Parenter Enter Nutr.* 1990;14:448–453.

152. Borum P. Carnitine in neonatal nutrition. *J Child Neurol.* 1995;10(suppl 2):S25–S31.

153. Winter SC, Szabo-Aczel S, Curry CJR, et al. Plasma carnitine deficiency: Clinical observations in 51 pediatric patients. *Am J Dis Child.* 1987;141:660–665.

154. Coran AG, Drongowshi RA, Baker PJ. The metabolic effects of oral L-carnitine administration in infants receiving total parenteral nutrition with fat. *J Pediatr Surg.* 1985;20:758–764.

155. Crill CM, Wang B, Storm MC, et al. Carnitine: A conditionally essential nutrient in the neonatal population? *J Pediatr Pharmacol Ther.* 2001;6:225.

156. Cairns PA, Stalker DJ. Carnitine supplementation of parenterally fed neonates. *Cochrane Database Syst Rev.* 2000;4:CD000950.

157. American Medical Association, Nutrition Advisory Group. Multivitamin preparations for parenteral use. *J Parenter Enter Nutr.* 1979;3:258–262.

158. Greer FR. Vitamin metabolism and requirements in the micropremie. *Clin Perinatol.* 2000;27:95–118.

159. Kumar D, Greer FR, Super DM, et al. Vitamin K status of premature infants: Implications for current recommendations. *Pediatr.* 2001;108:1117–1122.

160. Brion LP, Bell EF, Raghuveer TS, et al. What is the appropriate intravenous dose of vitamin E for very-low-birth-weight infants? *J Perinatol.* 2004;24:205–207.

161. Darlow BA, Graham PJ. Vitamin A supplementation for preventing morbidity and mortality in very low birth-weight infants. *Cochrane Database Syst Rev.* 2002;4: CD000501.

162. Moore MC, Greene HL, Phillips B, et al. Evaluation of a pediatric multiple vitamin preparation for total parenteral nutrition in infants and children. I. Blood levels of water-soluble vitamins. *Pediatrics.* 1986;77:530–538.

163. Greene HL, Moore MC, Phillips B, et al. Evaluation of a pediatric multivitamin preparation for total parenteral nutrition. II. Blood levels of vitamins A, D, and E. *Pediatr.* 1986;77:539.

164. Hahn JS, Berquist W, Alcorn DM, et al. Wernicke encephalopathy and beriberi during total parenteral nutrition attributable to multivitamin infusion shortage. *Pediatr.* 1998;101:E10.

165. Intravenous nutritional therapy. Vitamins, parenteral. *Drug Facts and Comparisons.* 2000;111.

166. Greer FR, Tsang RC. Calcium and vitamin D metabolism in term and low-birth-weight infants. *Perinatol Neonatol.* 1986;Jan/Feb:14.

167. Koo WWK, Tsang RC. Mineral requirements for low-birth-weight infants. *J Amer Coll Nutr.* 1991;10:474–486.

168. Changaris DG, Purohit DM, Balentine JD, et al. Brain calcification in severely stressed neonates receiving parenteral calcium. *J Pediatr.* 1984;104:941–946.

169. Goldsmith MA, Bhatia SS, Kanto AP, et al. Gluconate calcium therapy and neonatal hypercalciuria. *Am J Dis Child.* 1981;135:538–543.

170. Hufnagle KF, Khan SN, Penn D, et al. Renal calcifications: A complication of long-term furosemide therapy in preterm infants. *Pediatrics.* 1982;70:360–363.

171. Wood RJ, Bengoa JM, Sitrin MD, Rosenberg IH. Calciuretic effect of cyclic versus continuous total parenteral nutrition. *Am J Clin Nutr.* 1985;41:614–619.

172. Koo WWK, Kaplan LA, Horn J, Tsang RC, Steichen JJ. Aluminum in parenteral nutrition solution—sources and possible alternatives. *J Parenter Enter Nutr.* 1986; 10:591–595.

173. Moreno A, Dominguez C, Ballabriga A. Aluminum in the neonate related to parenteral nutrition. *Acta Paediatr.* 1994;83:25–29.

174. Vileisis RA. Effect of phosphorus intake in total parenteral nutrition infusates in premature neonates. *J Pediatr.* 1987;110:586–590.

175. Aladjem M, Lotan D, Biochis H, et al. Changes in the electrolyte content of serum and urine during total parenteral nutrition. *J Pediatr.* 1980;97:437–439.

176. Kimura S, Nose O, Seino Y, et al. Effects of alternate and simultaneous administrations of calcium and phosphorus on calcium metabolism in children receiving total parenteral nutrition. *J Parenter Enter Nutr.* 1986; 10:513–516.

177. Pelegano JF, Rowe JC, Carey DE, et al. Effect of calcium/phosphorus ratio on mineral retention in parenterally fed premature infants. *J Pediatr Gastroenterol Nutr.* 1991;12:351–355.

178. Hoehn GJ, Carey DE, Rowe JC, et al. Alternate day infusion of calcium and phosphate in very low birth weight infants: Wasting of the infused mineral. *J Pediatr Gastroenterol Nutr.* 1987;5:752–757

179. Department of Health and Human Services. *FDA Safety Alert: Hazards of Precipitation Associated with Parenteral Nutrition.* Rockville, MD: Food and Drug Administration; 1994.

180. Fitzgerald KA, MacKay MW. Calcium and phosphate solubility in neonatal parenteral nutrient solutions containing Trophamine. *Am J Hosp Pharm.* 1986;43:88.

181. Fitzgerald KA, MacKay MW. Calcium and phosphate solubility in neonatal parenteral nutrient solutions containing Aminosyn PF. *Am J Hosp Pharm.* 1987;44:1396.

182. Shils ME, Burke AW, Greene HL, et al. Guidelines for essential trace element preparations for parenteral use: A statement by an expert panel. *JAMA.* 1979;241: 2051–2054.

183. Pyati SP, Ramamurthy RS, Krauss MT, Pildes RS. Absorption of iodine in the neonate following topical use of povidone iodine. *J Pediatr.* 1977;91:825–828.

184. Shaw JC. Trace elements in the fetus and young infant II. Copper, manganese, selenium and chromium. *Am J Dis Child.* 1980;134:74–81.

185. Triplett WC. Clinical aspects of zinc, copper, manganese, chromium and selenium metabolism. *Nutr Int.* 1985;1:60.

186. American Academy of Pediatrics, Committee on Nutrition. Zinc. *Pediatr.* 1978;62:408–412.

187. Reynolds AP, Keily E, Meadows N. Manganese in long term paediatric parenteral nutrition. *Arch Dis Child.* 1994;71:527–528.

188. Fuhrman MP, Herrmann V, Masidonski P, et al. Pancytopoenia after removal of copper from total parenteral nutrition. *JPEN.* 2000;24:361–366.

189. Fok TF, Chui KK, Cheung R, et al. Manganese intake and cholestatic jaundice in neonates receiving parenteral nutrition: A randomized controlled study. *Acta Paediatr.* 2001;90:1009–1115.

190. Reed MD, Bertino JS, Halpin TC. Use of intravenous iron dextran injection in children receiving total parenteral nutrition. *Am J Dis Child.* 1981;135:829–831.

191. Seashore JH. Metabolic complications of parenteral nutrition in infants and children. *Surg Clin North Am.* 1980;60:1239.

192. Wan KK, Tsallas G. Dilute iron dextran formulation for addition to parenteral nutrient solutions. *Am J Hosp Pharm.* 1980;37:206.

193. Halpin T, Reed M, Bertino J. Use of intravenous iron dextran in children receiving TPN for nutritional support of inflammatory bowel disease. *J Parenter Enter Nutr.* 1980;4:600.

194. Ehrenkranz RA. Iron requirements of preterm infants. *Nutrition.* 1994;10:77.

195. Ohls RK, Harcum J, Schibler KR, Christensen RD, et al. The effect of erythropoietin on the transfusion requirements of preterm infants weighing 750 grams or less: A randomized, double-blind, placebo-controlled study. *J Pediatr.* 1995;126:421–426.

196. Meyer MP, Haworth C, Meyer JH, et al. A comparison of oral and intravenous iron supplementation in preterm infants receiving recombinant erythropoietin. *J Pediatr.* 1996;129:258–263.

197. Ng PC, Lam CWK, Lee CH, et al. Hepatic iron storage in very low birthweight infants after multiple blood transfusions. *Arch Dis Child Fetal Neonatal Ed.* 2001; 84:F101–105.

198. Bastian C, Driscoll R. Enteral tube feeding at home. In: Rombeau JL, Caldwell MD, eds., *Enteral and Tube Feeding.* Philadelphia: WB Saunders; 1984:494–512.

199. Beghin L, Michaud L. Total energy expenditure and physical activity in children treated with home parenteral nutrition. *Pediatr Res.* 2003;53:684–690.

200. Puntis JW. Nutritional support at home and in the community. *Arch Dis Child.* 2001;84:295–298.

201. Illingworth RS, Lister J. The critical or sensitive period, with special reference to certain feeding problems in infants and children. *J Pediatr.* 1964;65:839–848.

202. Nelson JK. Economics of nutrition support. In: Matarese LE, Gottschlich MM, eds., *Contemporary Nutrition Support Practice.* Philadelphia: WB Saunders Company;1998:643.

CHAPTER 26

Botanicals in Pediatrics

John Westerdahl

INTRODUCTION

Since the beginning of time, botanicals have played an important part in the diet and well-being of every major culture. The people of the ancient world relied heavily on various herbs for their medicines. Used by both adults and children, many of these plants were their chief therapy, offering comfort and healing during illness and disease. Botanicals were once the conventional medicines used in treating common health problems such as colds, flu, nausea, heart disease, depression, and most other conditions. Written historical records list many medicinal plants in early *materia medica* from ancient China, Babylon, Egypt, India, Greece, and other parts of the world. The ancient Egyptian medical text *Papyrus Ebers*, written in 1550 BC, lists over 800 medicinal formulas using herbs. The Greek physician Hippocrates (468–377 BC), known as the "father of medicine," used herbs extensively with his patients and wrote about their healing benefits. In the first century, another Greek physician, Dioscorides, listed 500 plant medicines in his classic herbal guide, *De Materia Medica*. Many of the currently popular medicinal herbs were once listed in official monographs in the *United States Pharmacopoeia* (*USP*) and the *National Formulary* (*NF*) and were used extensively by physicians. Today, some 25% of prescription drugs now marketed in the United States are derived from plants.[1,2]

Table 26–1 lists the botanicals that are currently approved by the U.S. Food and Drug Administration (FDA) as effective over-the-counter (OTC) drug ingredients. However, the FDA does not regulate herbal supplements in the United States. From a global perspective, the World Health Organization (WHO) estimates that 80% of the world's population currently relies mainly on traditional medicines, most of which utilize medicinal plants.[3]

During the past two decades, the use of herbs and phytomedicines has increased as consumers have become more aware of their uses. This can be attributed both to increased published scientific research documenting the therapeutic efficacy of many medicinal herbs and to the passing of the Dietary Supplement Health and Education Act of 1994 (DSHEA), which created a regulatory framework for dietary supplement products. It allows herbal manufacturers to make truthful, nonmisleading claims about the herb's effect on the structure and function of the body. These claims are required to be accompanied by a disclaimer that states, "This statement has not been evaluated by the Food and Drug Administration.[4] This product is not intended to diagnose, treat, cure, or prevent any disease." It is wise to look for standardized versions with measured amounts of active ingredients as much as possible. Also, people interested in using herbs should seek reputable manufacturers' products and call companies to ascertain the source of their herbs and manufacturing procedures. As a precaution for

Table 26–1 Botanicals Approved as OTC Drug Ingredients

Herb	*Approved Use*
Capsicum (*Capsicum* spp.)	Counterirritant
Ipecac root (*Cephaelis ipecacuanha*)	Emetic
Peppermint oil (*Mentha piperita*)	Antitussive
Psyllium (*Plantago psyllium*)	Bulk laxative
Senna (*Senna alexandrina; Cassia senna*)	Stimulant laxative
Slippery elm (*Ulmus fulva*)	Demulcent
Witch hazel (*Hamamelis virginiana*)	Astringent

Source: OTC Drug Review Ingredient Status Report. Rockville, MD: Food and Drug Administration; July 2003.

the child, herbal supplements should not be used by pregnant or nursing women without first consulting a knowledgeable physician.

GROWTH OF THE HERBAL MARKET

Consumers have shown a growing interest in trying natural alternatives to synthetic drugs that address their health concerns.[5] As a result, the herbal market has experienced rapid growth. In 2000, the size of the botanical medicine market had grown to an estimated annual retail sales figure of $4.1 billion.[6] Table 26–2 identifies the best-selling herbal products sold in the United States in 2002.[7] This marketing information is helpful to the health professional to identify the types of herbs that are being used by many patients today.

With the growing interest in herbs, an increasing number of parents use botanical medicines with their children. Several herbal product companies now market phytomedicines especially formulated for children. More and more parents perceive herbal remedies as effective and having actions that are "gentler," with fewer side effects than those of most conventional drugs. In the United States, the majority of doctors and pharmacists recognize that there is a growing consumer interest in herbal medicine, but most of them have little or no knowledge and absolutely no training in this area. Doctors, pharmacists, registered dietitians, and other health care practitioners should know some basic information about herbal products to better assist their patients who use them.

DEFINITIONS

In the world of herbs and phytomedicines, there is some basic nomenclature that the health professional should be familiar with when working with patients who use these preparations. This starts with adequately defining the word herb. Depending on the context, the term herb can be defined in a few different ways.

An *herb* is defined botanically as a seed-producing, nonwoody plant that dies down to its roots at the end of its growing season. Others have described an herb simply as a useful plant. In the culinary arts field, the term herb is described as a vegetable product that is used in cooking to add flavor and/or aroma to foods.[1] However, in the field of herbal medicine, the term herb takes on a more medical meaning. Perhaps the most precise and accurate definition of the term herb as it pertains to medicinal values is the definition offered by the late Dr. Varro E. Tyler, former dean and distinguished professor emeritus of the School of Pharmacy and Pharmacal Sciences at Purdue University. In his book *Herbs of Choice: The Therapeutic Use of Phytomedicinals,* Dr. Tyler defines *medicinal herbs* as "crude drugs of vegetable origin utilized for the treatment of disease states, often of a chronic nature, or to attain or maintain a condition of improved health."[8] Commercial herbal

Table 26–2 The 2002 Top-Selling Herbal Supplements in Food, Drug, and Mass Market Retail Outlets

Rank	*Herb*
1.	Garlic
2.	Ginkgo
3.	Echinacea
4.	Soy
5.	Saw palmetto
6.	Ginseng
7.	St. John's wort
8.	Black cohosh
9.	Cranberry
10.	Valerian
11.	Milk thistle
12.	Evening primrose
13.	Kava kava
14.	Bilberry
15.	Grape seed
16.	Yohimbe
17.	Green tea
18.	Ginger
19.	Pycnogenol®
20.	Aloe vera

Note: 52 weeks ending January 6, 2003

Source: Information Resources, Inc., Chicago, IL. Used by permission.

and phytomedicine preparations are available in several different forms.

Some of the key forms are defined as follows:[1]

- *Extract*—An herbal concentrate that contains the phytochemical constituents found in the herb. Extracts are made when the plant constituents are extracted from the plant by physical and/or chemical means.
- *Standardized extract*—An herbal extract that is guaranteed to provide a "standardized" level of a particular phytochemical constituent. In many cases, this phytochemical constituent is considered to be the key active compound.
- *Infusion*—An herbal tea. An herbal extract prepared by steeping dried plant parts in hot water.
- *Decoction*—An herbal extract prepared by putting the plant material (usually hard or woody parts) in water and boiling the water, then allowing it to simmer gently for extended periods of time. The liquid is then cooled and strained for use.
- *Tincture*—An herbal extract prepared by mixing the herb with a solvent (usually an alcohol and water mixture) for a specified period of time (hours to days). The solvent extracts phytochemical constituents from the herb. Any remaining solids are removed, and the solution that results is used medicinally.
- *Glycerite*—An herbal extract that is similar to a tincture. However, glycerol is used as the solvent in preparation instead of alcohol. Because they are alcohol-free, glycerites have recently become very popular for use with children.
- *Fluid extract*—Liquid preparations that usually contain a ratio of one part solvent to one part herb. They are much more concentrated than tinctures, and their alcohol content can vary.
- *Solid extract*—Solid extracts (also called *powdered extracts*) are made by evaporating all the residual solvent or liquid used during the extraction process.
- *Powder*—A preparation in the form of finely divided sieved herbal particles made from dried and finely milled herbs for use in herbal preparations such as tablets and capsules.
- *Syrups*—Syrups are a water and sugar solution to which flavoring and an herbal extract may be added. They are often used to relieve coughs or to mask the unpleasant flavor of a tincture. Syrups are a popular form of herbal medicine in pediatrics.

THE USE OF HERBS AND PHYTOMEDICINES IN PEDIATRICS

Although herbs have been used for centuries, most controlled clinical trials using herbs have included only adults. The scientific data examining the use of herbs with children is limited. As a result, herbal medicine experts do not have a consensus of opinion as to the appropriate use of botanicals for children, particularly the very young. Although more conservative experts feel strongly that botanicals should not be used by children under the age of 12 until there is more research in the pediatric population to confirm their safety, other experts have less concern and recommend their use for young children and even infants. Nevertheless, there are growing numbers of parents who are using many herbal products to treat minor illnesses in small children. The concern among many health professionals, however, is the potential hazards of the inappropriate use of herbal preparations by parents treating their children for serious health conditions without the consultation of a pediatrician.

In general, the safety of most responsibly formulated commercial herb products has been well established. However, there are situations in which specific herbs should not be used. If a child has an allergy to a specific herb, it must be avoided. Certain plants in the *Asteraceae*, *Apiaceae*, and other plant families possess a high degree of allergenicity with some children. It is advised to observe caution in the consumption of plants classified as ragweeds, especially flowers found in the *Asteraceae* family, such as chamomile.

Parents should observe the child who takes an herbal preparation for the first time for several hours for any adverse reactions. Watery, itchy eyes; sneezing; wheezing; coughing; or hives could be signs of allergy. Pediatricians who utilize herbal remedies in their practice recommend to concerned parents of allergy-prone children that they introduce an herb in the same way they would introduce new foods to an infant. The pediatrician's advice is to try only one herb at a time, administered in very small doses.

Herbs should not be given by the parent to a child who is currently taking a medication without first consulting a doctor. The interaction of an herb with medicinal substances should always be considered. Although there is little data available today on herb-drug interactions, some important information in this area is known by the medical profession.

There is debate among herbal medicine experts as to which herbal remedies are safe and appropriate for use by children. In Germany, Commission E, an interdisciplinary expert committee on herbal medicines consisting of physicians, pharmacists, pharmacologists, toxicologists, representatives of the pharmaceutical industry, and laypersons, is responsible for evaluating the scientific data on the safety and efficacy of phytomedicines. Commission E members are appointed by the Federal Institute for Drugs and Medical Devices (formerly the German Federal Health Agency) and are assigned the task of preparing monographs on medicinal plants. Most experts regard these monographs as the most accurate scientific information available in the world on the safety and efficacy of herbs and phytomedicines. While the monographs describe the medicinal use of herbs primarily for adults, they also identify herbs that are contraindicated for children (Exhibit 26–1).[9] Table 26–3 gives an

Exhibit 26–1 Herbs and Herbal Products Contraindicated for Children According to the German Commission E Monographs

Aloe
Buckthorn bark and berry
Camphor
Cajeput oil
Cascara sagrada bark
Eucalyptus leaf
Eucalyptus oil
Fennel oil
Horseradish
Mint oil (external)
Nasturtium
Peppermint oil (external)
Rhubarb root
Senna leaf and pod
Watercress

Source: Blumenthal M, et al., eds., Klein S, Rister RS, trans., *The Complete German Commission E Monographs: Therapeutic Guide to Herbal Medicines* © 1998 American Botanical Council and Integrative Medicine Communications.

Table 26–3 Common Herbal Remedies Used in Pediatrics

HERB *Common and Latin Names*	*TRADITIONAL USAGE* *Internal and External Uses*	*Contraindications/Precautions*
Aloe (*Aloe vera*)	External use: wound healing, minor skin irritation, burns	Not recommended internally for pediatrics
Anise (*Pimpinella anisum*)	Internal use: common colds, coughs, bronchitis, indigestion	Rare allergic reactions to anise and its constituent anethole
Bilberry (*Vaccinium myrtillus*)	Internal use: diarrhea	None known
Calendula flowers (*Calendula officinalis*)	Internal use: inflammation of mouth and pharynx	Rare allergic reactions through frequent skin contact
	External use: wounds and burns	
Catnip (*Nepeta cataria*)	Internal use: nervous disorders, sleep aid, common colds, colic	None known
Chamomile flowers (*Matricaria chamomilla*)	Internal use: carminative, sleep aid	Rare allergic reactions
	External use: inflammation and irritations of the skin, wounds, burns	
Cherry bark (*Prunus sp.*)	Internal use: coughs, common colds	None known
Comfrey leaf (*Symphytum officinale*)	External use: minor wounds, ulcers, inflammations, bruises, and sprains. Used as poultice for skin disorder	Not to be taken internally. Internal use promotes hepatotoxic effects
Echinacea (*Echinacea angustifolia*) (*Echinacea purpurea*)	Internal use: common colds, flu, coughs, bronchitis, fever, immune stimulant	Allergic reactions may occur with some individuals. Not recommended for individuals with autoimmune diseases
	External use: wounds, burns	
Elder flowers (*Sambucus nigra*)	Internal use: common colds, antiviral, diaphoretic	None known

continues

Table 26–3 continued

HERB *Common and Latin Names*	*TRADITIONAL USAGE* *Internal and External Uses*	*Contraindications/Precautions*
Eucalyptus (*Eucalyptus globulus*)	Internal use: expectorant, coughs, congestion of the respiratory tract	Nausea, vomiting, and diarrhea may occur after ingestion in rare cases. Eucalyptus preparations should not be applied to the face or nose of infants and very young children
Fennel Seed (*Foeniculum vulgare*)	Internal use: carminative, indigestion, coughs, bronchitis, gastrointestinal afflictions	Allergic reactions may occur with some individuals
Garlic (*Allium sativum*)	Internal use: common colds, bronchitis, fever External use: antibacterial, antifungal, ear infections	Intake of large quantities can lead to stomach complaints. Rare allergic reactions
Ginger (*Zingiber officinale*)	Internal use: carminative, antinausea, indigestion	None known
Goldenseal (*Hydrastis canadensis*)	Internal use: common colds, flu, inflammation of mucous membranes External use: antiseptic, antimicrobial, cuts, wounds, ear infections	Internal use can cause nausea, vomiting, diarrhea, and may disrupt intestinal flora. Internal use is not recommended for young children by many experts due to the herb's alkaloid (berberine and hydrastine) content
Hops (*Humulus lupulus*)	Internal use: nervous disorders, sleep aid	Rare allergic reactions
Horehound (*Marrubium vulgare*)	Internal use: coughs, bronchitis	None known
Hyssop (*Hyssopus officinalis*)	Internal use: coughs, common colds	None known
Lemon balm (*Melissa officinalis*)	Internal use: nervous disorders, sleep aid	None known
Licorice root (*Glycyrrhiza glabra*)	Internal use: coughs, bronchitis	Prolonged use with high doses may promote hypertension, edema, and hypokalemia
Marshmallow root (*Althaea officinalis*)	Internal use: coughs, bronchitis, sore throat	None known
Mullein leaf (*Verbascum thapsus*)	Internal use: coughs, bronchitis, common colds, flu	None known

continues

Table 26–3 continued

HERB *Common and Latin Names*	*TRADITIONAL USAGE* *Internal and External Uses*	*Contraindications/Precautions*
Oat straw (*Avena sativa*)	External use: inflammation of the skin, itching	None known
Passion flower (*Passiflora incarnata*)	Internal use: nervous disorders, sleep aid	None known
Peppermint leaf (*Mentha piperita*)	Internal use: carminative, indigestion, nausea, gastrointestinal disorders, common colds, cough, bronchitis	Preparations containing peppermint oil should not be applied to the face or nose of infants or very young children
Pleurisy root (*Asclepias tuberosa*)	Internal use: coughs, pleurisy	Excessive amounts can be toxic due to the herb's cardioactive steroid content that can lead to digitalis-like poisonings. High doses can promote vomiting
St. John's wort (*Hypericum perforatum*)	Internal use: emotional upsets, including anxiety and depressive moods. External use: cuts and abrasions	Safety of internal use with children has not been established. The safety and ethics of the use of herbal antldepressants with children without the consultation of a doctor is questionable Should not be taken by children already taking prescription medications for depression without first consulting a doctor May cause sun sensitivity in some individuals.
Thyme (*Thymus vulgarus*)	Internal use: cough, bronchitis, common colds	None known
Valerian root (*Valeriana officinalis*)	Internal use: nervous disorders, sleep aid	The safety and ethics of the use of herbal sedatives with children without the consultation of a doctor is questionable

Note: Clinical efficacy for each of these herbs has not necessarily been established.

overview of several of the internal and external uses of many of the medicinal herbs commonly used in pediatrics.

Laxatives and Stimulants

Most herbal medicine experts caution against the use of herbal stimulant laxatives by children under the age of 12. Herbal stimulant laxatives include aloe (*Aloe ferox*), buckthorn bark (*Rhamnus frangula*), cascara sagrada bark (*Rhamnus purshiana*), and senna leaf or pod (*Cassia senna*). Stimulants such as caffeine-containing herbs are also generally contraindicated for young children.[9,10]

Herbs that are classified as stimulants include not only coffee and black and green tea (*Camellia sinensis*), but also cola nut (also called kola nut) (*Cola nitida*), guarana (*Paullina cupana*), and maté (*Ilex paraguariensis*). Ma huang (also known as ephedra herb) is also a potent stimulant and is contraindicated for young children. It has been taken off the U.S. market. Asian ginseng (*Panax ginseng*) and American ginseng (*Panax quinquefolium*), traditionally regarded as herbal stimulants, are also not recommended for young children by many herbal medicine authorities.[1,10]

Sedatives and Antidepressants

Many plants have traditionally been used for their sedative properties. There is controversy as to whether it is proper or even ethical to administer any sedative to young children without the consultation of a physician. Definitely, this is quite clear in regard to prescription drugs, but naturally derived herbal sedatives have not always been looked at in the same light. Most health authorities would agree that any sedative, herbal or otherwise, should be given to a child only under medical direction. Many herbal medicine experts would agree that strong sedative herbs such as valerian (*Valeriana officinalis*) should not be given to young children. There is no consensus of opinion on the use of some of the other popular traditional sedative herbs for children, despite the fact that many of them have been used with children for centuries. These herbs include catnip (*Nepeta cataria*), German chamomile (*Matricaria recutita*), hops (*Humulus lupulus*), lemon balm (*Melissa officinalis*), and passion flower (*Passiflora incarnata*). St. John's wort (*Hypericum perforatum*), an herb that has proven efficacy in treating mild and moderate depression in adults, has not been adequately studied for use by children.

Herbs Containing Alkaloids

Many herbal experts have concerns about children's use of herbs that contain powerful alkaloids. One of the alkaloids of concern is berberine. Berberine is a key principal phytochemical constituent found in several of the currently popular herbal products found in natural food and drug stores. Herbs containing berberine include goldenseal root (*Hydrastis canadensis*), Oregon grape root (*Mahonia aquifolium*), and barberry root (*Berberis vulgaris*). Berberine has antibacterial properties. Overuse of herbs containing this and other alkaloids could disrupt the normal flora in a child's gastrointestinal tract.[10]

Alkaloids that affect the central nervous system (caffeine, ephedrine, pseudoephedrine, and others) are generally not recommended for young children except under a doctor's direction.[10]

Traditional Herbal Remedies Used with Infants and Children

For centuries, medicinal herbs have been used with children worldwide with an apparently good record of safety. Clinical research has shown that many traditional herbal remedies appear to be effective.[10] However, more research is needed to confirm the safety and efficacy of the use of medicinal herbs in pediatric medicine.

Few studies have ever been done with infants using herbal preparations. In 1993, a prospective, randomized, double-blind, placebo-controlled study published in *The Journal of Pediatrics* examined the effects of an herbal tea in treating infantile colic.[11] The tea was made from herbs known to have antispasmodic activity and traditionally used to treat indigestion and colic in infants. The tea contained chamomile (*Matricaria chamomilla*), vervain (*Verbena officinalis*), licorice root (*Glycyrrhiza glabra*), fennel (*Foeniculum vulgare*), and lemon balm (*Melissa officinalis*). The use of the herbal tea eliminated the colic in 19 (57%) of the 33 infants, whereas the placebo was helpful in only 9 (26%) of 35 ($p < 0.01$). The mean colic score was significantly improved in the infants treated with herbal tea. None of the infants in the study experienced any adverse effects from the herbal tea.[11]

In recent years, additional studies demonstrating the effectiveness of herbal remedies with children have been published in the scientific literature. Standardized ginger root has been shown to be effective in treating motion sickness in children ages 4 to 8 years of age.[12] Enteric-coated peppermint oil capsules have been demonstrated to be safe and effective as a treatment for pain associated with the acute phases of irritable bowel syndrome (IBS) in older children and adolescents.[13] A study conducted on 171 children (ages 5 to 18 years) using herbal ear drops containing a combination of mullein, marigold (calendula), St. John's wort, lavender, and garlic in an olive oil base reduced ear pain associated with acute otitis media (AOM) as effectively as standard anesthetic eardrops.[14] A review of randomized controlled trials indicates that ivy leaf extract (*Hedra helix*) preparations show effects respective to improving the respiratory functions of children with chronic asthma.[15]

Heinz Schilcher, an expert in pharmacognosy at the Institute of Pharmaceutical Biology at Berlin's Independent University and a member of the German Commission E, points out the value of herbal remedies in pediatrics in his book *Phytotherapy in Paediatrics: Handbook for Physicians and Pharmacists*.[16] He notes that the benefits of many phytomedicines outweigh the risks because they have a relatively good benefit/risk ratio. In European studies, the actions of many combinations of naturally occurring compounds in herbs have been experimentally established and/or clinically confirmed, with minimal or negligible side effects. Other advantages of herbal remedies mentioned by Schilcher are that herbs have gentle medicinal actions, and their common methods of administration (inhalation, baths, ointments, syrups) are particularly appropriate for children. As a result, this can provide for good compliance. He points out that herbal medicines in pediatrics may be used at a preventive level and not just for the use of treating symptoms. Schilcher also notes that, as a general rule, phytomedicines are less expensive than conventional medicines.[16]

Determining Proper Pediatric Dosage for Medicinal Herbs

There is little scientific or even traditional information available on the proper dosage of herbs and phytomedicines in pediatrics. Because most clinical trials using herbs have been with adults, official dosages have been established for only the adult population. The posology in the German Commission E monographs refers to adults. A general pediatric guide used for determining the dosage of phytotherapeutic drugs is one third of the adult dose (as established in the Commission E monographs) for very young and young children and one half the adult dose for school-aged children.[12] Two classic pharmacy rules that are traditionally used in determining the dosages for drugs for children are sometimes used by herbal medicine experts as well. These rules are known as *Clark's Rule* and *Young's Rule*. Exhibit 26–2 illustrates how they are calculated. Because children have lower body weight than adults and do not have the sufficient development of liver enzymes necessary to metabolize many medications, their dosages of conventional as well as herbal medicines must be reduced. The proper pediatric dosage is best determined by an experienced and trained health professional. In recent years, some herbal product manufacturers have formulated their preparations for dosage levels appropriate for children.

CONCLUSION

Medicinal herbs have been used in pediatrics since ancient times. Today, there is a growing trend among parents to use botanical and other

Exhibit 26-2 How to Calculate a Child's Dosage for Herbal Medicines

The following are two classic rules used to calculate the approximate dosage for a child.

Clark's Rule: Divide the child's weight by 150. The example given is for a 50-lb child:

$$\frac{50}{150} = \frac{1}{3} \text{ adult dosage}$$

Young's Rule: Divide the child's age by child's age + 12. The example given is for a 4-year-old child:

$$\frac{4}{4+12} = \frac{4}{16} = \frac{1}{4} \text{ adult dosage}$$

natural medicines with their children as alternatives to conventional medicines. Increased public awareness of the therapeutic value of certain herbs and an increasing amount of scientific research in this area have led to an explosion in the marketplace of herbal medicine preparations and products. Several leading pharmaceutical companies are now adding herbal medicines to their product lines. Herbal medicine preparations specifically formulated for children are being sold in natural food stores. Based on current trends, herbal medicine will undoubtedly play a more prominent role in the pediatric medicine of the 21st century. As a result, there is an increasing need for pediatricians and other health professionals who work with pediatric patients to gain some basic knowledge about herbal medicine and its potential role in the health care of infants and children. More clinical research is needed to evaluate the safety and efficacy of medicinal herbs in the pediatric population.

REFERENCES

1. Westerdahl J. *Medicinal Herbs: A Vital Reference Guide.* Dallas, TX: Bruce Miller Enterprises; 1998.
2. Principe PP. The economic significance of plants and their constituents as drugs. *Econ Med Plant Res.* 1989;3: 1–17.
3. Farnsworth NR, Akerele O, Bingel AS, Soejarto DD, Guo Z. Medicinal plants in therapy. *Bull World Health Org.* 1985;63:965–981.
4. Dietary Supplement Health and Education Act of 1994 (DHEA), Pub.L No. 103-417, 108 Stat, 1994. US Dept Food and Drug Administration, Center for Food Safety and Applied Nutrition. Available at www.vm.cfsan.fda.gov/ndMS/dietsupp.html.
5. Eisenberg DM, Kessler RC, Foster C, et al. Unconventional medicine in the United States. *N Engl J Med.* 1993;328:246–252.
6. Molyneaux M. Consumer attitudes predict upward trends for the herbal marketplace. *HerbalGram.* 2002;54:64–65.
7. Blumenthal M. Herbs continue slide in mainstream market: Sales down 14 percent. *HerbalGram.* 2003;58:71.
8. Tyler VE. *Herbs of Choice: The Therapeutic Use of Phytomedicinals.* Binghamton, NY: Pharmaceutical Products Press; 1994:1.
9. Blumenthal M, Busse WR, Goldberg A, et al., eds. Klein S, Rister RS, translators. *The Complete German Commission E Monographs: Therapeutic Guide to Herbal Medicines.* Austin, TX: American Botanical Council; Boston, MA: Integrative Medicine Communications; 1998.
10. *PDR for Herbal Medicines,* 3rd ed. Montvale, NJ: Thomson Medical Economics; 2004.
11. Weizman Z, Alkrinawi S, Goldfarb D, Bitran C. Efficacy of herbal tea preparation in infantile cholic. *J Pediatr.* 1993;122:650–652.
12. Careddu P. Motion sickness in children: Results of a double-blind study with ginger (Zintona) and dimenhydrinate. *European Phytotherapy.* 1999;2:102–107.
13. Kline RM, Kline JJ, Di Palma J, Barbero GJ. Enteric-coated, pH-dependent peppermint oil capsules for the treatment of irritable bowel syndrome in children. *J Pediatr.* 2001;138:125–128.
14. Sarrel FM, Cohen HA, Kahan E. Naturopathic treatment for ear pain in children. *Pediatrics.* 2003;111:574–579.
15. Hofmann D, Hecker M, Volp A. Efficacy of dry extract of ivy leaves in children with bronchial asthma—a review of randomized controlled trials. *Phytomedicine.* 2003;10:213–220.
16. Schilcher H. *Phytotherapy in Pediatrics: Handbook for Physicians and Pharmacists.* Stuttgart, Germany: Med-Pharm Scientific Publishers; 1997.

RESOURCES

ASSOCIATIONS

American Botanical Council, P.O. Box 144345 Austin, TX 78714 Phone: (800) 373-7105 www.herbalgram.org

The Herb Research Foundation, 4140 15th Street, Suite 200, Boulder, CO 80304 Phone: 303-449-2265 www.herbs.org

BOOKS AND PERIODICALS

1. *HerbalGram.* Austin, TX: The Journal of the American Botanical Council.
2. *The Review of Natural Products.* St. Louis, MO: Facts and Comparisons.
3. Tyler VE. *Herbs of Choice: The Therapeutic Use of Phytomedicinals.* New York: Pharmaceutical Products Press, 1994.
4. Blumenthal M, Busse WR, Goldberg A, et al. *The Complete German Commission E Monographs: Therapeutic Guide to Herbal Medicines.* Austin, TX: American Botanical Council and Boston, MA: Integrative Medicine Communications; 1998.
5. *PDR for Herbal Medicines,* 3rd ed. Montvale, NJ: Thomson Medical Economics; 2004.
6. Blumenthal M. *The ABC Clinical Guide to Herbs.* Austin, TX: American Botanical Council, 2003.

APPENDIX A

Premature Infant Growth Charts

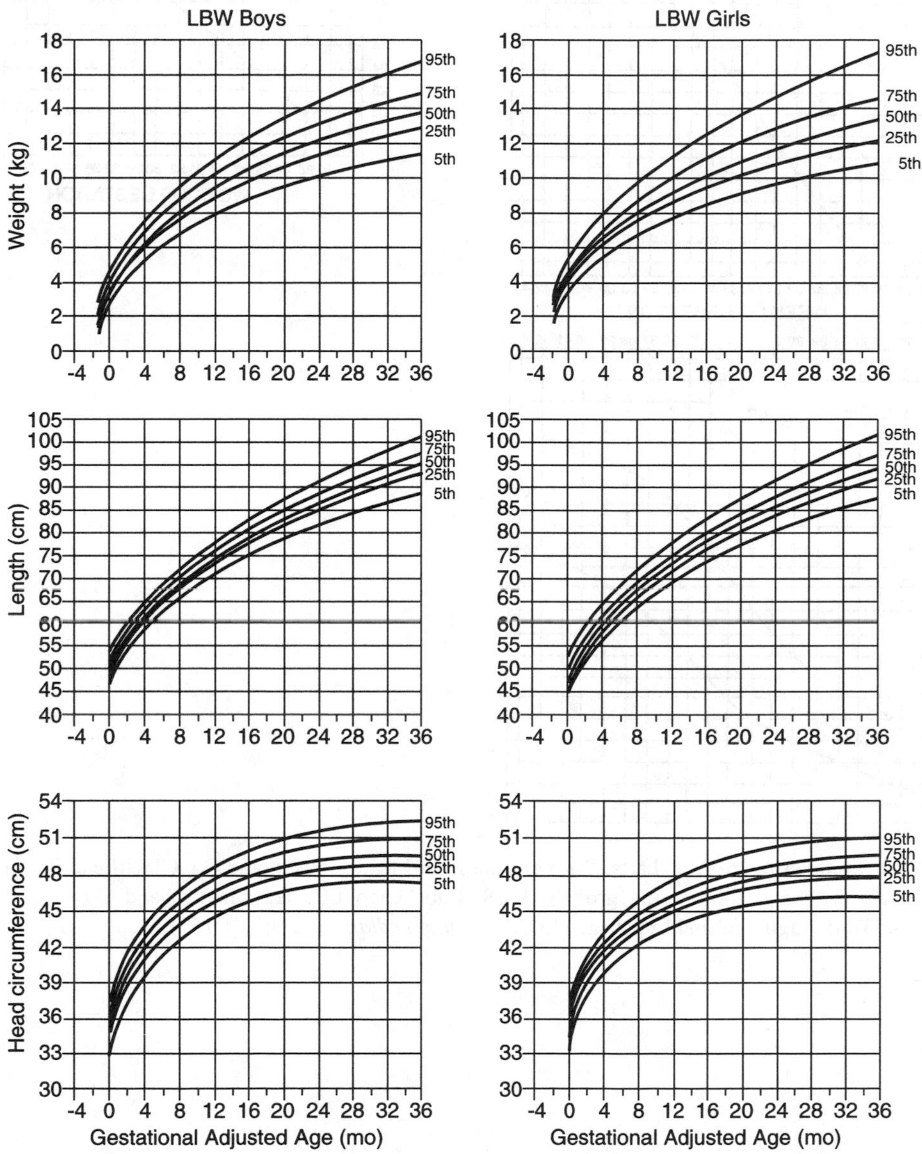

Figure A–1 Selected percentiles for status values of weight, length, and head circumference for very low birth weight (LBW) preterm infants in relation to gestation-adjusted ages. *Source:* Reprinted from Guo SS et al., Early Human Development, copyright 1997, pages 305–325, with permission from Elsevier Science.

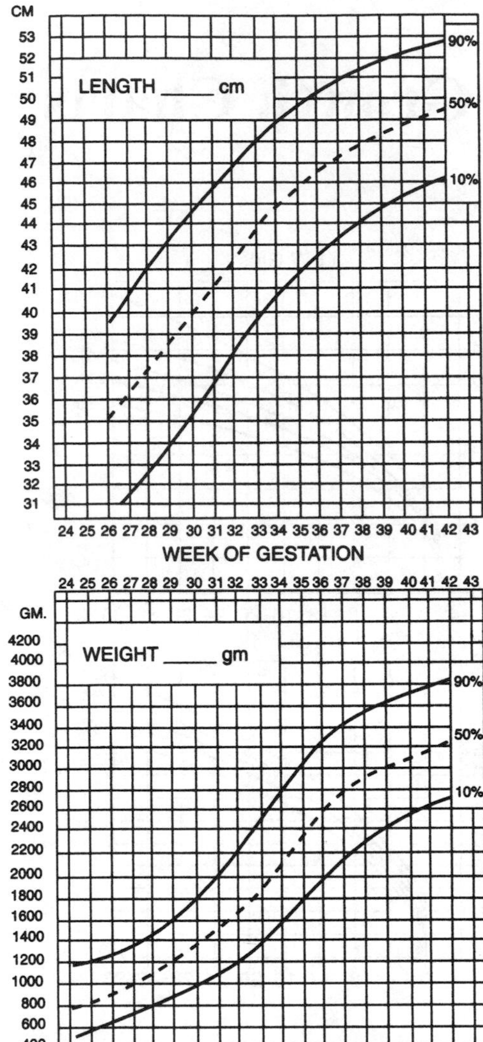

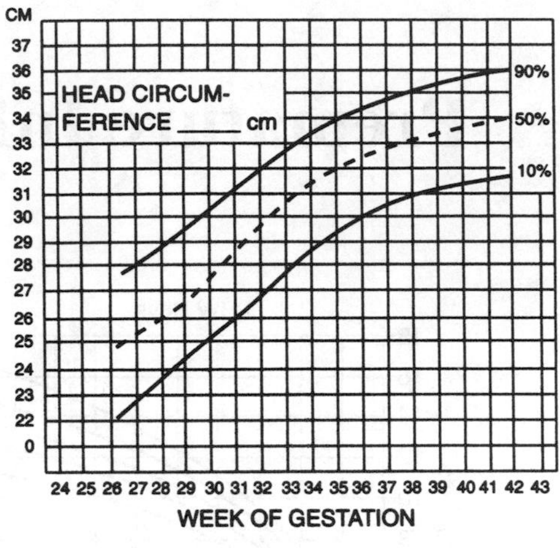

Figure A–2 Intrauterine growth charts. *Source:* Data from Mead Johnson and Co, Classification of newborns based on maturity and intrauterine growth, 1978; Lubchenco LC, Hansman C and Boyd E, *Pediatrics* (1966;37:403); Battaglia FC and Lubchenco LC, *Journal of Pediatrics* (1967;71:159).

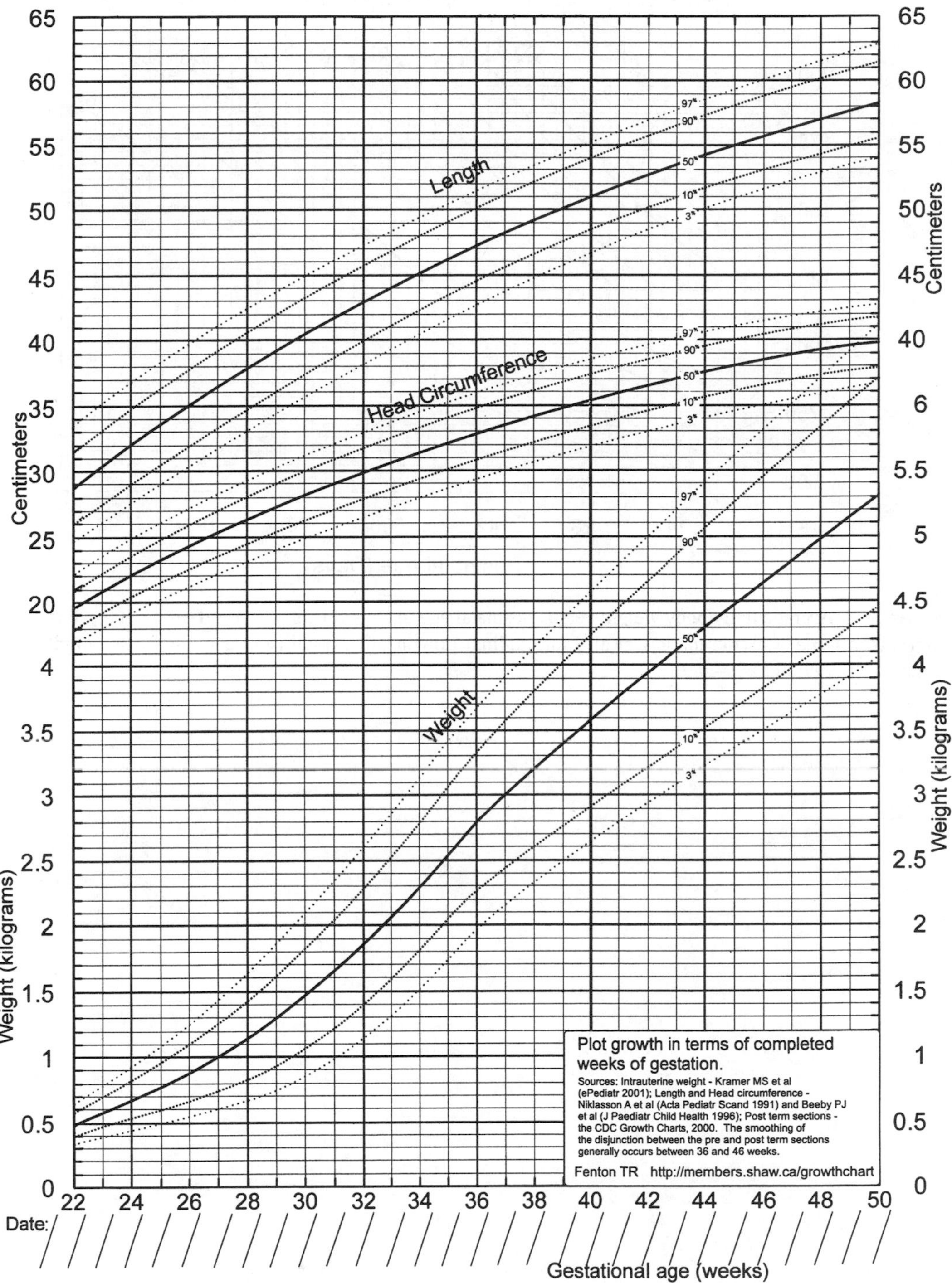

Figure A–3 A new growth chart for preterm babies: Babson and Benda's chart updated with recent data and a new format. *Pediatrics* (2003;3:13).

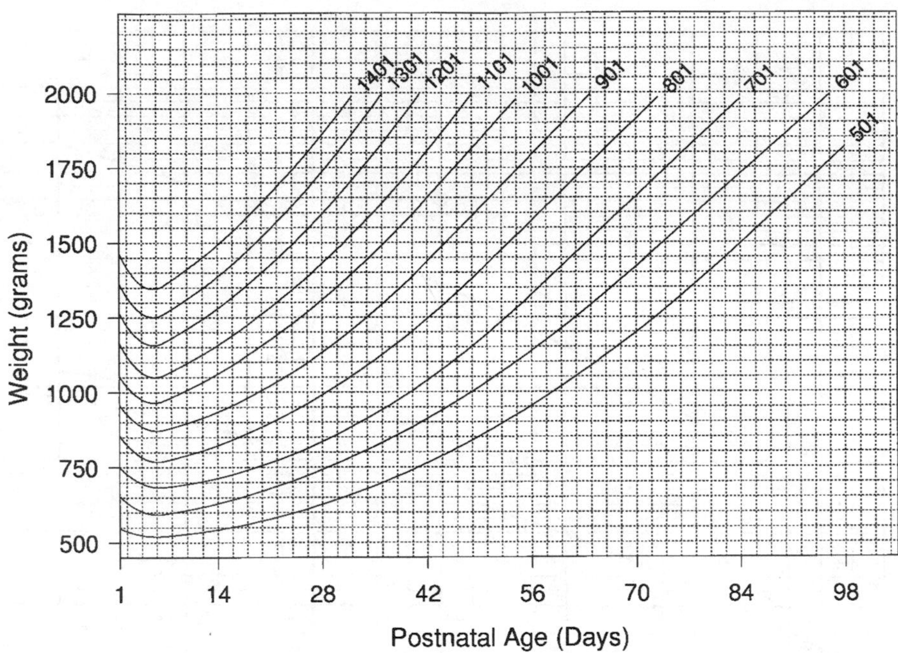

Figure A–4 Average daily body weight versus postnatal age in days for infants stratified by 100-g birth weight intervals. *Source:* Ehrenkranz RA et al. Longitudinal growth of hospitalized very low birth weight infants. *Pediatrics* (1999;104:280–289).

Appendix B

NCHS Growth Charts

Table B–1 Birth to 36 months: Boys. Length-for-age and Weight-for-age percentiles

Birth to 36 months: Boys
Length-for-age and Weight-for-age percentiles

NAME ______________________

RECORD # ______________

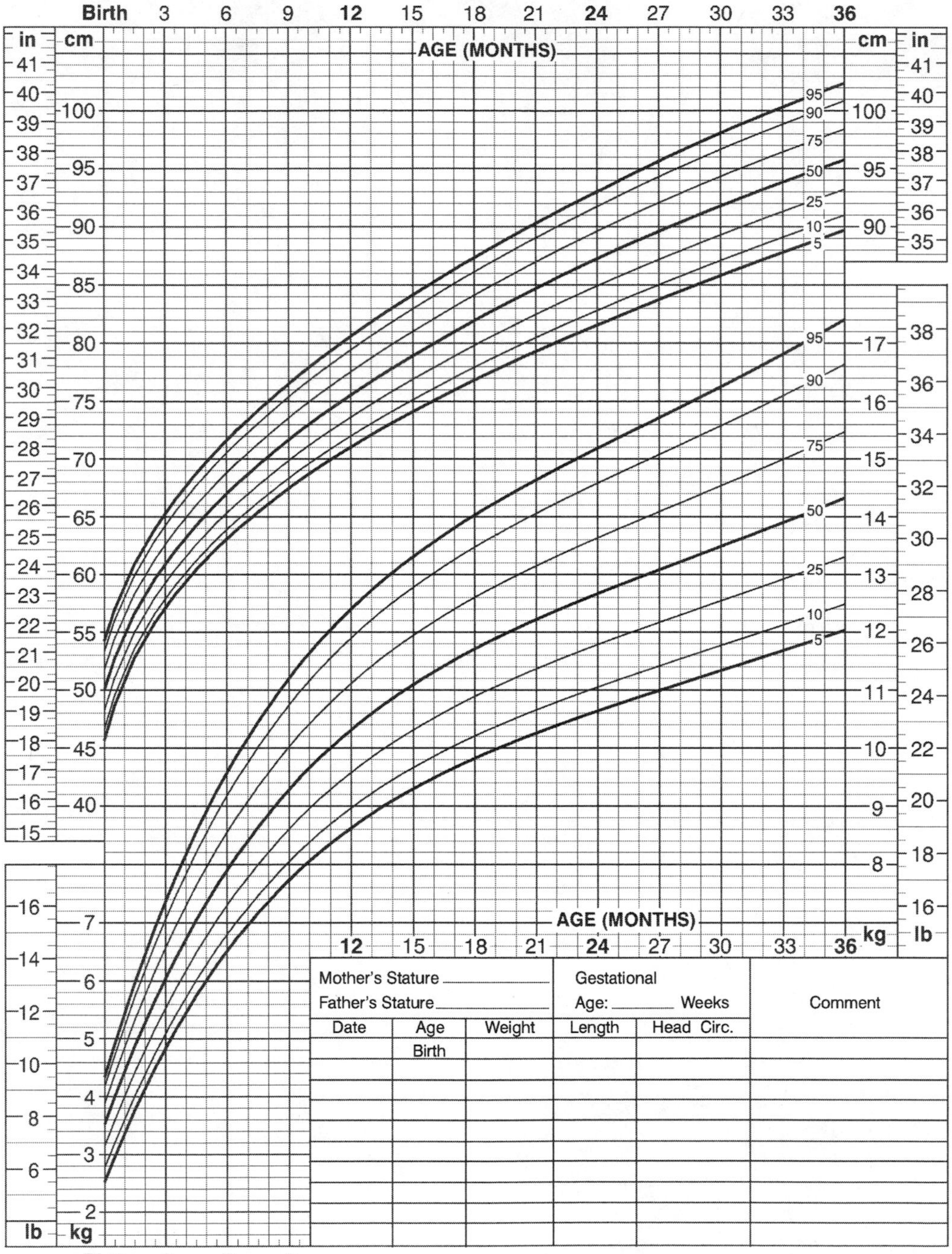

Mother's Stature			Gestational Age: ____ Weeks		Comment
Father's Stature					
Date	Age	Weight	Length	Head Circ.	
	Birth				

Published May 30, 2000 (modified 4/20/01).
SOURCE: Developed by the National Center for Health Statistics in collaboration with the National Center for Chronic Disease Prevention and Health Promotion (2000).
http://www.cdc.gov/growthcharts

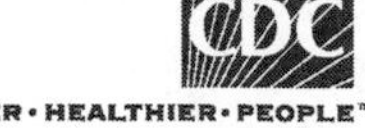

Table B–2 Birth to 36 months: Boys. Head circumference-for-age and Weight-for-length percentiles

Birth to 36 months: Boys
Head circumference-for-age and Weight-for-length percentiles

NAME ______________________

RECORD # ____________

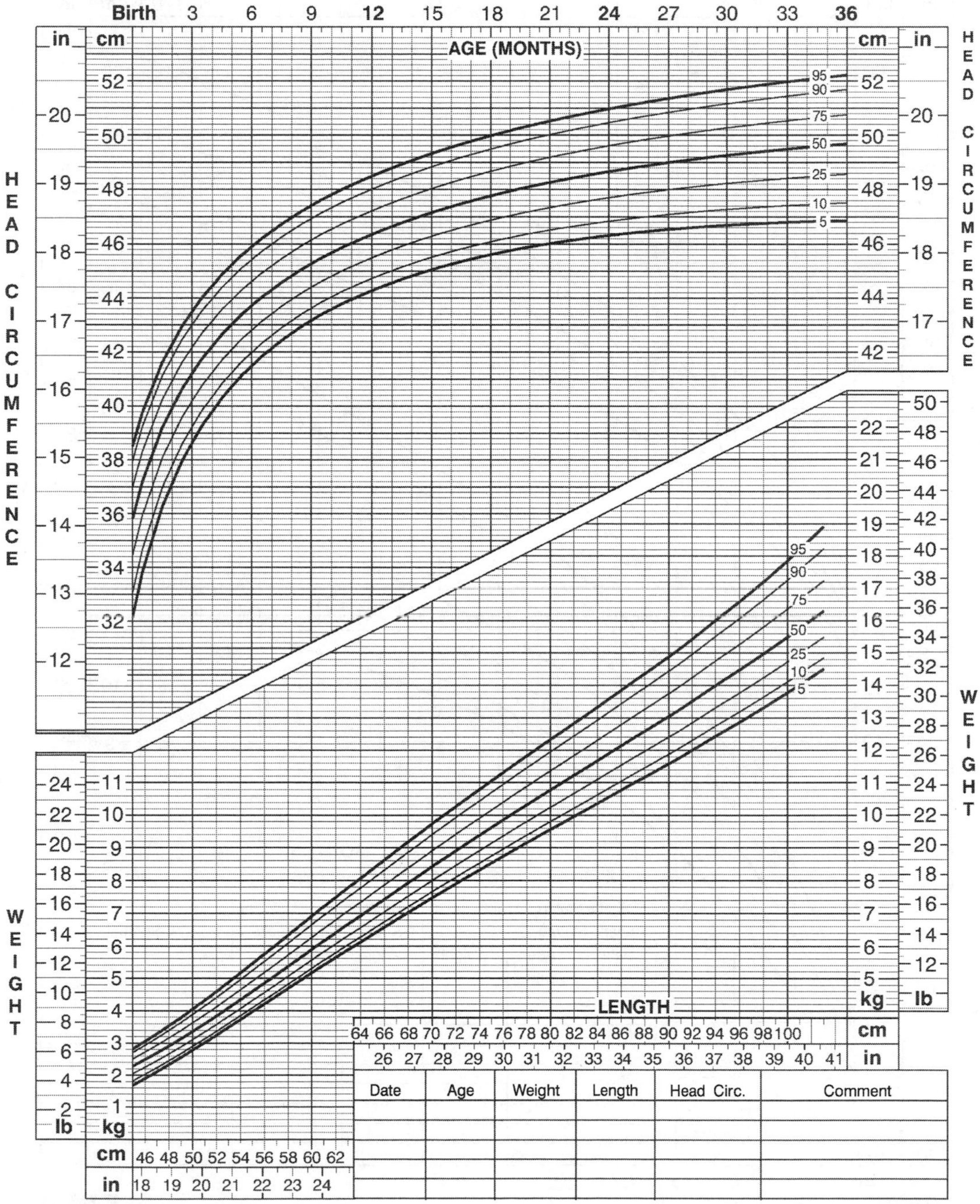

AGE (MONTHS)

Birth 3 6 9 12 15 18 21 24 27 30 33 36

HEAD CIRCUMFERENCE

in: 12 13 14 15 16 17 18 19 20

cm: 32 34 36 38 40 42 44 46 48 50 52

95 90 75 50 25 10 5

WEIGHT

kg: 1 2 3 4 5 6 7 8 9 10 11 12 13 14 15 16 17 18 19 20 21 22

lb: 2 4 6 8 10 12 14 16 18 20 22 24 26 28 30 32 34 36 38 40 42 44 46 48 50

LENGTH

cm: 46 48 50 52 54 56 58 60 62 64 66 68 70 72 74 76 78 80 82 84 86 88 90 92 94 96 98 100

in: 18 19 20 21 22 23 24 25 26 27 28 29 30 31 32 33 34 35 36 37 38 39 40 41

Date	Age	Weight	Length	Head Circ.	Comment

Published May 30, 2000 (modified 10/16/00).

SOURCE: Developed by the National Center for Health Statistics in collaboration with the National Center for Chronic Disease Prevention and Health Promotion (2000).
http://www.cdc.gov/growthcharts

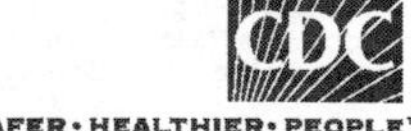

Table B–3 Birth to 36 months: Girls. Length-for-age and Weight-for-age percentiles

Birth to 36 months: Girls
Length-for-age and Weight-for-age percentiles

NAME ______________________

RECORD # __________

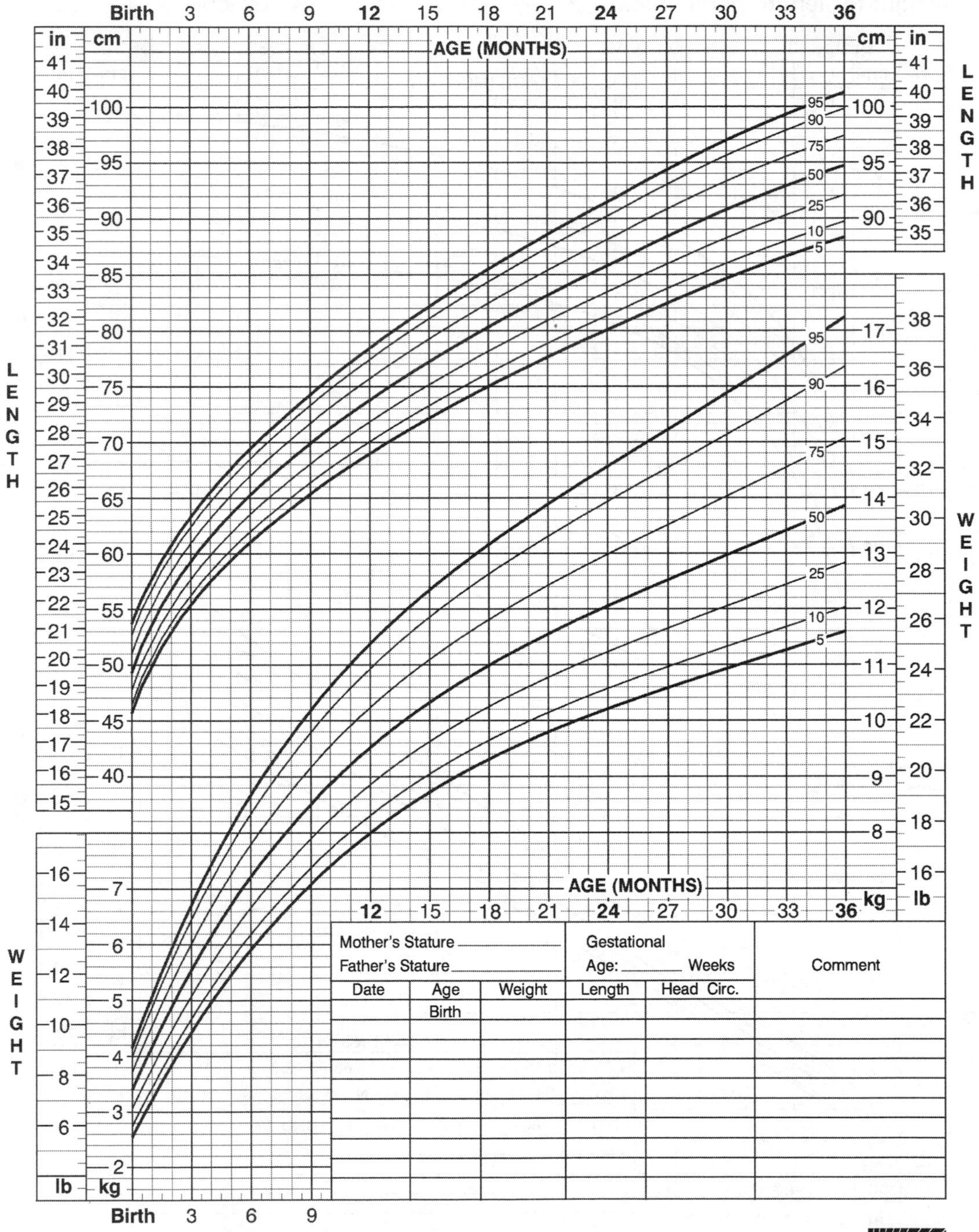

Birth 3 6 9 12 15 18 21 24 27 30 33 36

AGE (MONTHS)

LENGTH: in 15–41; cm 40–100

Percentiles: 95, 90, 75, 50, 25, 10, 5

WEIGHT: kg 2–17; lb 6–38

AGE (MONTHS)

12 15 18 21 24 27 30 33 36

Mother's Stature ______ Father's Stature ______			Gestational Age: ______ Weeks		Comment
Date	Age	Weight	Length	Head Circ.	
	Birth				

Birth 3 6 9

Published May 30, 2000 (modified 4/20/01).

SOURCE: Developed by the National Center for Health Statistics in collaboration with the National Center for Chronic Disease Prevention and Health Promotion (2000).
http://www.cdc.gov/growthcharts

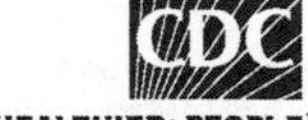

Table B–4 Birth to 36 months: Girls. Head circumference-for-age and Weight-for-length percentiles

Date	Age	Weight	Length	Head Circ.	Comment

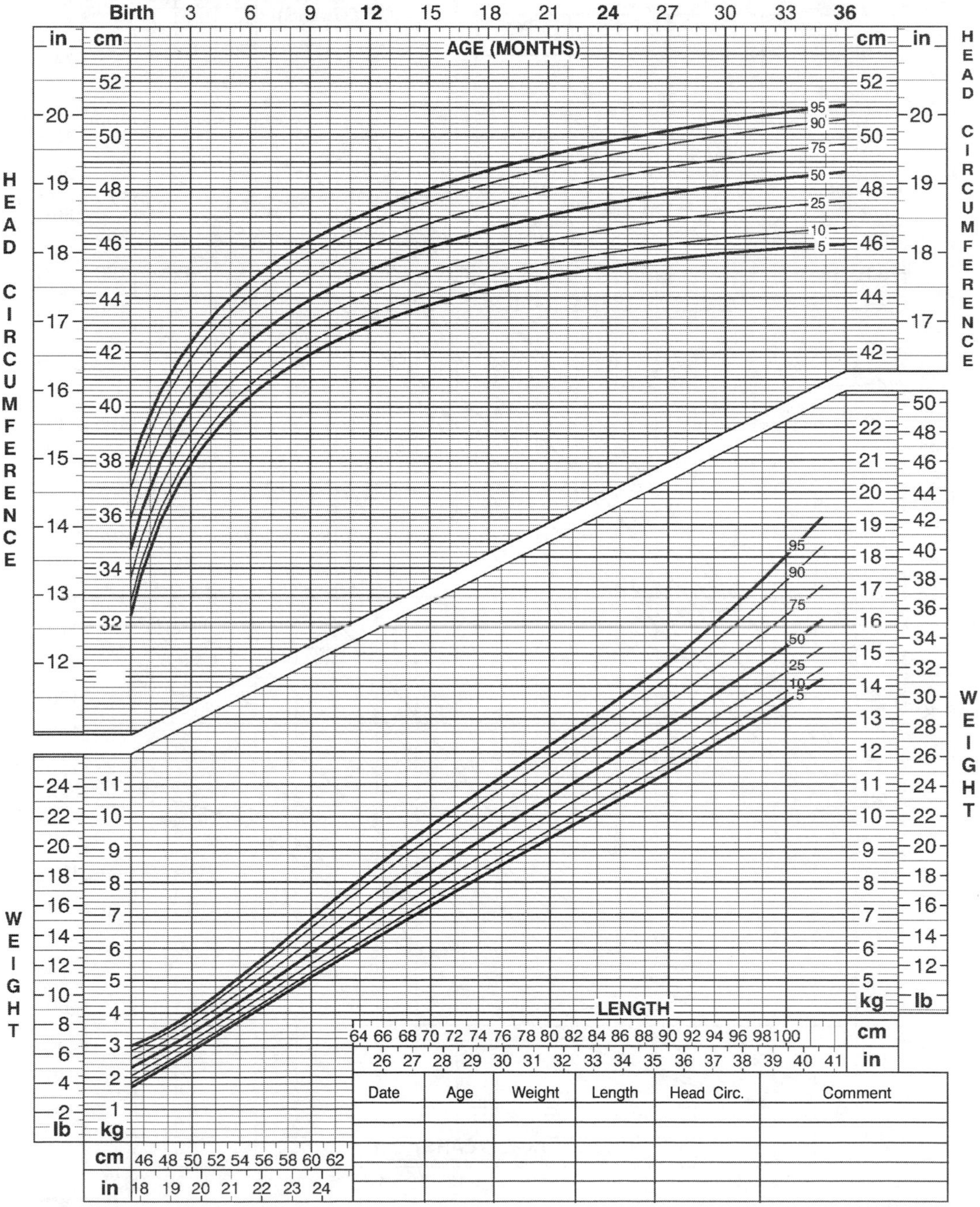

Published May 30, 2000 (modified 10/16/00).
SOURCE: Developed by the National Center for Health Statistics in collaboration with the National Center for Chronic Disease Prevention and Health Promotion (2000).
http://www.cdc.gov/growthcharts

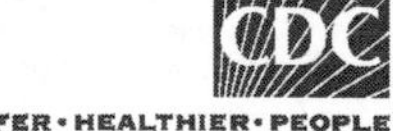

Table B–5 2 to 20 years: Boys. Stature-for-age and Weight-for-age percentiles

2 to 20 years: Boys
Stature-for-age and Weight-for-age percentiles

NAME ______________________

RECORD # ______________

Mother's Stature ____________ Father's Stature ____________

Date	Age	Weight	Stature	BMI*

***To Calculate BMI**: Weight (kg) ÷ Stature (cm) ÷ Stature (cm) x 10,000
or Weight (lb) ÷ Stature (in) ÷ Stature (in) x 703

AGE (YEARS)

STATURE

WEIGHT

Published May 30, 2000 (modified 11/21/00)..
SOURCE: Developed by the National Center for Health Statistics in collaboration with the National Center for Chronic Disease Prevention and Health Promotion (2000).
http://www.cdc.gov/growthcharts

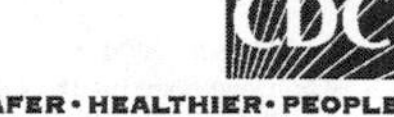

Table B–6 2 to 20 years: Boys. Body mass index-for-age percentiles

2 to 20 years: Boys
Body mass index-for-age percentiles

NAME ______________________

RECORD # ______________

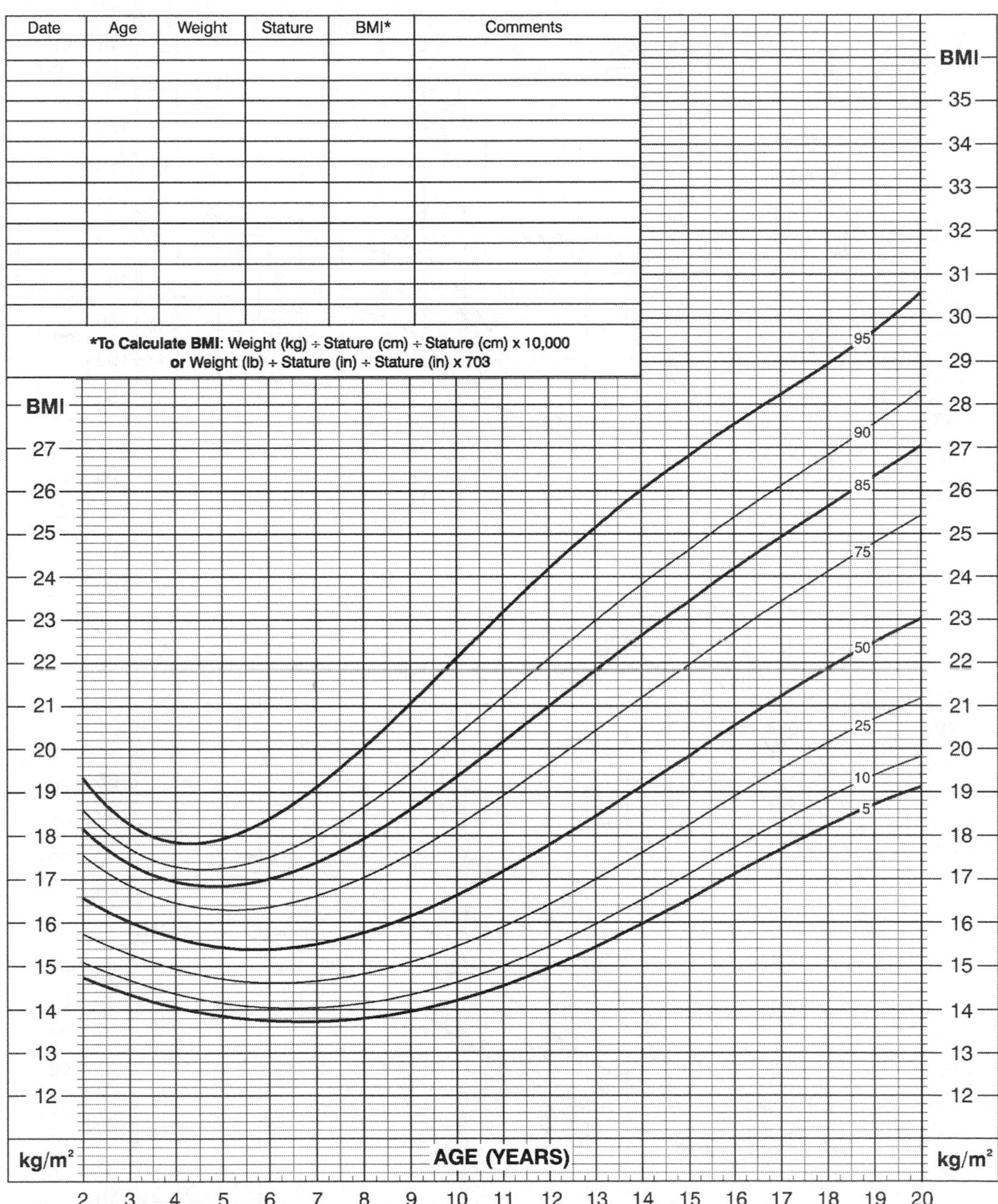

Published May 30, 2000 (modified 10/16/00).
SOURCE: Developed by the National Center for Health Statistics in collaboration with
the National Center for Chronic Disease Prevention and Health Promotion (2000).
http://www.cdc.gov/growthcharts

CDC
SAFER • HEALTHIER • PEOPLE™

Table B–7 2 to 20 years: Girls. Stature-for-age and Weight-for-age percentiles

2 to 20 years: Girls
Stature-for-age and Weight-for-age percentiles

NAME ______________________

RECORD # ______________

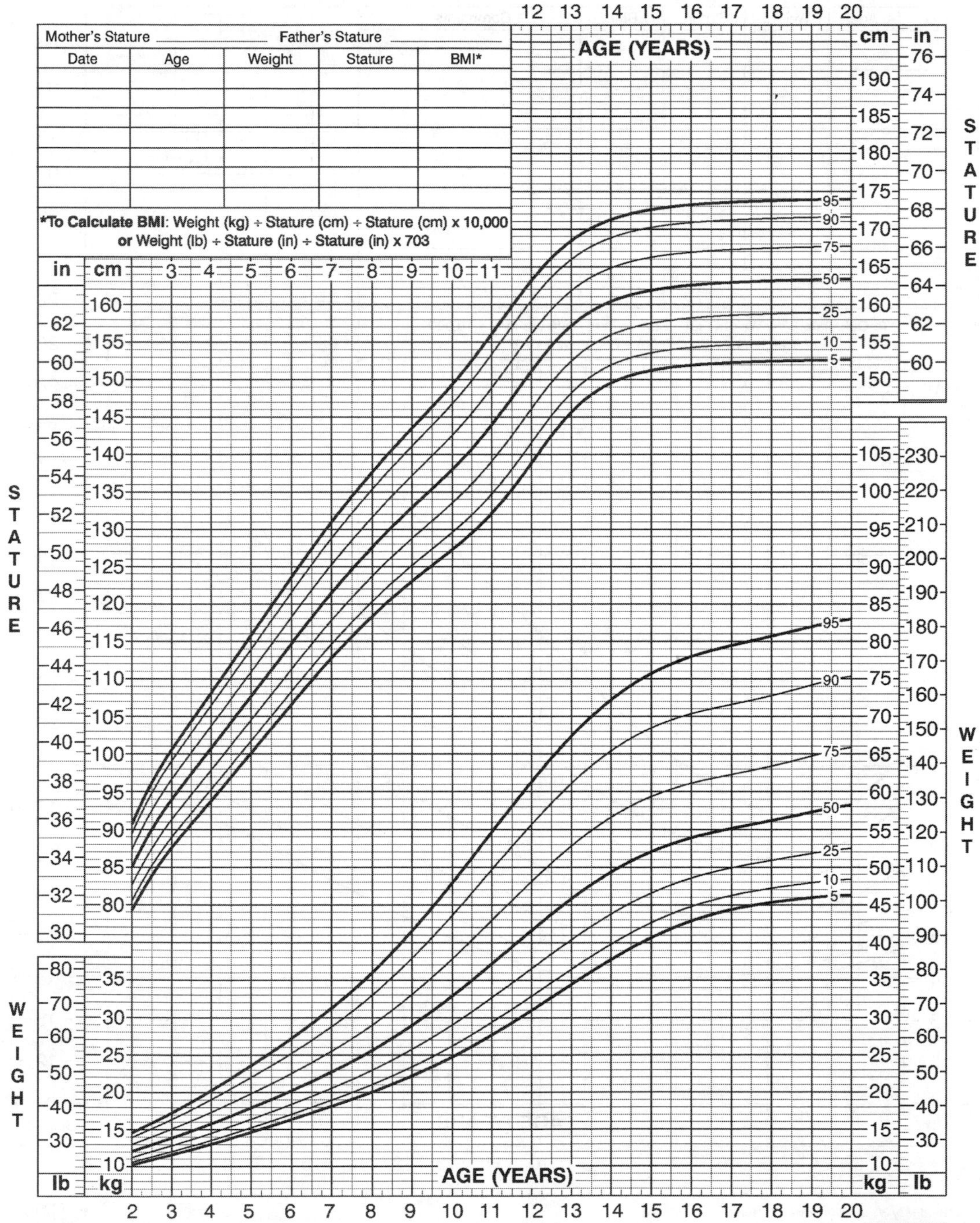

Mother's Stature ______________ Father's Stature ______________

Date	Age	Weight	Stature	BMI*

***To Calculate BMI**: Weight (kg) ÷ Stature (cm) ÷ Stature (cm) x 10,000
or Weight (lb) ÷ Stature (in) ÷ Stature (in) x 703

AGE (YEARS)

STATURE

WEIGHT

Published May 30, 2000 (modified 11/21/00).
SOURCE: Developed by the National Center for Health Statistics in collaboration with the National Center for Chronic Disease Prevention and Health Promotion (2000).
http://www.cdc.gov/growthcharts

CDC
SAFER • HEALTHIER • PEOPLE™

Table B–8 2 to 20 years: Girls. Body mass index-for-age percentiles

2 to 20 years: Girls
Body mass index-for-age percentiles

NAME ____________________

RECORD # ____________

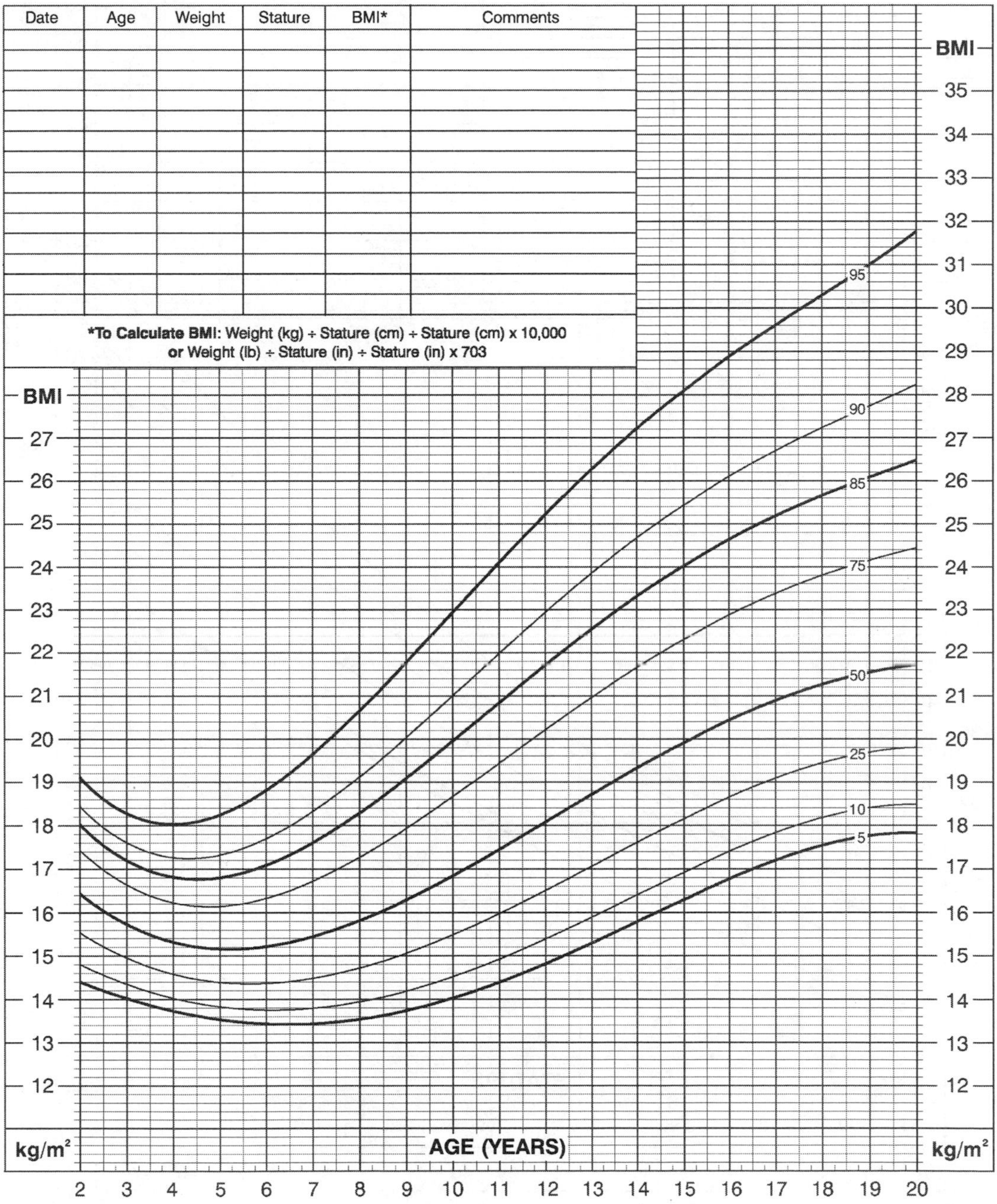
Date
Age
Weight
Stature
BMI*
Comments
*To Calculate BMI: Weight (kg) ÷ Stature (cm) ÷ Stature (cm) x 10,000
or Weight (lb) ÷ Stature (in) ÷ Stature (in) x 703
BMI
35
34
33
32
31
30
29
28
27
26
25
24
23
22
21
20
19
18
17
16
15
14
13
12
95
90
85
75
50
25
10
5
kg/m²
AGE (YEARS)
2 3 4 5 6 7 8 9 10 11 12 13 14 15 16 17 18 19 20

Published May 30, 2000 (modified 10/16/00).
SOURCE: Developed by the National Center for Health Statistics in collaboration with
the National Center for Chronic Disease Prevention and Health Promotion (2000).
http://www.cdc.gov/growthcharts

SAFER • HEALTHIER • PEOPLE™

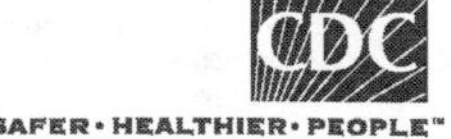

Table B–9 Weight-for-stature percentiles: Boys

NAME ______________________

Weight-for-stature percentiles: Boys

RECORD # ____________

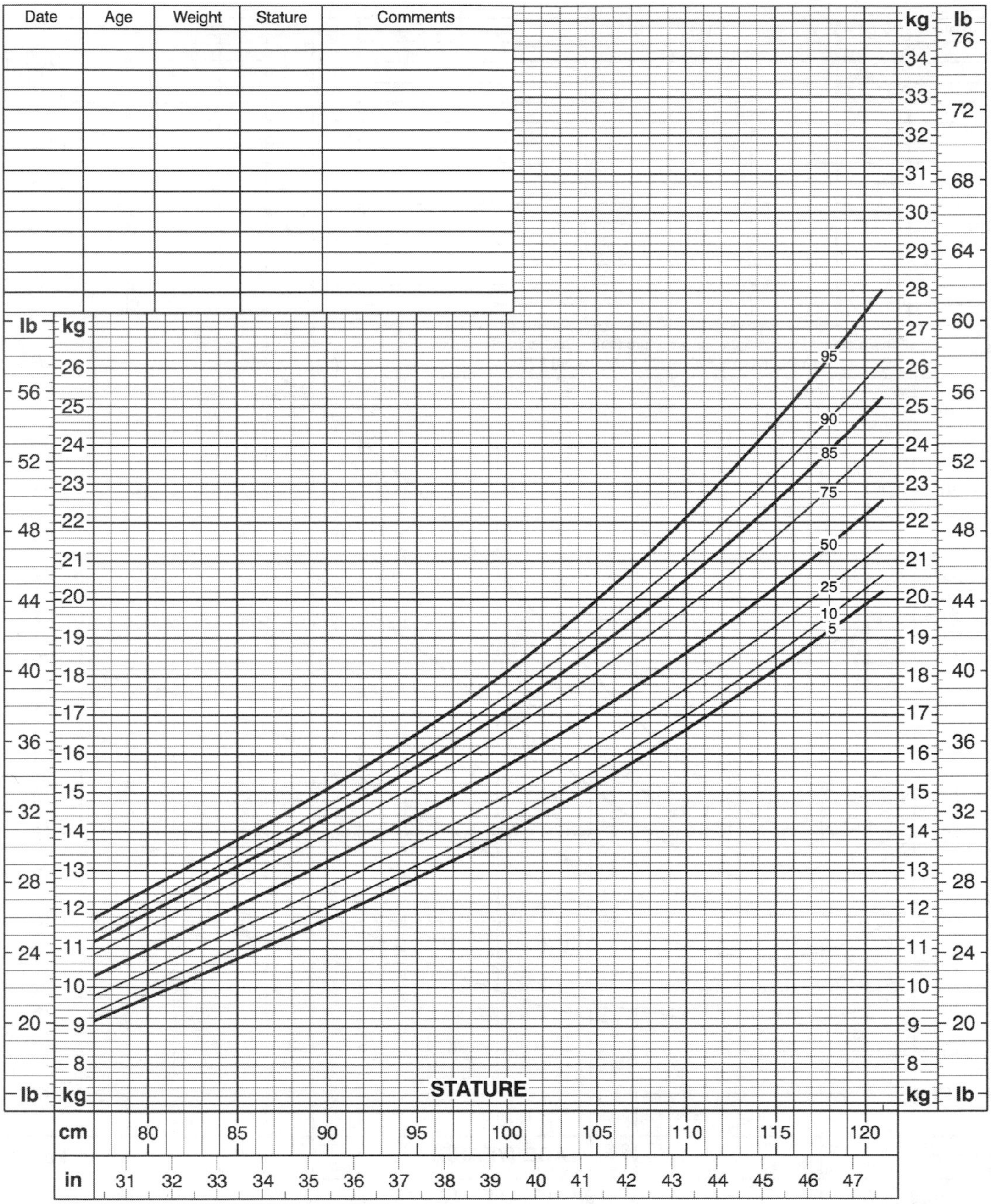

Date	Age	Weight	Stature	Comments

Published May 30, 2000 (modified 10/16/00).
SOURCE: Developed by the National Center for Health Statistics in collaboration with the National Center for Chronic Disease Prevention and Health Promotion (2000).
http://www.cdc.gov/growthcharts

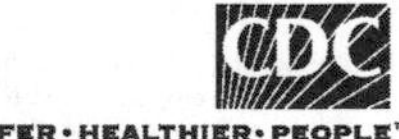

Table B–10 Weight-for-stature percentiles: Girls

NAME ____________________

Weight-for-stature percentiles: Girls

RECORD # ____________

Date	Age	Weight	Stature	Comments

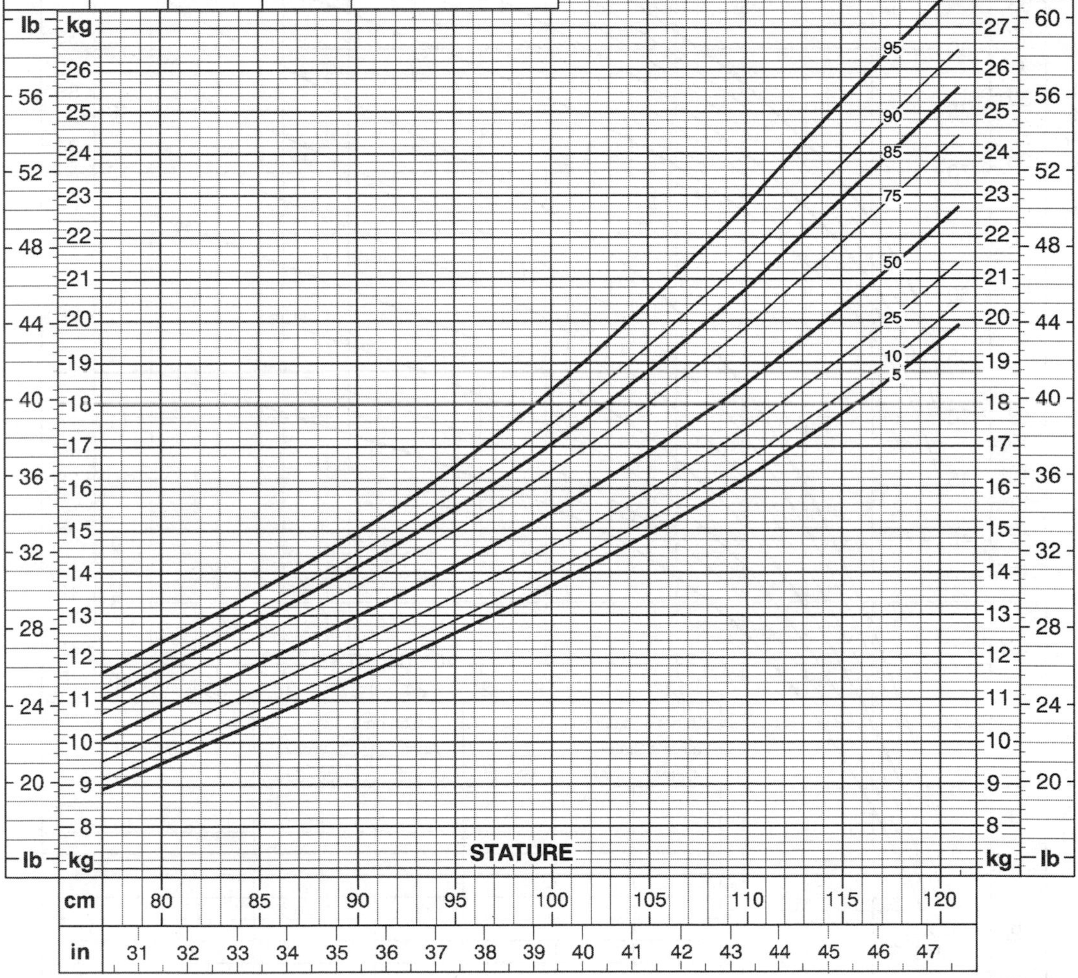

Published May 30, 2000 (modified 10/16/00).
SOURCE: Developed by the National Center for Health Statistics in collaboration with the National Center for Chronic Disease Prevention and Health Promotion (2000).
http://www.cdc.gov/growthcharts

CDC
SAFER • HEALTHIER • PEOPLE™

Table B–11 Birth to 36 months: Boys. Length-for-age and Weight-for-age percentiles

Birth to 36 months: Boys
Length-for-age and Weight-for-age percentiles

NAME ______________________

RECORD # ____________

Birth 3 6 9 12 15 18 21 24 27 30 33 36

AGE (MONTHS)

LENGTH (in / cm) — percentiles 97, 90, 75, 50, 25, 10, 3

WEIGHT (kg / lb) — percentiles 97, 90, 75, 50, 25, 10, 3

Mother's Stature ______ Father's Stature ______			Gestational Age: ______ Weeks		Comment
Date	Age	Weight	Length	Head Circ.	
	Birth				

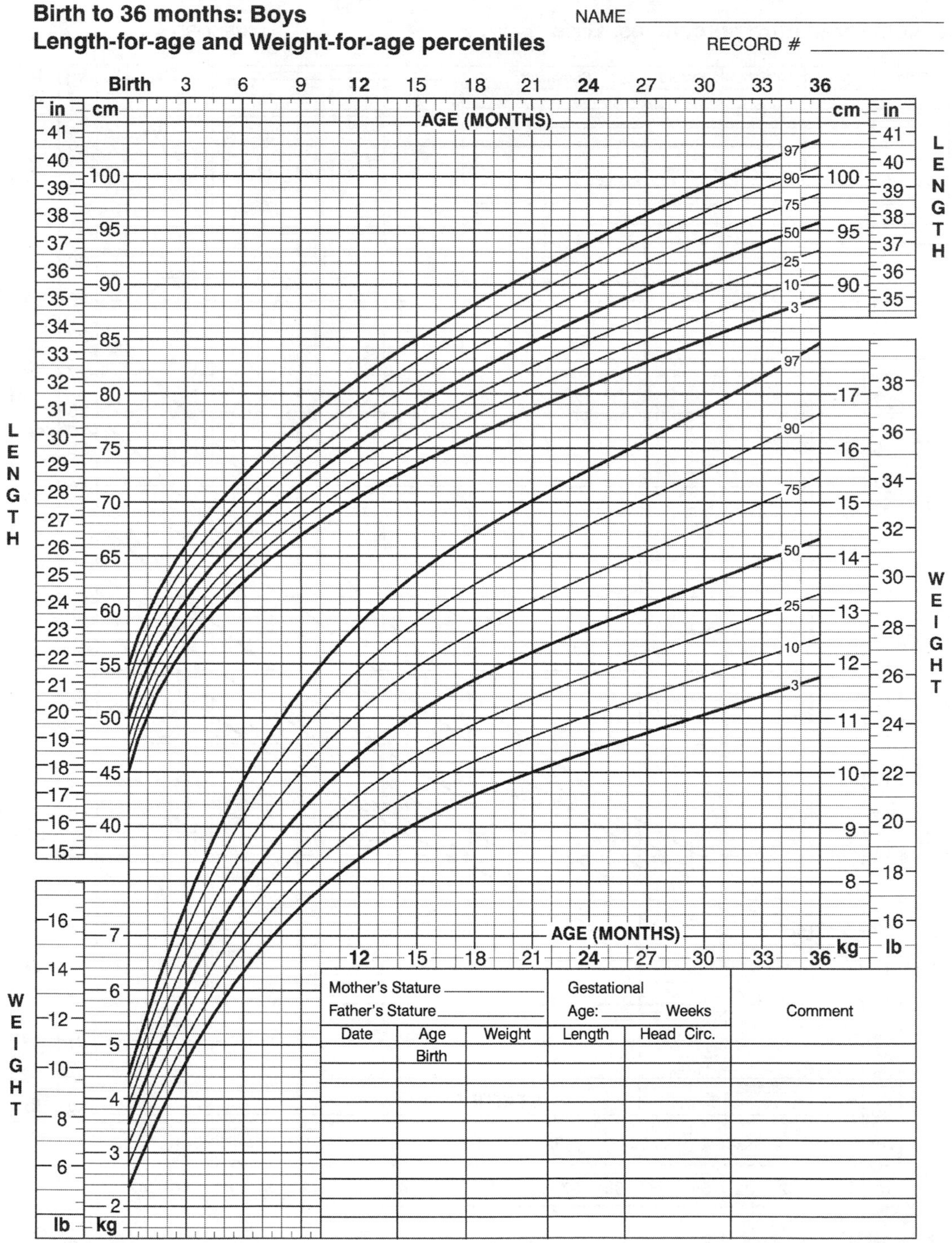

Published May 30, 2000 (modified 4/20/01).
SOURCE: Developed by the National Center for Health Statistics in collaboration with the National Center for Chronic Disease Prevention and Health Promotion (2000).
http://www.cdc.gov/growthcharts

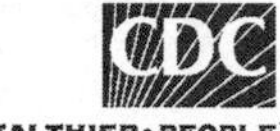

Table B–12 Birth to 36 months: Boys. Head circumference-for-age and Weight-for-length percentiles

Birth to 36 months: Boys
Head circumference-for-age and
Weight-for-length percentiles

NAME ______________________

RECORD # ______________

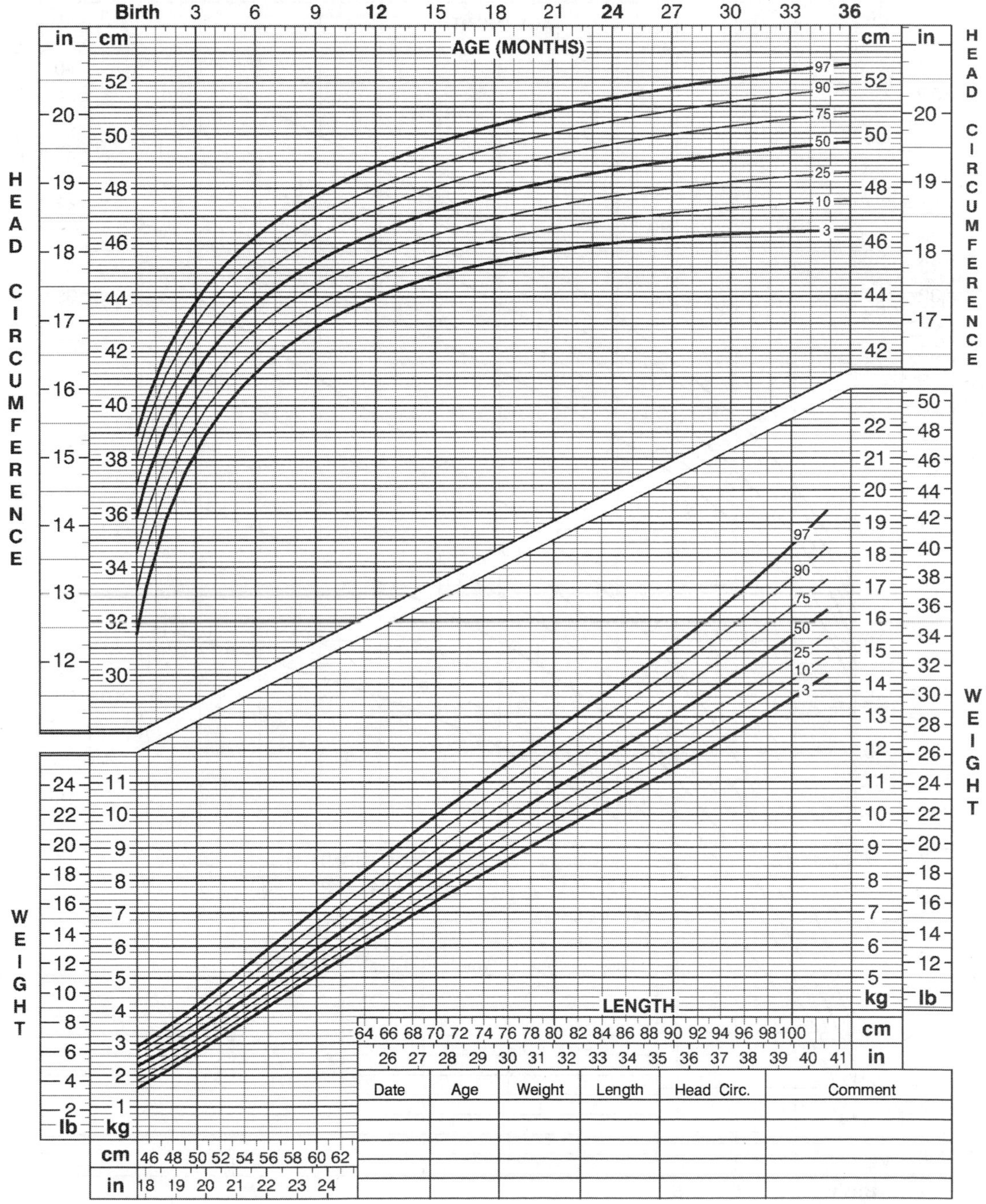

AGE (MONTHS): Birth 3 6 9 12 15 18 21 24 27 30 33 36

HEAD CIRCUMFERENCE — cm: 30 32 34 36 38 40 42 44 46 48 50 52; in: 12 13 14 15 16 17 18 19 20

Percentiles: 97 90 75 50 25 10 3

WEIGHT — kg: 1 2 3 4 5 6 7 8 9 10 11 12 13 14 15 16 17 18 19 20 21 22; lb: 2 4 6 8 10 12 14 16 18 20 22 24 26 28 30 32 34 36 38 40 42 44 46 48 50

LENGTH — cm: 46 48 50 52 54 56 58 60 62 64 66 68 70 72 74 76 78 80 82 84 86 88 90 92 94 96 98 100; in: 18 19 20 21 22 23 24 25 26 27 28 29 30 31 32 33 34 35 36 37 38 39 40 41

Date	Age	Weight	Length	Head Circ.	Comment

Published May 30, 2000 (modified 10/16/00).
SOURCE: Developed by the National Center for Health Statistics in collaboration with the National Center for Chronic Disease Prevention and Health Promotion (2000).
http://www.cdc.gov/growthcharts

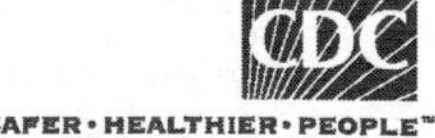

Table B–13 Birth to 36 months: Girls. Length-for-age and Weight-for-age percentiles

Birth to 36 months: Girls
Length-for-age and Weight-for-age percentiles

NAME ______________________

RECORD # ____________

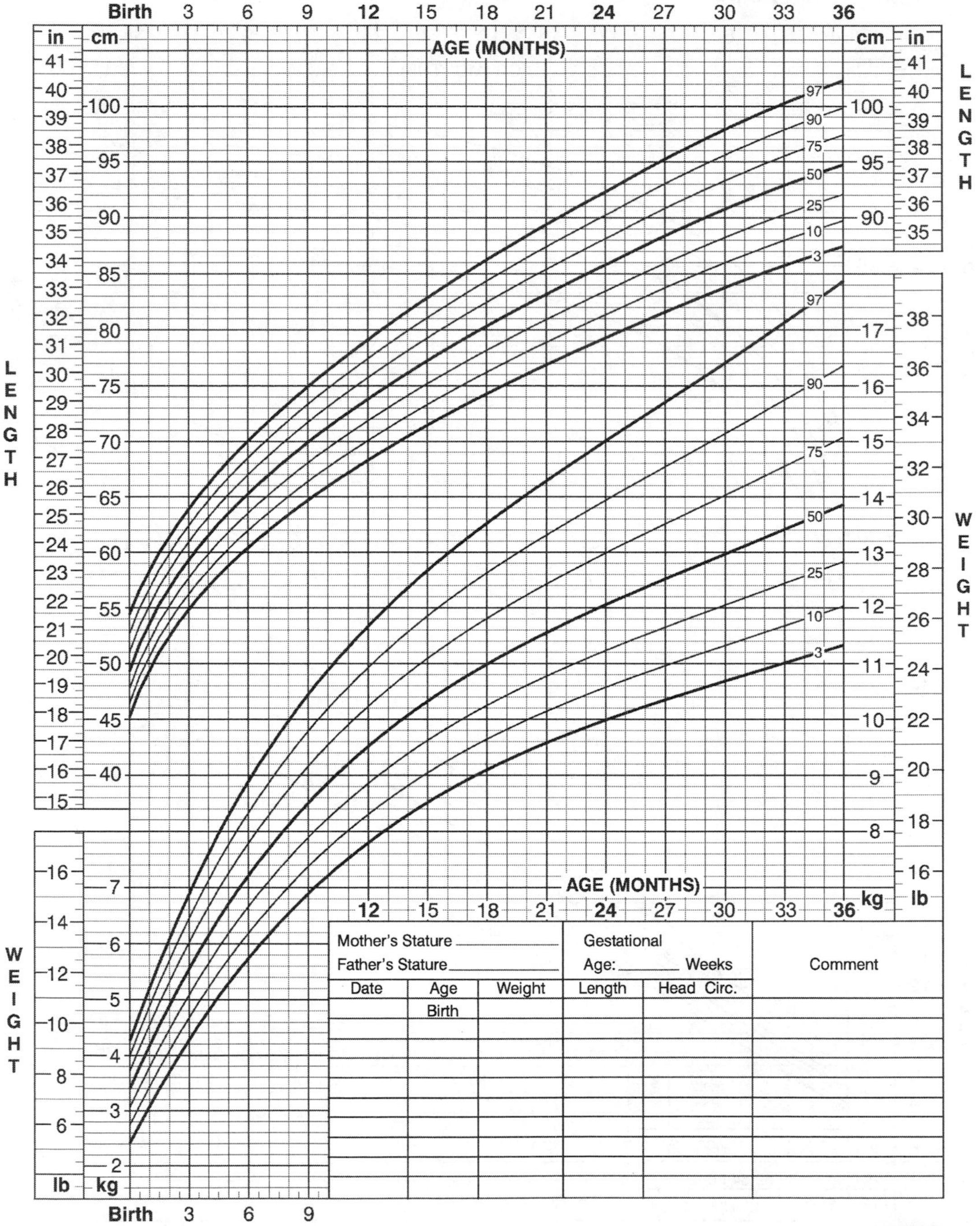

Birth 3 6 9 12 15 18 21 24 27 30 33 36

AGE (MONTHS)

LENGTH (in): 15 16 17 18 19 20 21 22 23 24 25 26 27 28 29 30 31 32 33 34 35 36 37 38 39 40 41

LENGTH (cm): 40 45 50 55 60 65 70 75 80 85 90 95 100

Length percentiles: 97 90 75 50 25 10 3

WEIGHT (kg): 2 3 4 5 6 7 8 9 10 11 12 13 14 15 16 17

WEIGHT (lb): 6 8 10 12 14 16 18 20 22 24 26 28 30 32 34 36 38

Weight percentiles: 97 90 75 50 25 10 3

AGE (MONTHS)

12 15 18 21 24 27 30 33 36

Birth 3 6 9

Mother's Stature ____________

Father's Stature ____________

Gestational Age: ________ Weeks

Date	Age	Weight	Length	Head Circ.	Comment
	Birth				

Published May 30, 2000 (modified 4/20/01).
SOURCE: Developed by the National Center for Health Statistics in collaboration with the National Center for Chronic Disease Prevention and Health Promotion (2000).
http://www.cdc.gov/growthcharts

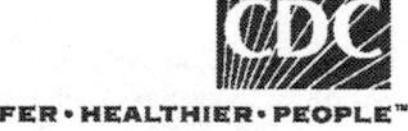

Table B–14 Birth to 36 months: Girls. Head circumference-for-age and Weight-for-length percentiles

Birth to 36 months: Girls
Head circumference-for-age and
Weight-for-length percentiles

NAME ______________________

RECORD # ____________

Birth 3 6 9 12 15 18 21 24 27 30 33 36

AGE (MONTHS)

HEAD CIRCUMFERENCE

in: 20 19 18 17 16 15 14 13 12

cm: 52 50 48 46 44 42 40 38 36 34 32 30

97 90 75 50 25 10 3

WEIGHT

kg: 22 21 20 19 18 17 16 15 14 13 12 11 10 9 8 7 6 5 4 3 2 1

lb: 50 48 46 44 42 40 38 36 34 32 30 28 26 24 22 20 18 16 14 12 10 8 6 4 2

97 90 75 50 25 10 3

LENGTH

cm: 46 48 50 52 54 56 58 60 62 64 66 68 70 72 74 76 78 80 82 84 86 88 90 92 94 96 98 100

in: 18 19 20 21 22 23 24 25 26 27 28 29 30 31 32 33 34 35 36 37 38 39 40 41

Date	Age	Weight	Length	Head Circ.	Comment

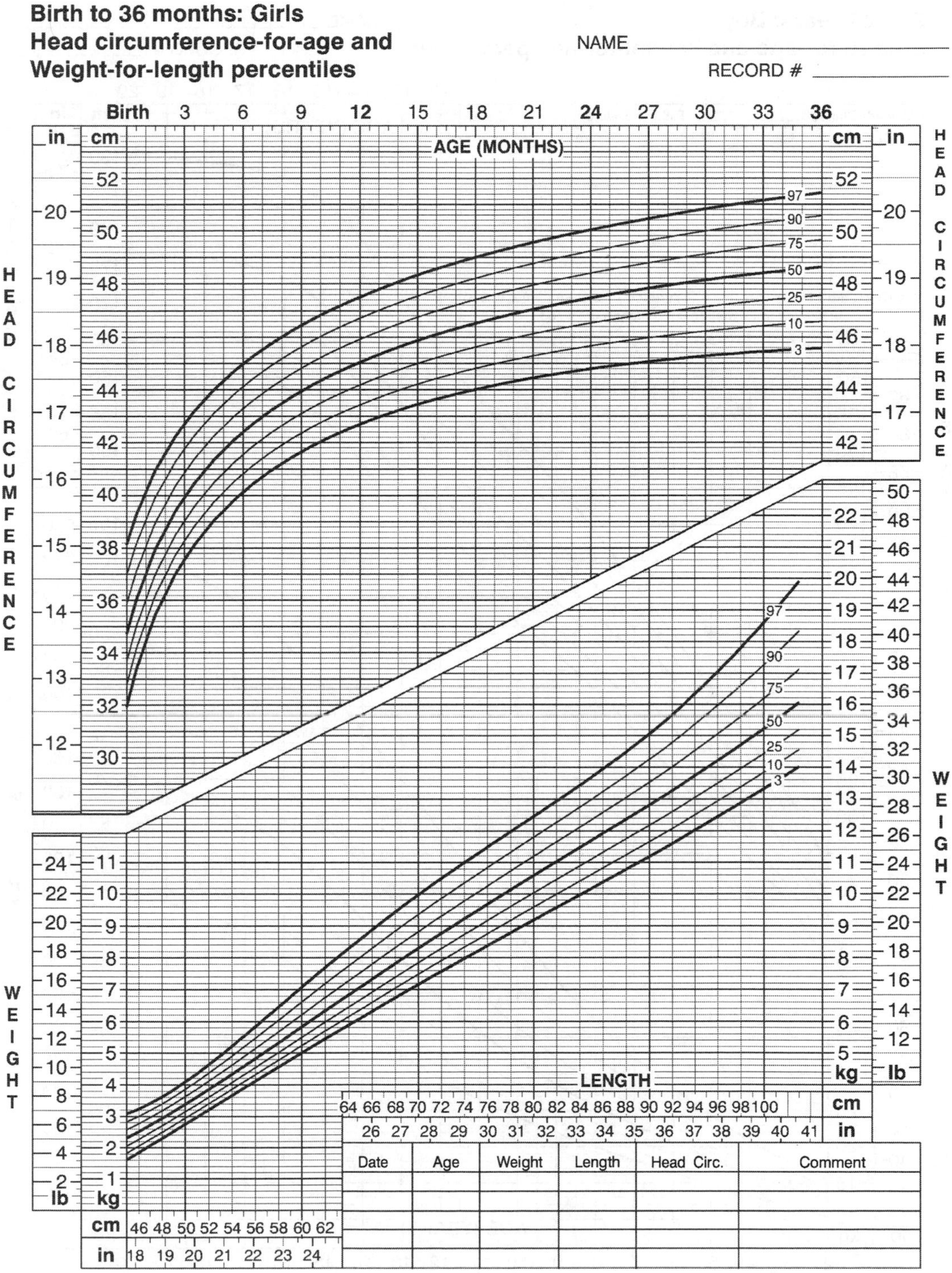

Published May 30, 2000 (modified 10/16/00).
SOURCE: Developed by the National Center for Health Statistics in collaboration with the National Center for Chronic Disease Prevention and Health Promotion (2000).
http://www.cdc.gov/growthcharts

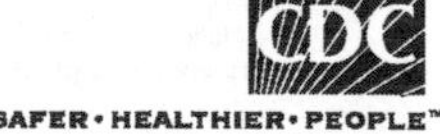

Table B–15 2 to 20 years: Boys. Stature-for-age and Weight-for-age percentiles

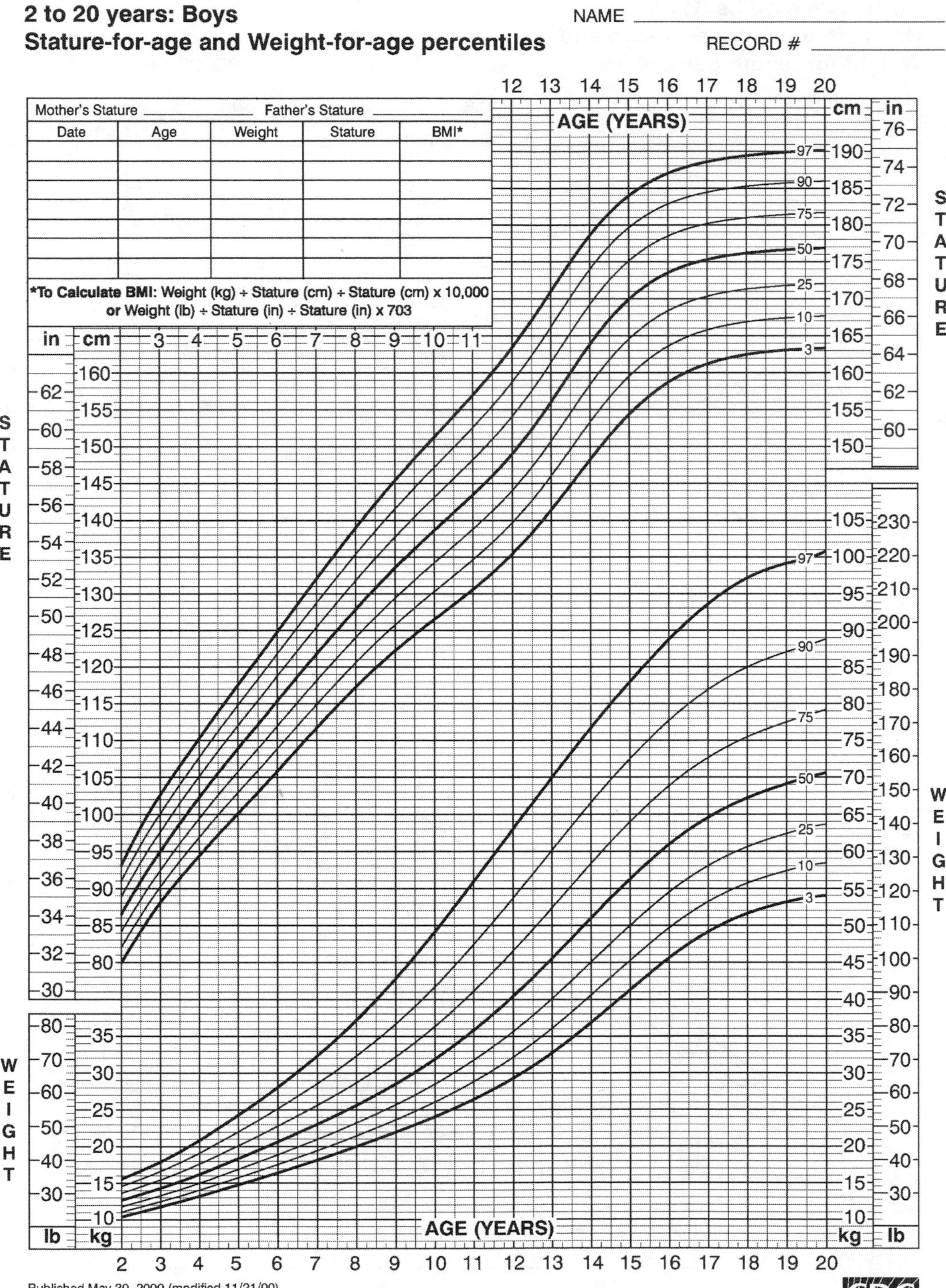

Table B–16 2 to 20 years: Boys. Body mass index-for-age percentiles

2 to 20 years: Boys
Body mass index-for-age percentiles

NAME ______________________

RECORD # ____________

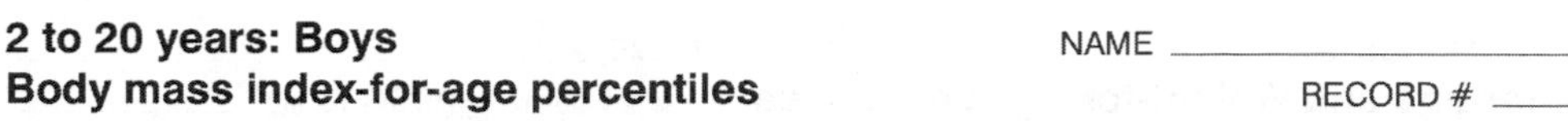

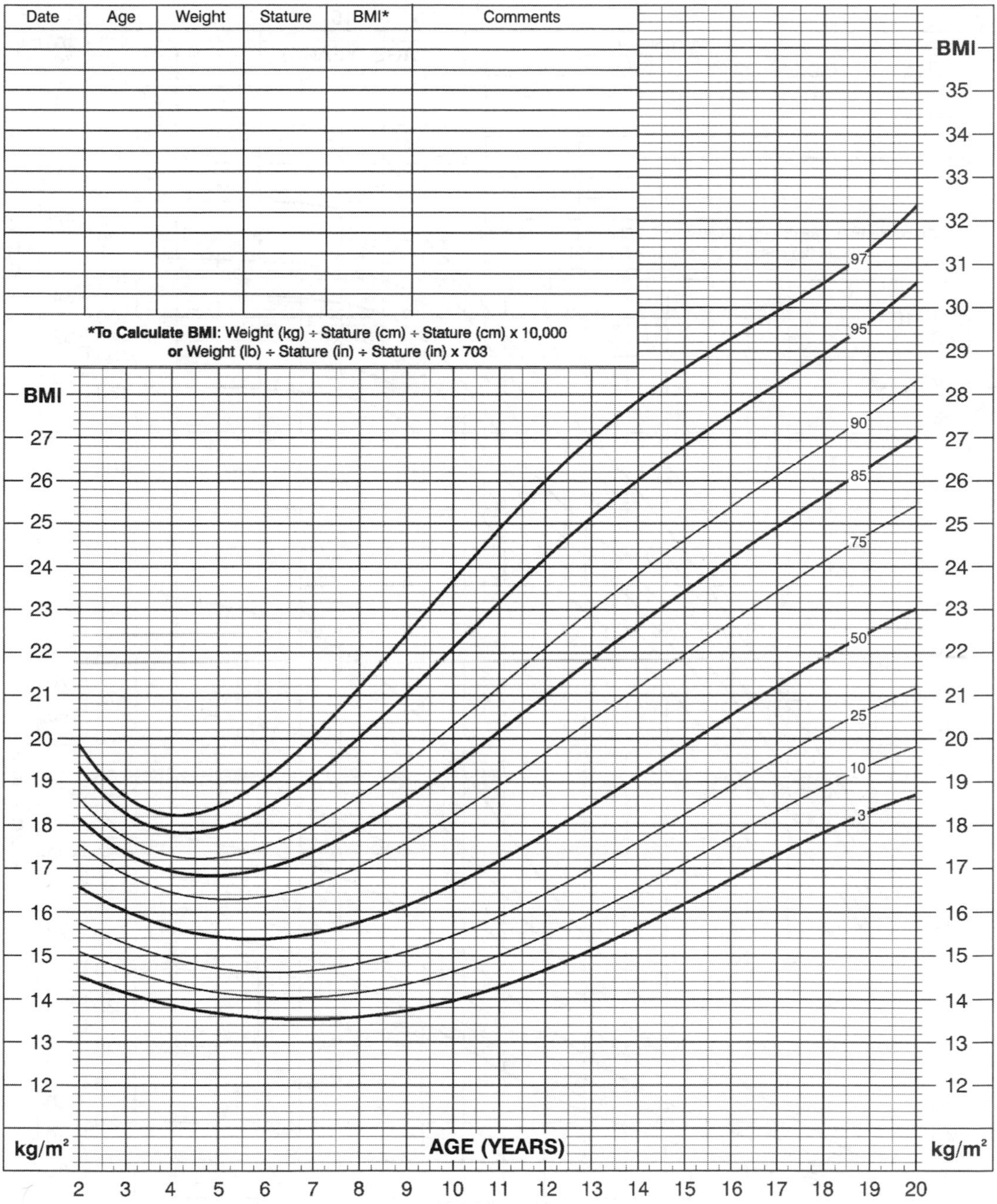
Date
Age
Weight
Stature
BMI*
Comments
*To Calculate BMI: Weight (kg) ÷ Stature (cm) ÷ Stature (cm) x 10,000
or Weight (lb) ÷ Stature (in) ÷ Stature (in) x 703
BMI
35
34
33
32
31
30
29
28
27
26
25
24
23
22
21
20
19
18
17
16
15
14
13
12
97
95
90
85
75
50
25
10
3
kg/m²
AGE (YEARS)
2 3 4 5 6 7 8 9 10 11 12 13 14 15 16 17 18 19 20

Published May 30, 2000 (modified 10/16/00).
SOURCE: Developed by the National Center for Health Statistics in collaboration with
the National Center for Chronic Disease Prevention and Health Promotion (2000).
http://www.cdc.gov/growthcharts

CDC
SAFER • HEALTHIER • PEOPLE™

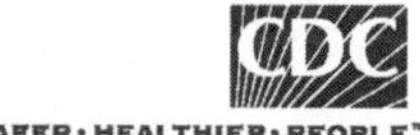

Table B–17 2 to 20 years: Girls. Stature-for-age and Weight-for-age percentiles

2 to 20 years: Girls
Stature-for-age and Weight-for-age percentiles

NAME ______________________

RECORD # ______________

Mother's Stature ______________ Father's Stature ______________

Date	Age	Weight	Stature	BMI*

***To Calculate BMI:** Weight (kg) ÷ Stature (cm) ÷ Stature (cm) x 10,000
or Weight (lb) ÷ Stature (in) ÷ Stature (in) x 703

AGE (YEARS)

2 3 4 5 6 7 8 9 10 11 12 13 14 15 16 17 18 19 20

STATURE (in / cm)

WEIGHT (lb / kg)

Percentiles: 97, 90, 75, 50, 25, 10, 3

Published May 30, 2000 (modified 11/21/00).
SOURCE: Developed by the National Center for Health Statistics in collaboration with
the National Center for Chronic Disease Prevention and Health Promotion (2000).
http://www.cdc.gov/growthcharts

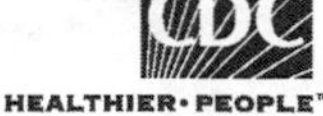

SAFER • HEALTHIER • PEOPLE™

Table B–18 2 to 20 years: Girls. Body mass index-for-age percentiles

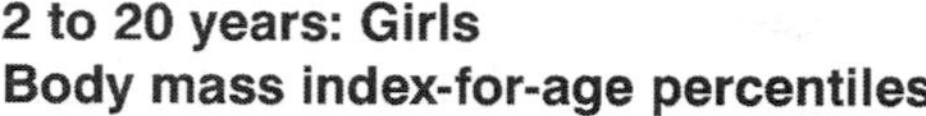

2 to 20 years: Girls
Body mass index-for-age percentiles

NAME ______________________

RECORD # ____________

Date	Age	Weight	Stature	BMI*	Comments

***To Calculate BMI:** Weight (kg) ÷ Stature (cm) ÷ Stature (cm) x 10,000
or Weight (lb) ÷ Stature (in) ÷ Stature (in) x 703

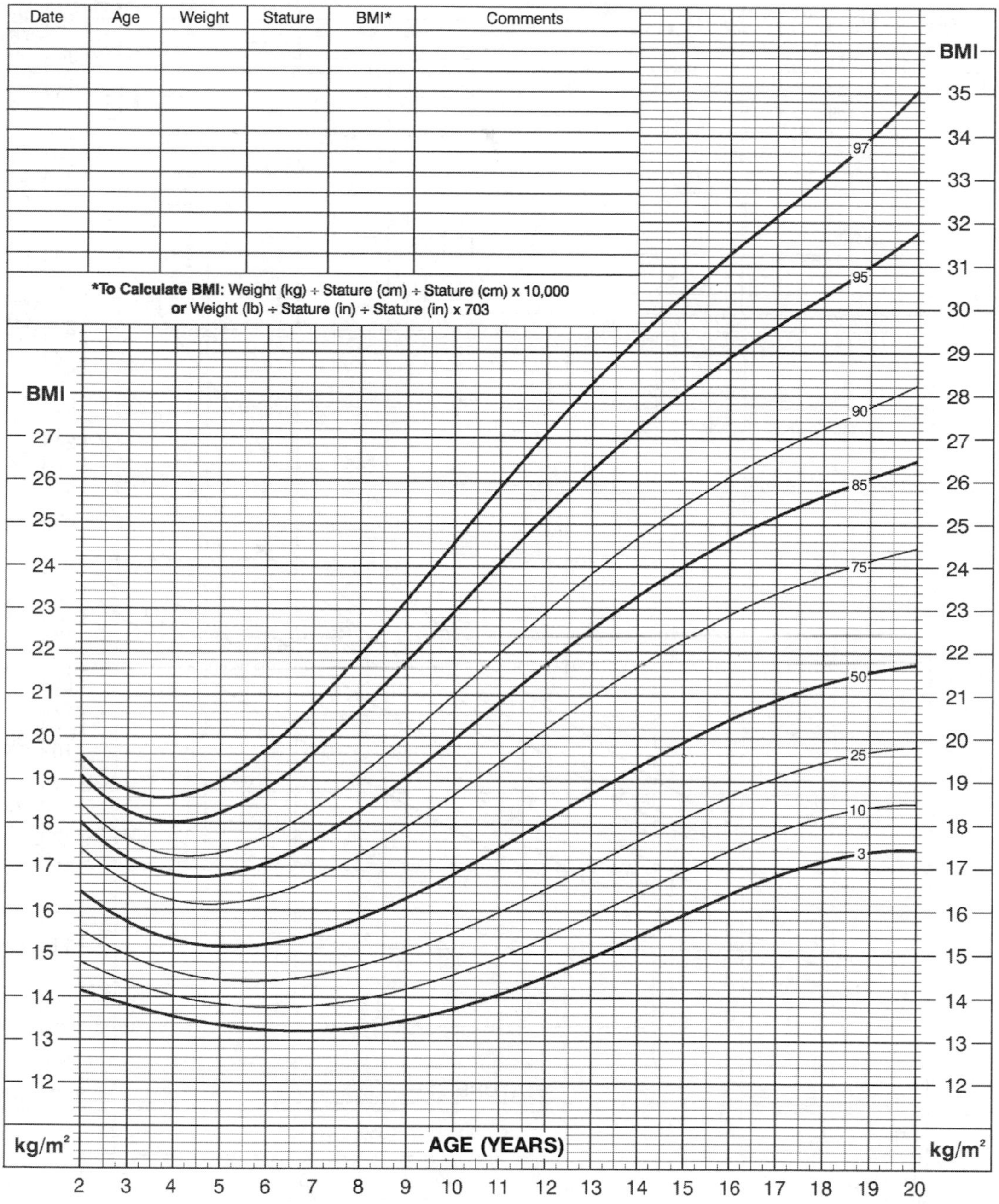

Published May 30, 2000 (modified 10/16/00).
SOURCE: Developed by the National Center for Health Statistics in collaboration with the National Center for Chronic Disease Prevention and Health Promotion (2000).
http://www.cdc.gov/growthcharts

CDC
SAFER • HEALTHIER • PEOPLE™

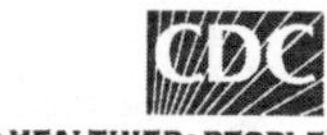

Table B–19 Weight-for-stature percentiles: Boys

NAME ______________________

Weight-for-stature percentiles: Boys

RECORD # ______________

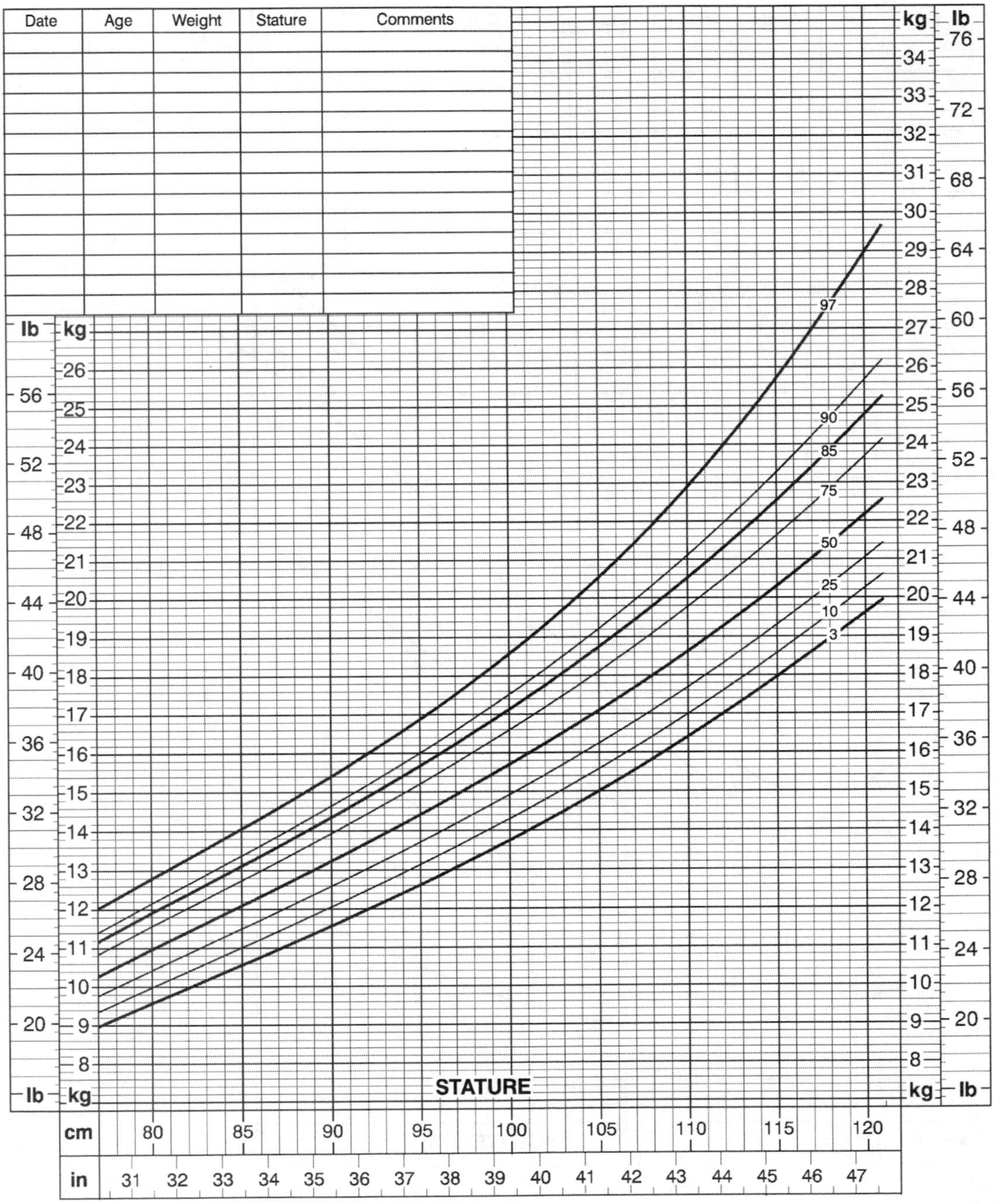

Date	Age	Weight	Stature	Comments

kg 34 33 32 31 30 29 28 27 26 25 24 23 22 21 20 19 18 17 16 15 14 13 12 11 10 9 8 kg

lb 76 72 68 64 60 56 52 48 44 40 36 32 28 24 20 lb

lb 56 52 48 44 40 36 32 28 24 20 lb

kg 26 25 24 23 22 21 20 19 18 17 16 15 14 13 12 11 10 9 8 kg

97 90 85 75 50 25 10 3

STATURE

cm 80 85 90 95 100 105 110 115 120

in 31 32 33 34 35 36 37 38 39 40 41 42 43 44 45 46 47

Published May 30, 2000 (modified 10/16/00).
SOURCE: Developed by the National Center for Health Statistics in collaboration with the National Center for Chronic Disease Prevention and Health Promotion (2000).
http://www.cdc.gov/growthcharts

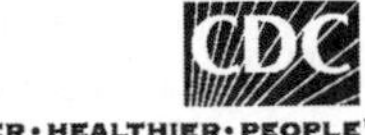

Table B–20 Weight-for-stature percentiles: Girls

NAME ____________

RECORD # ____________

Weight-for-stature percentiles: Girls

Date	Age	Weight	Stature	Comments

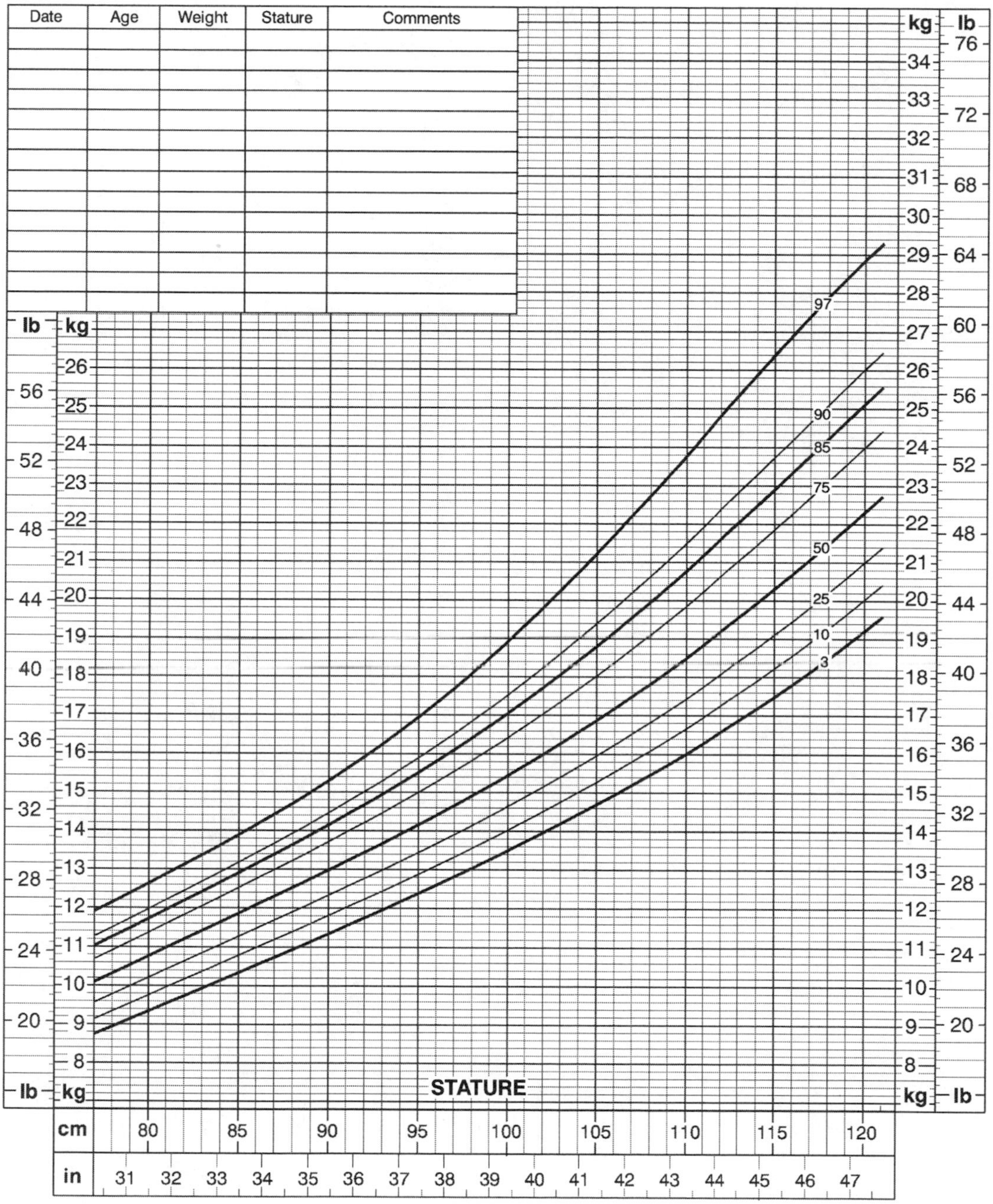

Published May 30, 2000 (modified 10/16/00).
SOURCE: Developed by the National Center for Health Statistics in collaboration with the National Center for Chronic Disease Prevention and Health Promotion (2000).
http://www.cdc.gov/growthcharts

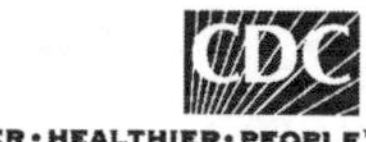

Appendix C

Incremental Growth Charts

Table C–1 Head circumference of boys: birth to 36 mo of age in 6-mo increments (Fels Longitudinal Study)

	Percentiles of 6-mo increments									
Age at end of interval	*3 (–2 SD)*	*5*	*10 (–1 SD)*	*25*	*50 (mean)*	*75*	*90 (+1 SD)*	*95*	*97 (+2 SD)*	*n*
mo					*cm/6 mo*					
6	5.97 (4.97)	6.21	6.51 (6.83)	7.50	8.58 (8.69)	9.77	10.62 (10.55)	11.13	11.50 (12.41)	263
9	3.58 (3.70)	4.07	4.30 (4.42)	4.67	5.13 (5.14)	5.57	6.02 (5.86)	6.27	6.56 (6.58)	263
12	2.05 (1.74)	2.13	2.40 (2.46)	2.72	3.09 (3.18)	3.54	3.98 (3.90)	4.44	4.68 (4.62)	271
18	0.46 (0.36)	0.61	0.88 (0.95)	1.14	1.51 (1.54)	1.92	2.19 (2.12)	2.47	2.60 (2.71)	270
24	0.03 (–0.08)	0.12	0.38 (0.42)	0.64	0.93 (0.93)	1.18	1.51 (1.43)	1.67	1.96 (1.94)	267
30	0.05 (–0.03)	0.21	0.32 (0.34)	0.52	0.70 (0.71)	0.92	1.07 (1.08)	1.26	1.52 (1.45)	213
36	–0.17 (–0.14)	–0.08	0.12 (0.16)	0.29	0.48 (0.46)	0.62	0.84 (0.76)	0.93	0.98 (1.06)	167

Source: Reprinted with permission from Baumgartner RN et al., "Incremental Growth Tables: Supplementary to Previously Published Charts," *The American Journal of Clinical Nutrition* 43, May 1986, pp. 711–722. Copyright © 1986 American Society for Clinical Nutrition.

Table C–2 Head circumference of girls: birth to 36 mo of age in 6-mo increments (Fels Longitudinal Study)

Age at end of interval	*Percentiles of 6-mo increments*									
	3 (–2 SD)	*5*	*10 (–1 SD)*	*25*	*50 (mean)*	*75*	*90 (+1 SD)*	*95*	*97 (+2 SD)*	*n*
mo	*cm/6 mo*									
6	5.53 (5.38)	5.80	6.17 (6.69)	7.14	8.05 (7.99)	8.84	9.48 (9.30)	10.11	10.41 (10.61)	249
9	3.10 (3.31)	3.53	4.03 (4.13)	4.48	4.96 (4.95)	5.40	5.95 (5.77)	6.14	6.44 (6.59)	243
12	1.60 (1.47)	2.08	2.30 (2.28)	2.68	3.12 (3.09)	3.51	3.79 (3.90)	4.02	4.13 (4.72)	252
18	0.34 (0.34)	0.71	0.96 (0.98)	1.34	1.60 (1.63)	1.91	2.34 (2.27)	2.55	2.78 (2.92)	240
24	0.03 (–0.56)	0.26	0.45 (0.23)	0.69	0.95 (1.03)	1.22	1.65 (1.81)	1.94	2.36 (2.61)	236
30	–0.15 (–0.21)	–0.06	0.22 (0.26)	0.50	0.71 (0.74)	0.96	1.23 (1.21)	1.63	1.80 (1.69)	191
36	–0.01 (–0.11)	0.09	0.15 (0.22)	0.34	0.52 (0.54)	0.71	0.94 (0.87)	1.17	1.35 (1.20)	151

Source: Reprinted with permission from Baumgartner RN et al., "Incremental Growth Tables: Supplementary to Previously Published Charts," *The American Journal of Clinical Nutrition* 43, May 1986, pp. 711–722.

Table C–3 Recumbent length of boys: birth to 36 mo of age in 6-mo increments (Fels Longitudinal Study)

	Percentiles of 6-mo increments									
Age at end of interval	*3 (–2 SD)*	*5*	*10 (–1 SD)*	*25*	*50 (mean)*	*75*	*90 (+1 SD)*	*95*	*97 (+2 SD)*	*n*
mo					*cm/6 mo*					
6	12.22 (12.00)	12.96	13.71 (14.49)	15.33	17.09 (16.98)	18.57	19.91 (19.47)	20.79	21.70 (21.96)	271
9	8.39 (8.19)	8.90	9.39 (9.72)	10.22	11.08 (11.25)	12.14	13.26 (12.77)	13.93	14.51 (14.30)	265
12	5.89 (5.64)	6.20	6.69 (7.06)	7.55	8.51 (8.48)	9.29	10.14 (9.90)	10.71	10.91 (11.32)	286
18	4.24 (4.03)	4.57	4.99 (5.29)	5.82	6.51 (6.56)	7.31	8.05 (7.82)	8.67	9.02 (9.08)	286
24	3.26 (2.94)	3.58	3.89 (4.17)	4.57	5.40 (5.41)	6.13	6.85 (6.64)	7.39	7.57 (7.88)	280
30	2.84 (2.73)	3.00	3.49 (3.70)	4.00	4.63 (4.67)	5.29	5.77 (5.63)	6.10	6.63 (6.60)	270
36	2.33 (2.23)	2.47	3.02 (3.18)	3.58	4.05 (4.12)	4.66	5.38 (5.07)	5.75	6.01 (6.01)	266

Source: Reprinted with permission from Baumgartner RN et al., "Incremental Growth Tables: Supplementary to Previously Published Charts," *The American Journal of Clinical Nutrition* 43, May 1986, pp. 711–722.

Table C–4 Recumbent length of girls: birth to 36 mo of age in 6-mo increments (Fels Longitudinal Study)

	Percentiles of 6-mo increments									
Age at end of interval	*3 (–2 SD)*	*5*	*10 (–1 SD)*	*25*	*50 (mean)*	*75*	*90 (+1 SD)*	*95*	*97 (+2 SD)*	*n*
mo					*cm/6 mo*					
6	12.00 (11.55)	12.36	13.26 (13.84)	14.51	16.06 (16.13)	17.66	18.85 (18.42)	19.76	20.34 (20.71)	254
9	8.18 (7.92)	8.40	9.10 (9.38)	9.78	10.82 (10.83)	11.77	12.58 (12.29)	13.22	13.53 (13.74)	248
12	5.94 (5.43)	6.20	6.76 (6.99)	7.41	8.49 (8.56)	9.43	10.34 (10.12)	10.87	11.32 (11.69)	263
18	3.94 (4.17)	4.61	5.19 (5.46)	6.00	6.79 (6.76)	7.50	8.15 (8.05)	8.81	9.17 (9.35)	262
24	3.72 (3.41)	4.00	4.40 (4.57)	4.95	5.59 (5.73)	6.45	7.09 (6.89)	7.60	7.87 (8.04)	259
30	2.90 (2.70)	3.19	3.54 (3.71)	4.02	4.66 (4.72)	5.23	6.00 (5.74)	6.39	6.77 (6.75)	245
36	2.54 (2.29)	2.72	2.99 (3.22)	3.62	4.13 (4.16)	4.67	5.25 (5.10)	5.78	6.16 (6.04)	246

Source: Reprinted with permission from Baumgartner RN et al., "Incremental Growth Tables: Supplementary to Previously Published Charts," *The American Journal of Clinical Nutrition* 43, May 1986, pp. 711–722. Copyright © 1986 American Society for Clinical Nutrition.

Table C–5 Stature of boys: 3 to 18 yr of age in 6-mo increments (Fels Longitudinal Study)

	Percentiles of 6-mo increments									
Age at end of interval	*3 (–2 SD)*	*5*	*10 (–1 SD)*	*25*	*50 (mean)*	*75*	*90 (+1 SD)*	*95*	*97 (+2 SD)*	*n*
yr					*cm/6 mo*					
3.5	2.54 (2.22)	2.64	2.84 (3.03)	3.36	3.81 (3.84)	4.33	4.72 (4.65)	5.00	5.32 (5.46)	208
4.0	2.14 (2.09)	2.49	2.69 (2.84)	3.11	3.59 (3.60)	4.02	4.41 (4.35)	4.77	4.86 (5.11)	233
4.5	2.27 (2.21)	2.52	2.73 (2.88)	3.05	3.53 (3.55)	4.03	4.40 (4.23)	4.59	4.77 (4.89)	244
5.0	2.08 (2.03)	2.34	2.67 (2.77)	3.05	3.53 (3.50)	3.92	4.41 (4.24)	4.66	4.93 (4.97)	262
5.5	2.25 (2.15)	2.33	2.67 (2.79)	3.02	3.45 (3.43)	3.79	4.20 (4.07)	4.51	4.62 (4.71)	241
6.0	1.99 (2.00)	2.07	2.43 (2.63)	2.93	3.35 (3.30)	3.67	4.10 (3.90)	4.23	4.48 (4.53)	240
6.5	2.00 (1.92)	2.07	2.31 (2.55)	2.76	3.21 (3.19)	3.60	3.96 (3.82)	4.22	4.39 (4.45)	233
7.0	1.99 (1.99)	2.24	2.45 (2.58)	2.70	3.19 (3.17)	3.53	3.93 (3.75)	4.11	4.26 (4.34)	235
7.5	1.83 (1.72)	2.01	2.20 (2.38)	2.62	2.99 (3.03)	3.45	3.88 (3.69)	4.11	4.29 (4.34)	229
8.0	1.69 (1.69)	1.86	2.18 (2.34)	2.51	3.02 (2.98)	3.45	3.75 (3.62)	3.90	4.18 (4.27)	226
8.5	1.80 (1.82)	2.01	2.23 (2.36)	2.59	2.96 (2.90)	3.21	3.56 (3.44)	3.79	3.86 (3.98)	214
9.0	1.77 (1.73)	1.89	2.11 (2.28)	2.45	2.84 (2.83)	3.21	3.52 (3.37)	3.67	3.70 (3.92)	212

continues

Table C–5 continued

Age at end of interval	Percentiles of 6-mo increments									
	3 (–2 SD)	*5*	*10 (–1 SD)*	*25*	*50 (mean)*	*75*	*90 (+1 SD)*	*95*	*97 (+2 SD)*	*n*
yr					*cm/6 mo*					
9.5	1.46 (1.43)	1.61	1.83 (2.02)	2.28	2.67 (2.62)	2.96	3.36 (3.22)	3.64	3.75 (3.82)	204
10.0	1.80 (1.56)	1.89	2.06 (2.15)	2.35	2.70 (2.73)	3.06	3.44 (3.31)	3.69	3.91 (3.89)	202
10.5	1.44 (1.30)	1.56	1.83 (1.94)	2.14	2.56 (2.57)	2.93	3.38 (3.20)	3.67	3.94 (3.84)	208
11.0	1.49 (1.31)	1.68	1.87 (1.96)	2.22	2.52 (2.61)	2.96	3.43 (3.26)	3.74	4.11 (3.91)	204
11.5	1.58 (1.22)	1.69	1.86 (1.96)	2.20	2.57 (2.70)	3.06	3.70 (3.44)	4.00	4.18 (4.18)	198
12.0	1.49 (0.99)	1.60	1.86 (1.93)	2.24	2.73 (2.86)	3.27	4.07 (3.79)	4.68	5.01 (4.72)	196
12.5	1.31 (0.67)	1.49	1.83 (1.85)	2.20	2.77 (3.03)	3.53	4.93 (4.20)	5.44	5.83 (5.38)	195
13.0	1.61 (1.05)	1.87	2.10 (2.28)	2.55	3.29 (3.52)	4.45	5.22 (4.75)	5.75	6.06 (5.98)	191
13.5	1.27 (1.26)	1.55	2.19 (2.42)	2.75	3.49 (3.58)	4.41	5.03 (4.74)	5.31	5.55 (5.89)	188
14.0	1.53 (1.49)	1.84	2.15 (2.65)	2.93	4.01 (3.81)	4.64	5.21 (4.97)	5.49	5.71 (6.13)	190
14.5	1.40 (1.00)	1.51	1.75 (2.28)	2.60	3.59 (3.57)	4.54	5.26 (4.85)	5.48	5.63 (6.13)	186
15.0	0.65 (0.67)	0.90	1.42 (1.90)	2.26	3.19 (3.13)	4.01	4.66 (4.36)	5.11	5.22 (5.59)	179
15.5	0.04 (–0.54)	0.32	0.66 (0.87)	1.24	2.05 (2.29)	3.26	4.28 (3.70)	4.66	4.95 (5.12)	178

continues

Table C–5 continued

Age at end of interval	3 (–2 SD)	5	10 (–1 SD)	25	50 (mean)	75	90 (+1 SD)	95	97 (+2 SD)	n
	Percentiles of 6-mo increments									
yr					*cm/6 mo*					
16.0	–0.28 (–0.62)	0.12	0.60 (0.58)	0.94	1.56 (1.78)	2.48	3.57 (2.98)	3.91	4.21 (4.18)	176
16.5	–0.67 (–1.07)	–0.50	0.03 (0.01)	0.44	0.94 (1.08)	1.50	2.44 (2.16)	2.98	3.81 (3.23)	155
17.0	–0.78 (–0.98)	–0.55	–0.16 (–0.04	0.25	0.83 (0.89)	1.33	1.94 (1.83)	2.85	3.24 (2.76)	153
17.5	–0.84 (–1.03)	–0.66	–0.37 (–0.23)	0.12	0.41 (0.57)	1.00	1.43 (1.37)	1.73	2.26 (2.17)	137
18.0	–0.87 (–0.83)	–0.55	–0.33 (–0.24)	–0.03	0.32 (0.36)	0.72	1.01 (0.96)	1.45	1.61 (1.56)	137

Source: Reprinted with permission from Baumgartner RN et al., "Incremental Growth Tables: Supplementary to Previously Published Charts," The *American Journal of Clinical Nutrition* 43, May 1986, pp. 711–722. Copyright © 1986 American Society for Clinical Nutrition.

Table C–6 Stature of girls: 3 to 18 yr of age in 6-mo increments (Fels Longitudinal Study)

Age at end of interval	*Percentiles of 6-mo increments*									
	3 (–2 SD)	*5*	*10 (–1 SD)*	*25*	*50 (mean)*	*75*	*90 (+1 SD)*	*95*	*97 (+2 SD)*	*n*
yr	*cm/6 mo*									
3.5	2.55 (2.31)	2.84	2.98 (3.09)	3.34	3.79 (3.87)	4.33	4.84 (4.65)	5.24	5.52 (5.43)	195
4.0	2.50 (2.37)	2.72	2.91 (3.04)	3.25	3.65 (3.71)	4.09	4.49 (4.38)	4.97	5.21 (5.05)	211
4.5	2.09 (2.07)	2.23	2.71 (2.82)	3.06	3.54 (3.57)	4.05	4.46 (4.31)	4.81	4.99 (5.06)	230
5.0	2.20 (2.06)	2.33	2.52 (2.80)	3.02	3.52 (3.54)	4.03	4.36 (4.27)	4.84	4.89 (5.01)	240
5.5	2.24 (2.08)	2.42	2.57 (2.74)	2.98	3.39 (3.39)	3.79	4.16 (4.05)	4.48	4.55 (4.71)	226
6.0	2.07 (1.99)	2.23	2.46 (2.64)	2.84	3.30 (3.29)	3.75	4.10 (3.95)	4.49	4.62 (4.60)	227
6.5	1.85 (1.76)	1.93	2.20 (2.42)	2.60	3.11 (3.08)	3.49	3.94 (3.74)	4.29	4.35 (4.41)	223
7.0	1.96 (1.86)	2.11	2.36 (2.48)	2.66	3.08 (3.09)	3.50	3.81 (3.71)	3.98	4.17 (4.33)	223
7.5	1.86 (1.81)	1.98	2.23 (2.42)	2.64	3.07 (3.02)	3.39	3.67 (3.63)	4.03	4.14 (4.23)	221
8.0	1.62 (1.64)	1.82	2.17 (2.31)	2.56	3.01 (2.98)	3.35	3.85 (3.65)	4.07	4.20 (4.32)	222
8.5	1.77 (1.58)	1.86	1.99 (2.22)	2.41	2.88 (2.86)	3.27	3.68 (3.50)	3.90	4.09 (4.14)	222
9.0	1.81 (1.70)	1.93	2.13 (2.28)	2.47	2.84 (2.85)	3.22	3.53 (3.43)	3.77	4.08 (4.01)	216

continues

Table C–6 continued

Age at end of interval	Percentiles of 6-mo increments: 3 (–2 SD)	5	10 (–1 SD)	25	50 (mean)	75	90 (+1 SD)	95	97 (+2 SD)	n
yr					*cm/6 mo*					
9.5	1.64 (1.50)	1.78	1.95 (2.16)	2.36	2.80 (2.83)	3.29	3.58 (3.49)	3.92	4.09 (4.16)	219
10.0	1.63 (1.31)	1.70	1.99 (2.11)	2.38	2.91 (2.90)	3.28	3.83 (3.70)	4.38	4.61 (4.49)	220
10.5	1.57 (1.13)	1.64	1.99 (2.07)	2.37	2.82 (3.01)	3.56	4.21 (3.95)	4.70	5.27 (4.90)	212
11.0	1.67 (1.38)	1.87	2.08 (2.27)	2.53	3.06 (3.16)	3.74	4.33 (4.05)	4.76	4.92 (4.94)	203
11.5	1.51 (1.41)	1.84	2.09 (2.38)	2.54	3.34 (3.35)	4.02	4.63 (4.32)	4.84	5.17 (5.29)	202
12.0	1.67 (1.22)	1.60	1.98 (2.25)	2.65	3.32 (3.28)	3.98	4.52 (4.31)	4.86	4.98 (5.34)	196
12.5	0.79 (1.04)	1.11	1.61 (2.07)	2.41	3.19 (3.10)	3.87	4.38 (4.13)	4.58	4.72 (5.16)	186
13.0	0.36 (0.37)	0.52	1.05 (1.52)	1.99	2.76 (2.67)	3.46	4.09 (3.82)	4.21	4.43 (4.97)	185
13.5	0.25 (–0.21)	0.35	0.57 (0.92)	1.20	1.98 (2.05)	2.90	3.56 (3.19)	3.92	4.24 (4.32)	184
14.0	–0.28 (–0.71)	–0.09	0.28 (0.43)	0.78	1.33 (1.58)	2.35	3.11 (2.72)	3.66	4.09 (3.86)	179
14.5	–0.32 (–0.79)	–0.21	0.04 (0.16)	0.47	0.88 (1.11)	1.65	2.77 (2.06)	2.97	3.32 (3.01)	154
15.0	–0.62 (–0.87)	–0.47	–0.16 (–0.04)	0.24	0.68 (0.78)	1.24	1.75 (1.60)	2.33	2.51 (2.43)	150
15.5	–0.88 (–0.88)	–0.67	–0.43 (–0.20)	0.07	0.49 (0.49)	0.83	1.27 (1.17)	1.62	1.91 (1.85)	143

continues

Table C–6 continued

Age at end of interval	3 (–2 SD)	5	10 (–1 SD)	25	50 (mean)	75	90 (+1 SD)	95	97 (+2 SD)	n
	Percentiles of 6-mo increments									
yr	*cm/6 mo*									
16.0	–0.53 (–0.68)	–0.48	–0.33 (–0.13)	0.04	0.46 (0.42)	0.75	1.08 (0.97)	1.42	1.54 (1.52)	139
16.5	–0.66 (–0.70)	–0.61	–0.37 (–0.21)	–0.05	0.23 (0.28)	0.63	0.91 (0.77)	1.02	1.19 (1.25)	132
17.0	–1.14 (–0.94)	–0.84	–0.65 (–0.38)	–0.13	0.19 (0.17)	0.56	0.81 (0.73)	0.94	1.08 (1.29)	133
17.5	–0.81 (–0.97)	–0.74	–0.51 (–0.41)	–0.21	0.04 (0.14)	0.38	0.97 (0.70)	1.25	1.42 (1.26)	126
18.0	–0.80 (–0.91)	–0.78	–0.64 (–0.39)	–0.15	0.09 (0.13)	0.46	0.83 (0.65)	1.05	1.08 (1.17)	123

Source: Reprinted with permission from Baumgartner RN et al., "Incremental Growth Tables: Supplementary to Previously Published Charts," *The American Journal of Clinical Nutrition* 43, May 1986, pp. 711–722. Copyright © 1986 American Society for Clinical Nutrition.

Table C–7 Weight of boys: birth to 18 yr of age in 6-mo increments (Fels Longitudinal Study)

Age at end of interval	3 (−2 SD)	5	10 (−1 SD)	25	50 (mean)	75	90 (+1 SD)	95	97 (+2 SD)	n
	Percentiles of 6-mo increments									
yr	*kg/6 mo*									
0.5	2.90 (2.84)	3.13	3.47 (3.66)	3.91	4.39 (4.47)	5.06	5.51 (5.29)	5.89	6.18 (6.11)	298
0.75	2.18 (1.86)	2.26	2.41 (2.56)	2.73	3.13 (3.26)	3.71	4.20 (3.96)	4.50	4.72 (4.66)	277
1.0	1.20 (0.93)	1.26	1.52 (1.61)	1.81	2.20 (2.28)	2.66	3.13 (2.96)	3.52	3.74 (3.63)	290
1.5	0.48 (0.20)	0.52	0.67 (0.78)	0.99	1.32 (1.36)	1.71	2.03 (1.93)	2.29	2.55 (2.51)	294
2.0	0.38 (0.27)	0.46	0.63 (0.71)	0.86	1.13 (1.15)	1.38	1.65 (1.59)	1.81	2.13 (2.03)	286
2.5	0.25 (0.19)	0.33	0.52 (0.61)	0.77	1.03 (1.03)	1.26	1.54 (1.45)	1.74	1.80 (1.87)	273
3.0	0.28 (0.21)	0.41	0.51 (0.61)	0.73	0.97 (1.00)	1.26	1.52 (1.40)	1.64	1.76 (1.79)	270
3.5	0.19 (0.00)	0.27	0.48 (0.49)	0.71	0.98 (0.99)	1.27	1.54 (1.48)	1.71	1.79 (1.98)	274
4.0	0.24 (0.07)	0.36	0.53 (0.53)	0.70	0.95 (0.98)	1.23	1.46 (1.43)	1.63	1.75 (1.88)	269
4.5	0.25 (0.08)	0.35	0.47 (0.58)	0.73	1.06 (1.07)	1.35	1.67 (1.57)	1.87	2.08 (2.06)	266
5.0	0.14 (−0.07)	0.25	0.48 (0.52)	0.78	1.06 (1.11)	1.38	1.76 (1.71)	2.03	2.21 (2.30)	268
5.5	0.21 (−0.02)	0.38	0.54 (0.59)	0.77	1.16 (1.19)	1.51	1.91 (1.80)	2.20	2.51 (2.40)	244

continues

Table C–7 continued

Age at end of interval	3 (–2 SD)	5	10 (–1 SD)	25	50 (mean)	75	90 (+1 SD)	95	97 (+2 SD)	n
	Percentiles of 6-mo increments									
yr					*kg/6 mo*					
6.0	0.07 (0.31)	0.24	0.45 (0.46)	0.82	1.18 (1.23)	1.54	2.01 (2.01)	2.23	2.40 (2.78)	243
6.5	0.09 (0.06)	0.21	0.51 (0.65)	0.90	1.16 (1.24)	1.54	2.07 (1.83)	2.34	2.44 (2.42)	232
7.0	0.21 (–0.32)	0.33	0.49 (0.52)	0.88	1.26 (1.37)	1.75	2.25 (2.22)	2.53	3.20 (3.06)	232
7.5	0.13 (–0.30)	0.40	0.60 (0.57)	0.92	1.38 (1.45)	1.79	2.40 (2.33)	2.87	3.29 (3.21)	224
8.0	0.20 (–0.28)	0.34	0.63 (0.66)	1.00	1.52 (1.61)	1.93	2.54 (2.55)	3.23	3.55 (3.50)	221
8.5	–0.10 (–0.49)	0.28	0.45 (0.54)	1.01	1.43 (1.57)	2.07	2.77 (2.60)	3.35	3.86 (3.63)	210
9.0	–0.46 (–0.77)	0.02	0.50 (0.43)	0.95	1.56 (1.64)	2.28	2.95 (2.84)	3.58	3.96 (4.05)	208
9.5	–0.02 (–0.70)	0.21	0.51 (0.50)	0.96	1.54 (1.71)	2.26	3.05 (2.91)	3.60	4.59 (4.12)	201
10.0	0.01 (–0.62)	0.08	0.38 (0.59)	1.18	1.70 (1.80)	2.38	3.14 (3.01)	3.92	4.36 (4.22)	199
10.5	–0.18 (–0.83)	0.22	0.56 (0.53)	1.09	1.61 (1.90)	2.65	3.63 (3.26)	4.30	4.60 (4.62)	205
11.0	0.15 (–0.47)	0.20	0.53 (0.72)	1.01	1.73 (1.91)	2.46	3.51 (3.10)	4.01	4.50 (4.29)	201
11.5	–0.10 (–0.70)	0.34	0.66 (0.76)	1.24	1.91 (2.22)	3.03	4.33 (3.68)	4.99	5.78 (5.14)	195
12.0	–0.36 (–0.93)	–0.21	0.54 (0.68)	1.30	2.00 (2.29)	3.27	4.24 (3.90)	4.85	5.04 (5.52)	193

continues

Table C–7 continued

Age at end of interval	3 (–2 SD)	5	10 (–1 SD)	25	50 (mean)	75	90 (+1 SD)	95	97 (+2 SD)	n
	Percentiles of 6-mo increments									
yr					*kg/6 mo*					
12.5	–0.39 (–1.03)	–0.01	0.60 (0.77)	1.35	2.45 (2.56)	3.47	4.79 (4.36)	5.36	6.12 (6.15)	192
13.0	0.10 (–0.55)	0.54	0.94 (1.20)	1.71	2.81 (2.95)	3.92	5.29 (4.70)	6.17	6.35 (6.46)	186
13.5	–0.04 (–0.69)	0.37	0.62 (1.19)	1.73	3.06 (3.06)	4.20	5.31 (4.94)	5.81	6.17 (6.81)	183
14.0	–0.61 (–0.59)	–0.06	0.95 (1.35)	2.20	3.33 (3.28)	4.23	5.71 (5.21)	6.56	7.04 (7.15)	187
14.5	–0.70 (–0.39)	–0.06	1.08 (1.58)	2.60	3.67 (3.54)	4.57	5.72 (5.51)	6.41	6.78 (7.47)	183
15.0	–2.99 (–2.08)	–0.72	0.44 (0.46)	1.87	3.24 (3.01)	4.48	5.73 (5.55)	6.34	6.51 (8.09)	176
15.5	–2.17 (–1.83)	–1.25	0.10 (0.41)	1.46	2.59 (2.65)	3.79	5.34 (4.89)	6.26	6.95 (7.12)	176
16.0	–2.58 (–2.49)	–1.36	–0.33 (–0.12)	1.03	2.18 (2.25)	3.54	5.07 (4.62)	6.18	6.92 (6.99)	174
16.5	–2.57 (–2.81)	–1.68	–0.73 (–0.54)	0.45	1.69 (1.73)	2.97	3.85 (4.00)	5.18	6.11 (6.27)	154
17.0	–3.42 (–3.33)	–2.32	–1.63 (–1.07)	–0.17	1.21 (1.19)	2.54	3.57 (3.45)	4.37	5.69 (5.71)	152
17.5	–3.00 (–3.38)	–2.57	–1.21 (–1.02)	–0.00	1.09 (1.35)	2.52	3.99 (3.71)	5.43	6.18 (6.08)	139
18.0	–3.86 (–3.83)	–3.05	–2.04 (–1.44)	–0.58	0.77 (0.94)	2.24	3.82 (3.32)	4.97	6.22 (5.71)	138

Source: Reprinted with permission from Baumgartner RN et al., "Incremental Growth Tables: Supplementary to Previously Published Charts," *The American Journal of Clinical Nutrition* 43, May 1986, pp. 711–722. Copyright © 1986 American Society for Clinical Nutrition.

Table C–8 Weight of girls: birth to 18 yr of age in 6-mo increments (Fels Longitudinal Study)

	Percentiles of 6-mo increments									
Age at end of interval	*3 (–2 SD)*	*5*	*10 (–1 SD)*	*25*	*50 (mean)*	*75*	*90 (+1 SD)*	*95*	*97 (+2 SD)*	*n*
yr					*kg/6 mo*					
0.5	2.61 (2.48)	2.75	2.96 (3.23)	3.41	4.00 (3.99)	4.54	4.97 (4.74)	5.12	5.31 (5.49)	284
0.75	1.85 (1.70)	1.98	2.21 (2.36)	2.55	3.01 (3.02)	3.46	3.88 (3.69)	4.17	4.26 (4.35)	259
1.0	1.30 (1.06)	1.37	1.51 (1.65)	1.83	2.19 (2.24)	2.59	3.02 (2.82)	3.29	3.40 (3.41)	271
1.5	0.42 (0.31)	0.43	0.68 (0.83)	1.03	1.33 (1.34)	1.63	1.94 (1.85)	2.08	2.18 (2.36)	269
2.0	0.41 (0.28)	0.50	0.61 (0.74)	0.88	1.21 (1.20)	1.45	1.80 (1.66)	1.97	2.18 (2.13)	266
2.5	0.21 (0.06)	0.36	0.51 (0.54)	0.75	0.97 (1.02)	1.27	1.60 (1.51)	1.87	2.09 (1.99)	251
3.0	0.24 (0.10)	0.37	0.48 (0.56)	0.69	1.02 (1.03)	1.31	1.59 (1.50)	1.83	1.98 (1.97)	249
3.5	0.34 (0.20)	0.42	0.55 (0.62)	0.76	1.00 (1.04)	1.29	1.56 (1.46)	1.80	1.92 (1.88)	249
4.0	0.11 (0.11)	0.30	0.50 (0.56)	0.73	0.98 (1.01)	1.26	1.54 (1.46)	1.73	1.84 (1.91)	242
4.5	0.13 (0.03)	0.22	0.43 (0.49)	0.67	0.94 (1.02)	1.29	1.78 (1.55)	1.88	2.14 (2.07)	241
5.0	0.05 (–0.18)	0.26	0.46 (0.46)	0.73	1.03 (1.09)	1.41	1.73 (1.72)	2.14	2.32 (2.36)	241
5.5	0.05 (–0.28)	0.22	0.36 (0.41)	0.68	0.97 (1.11)	1.44	2.06 (1.80)	2.37	2.56 (2.49)	221

continues

Table C–8 continued

Age at end of interval	3 (–2 SD)	5	10 (–1 SD)	25	50 (mean)	75	90 (+1 SD)	95	97 (+2 SD)	n
	Percentiles of 6-mo increments									
yr					*kg/6 mo*					
6.0	0.05 (–0.26)	0.23	0.44 (0.46)	0.78	1.12 (1.18)	1.44	1.97 (1.91)	2.49	2.88 (2.63)	221
6.5	0.18 (–0.25)	0.28	0.48 (0.52)	0.83	1.19 (1.29)	1.63	2.00 (2.06)	2.54	2.95 (2.82)	216
7.0	0.16 (–0.22)	0.28	0.44 (0.52)	0.80	1.18 (1.26)	1.59	2.27 (2.00)	2.52	2.74 (2.74)	216
7.5	0.25 (–0.28)	0.36	0.61 (0.60)	0.95	1.32 (1.48)	1.81	2.47 (2.36)	3.03	3.46 (3.24)	211
8.0	–0.08 (–0.42)	0.14	0.39 (0.53)	0.92	1.36 (1.48)	1.98	2.73 (2.43)	3.21	3.48 (3.38)	212
8.5	0.12 (–0.44)	0.26	0.53 (0.60)	1.00	1.48 (1.63)	2.06	2.87 (2.66)	3.36	4.06 (3.71)	214
9.0	0.14 (–0.29)	0.31	0.62 (0.68)	1.02	1.47 (1.65)	2.20	2.97 (2.61)	3.51	3.83 (3.58)	207
9.5	0.00 (–0.69)	0.37	0.58 (0.57)	1.02	1.53 (1.83)	2.48	3.27 (3.09)	3.90	4.77 (4.35)	209
10.0	–0.10 (–1.09)	0.14	0.44 (0.37)	1.05	1.57 (1.84)	2.36	3.48 (3.31)	4.35	5.05 (4.77)	210
10.5	–0.70 (–0.87)	0.23	0.53 (0.62)	1.17	1.96 (2.12)	2.87	4.04 (3.61)	4.80	5.22 (5.11)	202
11.0	–0.50 (–1.07)	–0.12	0.70 (0.57)	1.28	2.01 (2.22)	3.22	3.94 (3.87)	4.63	5.39 (5.51)	194
11.5	0.05 (–0.56)	0.28	0.88 (0.98)	1.39	2.48 (2.52)	3.44	4.39 (4.10)	4.97	5.78 (5.61)	194
12.0	–0.41 (–0.71)	0.31	0.68 (1.06)	1.68	2.74 (2.82)	3.90	5.11 (4.59)	5.47	5.91 (6.36)	187

continues

Table C–8 continued

Age at end of interval	3 (–2 SD)	5	10 (–1 SD)	25	50 (mean)	75	90 (+1 SD)	95	97 (+2 SD)	n
	Percentiles of 6-mo increments									
yr					*kg/6 mo*					
12.5	–0.42 (–0.67)	–0.09	0.51 (1.00)	1.43	2.76 (2.67)	3.69	4.79 (4.34)	5.63	6.14 (6.01)	177
13.0	–1.53 (–1.76)	–0.78	–0.03 (0.19)	1.40	2.15 (2.15)	3.26	4.15 (4.11)	4.76	5.10 (6.06)	175
13.5	–1.13 (–1.09)	–0.40	0.47 (0.68)	1.28	2.31 (2.45)	3.48	4.64 (4.22)	5.14	5.65 (5.99)	174
14.0	–2.15 (–2.02)	–1.52	–0.61 (–0.12)	0.51	1.83 (1.77)	3.11	4.13 (3.67)	4.61	5.21 (5.57)	169
14.5	–3.90 (–3.10)	–2.15	–1.12 (–0.86)	0.41	1.50 (1.38)	2.51	3.67 (3.62)	3.94	4.82 (5.86)	146
15.0	–3.61 (–3.05)	–1.94	–0.92 (–0.99)	–0.01	1.00 (1.07)	2.33	3.45 (3.13)	3.91	4.85 (5.18)	143
15.5	–2.61 (–2.60)	–2.01	–1.23 (–0.81)	–0.01	0.92 (0.97)	2.00	2.92 (2.76)	3.73	4.35 (4.54)	135
16.0	–3.13 (–3.49)	–2.85	–2.10 (–1.62)	–0.76	0.37 (0.25)	1.27	2.08 (2.11)	2.96	3.58 (3.98)	134
16.5	–3.17 (–2.98)	–2.48	–1.60 (–1.15)	–0.20	0.75 (0.68)	1.66	2.82 (2.52)	3.44	3.88 (4.35)	126
17.0	–3.92 (–3.25)	–2.51	–1.96 (–1.43)	–0.59	0.64 (0.40)	1.46	2.54 (2.22)	3.00	3.70 (4.04)	125
17.5	–2.98 (–3.16)	–2.52	–1.75 (–1.40)	–0.86	0.40 (0.36)	1.32	2.45 (2.12)	3.08	3.52 (3.88)	116
18.0	–3.84 (–3.21)	–3.11	–1.41 (–1.35)	–0.72	0.47 (0.50)	1.55	2.93 (2.35)	3.68	4.24 (4.21)	113

Source: Reprinted with permission from Baumgartner RN et al., "Incremental Growth Tables: Supplementary to Previously Published Charts," *The American Journal of Clinical Nutrition* 43, May 1986, pp. 711–722.

APPENDIX D

Down Syndrome Growth Charts

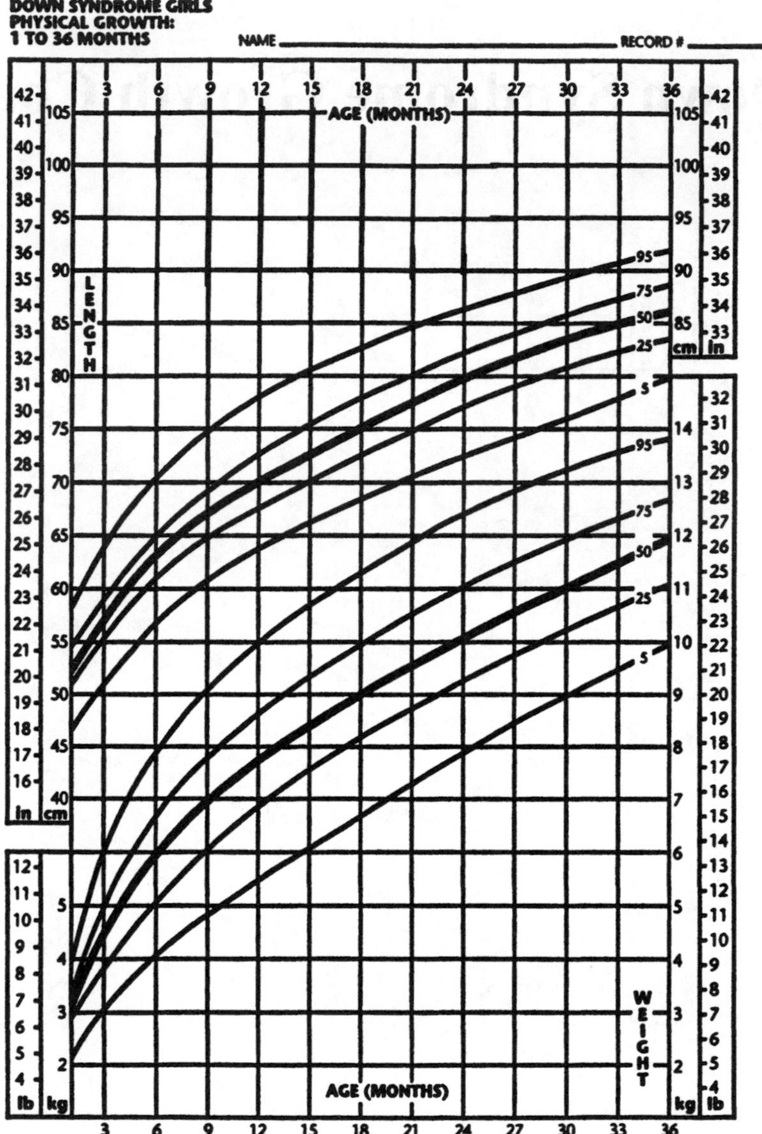

Figure D–1 Down syndrome, length and weight for girls, 1 to 36 months. *Source:* Reprinted with permission from Crocker CC et al, Growth Charts for Children with Down Syndrome: 1 Month to 18 Years of Age, *Pediatrics,* Vol. 81, pp. 102–110, © 1988, American Academy of Pediatrics.

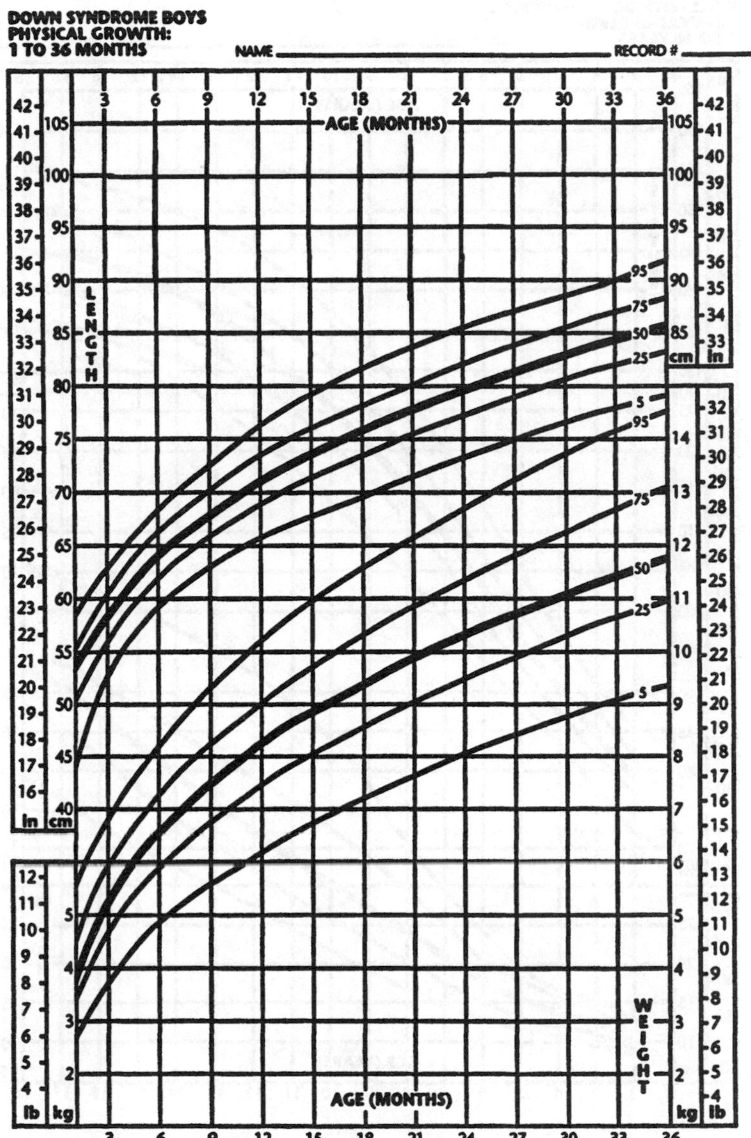

Figure D–2 Down syndrome, length and weight for boys, 1 to 36 months. *Source:* Reprinted with permission from Crocker CC et al, Growth Charts for Children with Down Syndrome: 1 Month to 18 Years of Age, *Pediatrics,* Vol. 81, pp. 102–110, © 1988, American Academy of Pediatrics.

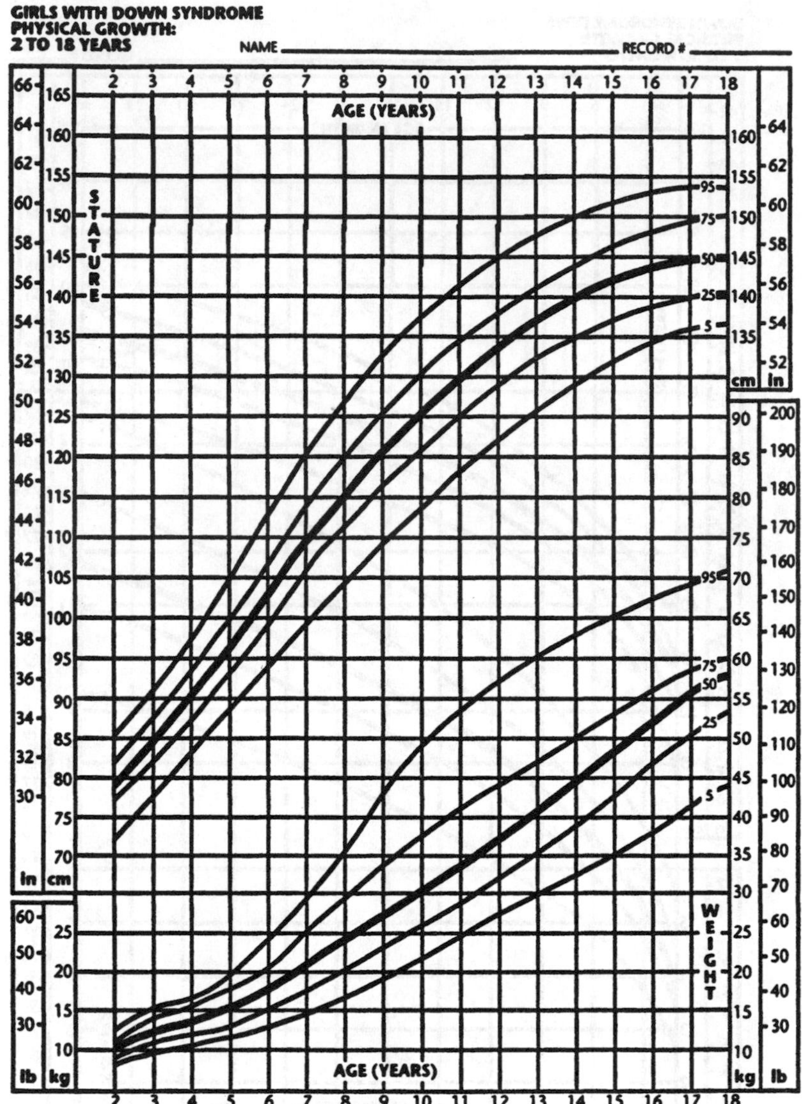

Figure D–3 Down syndrome, height and weight for girls, 2 to 18 years. *Source:* Reprinted with permission from Crocker CC et al, Growth Charts for Children with Down Syndrome: 1 Month to 18 Years of Age, *Pediatrics,* Vol. 81, pp. 102–110, © 1988, American Academy of Pediatrics.

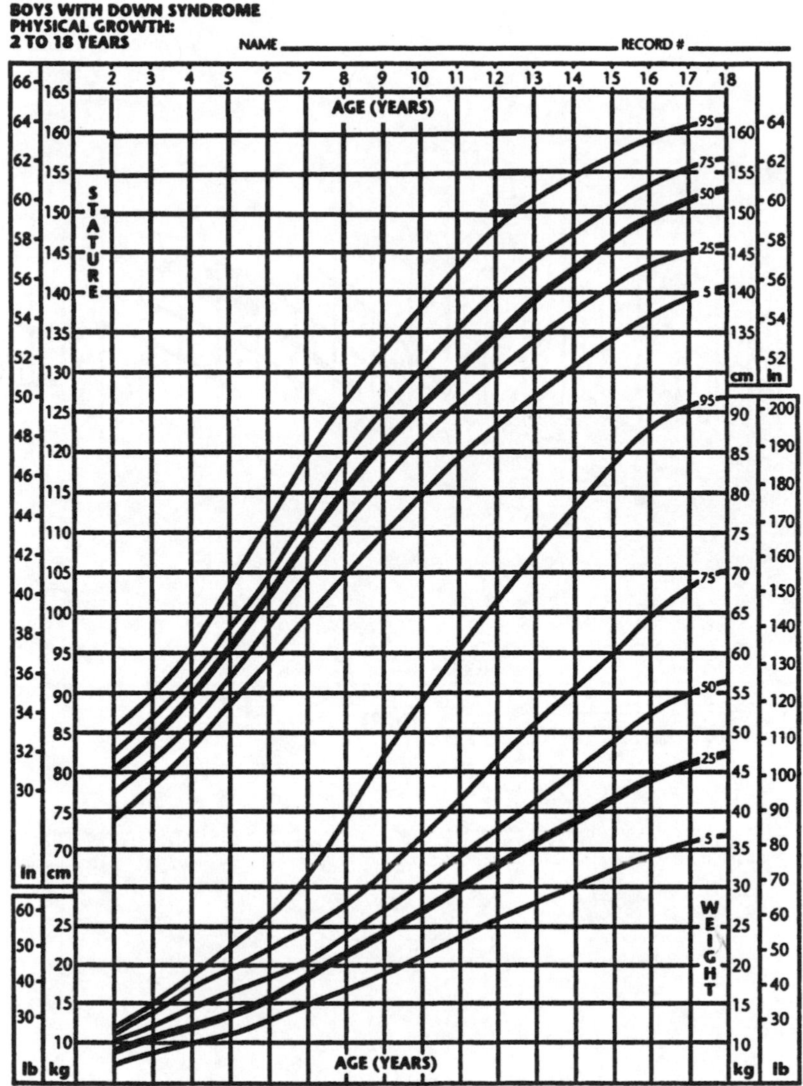

Figure D–4 Down syndrome, height and weight for boys, 2 to 18 years. *Source:* Reprinted with permission from Crocker CC et al, Growth Charts for Children with Down Syndrome: 1 Month to 18 Years of Age, *Pediatrics,* Vol. 81, pp. 102–110, © 1988, American Academy of Pediatrics.

APPENDIX E

Arm Measurements

Table E–1 Arm measurements, Mid-Upper-Arm-Circumference (MUAC) for Length or Height Reference Data

Length/ height (cm)*	*Boys*			*Combined sexes*			*Girls*			*Length/ height* (cm)*
	Median	*−2 SD*	*−3 SD*	*Median*	*−2 SD*	*−3 SD*	*Median*	*−2 SD*	*−3 SD*	
65.0	14.6	12.7	11.7	14.3	12.4	11.5	14.0	12.1	11.2	65.0
65.5	14.7	12.7	11.8	14.4	12.5	11.5	14.1	12.2	11.2	65.5
66.0	14.7	12.8	11.8	14.5	12.5	11.6	14.2	12.3	11.3	66.0
66.5	14.8	12.8	11.8	14.5	12.6	11.6	14.3	12.3	11.3	66.5
67.0	14.9	12.9	11.9	14.6	12.6	11.6	14.4	12.4	11.4	67.0
67.5	14.9	12.9	11.9	14.7	12.7	11.7	14.4	12.4	11.4	67.5
68.0	15.0	12.9	11.9	14.7	12.7	11.7	14.5	12.5	11.5	68.0
68.5	15.0	13.0	12.0	14.8	12.8	11.7	14.6	12.6	11.5	68.5
69.0	15.1	13.0	12.0	14.9	12.8	11.8	14.7	12.6	11.6	69.0
69.5	15.1	13.0	12.0	14.9	12.8	11.8	14.7	12.7	11.6	69.5
70.0	15.1	13.1	12.0	15.0	12.9	11.8	14.8	12.7	11.7	70.0
70.5	15.2	13.1	12.0	15.0	12.9	11.9	14.8	12.8	11.7	70.5
71.0	15.2	13.1	12.1	15.1	13.0	11.9	14.9	12.8	11.7	71.0
71.5	15.3	13.1	12.1	15.1	13.0	11.9	15.0	12.8	11.8	71.5
72.0	15.3	13.2	12.1	15.2	13.0	12.0	15.0	12.9	11.8	72.0
72.5	15.3	13.2	12.1	15.2	13.1	12.0	15.1	12.9	11.8	72.5
73.0	15.4	13.2	12.1	15.2	13.1	12.0	15.1	13.0	11.9	73.0
73.5	15.4	13.2	12.2	15.3	13.1	12.0	15.2	13.0	11.9	73.5
74.0	15.4	13.3	12.2	15.3	13.1	12.1	15.2	13.0	11.9	74.0
74.5	15.5	13.3	12.2	15.4	13.2	12.1	15.2	13.1	12.0	74.5
75.0	15.5	13.3	12.2	15.4	13.2	12.1	15.3	13.1	12.0	75.0
75.5	15.5	13.3	12.2	15.4	13.2	12.1	15.3	13.1	12.0	75.5
76.0	15.6	13.4	12.2	15.5	13.3	12.2	15.4	13.2	12.1	76.0
76.5	15.6	13.4	12.3	15.5	13.3	12.2	15.4	13.2	12.1	76.5
77.0	15.6	13.4	12.3	15.5	13.3	12.2	15.4	13.2	12.1	77.0
77.5	15.6	13.4	12.3	15.6	13.3	12.2	15.5	13.3	12.1	77.5
78.0	15.7	13.4	12.3	15.6	13.4	12.2	15.5	13.3	12.2	78.0
78.5	15.7	13.4	12.3	15.6	13.4	12.3	15.6	13.3	12.2	78.5
79.0	15.7	13.5	12.3	15.6	13.4	12.3	15.6	13.3	12.2	79.0
79.5	15.7	13.5	12.4	15.7	13.4	12.3	15.6	13.4	12.2	79.5
80.0	15.8	13.5	12.4	15.7	13.4	12.3	15.6	13.4	12.3	80.0
80.5	15.8	13.5	12.4	15.7	13.5	12.3	15.7	13.4	12.3	80.5
81.0	15.8	13.5	12.4	15.8	13.5	12.4	15.7	13.4	12.3	81.0
81.5	15.8	13.6	12.4	15.8	13.5	12.4	15.7	13.5	12.3	81.5
82.0	15.9	13.6	12.4	15.8	13.5	12.4	15.8	13.5	12.3	82.0
82.5	15.9	13.6	12.5	15.8	13.6	12.4	15.8	13.5	12.4	82.5
83.0	15.9	13.6	12.5	15.9	13.6	12.4	15.8	13.5	12.4	83.0
83.5	15.9	13.6	12.5	15.9	13.6	12.5	15.8	13.6	12.4	83.5
84.0	15.9	13.7	12.5	15.9	13.6	12.5	15.9	13.6	12.4	84.0
84.5	16.0	13.7	12.5	15.9	13.6	12.5	15.9	13.6	12.5	84.5
85.0	16.0	13.7	12.5	15.9	13.6	12.5	15.9	13.6	12.5	85.0
85.5	16.0	13.7	12.6	16.0	13.7	12.5	15.9	13.6	12.5	85.5
86.0	16.0	13.7	12.6	16.0	13.7	12.5	15.9	13.7	12.5	86.0
86.5	16.0	13.7	12.6	16.0	13.7	12.6	16.0	13.7	12.5	86.5
87.0	16.1	13.8	12.6	16.0	13.7	12.6	16.0	13.7	12.5	87.0
87.5	16.1	13.8	12.6	16.0	13.7	12.6	16.0	13.7	12.6	87.5
88.0	16.1	13.8	12.6	16.1	13.8	12.6	16.0	13.7	12.6	88.0
88.5	16.1	13.8	12.7	16.1	13.8	12.6	16.1	13.8	12.6	88.5
89.0	16.1	13.8	12.7	16.1	13.8	12.7	16.1	13.8	12.6	89.0
89.5	16.2	13.9	12.7	16.1	13.8	12.7	16.1	13.8	12.7	89.5
90.0	16.2	13.9	12.7	16.2	13.9	12.7	16.1	13.8	12.7	90.0
90.5	16.2	13.9	12.8	16.2	13.9	12.7	16.2	13.8	12.7	90.5
91.0	16.2	13.9	12.8	16.2	13.9	12.7	16.2	13.9	12.7	91.0
91.5	16.3	14.0	12.8	16.2	13.9	12.8	16.2	13.9	12.7	91.5
92.0	16.3	14.0	12.8	16.3	13.9	12.8	16.2	13.9	12.8	92.0

continues

Table E–1 continued

Length/ height (cm)*	*Boys*			*Combined sexes*			*Girls*			*Length/ height* (cm)*
	Median	*−2 SD*	*−3 SD*	*Median*	*−2 SD*	*−3 SD*	*Median*	*−2 SD*	*−3 SD*	
92.5	16.3	14.0	12.9	16.3	14.0	12.8	16.2	13.9	12.8	92.5
93.0	16.3	14.0	12.9	16.3	14.0	12.8	16.3	14.0	12.8	93.0
93.5	16.4	14.1	12.9	16.3	14.0	12.9	16.3	14.0	12.8	93.5
94.0	16.4	14.1	12.9	16.4	14.0	12.9	16.3	14.0	12.8	94.0
94.5	16.4	14.1	13.0	16.4	14.1	12.9	16.3	14.0	12.9	94.5
95.0	16.4	14.1	13.0	16.4	14.1	12.9	16.4	14.1	12.9	95.0
95.5	16.5	14.2	13.0	16.4	14.1	13.0	16.4	14.1	12.9	95.5
96.0	16.5	14.2	13.0	16.5	14.1	13.0	16.4	14.1	12.9	96.0
96.5	16.5	14.2	13.1	16.5	14.2	13.0	16.4	14.1	13.0	96.5
97.0	16.6	14.2	13.1	16.5	14.2	13.0	16.5	14.1	13.0	97.0
97.5	16.6	14.3	13.1	16.5	14.2	13.1	16.5	14.2	13.0	97.5
98.0	16.6	14.3	13.1	16.6	14.2	13.1	16.5	14.2	13.0	98.0
98.5	16.6	14.3	13.2	16.6	14.3	13.1	16.5	14.2	13.1	98.5
99.0	16.7	14.3	13.2	16.6	14.3	13.1	16.6	14.3	13.1	99.0
99.5	16.7	14.4	13.2	16.6	14.3	13.2	16.6	14.3	13.1	99.5
100.0	16.7	14.4	13.2	16.7	14.4	13.2	16.6	14.3	13.1	100.0
100.5	16.8	14.4	13.3	16.7	14.4	13.2	16.7	14.3	13.2	100.5
101.0	16.8	14.5	13.3	16.7	14.4	13.2	16.7	14.4	13.2	101.0
101.5	16.8	14.5	13.3	16.8	14.4	13.3	16.7	14.4	13.2	101.5
102.0	16.9	14.5	13.4	16.8	14.5	13.3	16.7	14.4	13.2	102.0
102.5	16.9	14.6	13.4	16.8	14.5	13.3	16.8	14.4	13.3	102.5
103.0	16.9	14.6	13.4	16.9	14.5	13.4	16.8	14.5	13.3	103.0
103.5	16.9	14.6	13.4	16.9	14.6	13.4	16.8	14.5	13.3	103.5
104.0	17.0	14.6	13.5	16.9	14.6	13.4	16.9	14.5	13.4	104.0
104.5	17.0	14.7	13.5	17.0	14.6	13.4	16.9	14.6	13.4	104.5
105.0	17.0	14.7	13.5	17.0	14.6	13.5	16.9	14.6	13.4	105.0
105.5	17.1	14.7	13.6	17.0	14.7	13.5	17.0	14.6	13.4	105.5
106.0	17.1	14.8	13.6	17.1	14.7	13.5	17.0	14.6	13.5	106.0
106.5	17.1	14.8	13.6	17.1	14.7	13.6	17.0	14.7	13.5	106.5
107.0	17.2	14.8	13.6	17.1	14.8	13.6	17.1	14.7	13.5	107.0
107.5	17.2	14.8	13.7	17.2	14.8	13.6	17.1	14.7	13.6	107.5
108.0	17.3	14.9	13.7	17.2	14.8	13.6	17.1	14.8	13.6	108.0
108.5	17.3	14.9	13.7	17.2	14.9	13.7	17.2	14.8	13.6	108.5
109.0	17.3	14.9	13.7	17.3	14.9	13.7	17.2	14.8	13.6	109.0
109.5	17.4	15.0	13.8	17.3	14.9	13.7	17.3	14.9	13.7	109.5
110.0	17.4	15.0	13.8	17.4	15.0	13.8	17.3	14.9	13.7	110.0
110.5	17.4	15.0	13.8	17.4	15.0	13.8	17.3	14.9	13.7	110.5
111.0	17.5	15.1	13.9	17.4	15.0	13.8	17.4	15.0	13.8	111.0
111.5	17.5	15.1	13.9	17.5	15.0	13.8	17.4	15.0	13.8	111.5
112.0	17.5	15.1	13.9	17.5	15.1	13.9	17.5	15.0	13.8	112.0
112.5	17.6	15.1	13.9	17.6	15.1	13.9	17.5	15.1	13.9	112.5
113.0	17.6	15.2	14.0	17.6	15.1	13.9	17.6	15.1	13.9	113.0
113.5	17.7	15.2	14.0	17.6	15.2	14.0	17.6	15.2	13.9	113.5
114.0	17.7	15.2	14.0	17.7	15.2	14.0	17.7	15.2	14.0	114.0
114.5	17.7	15.3	14.0	17.7	15.2	14.0	17.7	15.2	14.0	114.5
115.0	17.8	15.3	14.0	17.8	15.3	14.0	17.8	15.3	14.0	115.0
115.5	17.8	15.3	14.1	17.8	15.3	14.1	17.8	15.3	14.1	115.5
116.0	17.9	15.4	14.1	17.9	15.3	14.1	17.9	15.3	14.1	116.0
116.5	17.9	15.4	14.1	17.9	15.4	14.1	17.9	15.4	14.1	116.5
117.0	18.0	15.4	14.1	18.0	15.4	14.1	18.0	15.4	14.1	117.0
117.5	18.0	15.4	14.2	18.0	15.4	14.2	18.0	15.5	14.2	117.5
118.0	18.0	15.5	14.2	18.1	15.5	14.2	18.1	15.5	14.2	118.0
118.5	18.1	15.5	14.2	18.1	15.5	14.2	18.1	15.5	14.2	118.5
119.0	18.1	15.5	14.2	18.2	15.6	14.3	18.2	15.6	14.3	119.0
119.5	18.2	15.6	14.2	18.2	15.6	14.3	18.2	15.6	14.3	119.5

continues

Table E–1 continued

Length/ height (cm)*	*Boys Median*	*Boys −2 SD*	*Boys −3 SD*	*Combined sexes Median*	*Combined sexes −2 SD*	*Combined sexes −3 SD*	*Girls Median*	*Girls −2 SD*	*Girls −3 SD*	*Length/ height* (cm)*
120.0	18.2	15.6	14.3	18.3	15.6	14.3	18.3	15.7	14.3	120.0
120.5	18.3	15.6	14.3	18.3	15.7	14.3	18.4	15.7	14.4	120.5
121.0	18.3	15.6	14.3	18.4	15.7	14.4	18.4	15.7	14.4	121.0
121.5	18.4	15.7	14.3	18.4	15.7	14.4	18.5	15.8	14.4	121.5
122.0	18.4	15.7	14.3	18.5	15.8	14.4	18.5	15.8	14.5	122.0
122.5	18.5	15.7	14.4	18.5	15.8	14.4	18.6	15.9	14.5	122.5
123.0	18.5	15.8	14.4	18.6	15.8	14.5	18.7	15.9	14.5	123.0
123.5	18.6	15.8	14.4	18.6	15.9	14.5	18.7	16.0	14.6	123.5
124.0	18.6	15.8	14.4	18.7	15.9	14.5	18.8	16.0	14.6	124.0
124.5	18.7	15.8	14.4	18.8	15.9	14.5	18.9	16.1	14.6	124.5
125.0	18.7	15.9	14.5	18.8	16.0	14.6	18.9	16.1	14.7	125.0
125.5	18.8	15.9	14.5	18.9	16.0	14.6	19.0	16.1	14.7	125.5
126.0	18.8	15.9	14.5	19.0	16.1	14.6	19.1	16.2	14.7	126.0
126.5	18.9	16.0	14.5	19.0	16.1	14.6	19.2	16.2	14.8	126.5
127.0	18.9	16.0	14.5	19.1	16.1	14.7	19.2	16.3	14.8	127.0
127.5	19.0	16.0	14.5	19.2	16.2	14.7	19.3	16.3	14.8	127.5
128.0	19.1	16.1	14.6	19.2	16.2	14.7	19.4	16.4	14.9	128.0
128.5	19.1	16.1	14.6	19.3	16.3	14.7	19.5	16.4	14.9	128.5
129.0	19.2	16.1	14.6	19.4	16.3	14.8	19.5	16.5	14.9	129.0
129.5	19.3	16.2	14.6	19.4	16.3	14.8	19.6	16.5	15.0	129.5
130.0	19.3	16.2	14.6	19.5	16.4	14.8	19.7	16.6	15.0	130.0
130.5	19.4	16.2	14.6	19.6	16.4	14.9	19.8	16.6	15.1	130.5
131.0	19.5	16.3	14.7	19.7	16.5	14.9	19.9	16.7	15.1	131.0
131.5	19.5	16.3	14.7	19.8	16.5	14.9	20.0	16.7	15.1	131.5
132.0	19.6	16.3	14.7	19.8	16.6	14.9	20.1	16.8	15.2	132.0
132.5	19.7	16.4	14.7	19.9	16.6	15.0	20.2	16.8	15.2	132.5
133.0	19.8	16.4	14.7	20.0	16.7	15.0	20.2	16.9	15.2	133.0
133.5	19.8	16.5	14.8	20.1	16.7	15.0	20.3	17.0	15.3	133.5
134.0	19.9	16.5	14.8	20.2	16.8	15.0	20.4	17.0	15.3	134.0
134.5	20.0	16.5	14.8	20.3	16.8	15.1	20.5	17.1	15.3	134.5
135.0	20.1	16.6	14.8	20.4	16.9	15.1	20.6	17.1	15.4	135.0
135.5	20.2	16.6	14.9	20.5	16.9	15.1	20.7	17.2	15.4	135.5
136.0	20.3	16.7	14.9	20.6	17.0	15.2	20.8	17.2	15.5	136.0
136.5	20.4	16.7	14.9	20.7	17.0	15.2	20.9	17.3	15.5	136.5
137.0	20.5	16.8	14.9	20.8	17.1	15.2	21.1	17.4	15.5	137.0
137.5	20.5	16.8	15.0	20.9	17.1	15.3	21.2	17.4	15.6	137.5
138.0	20.7	16.9	15.0	21.0	17.2	15.3	21.3	17.5	15.6	138.0
138.5	20.8	16.9	15.0	21.1	17.2	15.3	21.4	17.6	15.7	138.5
139.0	20.9	17.0	15.0	21.2	17.3	15.4	21.5	17.6	15.7	139.0
139.5	21.0	17.0	15.1	21.3	17.4	15.4	21.6	17.7	15.7	139.5
140.0	21.1	17.1	15.1	21.4	17.4	15.4	21.7	17.8	15.8	140.0
140.5	21.2	17.2	15.2	21.5	17.5	15.5	21.9	17.8	15.8	140.5
141.0	21.3	17.2	15.2	21.7	17.6	15.5	22.0	17.9	15.9	141.0
141.5	21.5	17.3	15.2	21.8	17.6	15.6	22.1	18.0	15.9	141.5
142.0	21.6	17.4	15.3	21.9	17.7	15.6	22.2	18.0	15.9	142.0
142.5	21.7	17.5	15.3	22.0	17.8	15.7	22.4	18.1	16.0	142.5
143.0	21.9	17.5	15.4	22.2	17.9	15.7	22.5	18.2	16.0	143.0
143.5	22.0	17.6	15.4	22.3	17.9	15.8	22.7	18.3	16.1	143.5
144.0	22.1	17.7	15.5	22.5	18.0	15.8	22.8	18.4	16.1	144.0
144.5	22.3	17.8	15.5	22.6	18.1	15.9	22.9	18.4	16.2	144.5
145.0	22.4	17.9	15.6	22.8	18.2	15.9	23.1	18.5	16.2	145.0

*Length below 85 cm, height ≥ 85 cm. Reprinted with permission from: Mei Z et al. The development of a MUAC-for-height reference, including a comparison to other nutritional status screening indicators. *WHO Bull.* 1997;75:333–341.

Table E–2 Arm measurements. MUAC-for-Age Reference Data for Boys Aged 6–59 Months*

Age (months)	*−4 SD*	*−3 SD*	*−2 SD*	*−1 SD*	*Mean*	*+1 SD*	*+2 SD*	*+3 SD*
6	10.3	11.5	12.6	13.8	14.9	16.1	17.3	18.4
7	10.4	11.6	12.7	13.9	15.1	16.3	17.5	18.6
8	10.5	11.7	12.8	14.0	15.2	16.4	17.6	18.8
9	10.5	11.7	12.9	14.2	15.4	16.6	17.8	19.0
10	10.6	11.8	13.0	14.2	15.5	16.7	17.9	19.1
11	10.6	11.9	13.1	14.3	15.6	16.8	18.0	19.3
12	10.7	11.9	13.2	14.4	15.7	16.9	18.1	19.4
13	10.7	12.0	13.2	14.5	15.7	17.0	18.2	19.5
14	10.8	12.0	13.3	14.5	15.8	17.1	18.3	19.6
15	10.8	12.1	13.3	14.6	15.9	17.1	18.4	19.7
16	10.8	12.1	13.4	14.6	15.9	17.2	18.5	19.8
17	10.8	12.1	13.4	14.7	16.0	17.3	18.6	19.8
18	10.8	12.1	13.4	14.7	16.0	17.3	18.6	19.9
19	10.9	12.2	13.5	14.8	16.1	17.4	18.7	20.0
20	10.9	12.2	13.5	14.8	16.1	17.4	18.7	20.0
21	10.9	12.2	13.5	14.8	16.1	17.5	18.8	20.1
22	10.9	12.2	13.5	14.9	16.2	17.5	18.8	20.1
23	10.9	12.2	13.5	14.9	16.2	17.5	18.9	20.2
24	10.9	12.2	13.6	14.9	16.2	17.6	18.9	20.2
25	10.9	12.2	13.6	14.9	16.3	17.6	18.9	20.3
26	10.9	12.3	13.6	14.9	16.3	17.6	19.0	20.3
27	10.9	12.3	13.6	15.0	16.3	17.7	19.0	20.4
28	10.9	12.3	13.6	15.0	16.3	17.7	19.1	20.4
29	10.9	12.3	13.7	15.0	16.4	17.7	19.1	20.4
30	10.9	12.3	13.7	15.0	16.4	17.8	19.1	20.5
31	11.0	12.3	13.7	15.1	16.4	17.8	19.2	20.5
32	11.0	12.3	13.7	15.1	16.5	17.8	19.2	20.6
33	11.0	12.4	13.7	15.1	16.5	17.9	19.2	20.6
34	11.0	12.4	13.8	15.1	16.5	17.9	19.3	20.6
35	11.0	12.4	13.8	15.2	16.5	17.9	19.3	20.7
36	11.0	12.4	13.8	15.2	16.6	18.0	19.3	20.7
37	11.0	12.4	13.8	15.2	16.6	18.0	19.4	20.8
38	11.0	12.4	13.8	15.2	16.6	18.0	19.4	20.8
39	11.1	12.5	13.9	15.3	16.7	18.1	19.5	20.9
40	11.1	12.5	13.9	15.3	16.7	18.1	19.5	20.9
41	11.1	12.5	13.9	15.3	16.7	18.1	19.6	21.0
42	11.1	12.5	13.9	15.4	16.8	18.2	19.6	21.0
43	11.1	12.5	14.0	15.4	16.8	18.2	19.7	21.1
44	11.1	12.5	14.0	15.4	16.8	18.3	19.7	21.1
45	11.1	12.6	14.0	15.4	16.9	18.3	19.8	21.2
46	11.1	12.6	14.0	15.5	16.9	18.4	19.8	21.3
47	11.1	12.6	14.0	15.5	17.0	18.4	19.9	21.3
48	11.1	12.6	14.1	15.5	17.0	18.4	19.9	21.4
49	11.1	12.6	14.1	15.6	17.0	18.5	20.0	21.4
50	11.1	12.6	14.1	15.6	17.1	18.5	20.0	21.5
51	11.1	12.6	14.1	15.6	17.1	18.6	20.1	21.6
52	11.1	12.6	14.1	15.6	17.1	18.6	20.1	21.6
53	11.1	12.6	14.1	15.7	17.2	18.7	20.2	21.7
54	11.1	12.6	14.2	15.7	17.2	18.7	20.2	21.8
55	11.1	12.6	14.2	15.7	17.2	18.8	20.3	21.8
56	11.1	12.6	14.2	15.7	17.3	18.8	20.4	21.9
57	11.1	12.6	14.2	15.8	17.3	18.9	20.4	22.0
58	11.1	12.6	14.2	15.8	17.3	18.9	20.5	22.1
59	11.1	12.6	14.2	15.8	17.4	19.0	20.6	22.2

*Reprinted with permission from: de Onis M et al. The development of MUAC-for-age reference data recommended by a WHO expert committee. *WHO Bull.* 1997;75:11–18.

Table E–3 Arm measurements. MUAC-for-Age Reference Data for Boys Aged 6–59 Months*

Age (months)	*−4 SD*	*−3 SD*	*−2 SD*	*−1 SD*	*Mean*	*+1 SD*	*+2 SD*	*+3 SD*
6	9.2	10.4	11.5	12.7	13.9	15.0	16.2	17.4
7	9.4	10.6	11.8	13.0	14.1	15.3	16.5	17.7
8	9.6	10.8	12.0	13.2	14.4	15.6	16.8	18.0
9	9.8	11.0	12.2	13.4	14.6	15.8	17.0	18.2
10	9.9	11.1	12.3	13.6	14.8	16.0	17.2	18.4
11	10.0	11.3	12.5	13.7	15.0	16.2	17.4	18.6
12	10.1	11.4	12.6	13.9	15.1	16.4	17.6	18.8
13	10.2	11.5	12.7	14.0	15.2	16.5	17.7	19.0
14	10.3	11.6	12.8	14.1	15.4	16.6	17.9	19.2
15	10.4	11.7	12.9	14.2	15.5	16.7	18.0	19.3
16	10.4	11.7	13.0	14.3	15.6	16.8	18.1	19.4
17	10.5	11.8	13.1	14.4	15.7	16.9	18.2	19.5
18	10.5	11.8	13.1	14.4	15.7	17.0	18.3	19.6
19	10.6	11.9	13.2	14.5	15.8	17.1	18.4	19.7
20	10.6	11.9	13.2	14.5	15.8	17.2	18.5	19.8
21	10.6	11.9	13.3	14.6	15.9	17.2	18.5	19.8
22	10.7	12.0	13.3	14.6	15.9	17.3	18.6	19.9
23	10.7	12.0	13.3	14.7	16.0	17.3	18.6	20.0
24	10.7	12.0	13.4	14.7	16.0	17.4	18.7	20.0
25	10.7	12.0	13.4	14.7	16.1	17.4	18.7	20.1
26	10.7	12.1	13.4	14.7	16.1	17.4	18.8	20.1
27	10.7	12.1	13.4	14.8	16.1	17.5	18.8	20.2
28	10.7	12.1	13.4	14.8	16.1	17.5	18.9	20.2
29	10.7	12.1	13.5	14.8	16.2	17.5	18.9	20.3
30	10.8	12.1	13.5	14.8	16.2	17.6	18.9	20.3
31	10.8	12.1	13.5	14.9	16.2	17.6	19.0	20.3
32	10.8	12.1	13.5	14.9	16.3	17.6	19.0	20.4
33	10.8	12.2	13.5	14.9	16.3	17.7	19.0	20.4
34	10.8	12.2	13.6	14.9	16.3	17.7	19.1	20.5
35	10.8	12.2	13.6	15.0	16.3	17.7	19.1	20.5
36	10.8	12.2	13.6	15.0	16.4	17.8	19.2	20.5
37	10.8	12.2	13.6	15.0	16.4	17.8	19.2	20.6
38	10.9	12.2	13.6	15.0	16.4	17.8	19.2	20.6
39	10.9	12.3	13.7	15.1	16.5	17.9	19.3	20.7
40	10.9	12.3	13.7	15.1	16.5	17.9	19.3	20.7
41	10.9	12.3	13.7	15.1	16.6	18.0	19.4	20.8
42	10.9	12.3	13.8	15.2	16.6	18.0	19.4	20.8
43	10.9	12.4	13.8	15.2	16.6	18.1	19.5	20.9
44	10.9	12.4	13.8	15.2	16.7	18.1	19.5	21.0
45	11.0	12.4	13.8	15.3	16.7	18.1	19.6	21.0
46	11.0	12.4	13.9	15.3	16.7	18.2	19.6	21.1
47	11.0	12.4	13.9	15.3	16.8	18.2	19.7	21.2
48	11.0	12.4	13.9	15.4	16.8	18.3	19.8	21.2
49	11.0	12.5	13.9	15.4	16.9	18.3	19.8	21.3
50	11.0	12.5	14.0	15.4	16.9	18.4	19.9	21.4
51	11.0	12.5	14.0	15.5	17.0	18.4	19.9	21.4
52	11.0	12.5	14.0	15.5	17.0	18.5	20.0	21.5
53	11.0	12.5	14.0	15.5	17.0	18.6	20.1	21.6
54	11.0	12.5	14.0	15.6	17.1	18.6	20.1	21.7
55	11.0	12.5	14.1	15.6	17.1	18.7	20.2	21.7
56	11.0	12.5	14.1	15.6	17.2	18.7	20.3	21.8
57	11.0	12.5	14.1	15.7	17.2	18.8	20.3	21.9
58	11.0	12.5	14.1	15.7	17.3	18.8	20.4	22.0
59	11.0	12.5	14.1	15.7	17.3	18.9	20.5	22.1

*Reprinted with permission from: de Onis M et al. The development of MUAC-for-age reference data recommended by a WHO expert committee. *WHO Bull.* 1997;75:11–18.

Table E–4 Observed Means, Standard Deviations, and Smoothed Percentile Values of Triceps Skinfold (mm) by Sex and Age for Infants 7–13 Months Old

Age				Percentile						
(months)	*n*	*Mean*	*SD*	*5th*	*10th*	*25th*	*50th*	*75th*	*90th*	*95th*
Males										
7	45	9.2	3.1	—	5.9	7.1	7.5	8.0	11.0	—
8	80	8.8	2.2	5.0	5.9	7.2	8.4	9.2	11.1	11.8
9	95	8.8	2.1	5.2	5.8	7.2	8.6	9.6	11.1	12.1
10	124	9.3	2.3	5.4	6.2	7.4	8.6	9.7	10.8	12.6
11	103	9.3	3.1	5.6	6.8	7.6	8.8	10.3	13.3	15.0
12	68	10.0	3.5	5.6	7.0	7.6	9.3	10.3	13.1	15.9
13	30	9.5	2.5	—	—	—	9.5	—	—	—
Females										
7	46	8.2	2.5	—	3.0	5.2	7.5	9.0	11.0	—
8	88	8.6	2.7	3.0	3.5	5.5	7.5	9.3	10.8	12.0
9	109	8.4	2.5	3.7	4.2	5.6	7.5	9.2	10.8	12.0
10	120	8.7	2.3	3.9	4.6	5.8	7.7	9.5	11.1	13.3
11	95	9.4	3.5	4.4	5.0	6.0	8.3	9.7	11.1	13.8
12	70	9.2	2.7	5.2	5.4	6.4	8.9	10.2	11.1	12.3
13	27	9.5	1.9	—	—	—	9.2	—	—	—

Source: Reprinted with permission from Ryan AS and Martinez GA, Physical growth of infants 7 to 13 months of age: Results from a national survey, in *American Journal of Physical Anthropology* (1987;73:449), Copyright © 1987, Wiley-Liss, Inc., a subsidiary cf John Wiley & Sons, Inc.

Table E–5 Percentiles for Triceps Skinfold for Whites of the United States Health and Nutrition Examination Survey I of 1971–1974

Age Group	Triceps Skinfold Percentiles (mm²)															
	n	*5*	*10*	*25*	*50*	*75*	*90*	*95*	*n*	*5*	*10*	*25*	*50*	*75*	*90*	*95*
	Males								Females							
1–1.9	228	6	7	8	10	12	14	16	204	6	7	8	10	12	14	16
2–2.9	223	6	7	8	10	12	14	15	208	6	8	9	10	12	15	16
3–3.9	220	6	7	8	10	11	14	15	208	7	8	9	11	12	14	15
4–4.9	230	6	6	8	9	11	12	14	208	7	8	8	10	12	14	16
5–5.9	214	6	6	8	9	11	14	15	219	6	7	8	10	12	15	18
6–6.9	117	5	6	7	8	10	13	16	118	6	6	8	10	12	14	16
7–7.9	122	5	6	7	9	12	15	17	126	6	7	9	11	13	16	18
8–8.9	117	5	6	7	8	10	13	16	118	6	8	9	12	15	18	24
9–9.9	121	6	6	7	10	13	17	18	125	8	8	10	13	16	20	22
10–10.9	146	6	6	8	10	14	18	21	152	7	8	10	12	17	23	27
11–11.9	122	6	6	8	11	16	20	24	117	7	8	10	13	18	24	28
12–12.9	153	6	6	8	11	14	22	28	129	8	9	11	14	18	23	27
13–13.9	134	5	5	7	10	14	22	26	151	8	8	12	15	21	26	30
14–14.9	131	4	5	7	9	14	21	24	141	9	10	13	16	21	26	28
15–15.9	128	4	5	6	8	11	18	24	117	8	10	12	17	21	25	32
16–16.9	131	4	5	6	8	12	16	22	142	10	12	15	18	22	26	31
17–17.9	133	5	5	6	8	12	16	19	114	10	12	13	19	24	30	37
18–18.9	91	4	5	6	9	13	20	24	109	10	12	15	18	22	26	30
19–24.9	531	4	5	7	10	15	20	22	1060	10	11	14	18	24	30	34
25–34.9	971	5	6	8	12	16	20	24	1987	10	12	16	21	27	34	37
35–44.9	806	5	6	8	12	16	20	23	1614	12	14	18	23	29	35	38
45–54.9	898	6	6	8	12	15	20	25	1047	12	16	20	25	30	36	40
55–64.9	734	5	6	8	11	14	19	22	809	12	16	20	25	31	36	38
65–74.9	1503	4	6	8	11	15	19	22	1670	12	14	18	24	29	34	36

Source: Reprinted with permission from Frisancho AR, New norms of upper limb fat and muscle areas for assessment of nutritional status, in *American Journal of Clinical Nutrition* (1981;34:2540–2545), Copyright © 1981, American Society for Clinical Nutrition.

Table E–6 Percentiles of Upper Arm Circumference (mm) and Estimated Upper Arm Muscle Circumference (mm) for Whites of the United States Health and Nutrition Examination Survey I of 1971–1974

Males

	Arm Circumference (mm)							*Arm Muscle Circumference (mm)*						
Age Group	*5*	*10*	*25*	*50*	*75*	*90*	*95*	*5*	*10*	*25*	*50*	*75*	*90*	*95*
1–1.9	142	146	150	159	170	176	183	110	113	119	127	135	144	147
2–2.9	141	145	153	162	170	178	185	111	114	122	130	140	146	150
3–3.9	150	153	160	167	175	184	190	117	123	131	137	143	148	153
4–4.9	149	154	162	171	180	186	192	123	126	133	141	148	156	159
5–5.9	153	160	167	175	185	195	204	128	133	140	147	154	162	169
6–6.9	155	159	167	179	188	209	228	131	135	142	151	161	170	177
7–7.9	162	167	177	187	201	223	230	137	139	151	160	168	177	190
8–8.9	162	170	177	190	202	220	245	140	145	154	162	170	182	187
9–9.9	175	178	187	200	217	249	257	151	154	161	170	183	196	202
10–10.9	181	184	196	210	231	262	274	156	160	166	180	191	209	221
11–11.9	186	190	202	223	244	261	280	159	165	173	183	195	205	230
12–12.9	193	200	214	232	254	282	303	167	171	182	195	210	223	241
13–13.9	194	211	228	247	263	286	301	172	179	196	211	226	238	245
14–14.9	220	226	237	253	283	303	322	189	199	212	223	240	260	264
15–15.9	222	229	244	264	284	311	320	199	204	218	237	254	266	272
16–16.9	244	248	262	278	303	324	343	213	225	234	249	269	287	296
17–17.9	246	253	267	285	308	336	347	224	231	245	258	273	294	312
18–18.9	245	260	276	297	321	353	379	226	237	252	264	283	298	324
19–24.9	262	272	288	308	331	355	372	238	245	257	273	289	309	321
25–34.9	271	282	300	319	342	362	375	243	250	264	279	298	314	326
35–44.9	278	287	305	326	345	363	374	247	255	269	286	302	318	327
45–54.9	267	281	301	322	342	362	376	239	249	265	281	300	315	326
55–64.9	258	273	296	317	336	355	369	236	245	260	278	295	310	320
65–74.9	248	263	285	307	325	344	355	223	235	251	268	284	298	306

continues

Table E–6 continued

	Females													
	Arm Circumference (mm)							*Arm Muscle Circumference (mm)*						
Age Group	*5*	*10*	*25*	*50*	*75*	*90*	*95*	*5*	*10*	*25*	*50*	*75*	*90*	*95*
1–1.9	138	142	148	156	164	172	177	105	111	117	124	132	139	143
2–2.9	142	145	152	160	167	176	184	111	114	119	126	133	142	147
3–3.9	143	150	158	167	175	183	189	113	119	124	132	140	146	152
4–4.9	149	154	160	169	177	184	191	115	121	128	136	144	152	157
5–5.9	153	157	165	175	185	203	211	125	128	134	142	151	159	165
6–6.9	156	162	170	176	187	204	211	130	133	138	145	154	166	171
7–7.9	164	167	174	183	199	216	231	129	135	142	151	160	171	176
8–8.9	168	172	183	195	214	247	261	138	140	151	160	171	183	194
9–9.9	178	182	194	211	224	251	260	147	150	158	167	180	194	198
10–10.9	174	182	193	210	228	251	265	148	150	159	170	180	190	197
11–11.9	185	194	208	224	248	276	303	150	158	171	181	196	217	223
12–12.9	194	203	216	237	256	282	294	162	166	180	191	201	214	220
13–13.9	202	211	223	243	271	301	338	169	175	183	198	211	226	240
14–14.9	214	223	237	252	272	304	322	174	179	190	201	216	232	247
15–15.9	208	221	239	254	279	300	322	175	178	189	202	215	228	244
16–16.9	218	224	241	258	283	318	334	170	180	190	202	216	234	249
17–17.9	220	227	241	264	295	324	350	175	183	194	205	221	239	257
18–18.9	222	227	241	258	281	312	325	174	179	191	202	215	237	245
19–24.9	221	230	247	265	290	319	345	179	185	195	207	221	236	249
25–34.9	233	240	256	277	304	342	368	183	188	199	212	228	246	264
35–44.9	241	251	267	290	317	356	378	186	192	205	218	236	257	272
45–54.9	242	256	274	299	328	362	384	187	193	206	220	238	260	274
55–64.9	243	257	280	303	335	367	385	187	196	209	225	244	266	280
65–74.9	240	252	274	299	326	356	373	185	195	208	225	244	264	279

Source: Reprinted with permission from Frisancho AR, New norms of upper limb fat and muscle areas for assessment of nutritional status, in *American Journal of Clinical Nutrition* (1981;34:2540–2545), Copyright © 1981, American Society for Clinical Nutrition, Inc.

Table E–7 Percentiles for Estimates of Upper Arm Fat Area (mm²) and Upper Arm Muscle Area (mm²) for Whites of the United States Health and Nutrition Examination Survey I of 1971–1974

Males

Age Group	*Arm Muscle Area Percentiles (mm²)*							*Arm Fat Area Percentiles (mm²)*						
	5	*10*	*25*	*50*	*75*	*90*	*95*	*5*	*10*	*25*	*50*	*75*	*90*	*95*
1–1.9	956	1014	1133	1278	1447	1644	1720	452	486	590	741	895	1036	1176
2–2.9	973	1040	1190	1345	1557	1690	1787	434	504	578	737	871	1044	1148
3–3.9	1095	1201	1357	1484	1618	1750	1853	464	519	590	736	868	1071	1151
4–4.9	1207	1264	1408	1579	1747	1926	2008	428	494	598	722	859	989	1085
5–5.9	1298	1411	1550	1720	1884	2089	2285	446	488	582	713	914	1176	1299
6–6.9	1360	1447	1605	1815	2056	2297	2493	371	446	539	678	896	1115	1519
7–7.9	1497	1548	1808	2027	2246	2494	2886	423	473	574	758	1011	1393	1511
8–8.9	1550	1664	1895	2089	2296	2628	2788	410	460	588	725	1003	1248	1558
9–9.9	1811	1884	2067	2288	2657	3053	3257	485	527	635	859	1252	1864	2081
10–10.9	1930	2027	2182	2575	2903	3486	3882	523	543	738	982	1376	1906	2609
11–11.9	2016	2156	2382	2670	3022	3359	4226	536	595	754	1148	1710	2348	2574
12–12.9	2216	2339	2649	3022	3496	3968	4640	554	650	874	1172	1558	2536	3580
13–13.9	2363	2546	3044	3553	4081	4502	4794	475	570	812	1096	1702	2744	3322
14–14.9	2830	3147	3586	3963	4575	5368	5530	453	563	786	1082	1608	2746	3508
15–15.9	3138	3317	3788	4481	5134	5631	5900	521	595	690	931	1423	2434	3100
16–16.9	3625	4044	4352	4951	5753	6576	6980	542	593	844	1078	1746	2280	3041
17–17.9	3998	4252	4777	5286	5950	6886	7726	598	698	827	1096	1636	2407	2888
18–18.9	4070	4481	5066	5552	6374	7067	8355	560	665	860	1264	1947	3302	3928
19–24.9	4508	4777	5274	5913	6660	7606	8200	594	743	963	1406	2231	3098	3652
25–34.9	4694	4963	5541	6214	7067	7847	8436	675	831	1174	1752	2459	3246	3786
35–44.9	4844	5181	5740	6490	7265	8034	8488	703	851	1310	1792	2463	3098	3624
45–54.9	4546	4946	5589	6297	7142	7918	8458	749	922	1254	1741	2359	3245	3928
55–64.9	4422	4783	5381	6144	6919	7670	8149	658	839	1166	1645	2236	2976	3466
65–74.9	3973	4411	5031	5716	6432	7074	7453	573	753	1122	1621	2199	2876	3327

continues

Table E–7 continued

	Females													
	Arm Muscle Area Percentiles (mm²)							*Arm Fat Area Percentiles (mm²)*						
Age Group	*5*	*10*	*25*	*50*	*75*	*90*	*95*	*5*	*10*	*25*	*50*	*75*	*90*	*95*
1–1.9	885	973	1084	1221	1378	1535	1621	401	466	578	706	847	1022	1140
2–2.9	973	1029	1119	1269	1405	1595	1727	469	526	642	747	894	1061	1173
3–3.9	1014	1133	1227	1396	1563	1690	1846	473	529	656	822	967	1106	1158
4–4.9	1058	1171	1313	1475	1644	1832	1958	490	541	654	766	907	1109	1236
5–5.9	1238	1301	1432	1598	1825	2012	2159	470	529	647	812	991	1330	1536
6–6.9	1354	1414	1513	1683	1877	2182	2323	464	508	638	827	1009	1263	1436
7–7.9	1330	1441	1602	1815	2045	2332	2469	491	560	706	920	1135	1407	1644
8–8.9	1513	1566	1808	2034	2327	2657	2996	527	634	769	1042	1383	1872	2482
9–9.9	1723	1788	1976	2227	2571	2987	3112	642	690	933	1219	1584	2171	2524
10–10.9	1740	1784	2019	2296	2583	2873	3093	616	702	842	1141	1608	2500	3005
11–11.9	1784	1987	2316	2612	3071	3739	3953	707	802	1015	1301	1942	2730	3690
12–12.9	2092	2182	2579	2904	3225	3655	3847	782	854	1090	1511	2056	2666	3369
13–13.9	2269	2426	2657	3130	3529	4081	4568	726	838	1219	1625	2374	3272	4150
14–14.9	2418	2562	2874	3220	3704	4294	4850	981	1043	1423	1818	2403	3250	3765
15–15.9	2426	2518	2847	3248	3689	4123	4756	839	1126	1396	1886	2544	3093	4195
16–16.9	2308	2567	2865	3248	3718	4353	4946	1126	1351	1663	2006	2598	3374	4236
17–17.9	2442	2674	2996	3336	3883	4552	5251	1042	1267	1463	2104	2977	3864	5159
18–18.9	2398	2538	2917	3243	3694	4461	4767	1003	1230	1616	2104	2617	3508	3733
19–24.9	2538	2728	3026	3406	3877	4439	4940	1046	1198	1596	2166	2959	4050	4896
25–34.9	2661	2826	3148	3573	4138	4806	5541	1173	1399	1841	2548	3512	4690	5560
35–44.9	2750	2948	3359	3783	4428	5240	5877	1336	1619	2158	2898	3932	5093	5847
45–54.9	2784	2956	3378	3858	4520	5375	5964	1459	1803	2447	3244	4229	5416	6140
55–64.9	2784	3063	3477	4045	4750	5632	6247	1345	1879	2520	3369	4360	5276	6152
65–74.9	2737	3018	3444	4019	4739	5566	6214	1363	1681	2266	3063	3943	4914	5530

Source: Reprinted with permission from Frisancho AR, New norms of upper limb fat and muscle areas for assessment of nutritional status, in *American Journal of Clinical Nutrition* (1981;34:2540–2545), Copyright © 1981, American Society for Clinical Nutrition, Inc.

APPENDIX F

Progression of Sexual Development

Table F–1 Median ages at entry into each maturity stage and fiducial limits* in years for pubic hair and breast development in girls by race

Stage	Age at Entry for Girls					
	Non-Hispanic White		Non-Hispanic Black		Mexican-American	
	Median	FL	Median	FL	Median	FL
Pubic hair						
PH2	10.57†	10.29–10.85	9.43†	9.05–9.74	10.39	—
PH3	11.80†	11.54–12.07	10.57†	10.30–10.83	11.70†	11.14–12.27
PH4	13.00†	12.71–13.30	11.90†	11.38–12.42	13.19†	12.88–13.52
PH5	16.33†	15.86–16.88	14.70†	14.32–15.11	16.30†	15.90–16.76
Breast development						
B2	10.38†	10.11–10.65	9.48†	9.14–9.76	9.80	0–11.78
B3	11.75†	11.49–12.02	10.79†	10.50–11.08	11.43	8.64–14.50
B4	13.29†	12.97–13.61	12.24†	11.87–12.61	13.07†	12.79–13.36
B5	15.47†	15.04–15.94	13.92†	13.57–14.29	14.70†	14.37–15.04

FL indicates fiducial limit.
* Calculated 98.3% FLs to adjust for multiple comparisons between races for an overall α of 0.05.
† Significant pair-wise racial difference, $P < .05$.

Source: Reprinted with permission from Pediatrics, Vol. 110, pp. 911–918, Copyright 2002. Sun SS, Schuber CM, Chumlea WC, Roche AF, et al. National estimates of the timing of sexual maturation and racial differences among US children. *Pediatrics* 2002;110;911–918.

Tanner Stage, or sexual maturity rating: 1. Prepubertal; 2. First visible signs of pubertal change appear; 3. Pubic hair increases and becomes darker and coarser, breasts enlarge, and genitalia lengthen and enlarge; 4. Pubic hair becomes more abundant and coarse, genitalia and breasts increase in size; 5. Adult characteristics visible for breasts, pubic hair, and genitalia.

Table F–2 Mean ages in years and SEs for being in a stage for pubic hair and breast development in girls by race

Stage	Age in a Stage for Girls								
	Non-Hispanic White			Non-Hispanic Black			Mexican-American		
	N	Mean	SE	*N*	Mean	SE	*N*	Mean	SE
Pubic hair									
PH2	67	10.96*	0.23	85	10.25*	0.15	105	11.17*	0.21
PH3	61	12.41*	0.19	98	11.37*	0.23	108	12.84*	0.18
PH4	154	15.11*	0.18	184	13.69*	0.31	177	14.61*	0.26
PH5	133	16.53*	0.17	282	16.05*	0.14	161	16.61*	0.12
Breast development									
B2	82	11.05*	0.18	99	10.25*	0.20	129	10.70	0.21
B3	80	12.80*	0.19	106	11.94*	0.22	131	12.61*	0.20
B4	110	15.16*	0.32	112	13.61*	0.34	97	14.03*	0.27
B5	173	16.25*	0.18	338	15.78*	0.14	254	16.21*	0.12

SE indicates standard error.
* Significant pair-wise racial difference, $P < .05$.

Source: Reprinted with permission from Pediatrics, Vol. 110, pp. 911–918, Copyright 2002. Sun SS, Schuber CM, Chumlea WC, Roche AF, et al. National estimates of the timing of sexual maturation and racial differences among US children. *Pediatrics* 2002;110;911–918.

Tanner Stage, or sexual maturity rating: 1. Prepubertal; 2. First visible signs of pubertal change appear; 3. Pubic hair increases and becomes darker and coarser, breasts enlarge, and genitalia lengthen and enlarge; 4. Pubic hair becomes more abundant and coarse, genitalia and breasts increase in size; 5. Adult characteristics visible for breasts, pubic hair, and genitalia.

Table F–3 Median ages of entry into each stage and FLs* in years for pubic hair and genitalia development in boys by race

Stage	Age at Entry for Boys					
	Non-Hispanic White		Non-Hispanic Black		Mexican-American	
	Median	FL	Median	FL	Median	FL
Pubic hair						
PH2	11.98†	11.69–12.29	11.16†	10.89–11.43	12.30†	12.06–12.56
PH3	12.65	12.37–12.95	12.51†	12.26–12.77	13.06†	12.79–13.36
PH4	13.56	13.27–13.86	13.73	13.49–13.99	14.08	13.83–14.32
PH5	15.67	15.30–16.05	15.32	14.99–15.67	15.75	15.46–16.03
Genitalia development						
G2	10.03	9.61–10.40	9.20†	8.62–9.64	10.29†	9.94–10.60
G3	12.32	12.00–12.67	11.78†	11.50–12.08	12.53†	12.29–12.79
G4	13.52	13.22–13.83	13.40	13.15–13.66	13.77	13.51–14.03
G5	16.01†	15.57–16.50	15.00†	14.70–15.32	15.76†	15.39–16.14

FL indicates fiducial limit.

* Calculated 98.3% FLs to adjust for multiple comparisons between races for an overall of 0.05.

† Significant pair-wise racial difference, $P < .05$.

Source: Reprinted with permission from Pediatrics, Vol. 110, pp. 911–918, Copyright 2002. Sun SS, Schuber CM, Chumlea WC, Roche AF, et al. National estimates of the timing of sexual maturation and racial differences among US children. *Pediatrics* 2002;110;911–918.

Tanner Stage, or sexual maturity rating: 1. Prepubertal; 2. First visible signs of pubertal change appear; 3. Pubic hair increases and becomes darker and coarser, breasts enlarge, and genitalia lengthen and enlarge; 4. Pubic hair becomes more abundant and coarse, genitalia and breasts increase in size; 5. Adult characteristics visible for breasts, pubic hair, and genitalia.

Table F–4 Mean ages in years and SEs for being in a stage for pubic hair and genitalia development in boys by race

Stage	Age in a Stage for Boys								
	Non-Hispanic White			Non-Hispanic Black			Mexican-American		
	N	Mean	SE	*N*	Mean	SE	*N*	Mean	SE
Pubic hair									
PH2	42	11.81	0.16	106	11.48*	0.13	50	12.20*	0.24
PH3	39	13.03	0.27	86	12.79*	0.19	55	13.44*	0.26
PH4	75	14.89	0.18	94	15.21	0.26	93	15.25	0.16
PH5	133	16.84	0.13	238	16.67*	0.08	211	17.14*	0.10
Genitalia development									
G2	136	11.08	0.18	181	10.79	0.13	183	11.09	0.17
G3	63	12.55	0.29	113	12.03*	0.28	80	12.97*	0.28
G4	91	15.29	0.19	98	15.07	0.33	104	15.38	0.19
G5	120	16.64	0.15	253	16.42*	0.09	219	16.85*	0.13

* Significant pair-wise racial difference, $P < .05$.

Source: Reprinted with permission from Pediatrics, Vol. 110, pp 911–918, Copyright 2002. Sun SS, Schuber CM, Chumlea WC, Roche AF, et al. National estimates of the timing of sexual maturation and racial differences among US children. *Pediatrics* 2002;110;911–918.

Tanner Stage, or sexual maturity rating: 1. Prepubertal; 2. First visible signs of pubertal change appear; 3. Pubic hair increases and becomes darker and coarser, breasts enlarge, and genitalia lengthen and enlarge; 4. Pubic hair becomes more abundant and coarse, genitalia and breasts increase in size; 5. Adult characteristics visible for breasts, pubic hair, and genitalia.

Appendix G

Nomograms

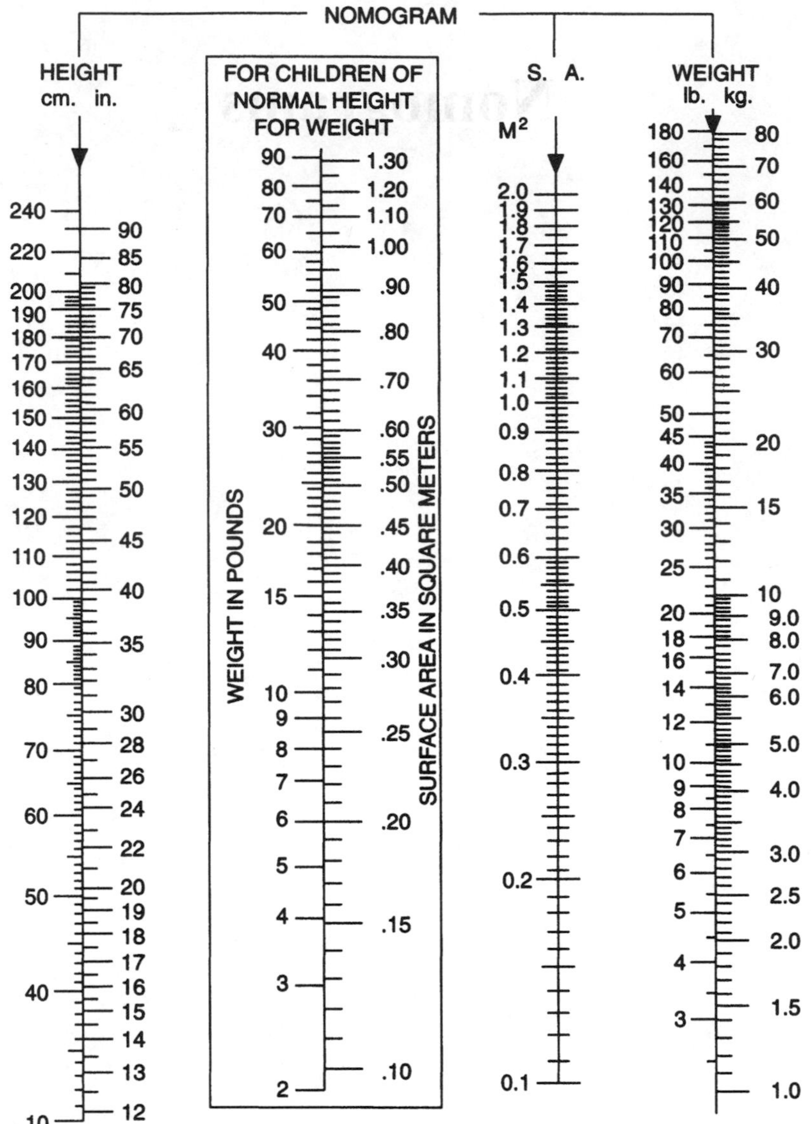

NOMOGRAM FOR ESTIMATION OF SURFACE AREA. THE SURFACE AREA IS INDICATED WHEN A STRAIGHT LINE THAT CONNECTS THE HEIGHT AND WEIGHT LEVELS INTERSECTS THE SURFACE AREA COLUMN: OR IF THE PATIENT IS ROUGHLY OF AVERAGE SIZE, FROM THE WEIGHT ALONE (ENCLOSED AREA). (NOMOGRAM MODIFIED FROM DATA OF E. BOYD BY C.D. WEST.)

Figure G–1 Nomogram for estimation of surface area. *Source:* Reprinted from *Nelson's Textbook of Medicine,* ed 13 (p 1521) by Behrman RE and Vaughan VC (eds) with permission of WB Saunders, © 1987.

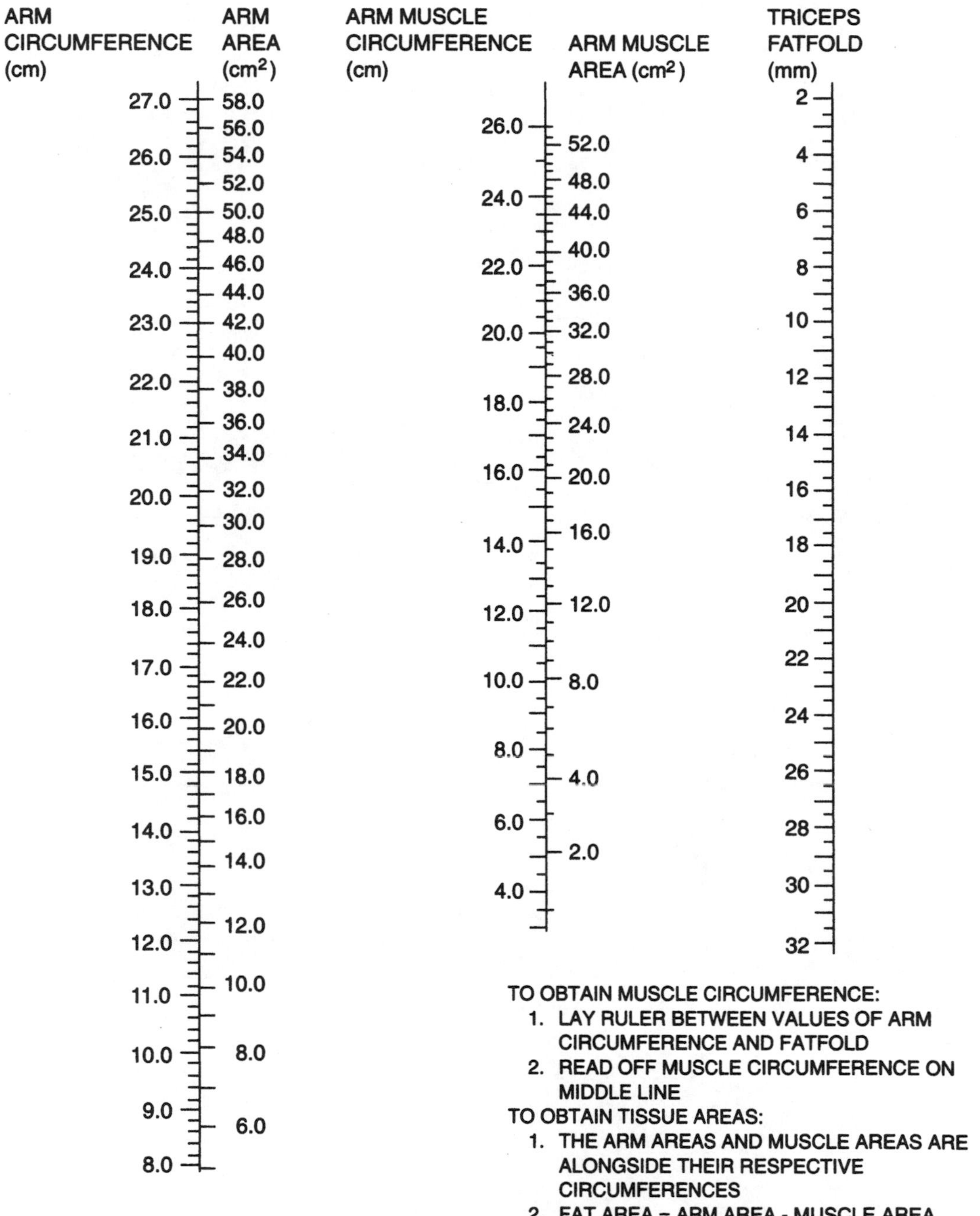

Figure G–2 Arm anthropometry nomogram for children. *Source:* Reprinted with permission from Gurney JM and Jeliffe DB, Arm anthropometry in nutritional assessment: nomogram for rapid calculation of muscle circumference and cross-sectional muscle and fat areas, in *American Journal of Clinical Nutrition* (1973;26: 912–915). Copyright © 1973, American Society for Clinical Nutrition.

Appendix H

Biochemical Evaluation of Nutritional Status

Table H–1 Biochemical Evaluation of Nutritional Status

Test	*Specimen*	*Reference Range*	
Albumin	Serum		*g/dl*
		Premature:	3.0–4.2
		Newborn:	3.6–5.4
		Infant:	4.0–5.0
		Thereafter:	3.5–5.0
Calcium, Ionized (iCa)	Serum, plasma or whole blood (heparin)		*mg/dl*
		Cord:	5.0–6.0
		Newborn: 3–24h:	4.3–5.1
		24–48h:	4.0–4.7
		Thereafter:	4.48–4.92
		Or	2.24–2.46 mEq/L
Calcium, total	Serum		*mg/dl*
		Cord:	9.0–11.5
		Newborn: 3–24h:	9.0–10.6
		24–48h:	7.0–12.0
		4–7 day:	9.0–10.9
		Child:	8.8–10.8
		Thereafter:	8.4–10.2
	Urine, 24h	Ca in Diet	*mg/day*
		Ca Free:	5–40
		Low to average:	50–150
		Average (20m/mold):	100–300
B-Carotene	Serum		*µg/dl*
		Infant:	20–70
		Child:	40–130
		Thereafter:	60–200

continues

Table H–1 continued

Test	*Specimen*	*Reference Range*	
Ceruloplasmin	Serum		*mg/dl*
		Newborn:	1–30
		6 mo–1 yr:	15–50
		1–12 yr:	30–65
		Thereafter:	14–40
Chloride	Serum or plasma (heparin)		*mmol/L*
		Cord:	96–104
		Newborn:	97–110
		Thereafter:	98–106
	CSF	118–132 mmol/L	
	Urine, 24h		*mmol/day*
		Infant:	2–10
		Child:	15–50
		Thereafter:	110–250
		(varies greatly with Cl intake)	
	Sweat		*mmol/L*
		Normal (homozygote):	0–35
		Marginal:	30–60
		Cystic fibrosis:	60–200
		Increases by 10 mmol/L during lifetime	
Cholesterol, total	Serum or plasma (EDTA or heparin)		*mg/dl*
		Cord:	45–100
		Newborn:	53–135
		Infant:	70–175
		Child:	120–200
		Adolescent:	120–210
		Adult:	140–310
		Recommended (desirable) range for	
		adults:	<200
		adolescents:	<170
Copper	Serum		*µg/dl*
		Birth–6 mo:	20–70
		6 yr:	90–190
		12 yr:	80–160
		Adult, M:	70–240
		F:	80–155
	Erythrocytes (heparin)	90–150 µg/dl	
	Urine (24h)	15–30 µg/day	

Table H–1 continued

Test	*Specimen*	*Reference Range*	
Creatinine			
Jaffe, kinetic or enzymatic	Serum or plasma		*mg/dl*
		Cord:	0.6–1.2
		Newborn:	0.3–1.0
		Infant:	0.2–0.4
		Child:	0.3–0.7
		Adolescent:	0.5–1.0
		Adult, M:	0.6–1.2
		F:	0.5–1.1
	Urine 24h		*mg/kg/day*
		Infant	8–20
		Child:	8–22
		Adolescent:	8–30
		Adult:	14–26
		or:	*mg/day*
		Adult, M:	800–2000
		F:	600–1800
Disaccharide absorption test	Serum		*mg/dl*
		Changes in glucose from fasting value:	
		Normal	>30
		Inconclusive	20–30
		Abnormal:	<20
Erythrocyte count	White blood (EDTA)	*millions of cells/mm³ (µl)*	
		Cord blood:	3.9–5.5
		1–3 d (cap):	4.0–6.6
		1 wk:	3.9–6.3
		2 wk:	3.6–6.2
		1 mo:	3.0–5.4
		2 mo:	2.7–4.9
		3–6 mo:	3.1–4.5
		0.5–2 yr:	3.7–5.3
		2–6 yr	3.9–5.3
		6–12 yr:	4.0–5.2
		12–18 yr, M:	4.5–5.3
		F:	4.1–5.1
		18–49 yr, M:	4.5–5.9
		F:	4.0–5.2
Fat, fecal	Feces, 72 h	Coefficient of fat absorption (%)	
		Infant, breast-fed:	>93
		Infant, formula-fed:	>83
		>1 yr:	≥95

continues

Table H–1 continued

Test	*Specimen*	*Reference Range*		
Fatty acids Nonesterified (Free)	Serum or plasma (heparin)	Adults: Children and obese adults: <31	8–25 mg/dl	
Ferritin	Serum	 Newborn: 1 mo: 2–5 mo: 6 mo–15 yr: Adult, M: F:	*ng/ml* 25–200 200–600 50–200 7–140 15–200 12–150	
Folate	Serum Erythrocytes (EDTA)	 Newborn: Thereafter: 150–450 ng/ml cells	*ng/ml* 7.0–32 1.8–9	
Glucose	Serum	 Cord: Premature: Neonate: Newborn, 1 d: >1 d: Child: Adult:	*mg/dl* 45–96 20–60 30–60 40–60 50–90 60–100 70–105	
Glucose Tolerance Test Serum (GTT) Oral Dose: Adult: 75 g Child: 1.75 g/kg of ideal weight up to maximum of 75 g		 Fasting: 60 min: 90 min: 120 min:	*mg/dl* *Normal* 70–105 120–170 100–140 70–120	 *Diabetic* >115 >200 >200 >140
Growth Hormone (hGH) (Somatotropin)	Serum or plasma (EDTA, heparin) fasting at rest	 Cord: Newborn: Child: Adult, M: F:	*ng/ml* 10–50 10–40 <5 <5 <8	

Table H–1 continued

Test	*Specimen*	*Reference Range*		
HDL-Cholesterol (HDLC)	Serum or plasma (EDTA)		*mg/dl*	
			Male	*Female*
		Mean	45	55
		Range		
		Cord blood:	5–50	5–50
		0–12 yr:	30–65	30–65
		15–19 yr:	30–65	30–70
		20–29 yr:	30–70	30–75
		30–39 yr:	30–70	30–80
		40+ yr.	30–70	30–85
		Values for blacks—20 mg/dl higher		
Hematocrit	Whole blood (EDTA)	*% of packed red cells (V red cells/V whole blood × 100)*		
Calculated from MCV and RBC (electronic displacement or laser)		1 d (cap):	48–69	
		2 d:	48–75	
		3 d:	44–72	
		2 mo:	28–42	
		6–12 yr:	35–45	
		12–18 yr, M:	37–49	
		F:	36–46	
		18–49 yr, M:	41–53	
		F:	36–46	
Hemoglobin (Hb)	Whole blood (EDTA)		*g/dl*	
		1–3 day (cap):	14.5–22.5	
		2 mo:	9.0–14.0	
		6–12 yr:	11.5–15.5	
		12–18 yr, M:	13.0–16.0	
		F:	12.0–16.0	
		18–49 yr, M:	13.5–17.5	
		F:	12.0–16.0	
	Serum or plasma (heparin, ACD)	< 10 mg/dl < 3 mg/dl with butterfly set-up and 18 g needle		
	Urine, fresh random	Negative		
Hemoglobin, glycosated	Whole blood (heparin, EDTA, or oxalate)			
Electrophoresis		5.6–7.5% of total Hb		
Column		6.9% of total Hb		
HPLC		HbA_{1a} 1.6% total Hb		
		HbA_{1b} 0.8		
		HbA_{1c} 3–6		

continues

Table H–1 continued

Test	*Specimen*	*Reference Range*		
Iron	Serum		*µg/dl*	
		Newborn:	100–250	
		Infant:	40–100	
		Child:	50–120	
		Thereafter, M:	50–160	
		F:	40–150	
		Intoxicated child:	280–2250	
		Fatally posioned child:	>1800	
Iron-binding capacity total (TIBC)	Serum	Infant:	100–400 µg/dl	
		Thereafter:	250–400	
LDL-Cholesterol (LDLC)	Serum or plasma (EDTA)		*mg/dl*	
			Male	*Female*
		Cord blood:	10–50	10–50
		0–19 yr:	60–140	60–150
		20–29 yr:	60–175	60–160
		30–39 yr:	80–190	70–170
		40–49 yr:	90–205	80–190
		Recommended (desirable range for adults: 65–175 mg/dl		
Lead	Whole blood (heparin)		*µg/dl*	
		Child:	< 30	
		Adult:	< 40	
		Acceptable for industrial exposure:	< 60	
		Toxic:	≥ 100	
	Urine 24 h	< 80 µg/dl		
Mean corpuscular hemoglobin (MHC)	Whole blood (EDTA)		*pg/cell*	
		Birth:	31–37	
		1–3 day (cap):	31–37	
		1 wk–1 mo:	28–40	
		2 mo:	26–34	
		3–6 mo:	25–35	
		0.5–2 yr:	23–31	
		2–6 yr:	23–31	
		6–12 yr:	25–33	
		12–18 yr:	25–35	
		18–49 yr:	26–34	

Table H–1 continued

Test	*Specimen*	*Reference Range*	
Mean corpuscular hemoglobin concentration (EDTA)	Whole blood (EDTA)		*% Hb.cell or g Hb/dl RBC*
		Birth:	30–60
		1–3 (cap):	29–37
		1–2 wk:	28–38
		1–2 mo:	29–37
		3 mo–2 yr:	30–36
		2–18 yr:	31–37
		> 18 yr:	31–37
Mean corpuscular volume	Whole blood (EDTA)		*μm^3*
		1–3 day (cap):	95–121
		0.5–2 yr:	70–86
		6–12 yr:	77–95
		12–18 yr, M:	78–98
		F:	78–102
		18–49 yr, M:	80–100
		F:	80–100
Niacin (nicotine acid)	Urine 24 h	0.3–1.5 mg/day	
Phenylalanine	Serum		*mg/dl*
		Premature:	2.0–7.5
		Newborn:	1.2–3.4
		Thereafter:	0.8–1.8
			mg/day
	Urine 24 h	10 day–2 wk:	1–2
		3–12 yr:	4–18
		Thereafter:	trace–17
Phosphatase, Alkaline (p-nitrophenyl phosphatase)	Serum		
SKI method 30ºC			*U/L*
		Infant:	50–155
		Child:	20–150
		Adult:	20–70
Bowers and McComb, 30ºC		25–90 U/L	
Phospholipid, total	Serum or plasma (EDTA)		*mg/dl*
		Newborn:	75–170
		Infant:	100–275
		Child:	180–295
		Adult:	125–275

continues

Table H–1 continued

Test	*Specimen*	*Reference Range*	
Phosphorus, inorganic	Serum		*mg/dl*
		Cord:	3.7–8.1
		Premature (1 wk):	5.4–10.9
		Newborn:	4.3–9.3
		Child:	4.5–6.5
		Thereafter:	3.0–4.5
Potassium	Serum		*mmol/l*
		Newborn:	3.9–5.9
		Infant:	4.1–5.3
		Child:	3.4–4.7
		Thereafter:	3.5–5.1
	Plasma (heparin)	3.5–4.5 mmol/L	
	Urine, 24 h	2.5–125 mmol/day varies with diet	
Prealbumin (PA, tryptophan-rich, thyroxine-binding TBPA) R/D	Serum		*mg/dl*
		Cord:	13
		1 yr:	10
		Maternal:	23
		Adult:	10–40
Protein, total	Serum		*g/dl*
		Premature:	4.3–7.6
		Newborn:	4.6–7.4
		Child:	6.2–8.0
		Adult	
		Recumbent:	6.0–7.8
		0.5 g higher in ambulatory patients	
Electrophoresis			*g/dl*
		Albumin	
		Premature:	3.0–4.2
		Newborn:	3.6–5.4
		Infant:	4.0–5.0
		α_1–Globulin	
		Premature:	0.1–0.5
		Newborn:	0.1–0.3
		Infant:	0.2–0.4
		Thereafter:	0.2–0.3
		α_2–Globulin	
		Premature:	0.3–0.7
		Newborn:	0.5–0.5
		Infant:	0.5–0.8
		Thereafter:	0.4–1.0

Table H–1 continued

Test	*Specimen*	*Reference Range*	
		β–Globulin	
		Premature:	0.3–1.2
		Newborn:	0.2–0.6
		Infant:	0.5–0.8
		Thereafter:	0.5–1.1
		γ–Globin	
		Premature:	0.3–1.4
		Newborn:	0.2–1.0
		Infant:	0.3–1.2
		Thereafter:	0.7–1.2
		Higher in blacks	
Total	Urine, 24 h	1–14 mg/dl	
		50–80 mg/dl (at rest)	
		< 250 mg/d after intense exercise	
Prothrombin time (PT) one-stage (quick)	Whole blood (Na citrate)	In general: 11–15s (varies with type of thromboplastin)	
		Newborn: prolonged by 2–3s	
Retinol-binding protein (RBP)	Serum plasma		*mg/dl*
		2–10 yr:	2.5–4.5
		16 yr and older, M:	4.5–9.0
		F:	2.5–9.0
Riboflavin (vitamin B2)	Urine, random, fasting		*µg/g* Creatinine
		1–3 yr:	500–900
		4–6 yr:	300–600
		7–9 yr:	270–500
		10–15 yr:	200–400
		Adult:	80–269
Sodium	Serum or plasma (heparin)		*mmol/L*
		Newborn:	134–146
		Infant:	139–146
		Child:	138–145
		Thereafter:	136–146
	Sweat		10–40
		Cystic fibrosis > 70	

continues

Table H–1 continued

Test	*Specimen*	*Reference Range*
Somatomedin C	Plasma	Vary with laboratory, e.g., Nichols Institute *U/L* *M* *F* 0–2 yr: 0.10–0.72 0.10–1.7 3–5 yr: 0.12–1.5 0.15–2.3 6–10 yr: 0.19–2.2 0.44–3.6 11–12 yr: 0.22–3.6 1.50–6.9 13–14 yr: 0.79–5.5 0.81–7.4 15–17 yr: 0.76–3.3 0.59–3.1 18–64 yr: 0.34–1.9 0.45–2.2 *Endocrine Sciences* Cord: 0.25–0.66 0–1 yr: 0.17–0.62 1–5 yr: 0.14–0.94 6–12 yr: 0.87–2.06 13–17 yr: 1.35–3.00 18–25 yr: 0.92–2.06 Thereafter: 0.70–2.04
Thiamine (vitamin B1)	Serum Urine, acidified with HCl	0–2.0 μg/dl μg/g creatinine 1–3 yr: 176–200 4–6 yr: 121–400 7–9 yr: 181–350 10–12 yr: 181–300 13–15 yr: 151–250 Thereafter: 66–129
Transferrin	Serum	Newborn: 130–275 mg/dl Adult: 200–400 mg/dl
Triglycerides (TG)	Serum, after ≥12 h fast	*mg/dl* Male Female Cord blood: 10–98 10–98 0–5 yr: 30–86 32–99 6–11 yr: 31–108 35–114 12–15 yr: 36–138 41–138 16–19 yr: 40–163 40–128 20–29 yr: 44–185 40–128 Recommended (desirable) levels for adults: Male: 40–160 mg/dl Female: 35–135 mg/dl

Table H–1 continued

Test	*Specimen*	*Reference Range*	
Tyrosine	Serum		*mg/dl*
		Premature:	7.0–24.0
		Newborn:	1.6–3.7
		Adult:	0.8–1.3
Urea nitrogen	Serum or plasma		*mg/dl*
		Cord:	21–40
		Premature (1 wk):	3–25
		Newborn:	3–12
		Infant/Child:	5–18
		Thereafter:	7–18
Vitamin A	Serum		*μg/dl*
		Newborn:	35–75
		Child:	30–80
		Thereafter:	30–65
Vitamin B1, see Thiamine			
Vitamin B2, see Riboflavin			
Vitamin B6	Plasma (EDTA)	3.6–18 ng/ml	
Vitamin B12	Serum	Newborn:	175–800 pg/ml
		Thereafter:	140–700
Vitamin C	Plasma (oxalate, heparin, or EDTA)	0.6–2.0 mg/dl	
Vitamin D2, 25 Hydroxy	Plasma (heparin)	Summer:	15–80 ng/ml
		Winter:	14–42
Vitamin D3, 1,25 Dihydroxy	Serum	25–45 pg/ml	
Vitamin E	Serum	5.0–20 μg/ml	
Zinc	Serum	70–150 μg/dl	

Source: Adapted with permission from Nelson's Textbook of Pediatrics, 13th ed., pp. 1535–1558, © 1989, W.B. Saunders Company.

Appendix I

Recommended Dietary Allowances/ Dietary Reference Intakes

Table I–1 Dietary reference intakes: Recommended intakes for individuals, Food and Nutrition Board, the National Academies of Sciences

	Infants 0–6 mo	*Infants 7–12 mo*	*Children 1–2 y*	*Children 3–8 y*	*Males 9–13 y*	*Males 14–18 y*	*Females 9–13 y*	*Females 14–18 y*	*Pregnancy 14–18*	*Lactation 14–18*
Active PAL[k] EER (kcal/d)	Male 570 Female 520 (3 mo)	Male 743 Female 676 (9 mo)	Male 1046 Female 992 (24 mo)	Male 1742 Female 1642 (6 y)	2279 (11 y)	3152 (16 y)	2071 (11 y)	2368 (16 y)	1st trimester 2368 2nd trimester 2708 3rd trimester 2820 (16 y)	1st 6 mo 2698 2nd 6 mo 2768
Carbohydrates			130	130	130	130	130	130	175	210
Total Fiber	ND[n]	ND	19	25	31	48	26	26	28	29
AI (g/d)[m] Fat	31	30	ND	ND	ND	ND	ND	ND	ND	ND
***n*-6 Polyunsaturated Fatty Acids (g/d) (Linoleic Acid)**	4.4	4.6	7	10	12	16	10	11	13	13
***n*-3 Polyunsaturated Fatty Acids (g/d) (α-Linoleic Acid)**	0.5	0.5	0.7	0.9	1.2	1.6	1.0	1.1	1.4	1.3
Protein (g/kg/d)		1.5	1.10	0.95	0.95	0.85	0.95	.085		
Vitamin A (μg/d)[a]	400*	500*	**300**	**400**	**600**	**900**	**600**	**700**	**750**	**1200**
Vitamin C (mg/d)	40*	50*	**15**	**25**	**45**	**75**	**45**	**65**	**80**	**115**
Vitamin D (μg/d)[b,c]	5*	5*	5*	5*	5*	5*	5*	5*	5*	5*
Vitamin E (mg/d)[d]	4*	5*	6	7	**11**	**15**	**11**	**15**	**15**	**19**
Vitamin K (μg/d)	2.0*	2.5*	30*	55*	60*	75*	60*	75*	75*	75*
Thiamin (mg/d)	0.2*	0.3*	**0.5**	**0.6**	**0.9**	**1.2**	**0.9**	**1.0**	**1.4**	**1.4**
Riboflavin (mg/d)	0.3*	0.4*	**0.5**	**0.6**	**0.9**	**1.3**	**0.9**	**1.0**	**1.4**	**1.6**
Niacin (mg/d)[e]	2*	4*	**6**	**8**	**12**	**16**	**12**	**14**	**18**	**17**
Vitamin B6 (mg/d)	0.1*	0.3*	**0.5**	**0.6**	**1.0**	**1.3**	**1.0**	**1.2**	**1.9**	**2.0**
Folate (μg/d)[f]	65*	80*	**150**	**200**	**300**	**400**	**300**	**400[g]**	**600[h]**	**500**
Vitamin B12 (mg/d)	0.4*	0.5*	0.9	1.2	1.8	2.4	1.8	2.4	2.6	2.8
Pantothenic Acid (mg/d)	1.7*	1.8*	2*	3*	4*	5*	4*	5*	6*	7*

Table I–1 continued

	Infants 0–6 mo	*Infants 7–12 mo*	*Children 1–2 y*	*Children 3–8 y*	*Males 9–13 y*	*Males 14–18 y*	*Females 9–13 y*	*Females 14–18 y*	*Pregnancy 14–18*	*Lactation 14–18*
Biotin (μg/d)	5*	6*	8*	12*	20*	25*	20*	25*	30*	35*
Choline[j] (mg/d)	125*	125*	200*	250*	375*	550*	375*	400*	450*	550*
Calcium (mg/d)	210*	270*	500*	800*	1300*	1300*	1300*	1300*	1300*	1300*
Chromium (μg/d)	0.2*	5.5*	11*	15*	25*	35*	21*	24*	29*	44
Copper (μg/d)	200*	220*	**340**	**440**	**700**	**890**	**700**	**890**	**1000**	**1300**
Fluoride (mg/d)	0.01*	0.5*	0.7*	1*	2*	3*	2*	2*	3*	3*
Iodine (μg/d)	110*	130*	**90**	**90**	**120**	**150**	**120**	**150**	**220**	**290**
Iron (mg/d)	0.27*	**11**	**7**	**10**	**8**	**11**	**8**	**15**	**27**	**10**
Magnesium (mg/d)	30*	75*	**80**	**130**	**240**	**410**	**240**	**360**	**400**	**360**
Manganese (mg/d)	0.003*	0.6*	1.2*	1.5*	1.9*	2.2*	1.6*	1.6*	2.0*	2.6*
Molybdenum (μg/d)	2*	3*	**17**	**22**	**34**	**43**	**34**	**43**	**50**	**50**
Phosphorus (mg/d)	100*	275*	**460**	**500**	**1250**	**1250**	**1250**	**1250**	**1250**	**1250**
Selenium (μg/d)	15*	20*	**20**	**30**	**40**	**55**	**40**	**55**	**60**	**70**
Zinc (mg/d)	2*	**3**	**3**	**5**	**8**	**11**	**8**	**9**	**13**	**14**

Note: This table (taken from the DRI reports, see www.nap.edu) presents Recommended Dietary Allowances (RDAs) in **bold type** and Adequate Intakes (AIs) in ordinary type followed by an asterisk (*). RDAs and AIs may both be used as goals for individual intake. RDAs are set to meet the needs of almost all individuals in a group. For healthy breastfed infants, the AI is the mean intake. The AI for other life stage and gender groups is believed to cover needs of all individuals in the group, but lack of data or uncertainty in the data prevent being able to specify with confidence the percentage of individuals covered by this intake.

[a] As retinol activity equivalents (RAEs). 1 RAE = 1 μg retinol, 12 μg β-carotene, 24 μg α-carotene, or 24 μg β-cryptoxanthin in foods. To calculate RAEs from retinol equivalents (REs) of provitamin A carotenoids in foods, divide the REs by 2. For preformed vitamin A in foods or supplements and for provitamin A carotenoids in supplements, 1 RE = 1 RAE.

[b] Cholecalciferol, 1 μg cholecalciferol = 40 IU vitamin D.

[c] In the absence of adequate exposure to sunlight.

[d] As α-tocopherol. α-Tocopherol includes RRR-α-tocopherol, the only form of α-tocopherol that occurs naturally in foods, and the 2R-stereoisomeric forms of α-tocopherol (RRR-, RSR-, RRS-, and RSS-α-tocopherol) that occur in fortified foods and supplements. It does not include the 2S-stereoisomeric forms of α-tocopherol (SRR-, SSR-, SRS-, and SSS-α-tocopherol), also found in fortified foods and supplements.

[e] As niacin equivalents (NE). 1 mg of niacin = 60 mg of tryptophan; 0–6 months=preformed niacin (not NE).

[f] As dietary folate equivalents (DFE). 1 DEF=1 μg food folate=0.6 μg of folic acid from fortified food or as a supplement consumed with food=0.5 μg of a supplement taken on an empty stomach.

continues

Table I–1 continued

[g] In view of evidence linking folate intake with neural tube defects in the fetus, it is recommended that all women capable of becoming pregnant consume 400 μg from supplements or fortified foods in addition to intake of food folate from the diet.

[h] It is assumed that women will continue consuming 400 μg from supplements or fortified food until their pregnancy is confirmed and they enter prenatal care, which ordinarily occurs after the end of the preconceptional period—the critical time for formation of the neural tube.

[i] Although AIs have been set for choline, there are few data to assess whether a dietary supply of choline is needed at all stages of the life cycle, and it may be that the choline requirement can be met by endogenous synthesis at some of these stages.

[j] For healthy moderately active American and Canadians.

[k] PAL = physical activity letter, EER = estimated energy requirement, TEE = total energy expenditure. The intake that meets the average energy expenditure of individuals at the reference height, weight, and age.

[l] RDA = Recommended Dietary Allowance. The intake that meets the nutrient need of almost all (97–98 percent) individuals in a group.

[m] AI = Adequate Intake. The observed average or experimentally determined intake by a defined population or subgroup that appears to sustain a defined nutritional status, such as growth rate, normal circulating nutrient values, or other functional indicators of health. The AI is used if sufficient scientific evidence is not available to derive an Estimated Average Requirement (EAR). For healthy infants receiving human milk, the AI is the mean intake. The AI is not equivalent to an RDA. Based on 14g/1000 kcal of required energy.

[n] ND = not determined. The observed average of experimentally determined intake by a defined population or subgroup that appears to sustain a defined nutritional status, such as growth rate, normal circulating nutrient values, or other functional indicators of health. The AI is used if sufficient scientific evidence is not available to derive an EAR. For healthy infants receiving human milk, the AI is the mean intake. The AI is not equivalent to an RDA.

No determined biological function in humans has been identified for the nutrients silicon and vanadium.

Table I–2 Dietary Reference Intakes (DRIs): Tolerable Upper Intake Levels (UL[a]), Food and Nutrition Board, the National Academies of Sciences

	Infants 0–6 mo	*Infants 7–12 mo*	*Children 1–3 y*	*Children 4–8 y*	*Males/ Females 9–13 y*	*Males/ Females 14–18 y*	*Pregnancy ≤18*	*Lactation ≤18*
Vitamin A (μg/d)[b]	600	600	600	900	1700	2800	2800	2800
Vitamin C (mg/d)	ND[f]	ND	400	650	1200	1800	1800	1800
Vitamin D (μg/d)	25	25	50	50	50	50	50	50
Vitamin E (mg/d)[c,d]	ND	ND	200	300	600	800	800	800
Vitamin K (μg/d)	ND	ND	ND	ND	ND	ND	ND	ND
Thiamin (mg/d)	ND	ND	ND	ND	ND	ND	ND	ND
Riboflavin (mg/d)	ND	ND	ND	ND	ND	ND	ND	ND
Niacin (mg/d)[d]	ND	ND	10	15	20	30	30	30
Vitamin B_6 (mg/d)	ND	ND	30	40	60	80	80	80
Folate (μg/d)[d]	ND	ND	300	400	600	800	800	800
Vitamin B_{12} (mg/d)	ND	ND	ND	ND	ND	ND	ND	ND
Pantothenic Acid (mg/d)	ND	ND	ND	ND	ND	ND	ND	ND
Biotin (μg/d)	ND	ND	ND	ND	ND	ND	ND	ND
Choline (mg/d)	ND	ND	1.0	1.0	2.0	3.0	3.0	3.0
Carotenoids[e]	ND	ND	ND	ND	ND	ND	ND	ND
Arsenic	ND	ND	ND	ND	ND	ND	ND	ND
Boron (mg/d)	ND	ND	3	6	11	17	17	17
Calcium (mg/d)	ND	ND	2.5	2.5	2.5	2.5	2.5	2.5
Chromium (μg/d)	ND	ND	ND	ND	ND	ND	ND	ND
Copper (μg/d)	ND	ND	1000	3000	5000	8000	8000	8000
Fluoride (mg/d)	.07	.09	1.3	2.2	10	10	10	10
Iodine (μg/d)	ND	ND	200	300	600	900	900	900

continues

Table I–2 continued

	Infants 0–6 mo	*Infants 7–12 mo*	*Children 1–3 y*	*Children 4–8 y*	*Males/ Females 9–13 y*	*Males/ Females 14–18 y*	*Pregnancy ≤18*	*Lactation ≤18*
Iron (mg/d)	40	40	40	40	40	45	45	45
Magnesium (mg/d)[c]	ND	ND	65	110	350	350	350	350
Manganese (mg/d)	ND	ND	2	3	6	9	9	9
Molybdenum (μg/d)	ND	ND	300	600	1100	1700	1700	1700
Nickel (mg/d)	ND	ND	0.2	0.3	0.6	1.0	1.0	1.0
Phosphorus (mg/d)	ND	ND	3	3	4	4	3.5	4
Selenium (μg/d)	45	60	90	150	280	400	400	400
Silicon[d]	ND	ND	ND	ND	ND	ND	ND	ND
Vanadium (mg/d)[e]	ND	ND	ND	ND	ND	ND	ND	ND
Zinc (mg/d)	4	5	7	12	23	34	34	34

[a] UL = The maximum level of daily nutrient intake that is likely to pose no risk of adverse effects. Unless otherwise specified, the UL represents total intake from food, water, and supplements. Due to lack of suitable data, ULs could not be established for vitamin K, thiamin, riboflavin, vitamin B_{12}, pantothenic acid, biotin, or carotenoids. In the absences of ULs, extra caution may be warranted in consuming levels above recommended intakes.

[b] As preformed vitamin A only.

[c] As α-tocopherol; applies to any form of supplemental α-tocopherol.

[d] The ULs for vitamin E, niacin, and folate apply to synthetic forms obtained from supplements, fortified foods, or a combination of the two.

[e] β-Carotene supplements are advised only to serve as a provitamin A source for individuals at risk of vitamin A deficiency.

[f] ND = Not determinable due to lack of data of adverse effects in this age group and concern with regard to lack of ability to handle excess amounts.

Source: This table is taken from the DRI report: see www.nap.edu.

Table I–3 Dietary Reference Intakes (DRIs) During Pregnancy[1]

	Females			*Pregnancy*		
Life Stage Group	*14–18 y*	*19–30 y*	*31–50 y*	*≤18y*	*19–30 y*	*31–50 y*
Calcium (mg/d)	1300*	1000*	1000*	1300*	1000*	1000*
Phosphorus (mg/d)	1250	700	700	1250	700	700
Magnesium (mg/d)	360	310	320	400	350	360
Vitamin A (μg/d)	700	700	700	750	770	770
Vitamin D (μg/d)[a,b]	5*	5*	5*	5*	5*	5*
Fluoride (mg/d)	3*	3*	3*	3*	3*	3*
Thiamin (mg/d)	1.0	1.1	1.1	1.4	1.4	1.4
Riboflavin (mg/d)	1.0	1.1	1.1	1.4	1.4	1.4
Niacin (mg/d)[c]	14	14	14	18	18	18
Vitamin B6 (mg/d)	1.2	1.3	1.3	1.9	1.9	1.9
Folate (μg/d)[d]	400[g]	400[g]	400[g]	600[h]	600[h]	600[h]
Vitamin B12 (μg/d)	2.4	2.4	2.4	2.6	2.6	2.6
Pantothenic Acid (mg/d)	5*	5*	5*	6*	6*	6*
Biotin (μg/d)	25*	30*	30*	30*	30*	30*
Choline[e] (mg/d)	400*	425*	425*	450*	450*	450*
Vitamin C (mg/d)	65	75	75	80	85	85
Vitamin E[f] (mg/d)	15	15	15	15	15	15
Iron (mg/d)	15	18	18	27	27	27
Zinc (mg/d)	9	8	8	13	11	11
Copper (μg/d)	890	900	900	1000	1000	1000
Selenium (μg/d)	55	55	55	60	60	60
Iodine (μg/d)	150	150	150	220	220	220

1. Institute of Medicine.

*Adequate Intakes (AI).

[a] As cholecalciferol. 1 μg cholecalciferol = 40 IU vitamin D.

[b] In the absence of adequate exposure to sunlight.

[c] As niacin equivalents (NE). 1 mg of niacin = 60 mg of tryptophan.

[d] As dietary folate equivalents (DFE). 1 DFE = 1 μg food folate = 0.6 μg of folic acid from fortified food or as a supplement consumed with food = 0.5 μg of a supplement taken on an empty stomach.

[e] Although AIs have been set for choline, there are few data to assess whether a dietary supply of choline is needed at all stages of the life cycle, and it may be that the choline requirement can be met by endogenous synthesis at some of these stages.

[f] As α-tocopherol. α-Tocopherol includes *RRR*-α-tocopherol, the only form of α-tocopherol that occurs naturally in foods, and the 2*R*-stereoisomeric forms of α-tocopherol (*SRR-, SSR-, SRS-*, and *SSS*-α-tocopherol), also found in fortified foods and supplements.

[g] In view of evidence linking folate intake with neural tube defects in the fetus, it is recommended that all women capable of becoming pregnant consume 400 μg from supplements or fortified foods in addition to intake of food folate from a varied diet.

[h] It is assumed that women will continue consuming 400 μg from supplements or fortified food until their pregnancy is confirmed and they enter prenatal care, which ordinarily occurs after the end of the periconceptional period—the critical time for formation of the neural tube.

1a. Institute of Medicine. Vitamin A. In: ***Dietary Intakes for Vitamin A, Vitamin K, Arsenic, Boron, Chromium, Copper, Iodine, Iron, Manganese, Molybdenum, Nickel, Silicon, Vanadium, and Zinc.*** National Academy Press; 2001:65–126

1b. Institute of Medicine FNB. Dietary Reference Intakes for Calcium, Phosporus, Magnesium, Vitamin D, and Fluoride. Washington, DC: Institute of Medicine; 1997

1c. Institute of Medicine FNB. Dietary Reference Intakes for Thiamin, Riboflavin, Niacin, Vitamin B_6, Folate, Vitamin B_{12}, Pantothenic Acid, Biotin, and Choline. Washington, DC: Institute of Medicine; 1998

1d. Institute of Medicine FNB. Dietary Reference Intakes for Vitamin C, Vitamin E, Selenium, and Carotenoids. Washington, DC: Institute of Medicine; 2000

Source: This table is taken from the DRI report: see www.nap.edu.

APPENDIX J

2005 Dietary Guidelines

DIETARY GUIDELINES FOR AMERICANS 2005

ADEQUATE NUTRIENTS WITHIN CALORIE NEEDS

Key Recommendations

- Consume a variety of nutrient-dense foods and beverages within and among the basic food groups while choosing foods that limit the intake of saturated and *trans* fats, cholesterol, added sugars, salt, and alcohol.
- Meet recommended intakes within energy needs by adopting a balanced eating pattern, such as the USDA Food Guide or the DASH Eating Plan.

WEIGHT MANAGEMENT

Key Recommendations

- To maintain body weight in a healthy range, balance calories from foods and beverages with calories expended.
- To prevent gradual weight gain over time, make small decreases in food and beverage calories and increase physical activity.

PHYSICAL ACTIVITY

Key Recommendations

- Engage in regular physical activity and reduce sedentary activities to promote health, psychological well-being, and a healthy body weight.
- To reduce the risk of chronic disease in adulthood: Engage in at least 30 minutes of moderate-intensity physical activity, above usual activity, at work or home on most days of the week.
- For most people, greater health benefits can be obtained by engaging in physical activity of more vigorous intensity or longer duration.
- To help manage body weight and prevent gradual, unhealthy body weight gain in adulthood: Engage in approximately 60 minutes of moderate- to vigorous-intensity activity on most days of the week while not exceeding caloric intake requirements.
- To sustain weight loss in adulthood: Participate in at least 60 to 90 minutes of daily moderate-intensity physical activity while not exceeding caloric intake requirements. Some people may need to consult with a healthcare provider before participating in this level of activity.
- Achieve physical fitness by including cardiovascular conditioning, stretching exercises for flexibility, and resistance exercises or calisthenics for muscle strength and endurance.

FOOD GROUPS TO ENCOURAGE

Key Recommendations

- Consume a sufficient amount of fruits and vegetables while staying within energy needs. Two cups of fruit and 21/2 cups of vegetables per day are recommended for a reference 2,000-calorie intake, with higher or lower amounts depending on the calorie level.
- Choose a variety of fruits and vegetables each day. In particular, select from all five vegetable subgroups (dark green, orange, legumes, starchy vegetables, and other vegetables) several times a week.
- Consume 3 or more ounce-equivalents of whole-grain products per day, with the rest of the recommended grains coming from enriched or whole-grain products. In general, at least half the grains should come from whole grains.
- Consume 3 cups per day of fat-free or low-fat milk or equivalent milk products.

FATS

Key Recommendations

- Consume less than 10 percent of calories from saturated fatty acids and less than 300 mg/day of cholesterol, and keep *trans* fatty acid consumption as low as possible.
- Keep total fat intake between 20 to 35 percent of calories, with most fats coming from sources of polyunsaturated and monounsaturated fatty acids, such as fish, nuts, and vegetable oils.
- When selecting and preparing meat, poultry, dry beans, and milk or milk products, make choices that are lean, low-fat, or fat-free.
- Limit intake of fats and oils high in saturated and/or *trans* fatty acids, and choose products low in such fats and oils.

CARBOHYDRATES

Key Recommendations

- Choose fiber-rich fruits, vegetables, and whole grains often.
- Choose and prepare foods and beverages with minimal added sugars or caloric sweeteners, in keeping with amounts suggested by the USDA Food Guide and the DASH Eating Plan.
- Reduce the incidence of dental caries by practicing good oral hygiene and consuming sugar- and starch-containing foods and beverages less frequently.

SODIUM AND POTASSIUM

Key Recommendations

- Consume less than 2,300 mg (approximately 1 tsp of salt) of sodium per day
- Choose and prepare foods with little salt. At the same time, consume potassium-rich foods, such as fruits and vegetables.

ALCOHOLIC BEVERAGES

Key Recommendations

- Those who choose to drink alcoholic beverages should do so sensibly and in moderation—defined as the consumption of up to one drink per day for women and up to two drinks per day for men.
- Alcoholic beverages should not be consumed by some individuals, including those who cannot restrict their alcohol intake, women of childbearing age who may become pregnant, pregnant and lactating women, children and adolescents, individuals taking medications that can interact with alcohol, and those with specific medical conditions.
- Alcoholic beverages should be avoided by individuals engaging in activities that require attention, skill, or coordination, such as driving or operating machinery.

FOOD SAFETY

Key Recommendations

- To avoid microbial food-borne illness:
- Clean hands, food contact surfaces, and fruits and vegetables. Meat and poultry should not be washed or rinsed.
- Separate raw, cooked, and ready-to-eat foods while shopping, preparing, or storing foods.
- Cook foods to a safe temperature to kill microorganisms.
- Chill (refrigerate) perishable food promptly and defrost foods properly.
- Avoid raw (unpasteurized) milk or any products made from unpasteurized milk, raw or partially cooked eggs or foods containing raw eggs, raw or undercooked meat and poultry, unpasteurized juices, and raw sprouts.

Figure J–1 Sample of USDA Food Guide and the DASH Eating Plan at the 2,000-Calorie Level[a]

Amounts of various food groups that are recommended each day or each week in the USDA Food Guide and in the DASH Eating Plan (amounts are daily unless otherwise specified) at the 2,000-calorie level. Also identified are equivalent amounts for different food choices in each group. To follow either eating pattern, food choices over time should provide these amounts of food from each group on average.

<table>
<tr><th>Food Groups and Subgroups</th><th>USDA Food Guide Amount[b]</th><th>DASH Eating Plan Amount</th><th>Equivalent Amounts</th></tr>
<tr><td>Fruit Group</td><td>2 cups (4 servings)</td><td>2 to 2.5 cups (4 to 5 servings)</td><td>½ cup equivalent is:
• ½ cup fresh, frozen, or canned fruit
• 1 med fruit
• ¼ cup dried fruit
• USDA: ½ cup fruit juice
• DASH: ¾ cup fruit juice</td></tr>
<tr><td>Vegetable Group
• Dark green vegetables
• Orange vegetables
• Legumes (dry beans)
• Starchy vegetables
• Other vegetables</td><td>2.5 cups (5 servings)
3 cups/week
2 cups/week
3 cups/week
3 cups/week
6.5 cups/week</td><td>2 to 2.5 cups (4 to 5 servings)</td><td>½ cup equivalent is:
• ½ cup of cut-up raw or cooked vegetable
• 1 cup raw leafy vegetable
• USDA: ½ cup vegetable juice
• DASH: ¾ cup vegetable juice</td></tr>
<tr><td>Grain Group
• Whole grains
• Other grains</td><td>6 ounce-equivalents
3 ounce-equivalents
3 ounce-equivalents</td><td>7 to 8 ounce-equivalents
(7 to 8 servings)</td><td>1 ounce-equivalent is:
• 1 slice bread
• 1 cup dry cereal
• ½ cup cooked rice, pasta, cereal
• DASH: 1 oz dry cereal (½–1¼ cup depending on cereal type—check label)</td></tr>
<tr><td>Meat and Beans Group</td><td>5.5 ounce-equivalents</td><td>6 ounces or less
meat, poultry, fish</td><td rowspan="2">1 ounce-equivalent is:
• 1 ounce of cooked lean meats, poultry, fish
• 1 egg
• USDA: ¼ cup cooked dry beans or tofu, 1 Tbsp peanut butter, ½ oz nuts or seeds
• DASH: 1½ oz nuts, ½ oz seeds, ½ cup cooked dry beans</td></tr>
<tr><td></td><td></td><td>4 to 5 servings per week
nuts, seeds, and dry beans[c]</td></tr>
<tr><td>Milk Group</td><td>3 cups</td><td>2 to 3 cups</td><td>1 cup equivalent is:
• 1 cup low-fat/fat-free milk, yogurt
• 1½ oz of low-fat or fat-free natural cheese
• 2 oz of low-fat or fat-free processed cheese</td></tr>
<tr><td>Oils</td><td>24 grams (6 tsp)</td><td>8 to 12 grams (2 to 3 tsp)</td><td>1 tsp equivalent is:
• DASH: 1 tsp soft margarine
• 1 Tbsp low-fat mayo
• 2 Tbsp light salad dressing
• 1 tsp vegetable oil</td></tr>
<tr><td>Discretionary Calorie Allowance
• Example of distribution:
Solid fat[d]
Added sugars</td><td>267 calories

18 grams
8 tsp</td><td>

~2 tsp (5 Tbsp per week)</td><td>1 Tbsp added sugar equivalent is:
• DASH: 1 Tbsp jelly or jam
• ½ oz jelly beans
• 8 oz lemonade</td></tr>
</table>

a All servings are per day unless otherwise noted. USDA vegetable subgroup amounts and amounts of DASH nuts, seeds, and dry beans are per week.

b The 2,000-calorie USDA Food Guide is appropriate for many sedentary males 51 to 70 years of age, sedentary females 19 to 30 years of age, and for some other gender/age groups who are more physically active.

c In the DASH Eating Plan, nuts, seeds, and dry beans are a separate food group from meat, poultry, and fish.

d The oils listed in this table are not considered to be part of discretionary calories because they are a major source of the vitamin E and polyunsaturated fatty acids, including the essential fatty acids, in the food pattern. In contrast, solid fats (i.e., saturated and *trans* fats) are listed separately as a source of discretionary calories.

DIETARY GUIDELINES FOR AMERICANS, 2005

Figure J–2 Adult BMI Chart

Locate the height of interest in the left-most column and read across the row for that height to the weight of interest. Follow the column of the weight up to the top row that lists the BMI. BMI of 19–24 is the healthy weight range, BMI of 25–29 is the overweight range, and BMI of 30 and above is in the obese range.

BMI	19	20	21	22	23	24	25	26	27	28	29	30	31	32	33	34	35
Height	Weight in Pounds																
4'10"	91	96	100	105	110	115	119	124	129	134	138	143	148	153	158	162	167
4'11"	94	99	104	109	114	119	124	128	133	138	143	148	153	158	163	168	173
5'	97	102	107	112	118	123	128	133	138	143	148	153	158	163	158	174	179
5'1"	100	106	111	116	122	127	132	137	143	148	153	158	164	169	174	180	185
5'2"	104	109	115	120	126	131	136	142	147	153	158	164	169	175	180	186	191
5'3"	107	113	118	124	130	135	141	146	152	158	163	169	175	180	186	191	197
5'4"	110	116	122	128	134	140	145	151	157	163	169	174	180	186	192	197	204
5'5"	114	120	126	132	138	144	150	156	162	168	174	180	186	192	198	204	210
5'6"	118	124	130	136	142	148	155	161	167	173	179	186	192	198	204	210	216
5'7"	121	127	134	140	146	153	159	166	172	178	185	191	198	204	211	217	223
5'8"	125	131	138	144	151	158	164	171	177	184	190	197	203	210	216	223	230
5'9"	128	135	142	149	155	162	169	176	182	189	196	203	209	216	223	230	236
5'10"	132	139	146	153	160	167	174	181	188	195	202	209	216	222	229	236	243
5'11"	136	143	150	157	165	172	179	186	193	200	208	215	222	229	236	243	250
6'	140	147	154	162	169	177	184	191	199	206	213	221	228	235	242	250	258
6'1"	144	151	159	166	174	182	189	197	204	212	219	227	235	242	250	257	265
6'2'	148	155	163	171	179	186	194	202	210	218	225	233	241	249	256	264	272
6'3'	152	160	168	176	184	192	200	208	216	224	232	240	248	256	264	272	279
	Healthy Weight						Overweight					Obese					

Source: Evidence Report of Clinical Guidelines on the Identification, Evaluation, and Treatment of Overweight and Obesity in Adults, 1998. NIH/National Heart, Lung, and Blood Institute (NHLBI).

APPENDIX K

Conversion Tables

Exhibit K–1 Conversion tables

Volume

1 t	= 1/3 T	= 1/6 fl oz	= 4.9 ml
3 t	= 1 T	= 1/2 fl oz	= 14.8 ml
2 T	= 1/8 cup	= 1 fl oz	= 29.6 ml
4 T	= 1/4 cup	= 2 fl oz	= 59.1 ml
5 1/3 T	= 1/3 cup	= 2 2/3 fl oz	= 78.9 ml
8 T	= 1/2 cup	= 4 fl oz	= 118.3 ml
10 2/3 T	= 2/3 cup	= 5 1/3 fl oz	= 157.7 ml
12 T	= 3/4 cup	= 6 fl oz	= 177.4 ml
14 T	= 7/8 cup	= 7 fl oz	= 207.0 ml
16 T	= 1 cup	= 8 fl oz	= 236.6 ml
1 ml	= 0.034 fl oz	= 1 ml	= 0.001 liter
1 liter	= 34 fl oz	= 1000 ml	
1 pint (pt)	= 2 cups	= .473 liter	= 473 ml
1 quart (qt)	= 2 pt	= .946 liter	= 946 ml
1 gallon	= 4 qts	= 3.785 liter	= 3785 ml
1 liter	= 1.057 qts	= 0.264 gallon	= 1000 ml

To convert mls to oz divide by 30
To convert oz to mls multipy by 30

Weight

1 gram (g) = 0.035 oz = .001 kg = 1000 mg = 1,000,000 mcg
1 mg = .001 g = 1000 mcg
1 oz = 28.35 g (often rounded to 28 g)
1 lb = 16 oz = 453.59 g = .454 kg
1 kg = 2.21 lb = 1000 g

Length

1 inch = 2.54 centimeters
1 foot = 30.5 centimeters
1 yard = 0.91 meters
1 mile = 1.61 kilometers
1 centimeter = 0.4 inches
1 meter = 3.3 feet
1 meter = 1.1 yard
1 kilometer = 0.6 miles

To convert inches to centimeters, multiply by 2.54; centimeters to inches, multiply by 0.4

Area

1 square inch = 6.5 square centimeters
1 square foot = 9.29 square meters
1 square yard = 0.84 square meters
1 square centimeter = 0.16 square inches
1 square meter = 1.2 square yards

Exhibit K–1 continued

Heat Measures
1 kilojoule = 0.239 kilocalories
1 kilocalorie = 4.184 kilojoules

Temperatures

Water freezes	0°C	32°F
Room temperature	27°C	72°F
Body temperature	37°C	98.6°F
Water boils	100°C	212°F

To convert Fahrenheit to Celsius (centigrade), subtract 32, multiply by 5, divide by 9; Celsius (centigrade) to Fahrenheit, multiply by 9, divide by 5, and add 32.

Milliequivalent-milligram conversion table

Mineral element	Chemical symbol	Atomic weight	Valence
Calcium	Ca	40	2
Choline	Cl	35.4	1
Magnesium	Mg	24.3	2
Phosphorus	P	31	2
Potassium	K	39	1
Sodium	Na	23	1
Sulfate	SO_4	96	2
Sulfur	S	32	2
Zinc	Zn	65.4	2

$$\text{Milliequivalents} = \frac{\text{milligrams}}{\text{Atomic weight}} \times \text{valence}$$

1 g. NaCl= 0.4 g Na
(Na+ = 40% of weight of NaCl)
1 g Na+ = 2.5g NaCl

Example: convert 1000 mg sodium to MEq of sodium

$$\frac{1000}{23} \times 1 = 43 \text{ Meq sodium}$$

To change milliequivalents back to milligrams, multiply the milliequivalents by the atomic weight and divide by the valence.

Example: convert 10 Meq sodium to mg sodium

$$\frac{10 \times 23}{1} = 230 \text{ mg sodium}$$

Exhibit K–2 Pound to Kilogram Conversion Chart

lb	*kg*	*lb*	*kg*	*lb*	*kg*	*lb*	*kg*	*lb*	*kg*
85.0	38.6	108.0	49.1	131.0	59.5	154.0	70.0	177.0	80.5
85.5	38.9	108.5	49.3	131.5	59.8	154.5	70.2	177.5	80.7
86.0	39.1	109.0	49.5	132.0	60.0	155.0	70.5	178.0	80.9
86.5	39.3	109.5	49.8	132.5	60.2	155.5	70.7	178.5	81.1
87.0	39.5	110.0	50.0	133.0	60.5	156.0	70.9	179.0	81.4
87.5	39.8	110.5	50.2	133.5	60.7	156.5	71.1	179.5	81.6
88.0	40.0	111.0	50.5	134.0	60.9	157.0	71.4	180.0	81.8
88.5	40.2	111.5	50.7	134.5	61.1	157.5	71.6	180.5	82.0
89.0	40.5	112.0	50.9	135.0	61.4	158.0	71.8	181.0	82.3
89.5	40.7	112.5	51.1	135.5	61.6	158.5	72.0	181.5	82.5
90.0	40.9	113.0	51.4	136.0	61.8	159.0	72.3	182.0	82.7
90.5	41.1	113.5	51.6	136.5	62.0	159.5	72.5	182.5	83.0
91.0	41.4	114.0	51.8	137.0	62.3	160.0	72.7	183.0	83.2
91.5	41.6	114.5	52.0	137.5	62.5	160.5	73.0	183.5	83.4
92.0	41.8	115.0	52.3	138.0	62.7	161.0	73.2	184.0	83.6
92.5	42.0	115.5	52.5	138.5	63.0	161.5	73.4	184.5	83.9
93.0	42.3	116.0	52.7	139.0	63.2	162.0	73.6	185.0	84.1
93.5	42.5	116.5	53.0	139.5	63.4	162.5	73.9	185.5	84.3
94.0	42.7	117.0	53.2	140.0	63.6	163.0	74.1	186.0	84.5
94.5	43.0	117.5	53.4	140.5	63.9	163.5	74.3	186.5	84.8
95.0	43.2	118.0	53.6	141.0	64.1	164.0	74.5	187.0	85.0
95.5	43.4	118.5	53.9	141.5	64.3	164.5	74.8	187.5	85.2
96.0	43.6	119.0	54.1	142.0	64.5	165.0	75.0	188.0	85.5
96.5	43.9	119.5	54.3	142.5	64.8	165.5	75.2	188.5	85.7
97.0	44.1	120.0	54.5	143.0	65.0	166.0	75.5	189.0	85.9
97.5	44.3	120.5	54.8	143.5	65.2	166.5	75.7	189.5	86.1
98.0	44.5	121.0	55.0	144.0	65.5	167.0	75.9	190.0	86.4
98.5	44.8	121.5	55.2	144.5	65.7	167.5	76.1	190.5	86.6
99.0	45.0	122.0	55.5	145.0	65.9	168.0	76.4	191.0	86.8
99.5	45.2	122.5	55.7	145.5	66.1	168.5	76.6	191.5	87.0
100.0	45.5	123.0	55.9	146.0	66.5	169.0	76.8	192.0	87.3
100.5	45.7	123.5	56.1	146.5	66.6	169.5	77.0	192.5	87.5
101.0	45.9	124.0	56.4	147.0	66.8	170.0	77.3	193.0	87.7
101.5	46.1	124.5	56.6	147.5	67.0	170.5	77.5	193.5	88.0
102.0	46.4	125.0	56.8	148.0	67.3	171.0	77.7	194.0	88.2
102.5	46.6	125.5	57.0	148.5	67.5	171.5	78.0	194.5	88.4
103.0	46.8	126.0	57.3	149.0	67.7	172.0	78.2	195.0	88.6
103.5	47.0	126.5	57.5	149.5	68.0	172.5	78.4	195.5	88.9
104.0	47.3	127.0	57.7	150.0	68.2	173.0	78.6	196.0	89.1
104.5	47.5	127.5	58.0	150.5	68.4	173.5	78.9	196.5	89.3
105.0	47.7	128.0	58.2	151.0	68.6	174.0	79.1	197.0	89.5
105.5	48.0	128.5	58.4	151.5	68.9	174.5	79.3	197.5	89.8
106.0	48.2	129.0	58.6	152.0	69.1	175.0	79.5	198.0	90.0
106.5	48.4	129.5	58.9	152.5	69.3	175.5	79.8	198.5	90.2
107.0	48.6	130.0	59.1	153.0	69.5	176.0	80.0	199.0	90.5
107.5	48.9	130.5	59.3	153.5	69.8	176.5	80.2	199.5	90.7

Index

A

B

C

D

E

F

H

I

J

K

L

O

Q

R

S

T

U

V

W

X

Y

Z

HARFORD COMMUNITY COLLEGE LIBRARY
401 THOMAS RUN ROAD
BEL AIR, MARYLAND 21015-1698